The Divine Prescription
and Science of Health and Healing

By

Gunther B. Paulien, Ph.D.

TEACH Services, Inc.
PUBLISHING
www.TEACHServices.com • (800) 367-1844

World rights reserved. This book or any portion thereof may not be copied or reproduced in any form or manner whatever, except as provided by law, without the written permission of the publisher, except by a reviewer
who may quote brief passages in a review.

The author assumes full responsibility for the accuracy of all facts and quotations as cited in this book. The opinions expressed in this book are the author's personal views and interpretations, and do not necessarily reflect those of the publisher.

This book is provided with the understanding that the publisher is not engaged in giving spiritual, legal, medical, or other professional advice. If authoritative advice is needed, the reader should seek the counsel of a competent professional.

Copyright © 1995, 1997, 2017 TEACH Services, Inc.
ISBN-13: 978-1-4796-0829-4 (Paperback)
ISBN-13: 978-1-4796-0830-0 (ePub)
ISBN-13: 978-1-4796-0831-7 (Mobi)
Library of Congress Control Number: 2017913162

Publisher

TEACH Services, Inc.
www.TEACHServices.com

INTRODUCTION

The author is endeavoring in this book to view the matter of health and healing from the standpoint of the Bible and the Spirit of Prophecy. God has bestowed upon us a physical organism which He Himself has made, and has bequeathed to us in all its beauty of form and features. He has made us custodians to keep it in the prime of health in which we were created. It is our responsibility to keep it that way.

In order for us to do so, God has also informed us of the knowledge and principles by means of which we can keep our bodies in perfect health as we apply this knowledge to ourselves. Who is it that can tell us more about ourselves, our physical, mental, and spiritual needs than the one who has created us? Who is it that can tell us more about how to maintain health, avoid disease, and maintain for ourselves a life of joy and happiness? Who knows more about the workings of our organism and the delicate interrelationships of all of its parts? Who knows more about all of our needs than the One who has given us life?

All of the principles of the Bible and the Spirit of Prophecy are designed to allow us to function in perfect harmony with God Himself. Hence, we maintain that the best way to treat this organism in health and in sickness is to treat it in harmony with the Health Manuel of our Creator, and the principles that God has outlined for us. Perfect health demands that we apply these principles to our own life.

The author feels that we have to a great extent moved away from these principles, methods, practices, and procedures. That we have ignored the blueprint and have followed worldly ways to our eternal detriment. We have used foods which were not beneficial to the upbuilding and maintenance of bodily functions. We have used poisonous drugs which are condemned by Inspiration, and which have poisoned our system and have defiled the temple of God. We have used medicines which have disappointed us in not restoring our health, but made our condition worse, because they acted contrary to the laws of nature and of the organism. God has given us the herbs of the field for our medicine, but we have rejected them as not being powerful enough to do us any good, and then have taken powerful chemicals to do ourselves harm.

We have not shown wisdom in this regard and as a result have been ill when we need not have been. God has been dishonored in our weakness, and we haven't shown to the world as good an example as we might have been. Our worldly habits have put the gospel of health to shame, and by our example we have said that we don't believe what we claim to believe. We have ourselves suffered because of our lack of discretion, and our mistakes, unintentional or otherwise. We have been sick when we could have been well, if we had done only as well as we knew, or as well as Inspiration has taught us.

This book discusses the methods and means of healthful living from which it appears that many have been drifting away. It deals with going back to First Things, and relying by faith upon the substances which God has established for our benefit. The Spirit of Prophecy has told us that if at all possible we should be our own doctors. Such a plan cannot be accomplished with the use of drugs which are rigidly controlled, but it can be accomplished if we have faith in the use of God's medicines, the herbs, which He has established for our health and healing, as well as with nature's doctors which He has established for our maintenance of health as well as for our restoration to health. If we study to learn to know about their qualities, we can help ourselves over physical difficulties with these harmless substances which have no poisonous side effects.

With God there are no incurable diseases. His medicines will surprise us in their ability to overcome difficulties which we did not think possible with such modest means.

This book is written mainly for Adventists, but the principles which it presents are considered to be scientifically sound so that anyone can apply them for their own greatest benefit.

KEY TO ABBREVIATIONS

AA	Acts of the Apostles
AH	The Adventist Home
1–12 BC	The Seventh-day Adventist Bible Commentary, vols. 1–12.
CG	Child Guidance
COL	Christ's Object Lessons
CD	Counsels on Diet and Foods
CH	Counsels on Health
CT	Counsels to Parents, Teachers, and Students
DA	The Desire of Ages
Ed	Education
EW	Early Writings
FE	Fundamentals of Christian Education
GW	Gospel Workers
HL	Healthful Living
LS	Life Sketches of Ellen G. White
MH	The Ministry of Healing
MM	Medical Ministry
SD	Sons and Daughters of God
1-3SM	Selected Messages, vols. 1-3
1-4SG	Spiritual Gifts, vols. 1-4
SOHM	The Story of our Health Message
Te	Temperance
1–9 T	The Testimonies, vols. 1–9
WM	Welfare Ministry
YI	Youth's Instructor

CONTENTS

INTRODUCTION iii
KEY TO ABBREVIATIONS v
THE DIVINE PHILOSOPHY OF HEALTH AND HEALING.. 1
    GOD'S HEALING PRINCIPLES 1
        God Created Man Perfect.. 1
        God's Healing Power Is In Nature 1
        God Heals Through The Laws He Has Established 2
        Disobedience To The Laws Of Health Brings Disease 3
        Our Body Is God's Temple 4
        Knowledge of God's Principles Of Health Is A Necessity 5
        Seek God's Help In Case Of Sickness 6
        Health Is Not A Matter Of Chance 8
        The Sin-Sickness Relation 8
        God Helps Those Who Help Themselves 9
GOD'S TRIUNE PHILOSOPHY OF HEALTH AND HEALING 11
    THE HYGIENIC PHILOSOPHY OF HEALTH 11
        Cleanliness Is Next To Godliness 11
        Disease Caused By Uncleanness 12
    THE NATUROPATHIC PHIILOSOPHY OF HEALTH 12
        Following Nature's Path 12
        The Principles Of Naturopathy 13
        The Power Within Us 16
    THE PSYCHOGENIC PHILOSOPHY OF HEALTH 17
        The Proper Mental Attitude 17
        No Mind Should Control Another Mind.. 18
        The Influence Of The Body Upon The Mind 19
        The Causes Of Mental Disease 19
        Healing Mental Disease 20
        Maintaining Proper Mental Health 22
CHRIST'S HEALING PRINCIPLES... 24
    Christ's Use Of Divine Power 24
    Christ's Purpose In Healing 27
    Christ's Use Of Remedies 29
    Bible Examples Of Health Principles Applied And Misapplied 32

SATAN, THE ORIGINATOR OF DISEASE 35
Satan The Destroyer 35
Satan Has Corrupted God's Creation 36
Christ's Warning To Us 39

PRAYER AND HEALING 40
Conditions Of Answered Prayer 40
Not all Are Healed 41
God Responds To Prayer According To His Will 43

THE DIVINE SCIENCE OF HEALTH AND HEALING 45
Disease As A Cleansing Crisis 45
Heredity 45
Accidents 47
Germs And Infections 47
Nutritional Causes 50
Sinful Habits 51

THE CAUSES OF DISEASE 53
The Definition Of Disease 53
Find The Basic Cause Of Disease In Order To Heal Disease 56
Germs As The Cause Of Disease 57
A Natural Treatment Maintains Body Energies 58
Why We Should Maintain Our Health 58
Disease Never Comes Without A Cause 58
Drugs Thwart The Body's Effort At Healing 59
Modern Medicine Looks For External Causes 60
A Hurt Organ Means A Hurt Body 61
Vaccinations 61

THE PREVENTION OF DISEASE 62
It Is Better To Prevent Than To Cure Disease 62
Physicians Are To Be Instructors In Health 63

THE USE OF DRUGS 65

DRUGS AND THE SPIRIT OF PROPHECY 65
Poisonous Substances 65
Drugs Themselves Cause Disease And Death 70
The Results Of Taking Drugs 70
Drugs Produce Side-Effects 71
Drugs Should Not Be Called Medicines 71
Present Benefit And Future Harm 72
Satan Temps Us To Take Poisons 72
The Plant Origin Of Drugs 72

OUR PERSONAL RESPONSIBILITY REGARDING DRUGS 73
We Should Accept God's Light On Drugs 73
Parents Sin Against Themselves And Their Children 73

- We Should Use Herbs Instead Of Drugs 73
- We Should Live Healthfully 74
- We Should Heal Without Drugs 74
- Drugs And Emergencies 75
- Substances Which Counteract Poisonous effects 75

HOW MEDICAL WORKERS SHOULD RELATE TO DRUGS 75
- They Should Understand The Needs Of The Human Body 75
- The Physician Should Use Rational Methods 76

THE ATTITUDE OF OUR INSTITUTIONS TOWARD DRUGS 76
- Mrs. White's Light Regarding Our Sanitariums 76
- Health Reform Should Be Taught 77
- How Nature Responds To Drugs 77
- Drugs Militate Against Patients Recovery 77

GOD'S ATTITUDE TOWARD DRUGS 77

GOD'S DOCTORS FOR THE RESTORATION TO HEALTH 79
GOD'S TRUE REMEDIES 79
- The Simple Agencies Of Nature 79
- We Must Know And Understand God's Remedies 79
- God's Natural Methods Are Superior To Man's Method 80

THE IMPORTANCE OF EXERCISE 81
- Adam And Eve In Eden 81
- It Is Necessary For Good Health 81
- It Quickens The Circulation Of The Blood 82
- Exercise In The Open Air 82
- Exercise Eliminates Impurities From The System 82
- Exercise And Disease 84
- Go Out Of Your Way To Exercise 85
- Exercise For Brain Workers 85
- The Results Of Inactivity 85
- Exercise Increases Bone Mass 85
- Exercise Under Normal Conditions 86
- Exercise And Aging 86
- The Miracle Of Walking 86
- Walking Is Everybody's Opportunity 87
- Walking is Good Medicine 87
- What Nature Lovers Say About Walking 88

THE NEED FOR AIR 88
- Air Is A Life Necessity 88
- Air For The Sick 89
- Indoor Air 90
- The Great Benefits Of Pure Air 90
- The Harmful Effects Of Impure Air 90

The Beneficial Effects Of Negative Ions	91
What We Can Do To Counter Air Pollution	92

WATER 94
- The Blessings Of Pure Water 94
- Making The Proper Use Of Water 95
- Water For Maintaining Health 95
- Types Of Water 95
- Water And Disease 97
- Internal And External Applications Of Water 98
- Impure Water 99
- Water And Diet 100

SUNLIGHT 101
- Sunlight As Healer 101
- Sunlight In Health 101
- Sunlight And Vitamin D 102
- Ultraviolet Light (UVL) 103
- Sunlight And Disease 104
- Sunlight And Skin Cancer 105
- Sunlight And Aging 105

REST 106
- Gods Example Of Rest 106
- Our Need For Rest 106
- The Best Scientific Principles Of Rest 108

TEMPERANCE, ABSTINENCE, AND FASTING 109
- Temperance In All Things 109
- Christ's Example Of Temperance 110
- Fasting And The Spirit Of Prophecy 110
- Fasting And Prayer 110
- Fasting As A Remedy For Disease 110

NUTRITION 115
- The Proper Diet 115
- Food In Natural State Represents Proper Diet 115
- Hygienic Principles Of Food Intake 118
- The Cooking Of Food 124
- The Acid-Alkaline Balance 129
- The Proper Combining Of Food 131
- The Digestion Of Food 132

HERBS ARE GOD'S MEDICINES 134
- God Gave Man The Herbs Of The Field For Food And Medicine 134
- God Gave Man No Flesh Food In The Beginning 134
- God Is Endeavoring To Lead Us Back To His Original Diet 135
- There Are No Incurable Diseases With God 135
- Herbs Of The Bible 135

- The History Of Herbs 137
- Common Herbs Used Today 139
- Flower Remedies—Aroma Therapy 154
- Mrs. White's Use Of Herbs 155
- Back To Eden—Jethro Kloss 157

THE HEALING FOODS 159
- What Is A Healing Substance 159
- Apple—The King Of Fruits 159
- Apricots 161
- Bananas 161
- Barley 162
- Beans And Peas 162
- Broccoli—The King Of The Cabbage Clan 163
- Brussels Sprouts—The Queen Of The Cabbage Family 163
- Cabbage 164
- Carrot 164
- Cherries 165
- Corn 166
- Celery 166
- Cranberry 166
- Date 167
- Figs 167
- Garlic 168
- Grapes 171
- Grapefruit 172
- Nuts 174
- Oats 174
- Olives 175
- Potatoes 177
- Rice 178
- Soybeans 179
- Spinach 180
- Tomatoes 180

SPECIAL FOODS 182
- Carob and Chocolate 182
- Honey 183
- Sugar 187
- Milk 192
- Bread 202

CHOLESTEROL, FATS, AND OILS 206
- Cholesterol—An Important Body Substance 206
- Vegetable Oils Verses Animal Fats 209
- Fish Oils 211

PROTEIN AND MEAT 213

INSPIRATION AND A MEAT DIET 213
God's Original Diet Did Not Include Meat 213
Meat is Secondhand Vegetables 213
The Composition Of Meat 213
What Meat Eating Does To Our Nature 213
Meat Eating And Disease 214
Why Meat Is Not A Good Food 214
A Tenfold Liability To Take Disease 215
The Use Of Eggs 215
Egg Yolk Contains Lecithin 215
Cholesterol Without Lecithin Can Be Harmful 216

MEAT EATING AND THE WORLD'S MORAL DILEMMA 216
Man Is Not Made For Meat Eating 216
Meat Is Low In Fiber 216
Vegetarians Live Longer 217
Vegetarianism Can Save The World 217
The American Attitude Toward Health is CURE-MINDED 217
Our View Of Health Is ADOLESCENT 218
Knowledge Is The Basis Of Prevention 218
Medical Facilities Created By Wealth Do Not Create Health 218
Pure Chemicals Do Not Develop And Maintain Health 219

THE BODY'S NEED FOR PROTEIN 219
The American Protein Craze 219
All Foods Contain Some Protein 219
Raw Protein Is Better Than Cooked Protein 220
Balancing The Amino Acids 220
How To Obtain Complete Proteins 220
The Benefits Of a Low Protein Diet 221
Excess Animal Protein Acidifies The Blood 221
Adventists Live Longer Than The General Population 221
Vegetarians Have More Endurance than Meat Eaters 221
Results Of A High Protein Diet 222
Protein From Soybeans 222
The Relation Between Protein, Carbohydrates, And Fluid Intake 222
Why Adventists Substitute Sweets For Meat 223
Protein Consumption And Aging 223

VITAMINS 224
Vitamins Are Organic Food Substances 224
The Sources Of Vitamins 225
The Daily Requirements Of Vitamins 225
Natural Versus Synthetic Vitamins 226
The Need For Vitamins In Disease 226

- The Need For Vitamins In Counteracting Poisons 227
- Vitamin Interrelationships 227
- Vitamin A 228
- Vitamin B 231
- Vitamin C—Ascorbic Acid 237
- Vitamin D—The Sunshine Vitamin 242
- Vitamin E 245

MINERALS 254
- The Body's Need Of Minerals 254
- Calcium (Ca) 254
- Phosphorus (P) 257
- Magnesium (Mg)—The Miracle Mineral 258
- Potassium (K) 260
- Sodium (Na) 262
- Chlorine (Cl) 262
- Sulfur (S) 263
- The Need For Trace Minerals 264
- Minerals And Other Poisonous Substances And Their Antidotes 267
- The Use Of Salt 270
- Salt And Disease 272
- Salt In Food 274
- Overcoming The Salt Habit 274
- Salt And Water Softeners 275
- Iodized Salt 275

HEALING DISEASE BY NATURAL MEANS 276
- How The Body Heals Disease 276
- Natural IMMUNITY 277
- Food, Vitamins, And Mineral Therapies 278

ACNE 278
- Acne Is An Adolescent Problem 278
- The Causes Of Acne 279
- Food, Vitamin, And Mineral Therapies For Acne 279
- Herbs 280
- General Detoxification 280

AIDS 281
- Nature Of The Disease 281
- Causes Of AIDS 281
- Successful Natural Treatments Of AIDS 282

ALLERGIES 283
- What Are Allergies 283
- The Causes Of Allergies 283
- Allergies From Various Substances 284

How To Prevent Allergies 285
How To Cure Allergies 285
How To Test For Food Allergens 286
ALZHEIMER'S DISEASE 286
Progressive Mental Deterioration 286
Possible Causes 286
Healing Substances For Alzheimer's Disease 287
Things To Do And Not To Do To Avoid Alzheimer's 289
ANEMIA 289
Nature Of The Disease 289
Causes Of Anemia 289
Dietary Considerations 290
Fruit And Vegetable Juices 290
Herbs 290
ARTHRITIS 290
Nature Of The Disease 290
The Causes Of Arthritis 291
Arthritis—An Acid Condition Of The Blood 293
Oxalic Acid 293
Uric Acid 294
How to Restore Arthritics to Health By Natural Means 294
Herbs 297
Other Methods That Have Been Found Beneficial 298
Steps To Strengthen The Immune System 299
ASTHMA 299
Nature Of The Disease 299
Causes Of Asthma 300
How Asthma Can Be Overcome 300
CANCER—A DISEASE OF CIVILIZATION 302
The General Causes Of Cancer 302
Enzymes And Cancer 305
Reduced Respiration Of The Cells 305
The Eating Of Meat And Cancer 305
Salt As A Cause Of Cancer 307
Toxins Cause Cancer 307
Acidity And Cancer 309
Aluminum And Cancer 310
Lack Of Cell Oxygenation As The Basic Cause Of Cancer 310
Cancer—A Deficiency Disease 311
Heat, Fats, And Cancer 312
Hormones And Cancer 313
Monosodium Glutamate—MSG 314

    Nitrates And Nitrites 315
    Overeating And Cancer 315
    Sunshine And Cancer 316
    Sugar, Tars, And Cancer 317
    Smallpox Vaccinations And Cancer 319
    Emotions And Cancer 319
    Radiation And Cancer 321
    Age And Cancer 321
    Types Of Cancer 321

HEALING OF CANCER BY NATURAL METHODS 325
    Methods Of Dealing With Cancer 325
    Hyperthermia—Fever 327
    Laetrile 327
    Vitamins And Cancer 328
    Raw Foods Can Fight And Cure Cancer 331
    Cancer Preventing Foods 332
    Herbs That Fight Cancer 334
    The Prevention Of Cancer 335
    An Anti-Cancer Diet 338
    Natural Professional Cancer Treatments 340

CANDIDA ALBICANS—CANDIDIASIS 344
    Candida Albicans Is Present In Every Person 344
    Causes Of Yeast Infection 344
    How To Heal Candida 345

CATARACTS 345
    Nature of The Disease 345
    The Diet For Cataracts 345

CIRCULATORY PROBLEMS 347
    The Purification Of The Blood 347
    How To Purify The Blood 348
    The Equalization Of The Blood 349

COLDS AND FLU 350
    The Nature Of The Diseases 350
    The Causes Of A Cold 350
    How A Cold Can Be Cured 352
    The Treatment Of A Cold And Flu 353
    How To Prevent A Cold 353

CRAMPS 354
    Causes Of Cramps 354
    How To Heal Cramps 354

CRIB DEATH—SUDDEN INFANT DEATH SYNDROME (SIDS) 355
    Crib Deaths Occur With Bottle-fed Babies 355

- SIDS Is An Allergic Reaction To Cow's Milk 356
- SIDS May Be Due To DPT Vaccinations 356

DIABETES 356
- Nature Of The Disease 356
- The Causes Of Diabetes 358
- Disease-Effects Of Diabetes 359
- Curing Diabetes Naturally 359
- Herbal Teas 362
- Dr. Lamar And Fructose 362

DIARRHEA 363
- Causes 363
- Preventing Diarrhea 363
- Curing Diarrhea 363

FEMALE PROBLEMS 364
- Breast Ailments 364
- Irregular Menstruation 365
- Causes Of Excessive Bleeding 365
- Premenstrual Syndrome (PMS) 366
- How To Cure Menstrual Problems 366
- The Uterus 367

FEVERS 367
- Fever And Inspiration 367
- What Fever Accomplishes In Disease 368
- The Causes Of Fever 369
- How To Cure A Fever 369
- Hay Fever 370
- Rheumatic Fever 370

GALLBLADDER DISEASE 370
- Nature Of The Disease 370
- The Cause Of Gallstones 371
- The Treatment Of Gallstones 372
- The Prevention Of Gallstones 373

GASTROINTESTINAL COMPLAINTS 373
- Stomach Problems 373
- Intestinal Problems 374
- Diet For Gastrointestinal Problems 376

GLAUCOMA 376
- Nature Of The Disease 376
- The Causes Of Glaucoma 377
- The Cure Of Glaucoma 377

HARDENING OF THE ARTERIES—ARTERIOSCLEROSIS—ATHEROSCLEROSIS 378
- Nature Of The Disease 378
- Causes Of Arteriosclerosis 378

 How To Heal Arteriosclerosis 379
HEART DISEASE 381
 Nature Of The Disease 381
 The Prevention Of Heart Disease 381
 Symptoms Of Heart Disease 383
 The Causes Of Heart Disease 383
 The Healing Of Heart Disease 385
HIGH BLOOD PRESSURE — HYPERTENSION (HBP) 386
 Nature Of The Disease 386
 Symptoms Of High Blood Pressure 387
 The Causes Of High Blood Pressure 387
 Results Of High Blood Pressure—Strokes 389
 Ways To Restore Normal Blood Pressure 389
 Herbs 391
 Vitamins 391
 Minerals 392
 Things To Avoid 392
HYPOGLYCEMIA—LOW BLOOD SUGAR 392
 Nature Of The Disease 392
 The Causes of Hypoglycemia 393
 The Effects of Hypoglycemia 394
 How To Heal Low Blood Sugar 394
INFECTIONS 395
 Nature Of The Disease 395
 What To Avoid 395
 How To Heal Infections 396
KIDNEY AND BLADDER DISEASES 397
 Nature Of The Disease 397
 Kidney Stones 397
 The Causes Of Kidney Stone Formation 397
 How to Heal Kidney Disease 399
 Bladder Problems 400
LIVER TROUBLES 401
 Nature Of The Disease 401
 Liver Troubles And Their Causes 401
 How To Heal Liver Troubles 402
MULTIPLE SCLEROSIS 403
 Nature Of The Disease 403
 The Cause Of Multiple Sclerosis 403
 The Cure Of Multiple Sclerosis 403
NERVE DISORDERS 404
 Nature Of The Disease 404

- The Causes Of Nerve Disorders...405
- How To Heal Nerve disorders 405

OSTEOPOROSIS...407
- Nature Of The Disease 407
- The Causes Of Osteoporosis 407
- How To Cure Osteoporosis 408
- What To Avoid 408

PNEUMONIA..409
- Nature Of The Disease 409
- The Symptoms Of Pneumonia..409
- The Causes Of Pneumonia 409
- How To Heal Pneumonia 409

PREMATURE AGING 410
- The Nature Of Aging 410
- Water—Nature's Life Extender..411
- The Causes Of Aging 414
- Effects Of Aging 416
- How To Lengthen The Lifespan...416

PROSTATE PROBLEMS 419
- Nature Of The Problem 419
- The Causes Of Prostate Problems 419
- How To Heal Prostate Disorders 419
- HERBS:..420

SKIN DISEASES 421
- Nature Of The Disease 421
- The Causes Of Skin Diseases 421
- Healing Skin Diseases 422

TUBERCULOSIS 424
- Nature Of The Disease 424
- Causes Of Tuberculosis 424
- How To Heal Tuberculosis 425

ULCERS 425
- Nature Of The Disease 425
- The Causes Of Ulcer 425
- Substances And Methods Used To Control Ulcers 426
- How To Heal Ulcers 427

VARIOUS AFFLICTIONS 429
- Alcoholism...429
- Bruises, Burns, Cuts, Sores, Wounds, And Stings 429
- Leprosy 431
- Headaches 432
- The Natural Elimination Of Pain..434

PSYCHOGENESIS — THE MENTAL CAUSE OF DISEASE 443
The Interrelations Of Mind And Emotions 443
The Mind-Body Unity 443
Emotions Suppress Or Enhance The Immune System 444
Emotional Factors That Lead To Disease 444
To Trust In God Means To Eliminate Our Bad Habits 453
Sinful Desires 453
All Negative Emotions Represent Stress 454
How To Overcome Mental Disease 454
Accept—Appreciation 455
Approve—Praise 455
Adore—Love 456

THE WORK OF OUR SANITARIUMS 457
PURPOSE OF OUR SANITARIUMS 457
To Reform The Medical Practices of Physicians 457
Established To Use Hygienic Methods 457
The Emphasis Is To Be On Sanitariums Rather Than Hospitals 457
The Functions Of Sanitariums 458
Drugs Were To Be Left Out Of Our Sanitariums 458
Sanitariums Were to Teach Self-treatment And Self-denial 459
Sanitariums Were To Advance Present Truth 459
The Sanitarium Diet 459
Healing Of Soul More Important Than Healing Of Body 460
Loma Linda 460
Medical Missionary Work 461

THE WORK OF THE DOCTOR 462
The Physician's Work Is To Cooperate With God 462
The Physician Should Be A Health Reformer 462
Doctors Are Not Well Trained In Nutrition 463
Physicians Should Teach Patients How To Prevent Disease 463
Physician Should Not Follow Practices Condemned By God 464
Physicians Should Teach By Means Of Cause And Effect 464
How The Doctor Treats Disease 466
Doctors And Nutrition 466
How The Doctor Treats The Patient 466
The "Cures" Of Medicine 467
Dealing With Symptoms 468
Surgery 469
Operations Are Not Without Danger 469
Treating Oneself — Self-Healing — Being Your Own Doctor 469

HEALTH REFORM 471
THE PRINCIPLES OF HEALTH REFORM 471
It Is Part Of The Third Angel's Message 471

 It Increases Spirituality 471
 The Need For Temperance 473
 The Results Of Intemperance 474
 Temperance Begins In The Home 475
 The Development Of Self-Control 476
 Reasoning From Cause To Effect... 479
 The Use Of Fiber 480
 Fiber And Disease 480
 Applying Self-Discipline 481
 Acting From Principle 482

BIBLIOGRAPHY 483

GLOSSARY OF TERMS 489

INDEX 490

THE DIVINE PHILOSOPHY OF HEALTH AND HEALING

GOD'S HEALING PRINCIPLES

God Created Man Perfect

◆ *Heir To No Disease*

God is the Creator of all mankind. He has made man what he is. He has designed his form, features and substance. He set all of his organs into action in their proper relationships. He knows what will keep them in healthful condition. It therefore represents prudent intelligence on the part of man to follow the plan that God has designed for our own good. We are told that "man came from the hand of his Creator perfect in organization and beautiful in form.... He possessed a body heir to no disease, and a soul bearing the impress of Deity." In the book of Genesis "we have no record of an infant's being born blind, deaf, crippled, deformed, or imbecile. There is not an instance upon record of a natural death in infancy, childhood, or early manhood. There is no account of men and women dying of disease" (CD117). Furthermore, "If Adam, at his creation, had not been endowed with twenty times as much vital force as men now have, the race, with their present habits of living in violation of natural law, would have become extinct" (3T138–9).

◆ *We Must Come Into Harmony With God's Original Plan*

"All the organs and faculties of his being were equally developed, and harmoniously balanced" (Te 11). "These He designs should work together in harmony. If we injure one all are affected" (HL195). They were all placed under law. If we want to maintain our health and not become sick, we must apply God's design to our daily life, for "the more nearly we come into harmony with God's original plan, the more favorable will be our position for the recovery and preservation of health"(CH174). Health begins with FAITH. Faith in God, without whom we can achieve nothing; Faith in His PRINCIPLES and LAWS of health and healing; faith in his HERBAL MEDICINES and NATURAL DOCTORS; and faith in our BODY'S POWER of SELF-HEALING.

God's Healing Power Is In Nature

◆ *God Is The Only Healer*

"God's healing power runs all through nature. If a human being cuts his flesh or breaks a bone, nature at once begins to heal the injury, and thus preserves the man's life. But man can place himself in a position where nature is trammeled so that she cannot do her work. It is God who has made the provision that nature shall work to restore the exhausted powers. The power is of God. He is the great Healer."(MM 11-12). "All life-giving power is from Him" (CH168).

"The religion of the Bible is not detrimental to the health of the body or of the mind. The influence of the SPIRIT OF GOD is the very best medicine that can be received by a sick man or woman. Heaven is all health; and the more deeply the heavenly influences are realized, the more sure will be the recovery of the believing invalid"(MM12). He says, "I am the Lord that healeth thee"(Ex. 15:26). This indicates that "God alone is the One who can heal" (MH243). It means that whenever one recovers from disease, "It is God who restores him"(MH113).

◆ *Nature The Effectual Restorer*

God constantly works through nature with His healing power. He is working day by day, hour by hour, moment by moment, to keep us alive

(MH112), for nature is God's physician (MH263). Nature alone is the effectual restorer (2SM451), and NATURE ALONE possesses CURATIVE POWERS (2SM452). "The things of nature are God's blessings, provided to give health to the body, mind, and soul. They are given to the well to KEEP THEM WELL, and to the sick to MAKE THEM WELL. Connected with water treatments, they are more effective in restoring health than all the DRUG MEDICATION in the world" (CH169).

Francis Bacon said: "We command nature only by obeying her." We are antagonizing nature by subduing symptoms. We must work with nature to restore health by using substances that are inherent to the chemistry of the body rather than using foreign chemicals with which to eliminate health warning signals.

◆ *God Wants Us Well*

God gives us health, maintains our health, and restores our health. "Who forgiveth all thine iniquities; and healeth all thine diseases" (Ps. 103:3). "He healeth the broken in heart, and bindeth up their wounds" (Ps. 147:3). God's words are health (Prov. 4:22), and departing from evil is health (Prov. 3:7, 8). The fear of the Lord is "health to thy navel, and marrow to thy bones" (Prov. 3:8). God has arranged conditions in such a way that with our desire to keep ourselves well, and with His willingness to make us well, we can maintain our organism in the highest possible condition of health. If by acts of indiscretion or ignorance we become ill, God is willing and able to heal us. As He said to Hezekiah, "I will heal thee" (2 Kings 20:5). Since God alone can heal, we are not to look to any HUMAN BEING as the source of our healing (MH242). Our dependence must be entirely in God, for man cannot heal (MM13). "It is not man who saves life; it is the GREAT RESTORER. NO TRADITION, CUSTOM, OR PRACTICE CONDEMNED BY GOD MUST BE FOLLOWED BY THE BELIEVING PHYSICIAN" (MM122).

◆ *Man Can Bring Health To His Fellow Man*

In the Bible we are told that man can bring health to his neighbor as he presents a pleasant favorable attitude to him. Prov. 12:18 tells us that "the tongue of the wise is health"; that "Pleasant words are as an honeycomb, sweet to the soul, and health to the bones" (Prov. 16:24). If we do welfare work for the poor and needy, then we are told that our "health shall spring forth speedily" (Isa 58:8).

God Heals Through The Laws He Has Established

◆ *The Laws Of Nature Are The Laws Of God*

God has established laws in the physical, spiritual, as well as in the biological sphere. The laws which God has established in nature are as much the laws of God as are the Ten Commandments. Hence, it is as much a sin to violate them as it is to violate the spiritual laws of God. To violate either is to break God's laws (CD17). "Obedience to them must be made a matter of personal duty. IGNORANCE in these things is SIN" (CD18). We must want to obey them for our own good. The person who is careless of the habits and practices that concern his physical life and health shows that he does not recognize, respect, or reverence God. He shows this through the injury done to the body in violation of physical law (HL17). Ignorance may be said to be the cause of much disease.

◆ *Disease Never Comes Without A Cause*

We are told that "disease never comes without a cause. The way is first prepared, and disease invited by disregarding the laws of health" (HL65). "We cannot expect the Lord to work a miracle for us while we neglect the simple remedies He has provided for our use, which, aptly and opportunely applied, will bring about a MIRACULOUS RESULT" (2SM346–7). "Health, strength, and happiness depend upon immutable laws; but these cannot be obeyed where there is not anxiety to become acquainted with them" (HL18). "The Lord will not work a miracle to preserve anyone in health who will not make an effort to obtain the KNOWLEDGE within his reach" (HL16). For this reason everyone has a responsibility to become intelligent in regard to disease and its causes (HL19). "All our enjoyment and suffering may be traced to obedience or transgression of natural law" (CD69).

◆ *The Laws Of Our Being Were Created For Our Good*

If the laws which God has established in our being "were never violated, if all acted in harmony with the divine will, health, peace, and happiness, instead of misery and continued evil would be the result" (CD20). This can be brought about most readily if we realized that "all the laws of nature are designed for our good" (CD464). "God in His wisdom has established natural laws for the proper control of our dress, our appetites, and our passions, and He requires of us obedience in every particular" (HL17). "Every 'Thou shalt not' whether in physical or moral law, contains or implies a promise. If it is obeyed blessings will attend our steps. If it is disobeyed, the result is danger and unhappiness"(Test. No. 32, p. 201). Whenever parents act contrary to the laws of their being, the harm done will be not only to themselves, but it will be repeated in FUTURE GENERATIONS (HL18).

◆ *Observance Of Health Laws Prevents Disease And Premature Death*

If we are to obtain any benefit from the laws of our being, then we must obey them, and follow them strictly. If we accept them as part of our daily living, they will keep us from disease and premature death (CD16). If people in general would obey them, it would eliminate NINE TENTHS of all misery and suffering in the world (Te164). God wants us to live as long as possible here on this earth so that through our service to humanity, we can do the greatest amount of good over the greatest length of time. A failure to live by the laws of our being will reduce that period of time available to us by producing disease and premature death (CD16).

A failure to care for our bodies is an insult to the Creator who has made us, and those who transgress the law of God in their physical being, will be inclined to violate the law of God as spoken from Sinai (CD17). We are told that the human family is suffering because of the transgression of the laws of God, and that "natures laws are not to be resisted but obeyed" (CH206, 127). Sometimes we think that disease is an accident which just happens, and for which there is no explanation. You caught something which you didn't want to catch. However, we are also told that health "is the result of obedience to law" (MH128). The lack of health means that we were in some way possibly disobedient to some law of health which disorganized some law of our being to make us sick.

◆ *Every Transgression Has A Penalty Attached To It*

For every law which God has established in our being, He has established a penalty for transgression. This penalty the individual transgressor must pay in his own body (CD142). Nature will protest every violation of these laws of life, and the penalty which is reaped will fall upon the mental as well as the physical powers (Te56). In spite of God's direct command, individuals will follow their inclinations, and will at times pray over the matter in order to allow God to approve their actions which are contrary to His expressed commands (CH109). However, we should realize that only obedience leads to happiness in life, and that disobedience leads to unhappiness and suffering (CD17).

"Those who have the light and do not follow it, but disregard the requirements of God, will find that their blessings will be changed to curses, and their mercies into judgments" (CD379). If we are not serious with regard to obeying the laws of health, if we will not eat and drink from principle, then we will not be strong to abide by principles in other matters (Te138). "A strict compliance with the requirements of God is beneficial to the health of body and mind" (CD32). We can become perfect only through SELF-DENIAL (CD36). If we consider these matters unimportant, we will find that God does not consider them so. A "thus said the Lord is to be our rule in all things" (CD57)

Disobedience To The Laws Of Health Brings Disease

◆ *Careless Inattention To The Laws Of Health Is Sin*

In the history of the world "the violation of physical law with its consequent suffering and premature death, has so long prevailed that these results are regarded as the appointed lot of humanity" (CD118). "The majority of diseases which the human family have been and are still suffering under they have created by IGNORANCE of their own organic laws. They seem indifferent in regard to the matter of health, and work perseveringly to tear themselves to pieces, and when broken down and debilitated in body and mind, send for the doctor and drug themselves to death" (CD19). But God did not bring about these conditions. It was the work of man that brought them about. It was brought about by the application of wrong habits to the daily affairs of life in eating, drinking, and working. We are told that if men had always been obedient to the laws of the Ten Commandments, "the curse of disease now flooding the world would not exist" (CD118). One cannot violate a single principle of nature without suffering for it. One will suffer for it whether one realizes it or not. One's body does not always make one immediately aware of the problems our BAD HABITS impose upon it. "God has claims upon your powers, therefore CARELESS INATTENTION to the laws of health is SIN. The better you observe the laws of health, the more clearly you can DISCERN TEMPTATIONS, and resist them, and the more clearly you can discern the VALUE OF ETERNAL THINGS" (Te188).

◆ *Neglect Does Not Glorify God*

Carelessness and inattention to health is shown by EATING AT ALL HOURS (GW241), by the LACK OF PHYSICAL AND MENTAL VIGOR (4T35), by MENTAL BREAKDOWN (SD172), and by APOPLEXY (4T502). Such results do not glorify God and bring his displeasure upon us (Te148). Such results are also seen in the offspring, and their tendencies toward physical weakness, disordered nerves, and unnatural cravings, which are transmitted to them as a legacy from parents to children to the third and fourth generations (Te56). "It is not possible for us to glorify God while living in violation of the laws of life and health" (Te148). "The only path of safety is for young and old to live in strict conformity to the principles of physical and moral law. The PATH OF OBEDIENCE is the only path that leads to HEAVEN" (Te60).

◆ *Obedience Brings Health*

The obedience that prevents illness is the obedience that brings health. There are many people who have asked Mrs. White for the best way to preserve their health. Her answer was, "Cease to transgress the laws of your being; cease to gratify a depraved appetite; eat simple food; dress healthfully, which will require modest simplicity; work healthfully; and you will not be sick" (CH37). She further says, "When men and women are truly converted, they will conscientiously regard the laws of life that God has established in their being, thus seeking to avoid physical, mental, and moral feebleness. Obedience to these laws must be made a matter of PERSONAL DUTY. We ourselves must suffer the ills of violated law" (CD18–19). Such obedience will bring us physical and mental vigor, and moral power for the warfare against Satan, against whom we may be more than conquerors on our own account (4T35–6).

Our Body Is God's Temple

◆ *We Are Made In God's Image*

God is the owner of the whole man. Body, soul, and spirit are His. Our life belongs to God to be consecrated to His service, that through the exercise of every faculty we may glorify Him. We are a specimen of God Himself, for we are made in His image. By the misuse of our powers we rob God of the honor due Him. We are God's workmanship and the Scriptures declare that we are "fearfully and wonderfully made" (Ps. 139:14). For this reason our HEALTH should be as carefully GUARDED AS OUR CHARACTER (ML144).

◆ *God Expects Us To Present Him A Living Sacrifice*

We are told "Know ye not that ye are the TEMPLE OF GOD, and that the Spirit of God dwelleth in you? If any man defile the temple of God, him shall God destroy; for the temple of God is holy, which temple ye are" (1 Cor. 3:16, 17). Paul says, "I beseech you therefore, brethren, by the mercies of God, that ye present your bodies a living sacrifice, holy, acceptable unto God, which is your reasonable service" (Rom. 12:1) "The Lord requires a LIVING SACRIFICE OF MIND, SOUL, BODY, AND STRENGTH" (HL42). "We were created so that every faculty might be the faculty of the divine mind" (ST May 31, 1896). In 3 John 2 John says, "Beloved, I wish above all things that thou mayest prosper and be in health, even as thy soul prospereth." For this reason we should not do anything with and to our bodies which will DEFILE them, for God has declared that if we do so He will destroy us. Disobedience to the physical laws of our being will defile the body temple, which is also the TEMPLE OF THE HOLY GHOST. Under these circumstances "It is impossible for a man to present his body a living sacrifice, holy and acceptable to God, while continuing in habits that are depriving him of physical, mental, and moral vigor" (CD119). Whatever injures the health not only lessens physical vigor, but tends to weaken the mental and moral powers. (MH128).

◆ *Health Makes Our Life Functions Useful*

Every function of life becomes more or less useless if we do not have health. Christ said that He came "that we might have life, and that we might have it more abundantly" (Jo. 10:10). If we do not have health, we have life only in a limited way. This means that we are bought with a price, and should therefore glorify God in our body and spirit which belong to Him (1 Cor. 6:20). It also means that our "body is the temple of the Holy Ghost which is in you, which ye have of God, and ye are not your own" (1 Cor. 6:19).

◆ *As God's Property We Are Not At Liberty To Do As We Please*

God wants us as active living beings to live for Him as long as life shall last. He wants us to live for Him even more than He wants us to die for Him. Even when we die an honorable martyr's death, our life of service for Him may be prematurely cut short. When we live for Him our influence can benefit the world for many years to come. "'Ye are not your own, for ye are bought with a price' should be hung in memory hall that we may ever recognize God's right to our talents, our property, our influence, our individual selves" (CD56), for "God is the owner of the whole man" (YI 9-7-1893). We should also recognize that "it is impossible for a man to present his body a living sacrifice, holy, acceptable to God, while continuing to indulge habits that are depriving him of physical, mental, and moral vigor" (CD119). We are all under obligation to preserve the living organism according to the laws of life and health. We are told that we can do the very BEST HOME MISSIONARY WORK BY TAKING CARE OF GOD'S TEMPLE, "for the health is to be as sacredly guarded as the character"(MM80; ML144).

◆ *The Wrong Food Defiles God's Temple*

When we take food into our body, we do so in order to nourish it, to maintain its health, and its integrity. The WRONG KIND OF FOOD, which may partially nourish the body and also harm bodily functions, WILL DEFILE the body and will lead it in the direction of disease and death. Daniel faced this fact when he said that he would not defile himself with the kings meat and wine (Dan. 1:8). If under these circumstances a person goes against his conscience, the inevitable result will follow. "If any man defile the temple of God, him shall God destroy" (1 Cor. 3:17)

Knowledge of God's Principles Of Health Is A Necessity

◆ *There Are Conditions To Be Observed To Maintain Health*

It is the Christian's responsibility to know and understand the laws of health, and to carefully observe them. This we owe to ourselves and to God. He considers it a sin for us to be ignorant of them when so much information has been made available to us. "There are CONDITIONS to BE OBSERVED by all who would preserve health. All should learn what these conditions are. The Lord is not pleased with IGNORANCE in regard to His laws, either natural or spiritual. We are to be workers together with God for the restoration of health to the body as well as to the soul" (CD121). The majority of the diseases which the human family is suffering under they have created by IGNORANCE of their own organic laws (CD19). In times past God may have winked at our ignorance of these laws, but now that we have so much knowledge on this subject he expects us to place ourselves in a right relation to these laws (CD20). This means that ignorance can no longer be claimed as an excuse for disobedience (CD70). God blesses those who make every effort to keep themselves free from disease and lead others to REGARD AS SACRED the HEALTH of the BODY as well as of the SOUL (6T302).

"Men and women should inform themselves in regard to the PHILOSOPHY OF HEALTH. The present generation have trusted their bodies with the doctors and their souls with the ministers. If they are sick, they send for the doctor—believe whatever He may tell, and swallow anything he may prescribe. They are not interested to learn how to keep their bodies in a healthy condition and prevent disease. A practical knowledge of the SCIENCE OF HUMAN LIFE is necessary in order to glorify God in our bodies. It is therefore of the highest importance that among the studies selected for childhood, PHYSIOLOGY should occupy THE FIRST PLACE" (CH37–8).

◆ *We Must Live Up To The Light Given*

It is our sacred duty to live up to the light which God has graciously given us. If we close our eyes to the light because we are afraid to face our wrong habits which we are unwilling to let go of, such WILLING IGNORANCE is still considered a sin (CD44). If we ignore the principles in one case, it is easier to ignore them in another case, and our sin is not thereby reduced (CD45). "Many are living in violation of the laws of health, and are ignorant of the relation their habits of eating, drinking, and working sustain to their health" (CD304). "Many are ignorant of the fact that DIET exerts a powerful influence upon the health" (MM77). Most people know better than they do, but they need to be impressed with the importance of making their knowledge a guide to life. (MH126). "A practical knowledge of the SCIENCE OF HUMAN LIFE is necessary in order to glorify God in our bodies" (CH38).

◆ *God Is Trying To Lead Us Back To His Original Design*

In this modern age we have strayed away from God's plan, and have adopted man's inventions as being superior to God's methods of retaining and restoring health. It seems that most of man's inventions work contrary to the laws, methods, and remedies which God has established for our good. This implies that some of the methods which man has established have not served man's best interest even though they were intended to do so. For this reason "God is trying to lead us back step by step to His original design—that man should SUBSIST UPON THE NATURAL PRODUCTS OF THE EARTH" (CD380). "God never forces us to do right, but He seeks to save us from the evil and lead us to the good" (MH114). "In His written word and in the book of nature He has revealed the principles of life. It is our work to obtain a knowledge of these principles, and by obedience cooperate with Him in restoring health to the body as well as to the soul" (MH115).

◆ *We Must Know Ourselves*

We are told that "The greatest cause of human suffering is IGNORANCE on the subject of how to treat our own bodies" (CD241). "Thousands of children die because of the IGNORANCE of parents and teachers.... In order to be in accordance with fashion and custom, many parents have sacrificed the health and lives of their children.... When parents allow children to eat irregularly and between meals of unhealthful food, they don't realize that they are sowing the seed which will bring forth disease and death " (CH176).

It is possible to know and understand the laws of health without applying them to our daily life. Every day we are forming habits. They may be for good or for evil. They may be habits of strict temperance or of self-gratification. We should remember that our FIRST DUTY to God and our fellow beings is that of SELF-DEVELOPMENT. Every faculty with which the Creator has endowed us should be cultivated to the highest degree of perfection so that we may be able to do the greatest amount of good of which we are capable (CD15). "The very best experience we can gain is to KNOW OURSELVES" (2SM289).

◆ *Sickness Represents A Draft Upon Others*

"Our first duty, one which we owe to God, to ourselves, and to our fellowmen, is to obey the laws of God, which include the laws of health. If we are sick, we impose a weary tax upon our friends, and unfit ourselves for discharging our duties to our families and to our neighbors. And when premature death is the result of our violation of nature's law, we bring sorrow and suffering to others; we deprive our neighbors of the help we ought to render them in living; we rob our families of the comfort and help we might render them, and rob God of the service He claims of us to advance His glory. Then, are we not, in the worst sense, transgressors of God's law?" (CD21).

Seek God's Help In Case Of Sickness

◆ *Seek God's Help First*

When we do get sick in spite of all that we have done to remain healthy, we should be ready to seek God's help first. We are told that God can heal all manner of disease by a touch, a word, or a look (5T196). In a moment of time He could heal the human race of all their diseases. But He knew that man must have something to do in order that life might be a blessing to him (4T472–3). When we seek God's help first, what we are saying is that we do want to live according to God's laws of life and health, and that we are appealing to God to help us maintain our status in that regard. It also means that we have, to the best of our knowledge, been trying to live up to God's principles in regard to this matter. It also indicates that we are willing to employ the simple means which God has ordained for the restoration of health. "Our Savior's words, 'Come unto me and I will give you rest', are a prescription for the healing of physical, mental, and spiritual ills" (MH115). "We are to do all in our power for the healing of the BODY, but we are to make the healing of the SOUL of far greater importance" (CH272).

When our sickness is due to the transgression of natural law, we are not as likely to CORRECT OUR MISTAKES and ask God's forgiveness for them, which we should do, but we instead seek out a physician to help us (5T194). If we do get better as a result, we do not then have a strong inclination to correct our mistakes, but instead we give the MEDICINE and the PHYSICIAN the CREDIT for healing us. What we are then doing is to idolize the wisdom and power of man. We should really give the GREAT PHYSICIAN, who is able to save us to the uttermost, all the glory and honor for correcting, through His physical laws, all of the mistakes that we have made. Otherwise, we will always be dependent upon the human physician and his medicines to bring us health, instead of perhaps modifying some of our habits in order to maintain our health ourselves in the future. If need be, God will lead us to a God-fearing physician who will further assist nature in her work of healing the injured body.

◆ *God's Pledge*

We are told that "God pledges Himself to keep this human machinery in healthful action if the human agent will obey His laws and cooperate with Him" (CD17). This is a pledge that we can rely upon. God will fulfill this pledge to us if we do our part. "All His promises are on condition of obedience" (4SpG 148). In the case of the Israelites, God said, "If thou wilt diligently harken to the voice of the Lord thy God, and wilt do that which is right in His sight, and wilt give ear to His commandments, and keep all His statutes, I will put none of these diseases upon thee which I have brought upon the Egyptians; for I am the Lord that healeth thee" (Ex. 15:26). We are told that "Christ gave to Israel definite instruction in regard to their habits of life, and He assured them 'The Lord will take away from thee all sickness' (Deut. 7:15). When they fulfilled the conditions, the promise was verified to them. 'There was not one feeble person among their tribes'" (Ps. 105:37; CD121).

However, Israel did not always obey the instruction they received, nor did they always profit from their advantages. If they had done so, "they would have been the WORLD'S OBJECT-LESSON of HEALTH and PROSPERITY. If as a people they had lived according to God's plan, they would have been preserved from the diseases that afflicted other nations. Above any other people they would have possessed physical strength, and vigor of intellect. They would have been the mightiest nation on the earth" (MH283). This shows that "nothing less than perfect obedience can meet the standard of God's requirements" (Te106). Individual servants of God such as Joseph, Daniel, Moses and Elisha followed God's principle, and we are told that if we follow their example, the same blessings would follow us (MH285).

◆ *God Always Takes The Blame*

The lesson to be learned here is for us also. This example does not necessarily imply that God would simply work a miracle to keep the Israelites in health, but rather that their obedience to His laws, upon which His blessing was placed, would keep them in health. "If they would obey Him in all things, He would preserve them from disease"(2SM412). By the statement "which I have brought upon the Egyptians" God did not mean that He had actually made them sick. What He meant was that they were made sick due to their disobedience to His laws of health. The principle involved in this statement is that in the Bible GOD MAKES HIMSELF RESPONSIBLE FOR THAT WHICH HE DOES NOT PREVENT, even if such responsibility is an indirect responsibility, for He has the omnipotent power to prevent anything that He wants to prevent. This is indicated in Isa 53:10 where it says that "it pleased the Lord to bruise Him," thereby indicating that He took the blame for His Son's crucifixion and death.

Health Is Not A Matter Of Chance

We are told that "health does not depend upon chance. It is a result of obedience to law" (MH128). Dr. Waerland of Sweden said: "Man brought disease upon himself by disobeying the God-given laws of nature. Eliminate the mistakes in your way of living and attune yourself with the laws of health and all diseases will disappear." The laws within our being are divinely appointed rules which, if observed, will allow us to live a normal lifetime of at least seventy years, and keep us from going off the stage of action before our time. He does not want us to shorten our lifetime due to lack of consideration of the laws of health. "Whatever injures the health not only lessens physical vigor, but tends to weaken the mental and moral powers. Indulgence in any unhealthful practice makes it more difficult for one to DISCRIMINATE BETWEEN RIGHT AND WRONG and hence more difficult to resist evil. It increases the danger of failure and defeat" (MH128). "If men strictly and conscientiously kept the law of God, there would be no drunkards, no tobacco inebriates, no distress, penury, and crime. Liquor saloons would be closed for want of patronage, and NINE-TENTHS of all misery existing in the world would come to an end" (Te164).

The Sin-Sickness Relation

◆ *Sickness Is Caused By Sin*

We are told that "there is a divinely appointed connection between sin and disease.... SIN AND DISEASE bear to each other the relationship of CAUSE AND EFFECT" (CH325). "It is a sin to be sick, for all sickness is the result of transgression. Many are suffering in consequence of the transgression of their parents. They cannot be censured for their parents' sin; but it is nevertheless their duty to ascertain wherein their parents violated the laws of their being, which has entailed upon their offspring so miserable an inheritance; and wherein their parents' habits were wrong they should change their course, and place themselves by correct habits in a better relation to health."(CH37).

◆ *Sin Is Our Own Act*

We should realize that it is not in the power of earth or hell to compel anyone to do evil. Satan attacks us at our WEAK POINTS, but we need not be overcome. However severe or unexpected the assault, God has provided help for us, and in his strength we may conquer (PP421). "No man without his own consent can be overcome by SATAN. The tempter HAS NO POWER TO CONTROL THE WILL OR FORCE THE SOUL TO SIN. He may distress but he cannot contaminate. He can cause agony but not defilement. The fact that Christ has conquered should inspire His followers with courage to fight manfully the battle against sin and Satan" (GC510), for EVERY SIN IS AN OFFENSE TO GOD (MH228). "Every man is tempted when he is drawn away of his own lusts and enticed.... It is Satan's act to tempt us, but it is our own act to yield. It is not in the power of all the host of Satan to force the tempted one to transgress" (4T623). "NO MAN CAN BE FORCED TO COMMIT SIN." "TEMPTATION, HOWEVER STRONG, IS NEVER AN EXCUSE FOR SIN" (5T177). "No matter how severe the pressure that is brought to bear upon us, SIN IS OUR OWN ACT" (AH331). Since the COMMISSION of sin is our own act, the EXPULSION of sin is also our own act, although this cannot be accomplished without divine help (DA466).

◆ *There Is Always A Reason For Disease*

"DISEASE NEVER COMES WITHOUT A CAUSE. The way is prepared, and disease invited, by disregard of the laws of health" (CD122). "The burden of sin, with its unrest and unsatisfied desires, lies at the very foundation of a large share of the maladies the sinner suffers"(CH202). "Sin has brought many of them where they are—to a state of feebleness of mind and debility of body" (CH373). The Jews weren't too far off when they considered disease to be the result of a life of sin, "an evidence of divine displeasure" (DA267). This idea, however, had become perverted in that they believed that disease and death proceeded from God as punishment arbitrarily inflicted on account of sin. They considered it as a JUDGMENT FROM GOD. It was falsely attributed to God's providence. So people who were suffering from an ailment had the additional burden of being regarded as great sinners. However, "the history of Job had shown that SUFFERING IS INFLICTED BY SATAN, and is OVERRULED BY GOD for purposes of mercy" (DA471).

The unregenerate heart will not consider the misuse of its physical powers as very important. It will regard such sin as a trivial thing, and will excuse it as a weakness in human nature. He will even cherish the wrong which should be condemned. But we are not to tamper with sin which is the source of every misery in our world (6T404). We should not lessen our guilt by excusing it. Familiarity with sin blinds one's eyes to its enormity (MYP398). The excuses which people give to their wrong action is that it was the circumstances that caused it (MH178). We should realize that NO SIN IS SMALL IN GOD'S SIGHT (SC30). Therefore we should never seek to cover it up (1SM390). We should have NO SOFT WORDS FOR SIN (Ev 368). Without God's help we cannot keep ourselves from sin for one moment (MH180). Sickness is caused by NEGLECT, IGNORANCE, and ABUSE of the BODY; through HARMFUL HABITS, and DEFICIENT FOOD. "Whatever injures the health not only lessens physical vigor, but tends to weaken the moral powers. Indulgence in any unhealthful practice makes it more difficult for one to discriminate between right and wrong, and hence more difficult to resist evil" (MH128).

◆ *Sin Can Be Overcome*

We are born with INHERENT TENDENCIES to sin (5BC1128), but we cannot say that we are born as sinners. If this were the case then we would have had to break the law before we were born. Each person has a close struggle with the problem of overcoming sin in his own life. Nevertheless, it is possible for every person to overcome every sin in his own life (1T144). It is a fatal mistake for anyone to believe that sin cannot be overcome. Such an idea is a deception of Satan (GC489). With God all things are possible (Mark 10:27), and we should never despair of accomplishing this task. In fact we must accomplish it, because God's law will excuse no sin (MH451). Here we must state that God and Christ will not excuse sin either, but they will not condemn the sinner. It is the law of God that will condemn the sinner (COL218).

God hates sin but loves the sinner (SC54). He is willing to do what is necessary to help the sinner overcome sin. The sinner cannot overcome sin in his own strength (PP717), but he must strive with all his might to do his part in the process of overcoming. WITH DIVINE HELP IT IS POSSIBLE TO OVERCOME EVERY SIN (MYP55). The power to overcome is given by Christ (AA306), with the help of his angels (1T346). The warfare against sin involves self-denial and cross-bearing (3T43), for the natural propensities of our being must be controlled (4T235). Sin is not to be given up a little at a time (1SM327), but must be cast out of the soul through confession and repentance (8T46). The worst thing about sin is that it separates the people from God (PP584).

God Helps Those Who Help Themselves

We are told that "the Lord helps those who help themselves" (CD35). There are many things which we can do for ourselves which others cannot do for us, or which they cannot do as well for us. We can take care of our bodies better than anyone else can do for us. We can get exercise, breathe fresh air, rest when needed, drink plenty of water, dress ourselves properly according to environmental conditions, and work moderately. We are also told that we can do for ourselves that which the most experienced physician can never do for us, and that is to REGULATE OUR DIET. (CD124). We can do these things while we are well, and some of them we can have control over while we are ill.

Mrs. White says that "We are working to educate our people how to treat the body in sickness, how to regain health, and how to keep well when health is restored" (MM63). This is the best home missionary work, and we are admonished that "All teachers and students should learn how to TREAT THEMSELVES" (MM81), and that "all should UNDERSTAND WHAT TO DO FOR THEMSELVES in case of sickness" (2SM290). People "may have every facility to develop a perfect character; but all will be in vain unless they are willing to HELP THEMSELVES. They must put forth their own God-given powers, or they will sink lower and lower, and be of no account for good, either in time or in eternity" (Te114–15). "The philosophy of health should compose one of the important studies for our children. It is all-important that the human organism be understood, and then intelligent men and women can be THEIR OWN PHYSICIANS" (2SM443).

GOD'S TRIUNE PHILOSOPHY OF HEALTH AND HEALING

HYGIENIC—NATUROPATHIC—PSYCHOGENIC

THE HYGIENIC PHILOSOPHY OF HEALTH

Cleanliness Is Next To Godliness

◆ *Perfect Cleanliness Means Perfect Health*

GOD'S PHILOSOPHY OF HEALTH is first of all a hygienic philosophy. This means that health depends upon cleanliness, both internal and external. It was John Wesley who coined the phrase "cleanliness is next to godliness." But such a phrase harmonizes with all Bible principles. We are told that "the mighty God of Israel is still a God of cleanliness" (CH82). "Order and cleanliness is the law of heaven" (4T142), therefore, "Strict habits of cleanliness should be observed" (CH61), and PERFECT CLEANLINESS is necessary for perfect health.

A knowledge of physiology and hygiene should be the basis of all educational effort, that every school should give such instruction, and that the health should thereby be as faithfully guarded as the character (Ed. 195, 196). In the study of hygiene students should also be taught the NUTRIENT VALUE of different foods (Ed. 204).

◆ *Cleanliness Required Of The Israelites*

In the time of Christ individuals suspected of a serious disease had to show themselves to the priests to be judged regarding the presence of such a disease. If they had the leprosy they were called unclean, were separated from the rest of society, and had to congregate with their own kind. The clothing which they wore was finally to be burnt. In all the affairs of daily life the distinction between clean and unclean was observed among the Israelites. The necessity of personal cleanliness was taught in the most impressive manner. Before they gathered at Mount Sinai to listen to the proclamation of the law they were to wash themselves and their clothing. This direction was enforced on pain of death. NO IMPURITY was to be tolerated in the presence of God.

Anyone who touched any sick person or anything that the sick person touched was to wash his clothes, bathe himself in water, and was to be unclean till the evening (MH279). "God commanded that the children of Israel should in no case allow impurities of their persons, or of their clothing. Those who had any PERSONAL UNCLEANNESS were shut out of the camp until evening, and then were required to cleanse themselves and their clothing before they could enter the camp. Also they were commanded of God to have no impurities upon their premises within a great distance of the encampment, lest the Lord should pass by and see their uncleanness" (2SM461)

◆ *God Requires Cleanliness From Us Today*

"If God was so particular to enjoin cleanliness upon those journeying in the wilderness, who were in the open air nearly all the time, He requires no less of us who live in ceiled houses, where impurities are more observable and have a more unhealthful influence" (CG106). "A great amount of SUFFERING might be SAVED if all would labor to PREVENT DISEASE, by strictly obeying the laws of health. Strict habits of cleanliness should be observed. Many, while well, will not take the trouble to keep in a healthy condition. They neglect personal cleanliness, and are not careful to keep their clothing pure. Impurities are constantly and imperceptibly passing from the body through the pores, and if the surface of the skin is not kept in a healthy condition, the system is burdened with impure matter. Its millions of pores are quickly clogged unless kept clean by frequent bathing, and the impurities which should pass off through the SKIN become an additional burden to the other eliminating organs" (MH276).

Disease Caused By Uncleanness

◆ *We Must Cleanse System Of Impurities*

We are told that "A NEGLECT OF CLEANLINESS WILL INDUCE DISEASE. Sickness and premature death do not come without a cause" (2SM461). The God of Israel is still the God of cleanliness. God says, "Be ye clean that bear the vessels of the Lord" (Isa 52:11). It is the function of all of GOD'S HEALTH AGENCIES to cleanse the system from IMPURITIES so as to establish healthful conditions within the body. This means that the causes of disease are largely to be found in the impurities that are produced within the body, or that are introduced there from without (CH52). In order for us to help God's agencies to do the cleansing, we must acquire an intelligent knowledge of their nature (CH503). If the clothing is not frequently cleaned, the pores of the skin REABSORB the WASTE MATTER thrown off. If the impurities of the body are not allowed to escape, they are taken back into the blood, and are forced upon the internal organs. Nature to relieve herself of POISONOUS IMPURITIES, makes an effort to free the system, which effort produces fevers, and what we call DISEASE (2SM460).

It has been recently determined that bacteria cannot live at FEVER TEMPERATURES. Also that IRON and ZINC stores, which bacteria need for growth, are lowered during a FEVER, so that bacteria are both BURNED and STARVED. Instead of being seen as an enemy, fever is acknowledged as an ally in the treatment of disease.

The impurities about their premises have brought upon families contagious diseases. Every family that prizes health should cleanse their houses and their premises of all decaying substances (2SM461). "DEATH-PRODUCING GERMS abound in dark, neglected corners, in decaying refuse, in dampness and mold and must. No waste vegetables or heaps of fallen leaves should be allowed near the house to decay and poison the air. Nothing unclean or decaying should be tolerated within the home. In towns or cities regarded perfectly healthful, many an epidemic of fever has been traced to decaying matter about the dwelling of some careless householder. Perfect cleanliness, plenty of sunlight, careful attention to sanitation in every detail of the home life, are essential to freedom from disease and to the cheerfulness and vigor of the inmates of the home" (CG108).

◆ *Hygienic Living*

Hygienic living is "clean living." In the process of everyday living, cells break down and die, and they become part of the refuse which must be eliminated from the body. In the metabolism of food, and food substances, even of the best of food, some of the products of digestion become waste products, which will clog the system if they are not eliminated from it. This means that even pure foods develop waste products. God in His wisdom has created herbs, plants, and fruit trees whose substances and fruits are compatible with man's organic makeup, so that they are food for man's organism. Such plants and fruits when eaten and assimilated, give strength to body and mind, and promote the highest degree of development of both. Besides being food, these substances have the property of keeping the body clean, and therefore in the best possible healthful condition. They also act as medicines, because they act to keep the body clean, thereby preventing disease. This is why some naturopathic doctors have written books entitled, "Food Is Your Best Medicine."

THE NATUROPATHIC PHILOSOPHY OF HEALTH

Following Nature's Path

◆ *God's Restoring Power Is In All Nature*

The second phase of God's philosophy of health is NATUROPATHY, which means "nature's path." This idea is exemplified in the statement, "NATURE'S PATH is the road He marks out and it is broad enough for any Christian" (CH74). In order for us to get well with God's blessing, we must make use of the agencies of nature which He has given us for our health and healing. Aristotle said: "If there is one way better than another, it is the WAY OF NATURE." This statement is as true today as when it was first uttered over 2000 years ago.

◆ *Nature Is God's Physician*

We are told that nature is God's physician. The PURE AIR, the GLAD SUNSHINE, the FLOWERS and TREES, the ORCHARDS and VINEYARDS, and OUTDOOR EXERCISE are health-giving, and life-giving. Physicians and nurses should encourage their patients to be much in the open air. OUTDOOR LIFE is the only remedy that many invalids need. It has a wonderful power to heal diseases caused by the excitements and excesses of fashionable life, a life that weakens and destroys the powers of body, mind, and soul. There are life-giving properties in the balsam of the PINE, in the fragrance of the CEDAR and the FIR, and other trees also have properties that are health-restoring. EXERCISE in the open air should be prescribed as a LIFE-GIVING NECESSITY, and no open air exercise is better than the CULTIVATION OF THE SOIL. (MH263–5).

◆ *What Modern Hygienists Are Saying*

Hygienist T. C. Fry makes the following statements: "All healing is the exclusive province of the body wisdom and power. RESTORATIVE POWER IS ONLY IN NATURE. You cannot violate a single principle of nature without suffering for it. You will suffer for it whether you realize it or not. Your body does not always make you consciously aware of the problems your bad habits impose upon you. Hygienists reject drugs, and they reject the theory of drug action. Drugs are in their very nature POISONOUS. This is their intrinsic quality. All current medical steps amount to harmful interference with the healing process. Because they do not understand disease, they do not understand health. Only the practice of SETTING BONES, REPAIRING THE RESULTS OF INJURIES, and the MECHANICAL CORRECTION OF PHYSICAL DEFECTS, can be said to be CONSTRUCTIVE PRACTICE."

◆ *God Blesses His Remedies In Nature*

It is only natural that God wants us to use His own remedies, for they are the ones, which, if rightly used, insure our well-being, and also restore our well-being. In reality we may say that God really blesses only His remedies, and not any remedies which He has not ordained. "When in faith the human agent does all He can to combat disease, using the simple methods of treatment that God has provided, his efforts will be blessed of God" (CD25). The remedies we are to use are, "PURE AIR, SUNLIGHT, ABSTEMIOUSNESS, REST, EXERCISE, PROPER DIET, THE USE OF WATER, TRUST IN DIVINE POWER, — these are the TRUE REMEDIES." (MH127) These are the remedies for the want of which thousands are dying. They do not tax or debilitate the system through their powerful properties, yet they are going out of date because their skillful use requires work that the people do not appreciate. God has made them easily available to everybody, and they are all available with little expense; but drugs are expensive, both in outlay of means, and in the injurious effect they have upon the system (CD301). In addition to these FOR MEDICINES GOD HAS GIVEN US THE HERBS OF THE FIELD, and other common substances (2SM279, 288, 289, 291–980). God wants us to use these for ourselves after we have gained knowledge of their medicinal properties through study and application. With their use God wants us to BE OUR OWN DOCTORS as far as that is possible.

◆ *Nature's Process Of Healing Is Gradual*

"Nature's process of healing and upbuilding is GRADUAL and to the impatient it seems slow. The surrender of hurtful indulgences requires sacrifice. But in the end it will be found that nature, untrammeled, does her work wisely and well. Those who persevere in obedience to her laws will reap the reward in health of body and health of mind. Sick people do not have to go to far away places to regain their health. If they would eat temperately, engage in healthful exercise with a cheerful spirit, they would, in NINE CASES OUT OF TEN, regain health and save time and money.(CD301, 302).

The Principles Of Naturopathy

In his book *Everybody's Guide To Nature Cure* by Harry Benjamin, the author gives us the principles of naturopathy, and we will now compare the health principles presented in the Spirit of Prophecy with the principles which he presents.

◆ Disease Is Due To Impurities In The System

A. Benjamin, p. 8. — "The first and most fundamental principle of Nature Cure is that all forms of disease are due to the same cause, namely, the accumulation in the system of WASTE MATERIALS and BODILY REFUSE, which has been steadily piling up in the body of the individual concerned through years of wrong habits of living, the chief of these being wrong feeding, improper care of the body, and habits tending to set up enervation and nervous exhaustion, such as worry, overwork, excesses and abuses of all kinds."

B. White, MH127 — "Disease is an effort of nature to free the system from conditions that result from a violation of the laws of health. In case of sickness, the cause should be ascertained. Unhealthful conditions should be changed, wrong habits corrected. Then nature is to be assisted in her effort to expel impurities and to re-establish right conditions in the system" "Nature to relieve herself of POISONOUS IMPURITIES, makes an effort to free the system, which effort produces fevers, and what is termed disease.... Only seek to assist nature in her efforts, by removing every obstruction, and then leave her to recover the exhausted energies of the system" (HL224, 225).

◆ The Body Is Always Striving For The Good Of The Individual

A. Benjamin, p. 9–10 —"The second principle of Nature Cure is that the body is always striving for the ultimate good of the individual, no matter how ill-treated it may be; and that all ACUTE diseases — such as FEVERS, COLDS, DIARRHEAS, SKIN ERUPTIONS OF ALL KINDS, INFLAMMATIONS, ETC. — are nothing more than self-initiated attempts on the part of the body to throw off the accumulations of waste material which are interfering with its proper functioning, and that all CHRONIC diseases — such as VALVULAR DISEASE of the heart, DIABETES, KIDNEY DISEASE, RHEUMATISM, BRONCHITIS, etc. are really the result of the continued SUPPRESSION of these same acute diseases by ORTHODOX MEDICAL METHODS of treatment."

B. White, HL211 — "Nature is burdened and endeavors to resist your efforts to cripple her. CHILLS and FEVERS are the result of those attempts to rid herself of the burden you lay upon her.... Nature bears abuse as long as she can without resisting, then she arouses, and makes a mighty effort to rid herself of the encumbrances and evil treatment she has suffered. Then come HEADACHE, CHILLS, FEVERS, NERVOUSNESS, PARALYSIS, and other evils too numerous to mention." "A practice that is laying the foundation of a vast amount of disease and of even more serious evils, is the free use of poisonous drugs" (MH126).

◆ Only Nature Possesses Restorative Powers

A. Benjamin, p. 10 — "The third principle of Nature Cure is that the body contains within itself the power to bring about a return to that condition of normal well-being known as health.... p. 40 — Within himself every individual possesses the POWER TO CURE HIMSELF of any disease from which he may be suffering, providing (1), the right means to bring this about are employed; and (2), the vitality of the individual has not sunk so low as to render recuperation impossible.... The natural healing powers latent within the body alone are capable of bringing about that return to normal functioning which is synonymous with health. Not man, but nature cures.... p. 42 — NATURE IS THE ONLY HEALER."

B. White, HL224 — "Nature alone possesses restorative powers. She alone can build up her exhausted energies, and repair the injuries she has received by inattention to her fixed laws.... NATURE ALONE IS THE EFFECTUAL RESTORER...." MH, p. 127 — "Let physicians teach the people that restorative power is not in drugs, but in nature." MM, p. 232 — "NATURE IS THE GREAT PHYSICIAN that will heal them of all their maladies, both spiritual and physical." GOD'S HEALING POWER RUNS THROUGH ALL NATURE, and He has made the provision that nature is to restore man's depleted and exhausted powers (MM11–12). This means that any ARTIFICIAL SUBSTANCE produced by man is to be avoided. God, being our Creator, knows what is best for the organism which He has created. If intelligently used, all of GOD'S AGENCIES ARE COMPATIBLE WITH THE HUMAN ORGANISM in the form in which He has created them. The manner in which God has put substances together in plants, fruits, and vegetables is supernatural. No one can artificially produce them with the same beneficial effect upon the organism. The natural means which God has provided must be used in the way He has intended them to be used, and they will then bring about supernatural results (2SM346).

Natural means are the real "wonder drugs." They are the ones that produce real miracles because the blessing of God is with them. "Through the AGENCIES OF NATURE, God is working day by day, hour by hour, moment by moment, to keep us alive" (MH112). They ARE GOD'S PHYSICIANS (2SM281).

◆ *Fasting, A Most Important Healing Method*

A. Benjamin, pp. 46–9 — "Of these natural curative agents, by far the most important is fasting. The first thing that one notices about all animals or birds when unwell—is that they immediately cease from taking food. They stop eating at once. By not eating—or fasting—the body is given an opportunity for self-cleansing which the daily ingestion of a regular quantity of food renders impossible.... For a really clean body internally means a healthy body; and fasting is the BODY CLEANSER SUPREME.... When food is withheld, as during the process of fasting, then assimilation stops, and the reverse or negative process of elimination takes place.... Fasting restores physiological balance."

B. White, CD189, — "In many cases of sickness, the very best remedy is for the patient to FAST for a meal or two, that the overworked organs of digestion may have an opportunity to rest. A fruit diet for a few days has often brought great relief to brain workers. Many times a short period of entire ABSTINENCE FROM FOOD, followed by simple moderate eating, has led to recovery through nature's own recuperative effort. An abstemious diet for a month or two would convince many sufferers that the PATH OF SELF-DENIAL IS THE PATH TO HEALTH. There are some who would be benefited more by ABSTINENCE FROM FOOD for a day or two every week than by any amount of treatment or medical advice. To fast one day a week would be of incalculable benefit to them." CD188 — "The true fasting which should be recommended to all, is abstinence from every stimulating kind of food, and the proper use of wholesome, simple food, which God has provided in abundance." (CD 90)

◆ *Self-Indulgence, The Basis of Nine-tenths Of All Disease*

A. Benjamin, p. 31 — Self-indulgence is at the bottom of NINE-TENTHS of the ills of today,.... and until one has learned self-control, how can one hope for the establishment of a proper mode of living.

B. White, MM225 — Thousands need to be educated patiently, kindly, tenderly, but decidedly, that NINE-TENTHS of their complaints are created by their own course of action. There is even among those who have intelligence in regard to the laws of life and health, a constant selfish indulgence in those things which are injurious to both soul and body. There is intemperance in eating and in the many varieties of food taken at one meal.

◆ *A Proper Diet Is Essential To Health*

A. Benjamin, pp. 56–66 — Proper diet is the essential factor in health production, and conversely, wrong feeding is the main attributive cause of disease. The medical profession have completely overlooked the part played by the MINERAL SALTS contained in all natural unspoiled foods. To them it has just been a matter of supplying the body with proteins, starches, sugars and fats, and that is all. They have reasoned that proteins are needed for body building, sugar and starches for energizing purposes, and fats for warmth. That the body should need the continued supply of the mineral salts for cleansing and purifying purposes, has never occurred to them. Our medical advisors see nothing wrong in a world refining and demineralizing its foods or boiling or cooking them, (all of them processes which ruthlessly remove these essential mineral elements from our food). That ill-health follows such practices is not connected in any way with the practices themselves. The root basis of foolish feeding habits lies in the inability to distinguish what is good for the body and what is not. DISEASE is nothing more than the manifestation within the body of a move toward SELF-CLEANSING, which, being misunderstood by the medical profession, is wrongly taken to be the result of germ action from without or other external cause. Through the SCIENCE OF NATURAL DIETETICS, the practitioners of natural therapeutics are achieving the most amazing results in the curative treatment of diseases as diverse as RHEUMATISM, DIA-

BETES, HEART DISEASE, NEURASTHENIA, KIDNEY DISEASE, ASTHMA, etc.... Many of the cases thus treated had been previously given up as INCURABLE by the leading lights of orthodox medication."

B. White, HL76 — "The diet question deserves careful study. A reform in eating would be a saving of expense and labor. The diet affects both physical and moral health. Learn for yourself what you should eat, what kinds of food best nourish the body, and then follow the dictates of reason and conscience. This is not a matter of trifling importance. Those who will not eat and drink from principle, will not be governed by principle in other things" p. 78 — "The Lord intends to bring His people back to live upon simple fruits, vegetables, and grains." (MM277). God provided fruit in its natural state for our first parents. All the elements of nutrition are contained in the fruits, vegetables, and grains. Grains and fruits prepared free from grease, and in AS NATURAL CONDITION AS POSSIBLE, should be the food for the tables of those who claim to be preparing for translation to heaven. They make with milk and cream the most healthful diet.

The Power Within Us

◆ *The Self-Healing Power that Maintains Our Health*

All living organisms are to a degree self-maintaining, self-constructing, self-repairing, self-directing. self-preserving, and self-healing. By divine law God has placed within our bodies the power to maintain them in health when in health, and to restore them to health when ill. This power is applied continuously, and will preserve us, if we cooperate with it, and give it the opportunity to do so.

To give this power the opportunity to maintain our physical being, we must cooperate with it and the principles that apply to it. This means that we must not allow the impurities that develop within the body, as well as the impure substances that come into the body from without to counteract or work against the processes that are endeavoring to maintain the body's integrity. It means keeping the body as clean as possible. We are all creatures of habit, and while we are developing habits, with a little extra effort it will be just as easy to develop good habits instead of bad habits. Unless we develop good habits from our earliest moments, we may be naturally inclined to develop those habits which are destructive of our life forces, and of our own existence.

◆ *The Body Heals Its Own Wounds*

To eliminate disease and recover health, we must cease to rely on unnatural destructive measures, agents, and processes, and rely on constructive natural agents, energies, and methods. THE BODY IS SELF-HEALING. Bruises vanish, cuts heal, broken bones mend. If the body can do all of these things, then it can also overcome the handicaps represented by illnesses. The healing power within the body is GOD-ORDAINED. It cannot be improved upon. In order to allow the healing power to heal, we must not work against it but cooperate with it.

◆ *Impurities Work Against The Body's Healing Power*

POISONOUS SUBSTANCES introduced into the body work against the healing process of the body. They do not remove impurities because they themselves are impurities. They do not remove the cause of ill health, because they themselves contribute to the cause of ill health. They harm the body rather than help it get over the disease, and they slow the healing process. They also work to override the body's healing process on the false premise that they themselves enhance the healing process. To avoid illness we must avoid the causes of illness. To heal disease we must remove the causes of disease. If you would be disease free, do not cause disease. To build health we must employ the agents of health. The popular methods of preventing and healing disease neither prevent disease nor restore health, because they do not REMOVE THE CAUSES OF DISEASE.

There is nothing outside of the body wisdom that can substitute for the body's healing functions. If we abuse the laws of our being, we must restore our health by giving our internal restoring forces the opportunity to do so. This can be done by giving them rest, giving them purifying substances, and avoiding to place added enervating loads upon it. All energies must concentrate upon the healing function, and all of God's remedies will do this. By means of WITHDRAWAL SYMPTOMS the body indicates its endeavor to heal itself. But if more unwelcome substances are introduced, these healing symptoms may disappear. Pains, headaches, swellings etc. are signs of the body's HEALING PROCESSES at work.

THE PSYCHOGENIC PHILOSOPHY OF HEALTH

The Proper Mental Attitude

◆ *The Influence Of The Mind Upon The Body*

GOD'S PHILOSOPHY OF HEALTH is also a PSYCHOGENIC PHILOSOPHY. By this we mean that many diseases originate in the mind, in the state of mind of the individual, and they can be cured only by changing this state of mind. This means that psychogenesis represents MENTAL HYGIENE as well as MIND-CURE. We are told that "The relation that exists between the mind and the body is very intimate. When one is affected, the other sympathizes. The condition of the mind affects the health to a far greater degree than many realize. Many of the diseases from which men suffer are the result of MENTAL DEPRESSION. Grief, anxiety, discontent, remorse, guilt, distrust, all tend to break down the life forces and to invite decay and death" (MH241). Many more people suffer from mental disease than we imagine. "Many are suffering from maladies of the soul far more than from diseases of the body, and they will find no relief until they come to Christ, the wellspring of life…. Complaints of weariness, loneliness, and dissatisfaction will then cease. Satisfying joys will give vigor to the mind and health and vital energy to the body"(CH502). (3T184).

It is a true saying that the action of the mind affects the body, and that the condition of the body affects the mind. But the body affects the mind largely only if we let it. The mind is to control the body, its feelings and emotions. However, if the mind is not strong enough to take control, then bodily influences will control mental processes to a large degree. "A great deal of the sickness which afflicts humanity has its origin in the mind and can only be cured by restoring the mind to health" (3T184).

◆ *The Imagination Can Aggravate Disease*

"Disease is sometimes produced, and is often greatly aggravated, by the imagination. Many are lifelong invalids who might be well if they only thought so. Many imagine that every slight exposure will cause illness, and the evil effect is produced because it is expected. Many die from disease, the cause of which is wholly imaginary" (MH241). "Thousands are sick and dying around us who might get well and live if they would; but their IMAGINATION holds them. They fear that they will be made worse if they labor or exercise, when this is just the change they need to make them well. Without this they never can improve" (MM105). "I frequently turn from the bedside of these self-made invalids, saying to myself, dying by inches, dying of indolence, a disease which no one but themselves can cure" (MM107). "The mind needs to be controlled, for it has a most powerful influence upon the body. The imagination often misleads, and when indulged, brings severe forms of disease upon the afflicted" (2T523). Courage, hope, faith, sympathy, love, promote health and prolong life. A contented mind, a cheerful spirit, is health to the body and strength to the soul. 'A MERRY HEART doeth good like a medicine'(Prov. 17:21). "In the treatment of the sick, the effect of mental influence should not be overlooked. Rightly used, this influence affords one of the most effective agencies for combating disease'(MH241).

◆ *Overcoming Mental-Emotional Problems*

If physical illness appears to have a mental cause, it is usually dismissed as something that is "unreal," and not really the true cause. For the true cause of disease we usually try to find a physical reason, something that is tangible. When we say that "its all in your mind," we mean that it is something which is not worthy of paying attention to. However, the influence of the body over the mind is real, and it is worthy of careful study. Prov. 23:7 says, "For as a man thinketh in his heart so is he." If a man thinks negative thoughts such that he believes that he is going to get worse, then he probably will. If he thinks that he is going to get well, then he has achieved one big step towards getting well. This indicates to us that the emphasis on POSITIVE THINKING has its merits.

The fundamental way to avoid mental-emotional problems is to live one's life according to the principles of righteousness. When one always does what is right, one will not have any problem with one's conscience, and there will be no harmful influence of the mind upon the body, and the body will also be kept in health. We are told that "Good deeds are twice a blessing, benefiting both the giver and the receiver of the kindness. The consciousness of RIGHT DOING is the best medicine for diseased bodies and minds"(CH628).

◆ *A Spirit Of Gratitude Promotes Health*

We are told that "Nothing tends more to promote health of body and of soul than does a spirit of gratitude and praise. It is a positive duty to resist melancholy, discontented thoughts and feelings, — as much a duty as it is to pray.... It is a law of nature that our thoughts and feelings are encouraged and strengthened as we give them utterance" (MH251). "In order to be healthy and happy, we must not allow our mind to place a burden upon our body which tends toward weakening the physical powers to the extent of causing physical disease." "Sickness of mind prevails everywhere.... remorse for sin sometimes undermines the constitution and unbalances the mind" (CH324). "Those who are always busy, and go cheerfully about the performance of their daily tasks, are the most happy and healthy"(2T529).

No Mind Should Control Another Mind

◆ *Don't Look To Man To Heal You.*

"It is not God's purpose that any human being should yield His mind and will to the control of another, becoming a passive instrument in his hands. No one is to merge His individuality in that of another. He is not to look to any other human being as the source of healing. His dependence must be in God. In the dignity of his God-given manhood, he is to be controlled by God Himself, not by any human intelligence. God desires to bring men into direct relation with Himself.... Satan works to thwart this purpose. He seeks to encourage dependence upon men.... The theory of mind controlling mind was originated by Satan, to introduce himself as the chief worker, to put human philosophy where divine philosophy should be. Of all the errors that are finding acceptance among professedly Christian people, none is a more dangerous deception, none more certain to separate man from God, than is this. Innocent though it may appear, if exercised upon patients it will tend to their destruction, not their restoration" (MH242, 243)

◆ *Look To God For Healing Of Mind And Body*

"There is something better for us to engage in than the control of humanity by humanity. The physician should educate the people to look from the human to the divine. Instead of teaching the sick to depend upon human beings for the cure of soul and body, he should direct them to the one who can save to the uttermost all who come unto Him. He who made man's mind knows what the mind needs. God alone is the one who can heal. Those whose minds and bodies are diseased are to behold Christ the restorer. 'Because I live', He says, 'ye shall live also' (Jo. 14:19)." (MH243–244) "We need never feel that we are alone. Angels are our companions. The Comforter that Christ promised to send in His name abides with us" (MH249). "This is the life we are to present to the sick, telling them that if they have faith in Christ as the restorer, if they cooperate with Him, obeying the laws of health, and striving to perfect holiness in His fear, He will impart to them life. When we present Christ to them in this way, we are imparting a power, a strength, that is of value; for it comes from above. This is the TRUE SCIENCE OF HEALING for body and soul." (MH244)

◆ *The Power Of The Will*

The power of the will is also a power for dealing with disease. The will is an organic function which, if rightly used and applied, can be a wonderful aid in the maintenance of health, as well as in dealing with, resisting, and overcoming disease of both mind and body by controlling the imagination. Many times the deciding factor in getting well is the WILL TO GET WELL, and THE WILL TO LIVE. We are told that "There are thousands who can recover health if they will. The Lord does not want them to be sick"(MH246). He wants them to be well, and to make up their minds to be well. They must resist the disease by rising above their aches and pains and engage in useful work suited to their strength. In this way many an invalid can recover health and strength. For every trial God has provided help. If we seek Him under these circumstances, Christ will give us help. We are told that "Those who surrender their lives to His guidance and to His service will never be placed in a position for which He has not made provision" (MH248).

The Influence Of The Body Upon The Mind

◆ *Physical Conditions Cause Mental States.*

Bodily conditions can affect mental and emotional states with great intensity. We are told that "Bodily disease accompanies mental disease" (6T301). Hunger can cause irritability, lack of sleep can cause inability to concentrate. Pills can cause depression, mental distress can come from physical imbalances. "A diseased body affects the brain" (4SpG146). Dr. Schoenthaler says that the brain often shows signs of undernutrition long before the rest of the body. "What is enough to prevent physical symptoms of VITAMIN DEFICIENCIES may not be enough to prevent impaired mental function," he says. For example, we have been told that a mental breakdown or mental debility can be caused by an improper diet (CD122), by eating too much (Ed205), by indulgence in appetite (CD135). Mental degeneracy or depravity is caused by the violation of the laws of health (4SpG124), by intemperance (CH49), by cherishing sin (COL281). Mental depression is caused by drinking tea and coffee (CG403), by physical disease (1T185). We are told that mental depression is SATAN'S WORK (1T702). Mental disease is caused by ERRONEOUS DOCTRINES (5T444). But the study of the Bible is a safeguard against all forms of mental disease (Ed124).

◆ *It Is Not Wise To Concentrate Our Attention On Our Feelings*

Some patients suffer from ungratified desires, disordered passions, and from the condemnation of their own consciences. They are always anticipating trouble. They are gradually losing their hold on life, and have no prospect of the life to come. But there is help for them in Christ when He said, "Come unto Me, all ye that labor and are heavy laden, and I will give you rest" (Matt. 11:28). "Those who surrender their lives to His guidance and to His service will never be placed in a position for which He has not made provision" (MH248). He also says, " 'Peace I leave with you, My peace I give unto you; not as the world giveth give I unto you'…. When the sunshine of God's love illuminates the darkened chambers of the soul, restless weariness and dissatisfaction will cease, and satisfying joys will give vigor to the mind, and health and energy to the body" (Jo. 14:27; MH247).

◆ *We Should Look Away From Self To Christ*

"It is not wise to look to ourselves, and study our emotions. If we do this, the enemy will present difficulties and temptations, that weaken faith and destroy courage. Closely to study our emotions and give way to our feelings is to entertain doubt, and entangle ourselves in perplexity. We are to LOOK AWAY FROM SELF TO JESUS" (MH249). To center our attention upon ourself is one of the surest hindrances to our recovery. We must forget self and concentrate our interest in others. We are not to talk of our lack of faith and our sorrows and sufferings. When we talk of these gloomy subjects we are GLORIFYING SATAN and the great power that he has to overcome us. It is our duty to give more expression to the blessings that result from appreciating the goodness and love of God. (MH253).

The Causes Of Mental Disease

◆ *Dissatisfied Feelings*

One of the causes of mental disease is the matter of dissatisfied feelings. One may be dissatisfied with world conditions, with the things in our environment, with confining conditions, with people who do not act according to our expectations, with a lack of money. They can all affect our minds in such a way as to unbalance them. That is why we are told that "that which brings sickness of body and mind to nearly all is dissatisfied feelings and discontented repinings" (1T566). Such people are creating a time of trouble before their time, they have anxiety stamped upon every feature, and are always looking for some awful evil that may happen to them in the future. The Bible gives us the solution to this problem. Luke 3:14 says, "be content with your wages." In Phil. 4:11 Paul tells us, "for I have learned, in whatever state I am, therewith to be content." Hebr. 13:5 says, "and be content with such things as ye have." The reason for such contentment is clear. God will never place the true Christian in a position for which he has not made provision(COL 173). So we must believe that for the true Christian any position he might find himself in, is God-arranged and God-supported.

Alexis De Toqueville was a young member of the French Assembly. He came to the U.S. in the eighteen twenties in order to study how the young American democracy had developed. He stayed three years and thereupon wrote the great classic *Democracy In America*. He compared what he saw in the U.S. with what he saw in Europe. He said that in the U.S. he saw people surrounded by the greatest prosperity with a constant frown upon their faces, while in Europe he saw people who were in the most abject poverty but with a smile upon their faces. The reason he gave for the frown was that in the U.S. people were always looking toward and desiring those things which they did not presently possess, while the attitude of the poor in Europe was that they were satisfied with their lot.

◆ *Specific Causes Of Mental Disease*

We have been told that "Sickness of the mind prevails everywhere. NINE TENTHS of the diseases from which men suffer have their foundation here. Perhaps some home trouble is, like a canker, eating to the very soul and weakening the life forces. Remorse for sin sometimes undermines the constitution and unbalances the mind. There are erroneous doctrines also, as that of an eternally burning hell and the endless torment of the wicked, that, by giving exaggerated and distorted views of the character of God, have produced the same result upon sensitive minds. Infidels have made the most of these unfortunate cases, attributing insanity to religion" (5T444).

We are also told that "The influence of worldly selfishness, which is carried about by some like a cloud, chilling the very atmosphere that others breathe, causes sickness of soul and frequently chills to death" (3T528). Furthermore, the reading of fiction in which impurity is portrayed, and passion aroused, harms the mind. In fact, we are told that "Even FICTION which contains no suggestion of impurity, and which may be intended to teach excellent principles, is harmful. It encourages the habit of hasty and superficial reading merely for the story. Thus it tends to destroy the power of connected thought; it unfits the soul to contemplate the great problems of duty and destiny" (MH445-6). For the lover of fiction total abstinence is his only safety. But the RELIGION OF CHRIST is one of the most effectual REMEDIES for mental disease.

Healing Mental Disease

◆ *Life In The Open Air*

"Proper periods of sleep and rest and an abundance of physical exercise are essential to health of body and mind" (7T247). The reason for establishing sanitariums in the country is so that patients can breathe the pure air of heaven. As they walk among the flowers and trees, joy and gladness fills their hearts. It is as if the smile of God were upon them, as they look upon the beautiful things He has created to bring joy to their hearts. "Life in the open air is good for body and mind. It is GOD'S MEDICINE for the restoration of health. Pure air, good water, sunshine, beautiful surroundings — these are the means for restoring the sick to health in NATURAL WAYS" (MM233). As the sick look upon the beautiful scenery, as they see the flowers in their loveliness, which are messengers of God's love to His family in affliction here below, they will find health, cheerfulness, and happy thoughts. Life in the open air is health-restoring. The PURE AIR has in it HEALTH AND LIFE. As it is breathed in, it has an invigorating effect upon the whole system. (MM232). Researchers in Holland have found that people who lovingly tend to their plants have fewer heart attacks, lower blood pressure, looser muscles, and a slower heart rate.

◆ *The Effect Of Color On Health*

Each color stimulates an aspect of the HYPOTHALAMUS, which in turn stimulates the PITUITARY GLAND. Artificial light does not have the color frequency of natural light. We can change the situation by allowing ourselves to spend a little time of the day in natural sunlight. COLOR THERAPY realizes that different colors have various effects on health.

✓ RED—The longest wavelength in the visible spectrum is related to vitality and glandular activity. It stimulates the nervous system and the circulatory system. It represents force and analogy and increases the activity of the liver. In the form of ROSE-PINK it results in a feeling of love and tenderness. PINK can raise the vibrations of the body, and can be a healing color except when people are inclined to be nervous. Then pink or red should be avoided, especially in the bedroom.

- ✓ ORANGE—is the color of learning and success. It is a mixture of red and yellow. GOLDEN ORANGE acts on the THYROID, THE LIVER. It releases nervous tension, strengthens the heartbeat, may help to lower the need for insulin in diabetics and increases glandular activity. Foods are: CARROTS, SWEET POTATOES, PUMPKIN, ORANGE, and APRICOTS.
- ✓ YELLOW—Purifies the blood, promotes action, self-confidence, and stimulates energy. PALE YELLOW helps to relieve tension, heals scars, and helps to activate the THYMUS gland.
- ✓ GREEN—Stimulates the PITUITARY gland, helps healing, and breaks up congestion.
- ✓ BLUE—Blue should be the bedroom color including the blankets. It has a calming effect, and acts on the PINEAL GLAND. If you cant sleep at night, change your pink blanket for a blue one, and prove to yourself the efficacy of color in your life.
- ✓ PURPLE—is a good color for MEDITATION. It has a calming effect, slows the heartbeat, and helps produce sleep.
- ✓ NEUTRAL COLORS—are green and magenta.
- ✓ COLD COLORS—are turquoise, blue, indigo, and violet.

◆ *Sympathy*

We are told that "few realize the power that the mind has over the body. A great deal of the sickness which afflicts humanity has its origin in the mind and can only be cured by restoring the mind to health.... Mental trouble has a paralyzing influence upon the digestive organs.... A sore, sick heart, a discouraged mind, needs mild treatment, and it is through tender sympathy that this class of minds can be healed" (3T184). "There are many from whom hope has departed. Bring back the sunshine to them. Many have lost their courage. Speak to them words of cheer. Pray for them. There are those who need the bread of life. Read to them from the word of God. Upon many is a soul sickness which no earthly balm can reach nor physician heal. Pray for these souls, bring them to Jesus. Tell them that there is a balm in Gilead and a physician there" (COL 418).

◆ *Doing Good*

Besides having sympathies for others, God's people themselves are equally in need of opportunities that draw out their sympathies, give efficiency to their prayers, and develop in them a character like that of the divine pattern. It is to provide these opportunities that God has placed among us the poor, the unfortunate, the sick, and the suffering. They are Christ's legacy to His church, and they are to be cared for as He would care for them. In this way God takes away the dross and purifies the gold, giving us that culture of heart and character which we need (6T261).

"Those who cultivate benevolence are not only doing a good work for others,.... but they are benefiting themselves by opening their hearts to the benign influence of true benevolence. Every ray of light shed upon others will be reflected upon our own hearts. Every kind and sympathizing word spoken to the sorrowful, every act to relieve the oppressed, and every gift to supply the necessities of our fellow beings, given or done with a eye to God's glory, will result in blessings to the giver.... The pleasure of doing good to others imparts a glow to the feelings which flashes through the nerves, quickens the circulation of the blood, and induces mental and physical health" (4T56).

◆ *Leading The Sick To Christ*

The prescription for the healing of all mental and physical and spiritual ills is Christ's statement, "Come unto Me, all ye that labor and are heavy-laden, and I will give you rest" It is Christ's gift to those who seek Him in sincerity and in truth. He is the Mighty Healer. Then comes another invitation: "Take my yoke upon you, and learn of Me; for I am meek and lowly in heart: and ye shall find rest unto your souls. For My yoke is easy, and my burden is light." Matt. 11:28–30). Wearing Christ's yoke and learning of Him the lesson of meekness and lowliness, we find rest in faith, and confidence and trust. We find that Christ's yoke is easy and His burden light. (9T124). "When the love and sympathy that Christ manifested for the sick is combined with the physician's knowledge, his very presence will be a blessing" (MH245). Never does our merciful God turn from the soul that in sincerity seeks Him for help.

Maintaining Proper Mental Health

◆ *Scientific Determinations Regarding Proper Mental Health*

✓ According to an Australian cardiologist, "For those who do not know how to deal with stress, LIFE IS A TERMINAL ILLNESS."

✓ People who blame themselves for misfortune are more susceptible to disease.

✓ Stress invites disease by assaulting the immune system, and thereby makes the development of disease more likely.

✓ Stress doesn't make you sick, but your interpretation of the stressful situation does. How you react to it determines how well you handle it.

✓ A friendly agreeable attitude helps reduce conflict in life and invites support from others. The feeling of being loved and cared for by friends and family goes a long way in protecting you from the negative effects of stress.

✓ By letting go of the resentment, and forgetting the idea of seeking revenge, the weight of anger lifts from your shoulder, easing your pain, and allowing you to forget the bad experience. "Vengeance is mine; I will repay, saith the Lord" (Rom. 12:19).

✓ If you are attacked your adrenal glands pour adrenaline into the bloodstream to give you supernatural strength. If this adrenaline is not used up, it becomes toxic and affects the internal organs and skin adversely. One may say that you are then eating yourself alive.

✓ Don't put yourself in situations that tend toward overeating such as: going shopping when you are hungry; buying food you shouldn't eat; leaving snacks on the kitchen counter; meeting friends in a restaurant. Go shopping right after dinner, on a full stomach. Also plan meals on a full stomach. A weekly meal plan is even better.

✓ In one study those who watched TV for more than three hours per day were more than twice as likely to be obese than those who watched TV for less than one hour per day.

✓ Eat to slow music. When slow classical music was played people took fewer bites per minute. Even though their meals were 15 minutes longer, they ate less.

✓ People who eat more soup eat less food and gain less weight, because soup takes longer to eat.

✓ Eat food from GRAY, GREEN, or BROWN plates. Studies show that these colors make you eat less. Also put your food on smaller plates, it will look like more. Eat from your own special plate, on your own special place mat.

✓ Don't thicken soup with flour or cream, but with mashed potato flour.

✓ Use YOGURT instead of sour cream. Yogurt has only 40% of the caloric value of sour cream.

✓ One study showed that people ate 44% more food when they dined out with others than when they ate alone, and they felt 30% less satisfied.

✓ To lose more excess fat, don't eat before you exercise. A study of two groups of women showed that in both cases you use up about the same number of calories, but when you exercise on an empty stomach, you burn up 50% more fat calories.

✓ Don't become overwhelmed by tasks and obligations, but see them in perspective. Accept what you can do, and don't worry about what you can't do. Simplifying your life and cutting your obligations will make you happier.

✓ Laugh more at life situations. It protects against the effects of negative stress by triggering the brain's release of ENDORPHINS, ENKEPHALINS, and DYNORPHINS, the body's natural pain killers. They are released by the PITUITARY GLAND, and are a kind of biological version of MORPHINE or HEROIN. They are more powerful than any man-made drug, in some instances up to 700 times more powerful in pain-killing ability than MORPHINE.

- ✓ Accept frustrations as part of the price for getting things done. Things are not going to be the way you want them to be all of the time.
- ✓ In times of stress, train yourself to look back and remember the pleasant experiences, and satisfying moments, and relive them.
- ✓ Exercise directly reduces anxiety and tensions, and produces an increase in psychological well-being.
- ✓ Talk of what is right in the relationship first, then discuss what would be helpful to change. Don't make the other person feel guilty. This won't solve any problems, but may create new ones.
- ✓ Stick to one romantic commitment at a time. Multiple commitments present such a severe psychological stress, as to accelerate the course of coronary artery disease.

CHRIST'S HEALING PRINCIPLES

Christ's Use Of Divine Power

◆ *Christ Came To Earth With Two Natures*

When Christ came to this earth and was born in Bethlehem, he came with two natures, one divine and one human, and in His person these two natures were blended (7BC904). His divine nature was covered so that only His human nature showed. When Christ said: "I can of mine own self do nothing" (Jo. 5:30), He was speaking from the standpoint of His humanity. When He said: "All power is given me in heaven and on earth" (Matt. 28:18), He was speaking from the standpoint of His divinity. When He said: "for without me ye can do nothing" (Jo. 15:5), He was again speaking from the standpoint of His divinity. Such divinity can never be taken from Him. It is part of His nature. Because of His divinity, He had the power of God within Himself. When He was on the mount of transfiguration we are told that "Divinity from within flashes through humanity, and meets the glory coming from above" (DA421).

◆ *As A Man Christ Laid Aside His Divine Authority*

When He came to earth, Christ temporarily abdicated His throne in heaven and the responsibility that went with it. When He stilled the storm DA336 states: "But He rested not in the possession of almighty power. It was not as the 'Master of earth and sea and sky' that He reposed in quiet. That power He had laid down. He trusted in the Father's might. It was in faith—faith in God's love and care—that Jesus rested, and the power of that word which stilled the storm was the power of God." When it says that Christ "rested not in the possession of almighty power," it means that while He had divine power He did not always utilize it. In this case He did not utilize His own divine power because, while He had the power of God within Himself, He Himself, as well as the disciples, were in danger on the sea of Galilee. Had He exercised His divine power under these circumstances, He would have used it for the disciples benefit as well as His own. This He could not do and still maintain His integrity within the plan of salvation that He was to follow.

◆ *While On Earth Christ At Times Made Use Of His Divine Power*

We are told that while on earth Christ "laid aside His divinity" (ST Mar. 17:1887). This is not to be interpreted to mean that while on earth Christ never made use of His divinity. He laid His divinity aside as a man first of all, and secondly, He laid it aside in His own behalf. As a man He could not utilize any part of it, because He had to show the world that His obedience to the law was accomplished as a human being with divine help obtained from outside of Himself, in a manner of which every human being can avail himself. On the other hand, Christ did make use of His divine power while here on earth, but not to accomplish a human task for Himself. He used it to accomplish a super-human task such as is involved in the performance of miracles.

◆ *Christ Used Divine Power For The Benefit Of Others Only*

We are told that "Christ was not to exercise divine power for His own benefit…Neither here nor at any subsequent time in His earthly life did He work a miracle in His own behalf. His wonderful works were all for the good of others" (DA119–20). "His divine miraculous power was to be exercised for the salvation of others, but not in His own benefit" (EW174). When He was before Herod, Herod asked Him to work a miracle for His own good. Christ refused, for He "had taken upon Himself man's nature. He must do as man must do under like circumstances. Therefore He would not work a miracle to save Himself the pain and humiliation that man must endure when placed in a similar position" (DA729).

When Christ was before Pilate, His enemies had demanded a miracle as evidence of His divinity. His claim to be the Son of God was ridiculed. "Satan led the cruel mob in its abuse of the Savior. It was his purpose to provoke Him to retaliation if possible, or to drive Him to perform a miracle to release Himself, and thus break the plan of salvation" (DA734). If Christ had done this, the plan of salvation would have been broken, for He then would have used His divine power to perform a miracle in His own behalf to save himself. This no other human being could have done, hence, He would have acted in His own behalf as more than a human being.

◆ *Christ's Miracles Are A Proof Of His Divinity*

"The miracles of Christ are a proof of His divinity" (DA799). "Every miracle that Christ performed was a sign of His divinity.... The greatest significance of His miracles is seen in the fact that they were for the blessing of humanity. The highest evidence that He came from God is, that His life revealed the character of God. He did the works and spoke the words of God" (DA406). We are told that at times Christ was tempted to use His divinity for the benefit of His humanity, but He never did.

◆ *Christ Used His Divinity When He Healed People*

"Jesus revealed His divinity by His mighty miracles, when He healed the sick and raised the dead" (DA608). "In every city He laid His hands upon the afflicted ones and healed them" (MH18). "Physical disease, however malignant and deep-seated, was healed by the power of Christ" (DA271). "Even though those who asked for healing had brought disease upon themselves, Christ did not refuse to heal them" (DA823). "He longed to exercise His healing power and make every sufferer whole" (MH81). "It was by His word that Christ healed disease and cast out demons. By His word He stilled the sea, and raised the dead; and the people bare witness that His word was with power" (MH122).

The people questioned whether or not He was the Son of David. But many of those who called Him the Son of David did not recognize His divinity. "They did not understand that the Son of David was also the Son of God" (DA609). In the experience of the raising of Lazarus from the dead, Christ had delayed His going to Bethany because He believed that by raising Lazarus from the dead instead of from the sickbed, He would give the stubborn unbelieving people another evidence that He was "the resurrection and the life." In His mercy He purposed to give them one more evidence that the priests could not misinterpret. This was the reason of His delay in going to Bethany. "This crowning miracle, the raising of Lazarus, was to set the seal of God on His work and on His claim to divinity" (DA529).

◆ *Christ Forgave Sins When He Healed*

Whenever Christ healed, He healed not only the body but the soul also. The paralytic found in Christ healing for both soul and the body. He needed health of soul before he could appreciate health of body. There are today thousands suffering from physical disease, who like the paralytic, are longing for the message 'Thy sins are forgiven'. They can find no relief until they come to the healer of the soul. The peace which He alone can impart, would restore vigor to the mind, and health to the body (MH77).

◆ *Power To Heal Goes With Power To Forgive Sins.*

Jesus declared that the sins of the paralytic were forgiven, and in saying this Christ showed Himself to be God. But the Pharisees said in their hearts that only God can forgive sins, and implied that this man could not be God. He looked too much like themselves. However, they realized that "Christ possessed a power which they had ascribed to God Alone."(DA270). Christ said to them "whether is it easier to say, 'Thy sins be forgiven thee'; or to say, 'Arise and walk?' But that ye may know that the Son of man hath power on earth to forgive sins, He said, turning to the paralytic, 'Arise, take up thy bed, and go unto thine house'" (DA269).

Christ had connected the power to heal with the power to forgive sins. The power to heal was as divine as the power to forgive sins. Since sickness was the result of sin, then the power to take away sickness was one with the power to take away sin. This is shown in the statement of Ps. 103:3 where the spiritual is also mentioned before the physical. It says: "Who forgiveth all thine iniquities; who healeth all thy diseases." No human agent has the power to heal, because he does not have the power to forgive sins.

◆ Christ Did Not Refuse To Heal Anyone Who Came To Him For Healing

"In every city He laid His hands upon the afflicted ones and healed them" (MH18). "Physical disease, however malignant and deep-seated, was healed by the power of Christ" (DA271). "Even though those who asked for healing had brought disease upon themselves, Christ did not refuse to heal them" (DA823). "He longed to exercise His healing power and make every sufferer whole" (MH81). "It was by His word that Christ healed disease and cast out demons. By His word He stilled the sea, and raised the dead; and the people bare witness that His word was with power" (MH122).

◆ The Tribute Money Revealed Christ's Glory

In the case of the payment of the tribute money, prophets were exempted from this payment, but when the rabbis required tribute from Christ, they were setting aside His claim as a prophet. If Christ refused to pay it, He would be charged with disloyalty to the temple. If He paid it without protest, He would admit their claim that He wasn't a prophet, and He would thereby deny His divinity. When He provided for the tribute from the fish's mouth, He neither denied His divinity, nor did He pay it out of His own pocket, which act would have denied His divinity. But the manner in which He obtained it "gave evidence of His divine character…. Though He had clothed His divinity with humanity, in this miracle He revealed His glory" (DA434).

◆ He Healed The Soul Before He Healed The Body

There were many who wanted to be healed, but they first needed to ask for forgiveness of the sins which brought on the disease. They were to repent of what they had done wrong and needed to desire not to do that wrong again. They were first to get rid of the SIN IN THEIR SOUL before they were helped to get rid of the DISEASE IN THEIR BODY. They must determine by the help of God to change their life accordingly. "Before the physical malady could be healed, Christ must bring relief to the mind, and cleanse the soul from sin"(MH77). "When virtue from Him entered into these souls, they were convicted of sin, and many were healed of their spiritual disease as well of their physical maladies" (MH73). "To many of the afflicted ones who received healing Christ said, 'Sin no more, lest a worse thing come unto thee' (Jo. 5:14). Thus He taught that disease is the result of violating God's laws, both natural and spiritual" (CH30).

In the case of the paralytic whom Christ healed, his disease was the result of a life of sin, and his sufferings were embittered by remorse. He had been pronounced incurable. However, he wanted relief from the burden of sin more than restoration of the body. "When he repented of his sins, and believed in the power of Jesus to make him whole, the mercy of the Savior had blessed his heart" (MH75). Then the burden of guilt, which he had borne so long, rolled off his shoulders, and he was a free man again. "It required nothing less than creative power to restore health to that decaying body. The same voice that spoke life to man created from the dust of the earth, had spoken life to the dying paralytic. And the same power that gave life to the body, had renewed the heart" (MH77)

◆ Christ's Disciples Performed Healing Miracles Through Christ's Power

When Christ was about to go to His father He told His disciples that they would do as great or greater works than He did (Jo. 14:12). Such works they would accomplish through the power given them by Christ. All power in heaven and on earth is derived from Christ. He gives to men power to live His life (COL314), to obey (SC70), and to overcome sin (1SM226). Measureless divine power is placed at our disposal (9T186–7). Divine power is not summoned to do what human power can do (DA535). Outside of and beyond himself man needs divine power (DA296). Christ is the source of spiritual power (TM390), and His Spirit endows men with power (6T306).

As man Christ had God dwelling within Him as is indicated in John 14:10 where it says: "The words that I speak unto you I speak not of myself, but the father that dwelleth in me, He doeth the works." Christ had the father dwelling within Him by means of the Holy Spirit. This every Christian can have and does have available to him. When it came to the performing of miracles, Christ acted through his own divinity, and performed them through His own divine power. Christ disciples performed the same miracles that He performed, but in their case those miracles were not a sign of their divinity, because they were not divine. God was working these miracles for them. Or we may say that the God who performed those miracles for them was the divine power of Christ Himself. This is implied in Christ's statement: "Without me ye can do nothing" (Jo. 5:30), and also in the statement that divine power is imparted by Christ to cooperate with human effort (PP64).

The disciples were given power to cast out unclean spirits and to heal all manner of sickness and diseases (Matt. 10:1). Luke 9:2 says; "And He sent them to preach the kingdom of God, and to heal the sick." Whenever they entered a city they were to "heal the sick that are therein, and say unto them, The kingdom of God is come nigh unto you" (Luke 10:9).

◆ *Christ Exercised His Divinity By Reading Peoples Minds And Hearts*

Christ also exercised His Divinity by reading the hearts and minds of people. He often knew what was going on at different times and in distant places. He knew, for example, that the Syro-Phoenician woman was looking for Him, and so "He placed Himself in her path"(DA400). Her daughter was vexed with a devil, and Christ made her whole at a distance. We are told that "it was for the performance of this act that He went to the borders of Tyre and Sidon" (DA402). In the case of Judas, Christ used His MIND-READING POWER as a sign of His divinity, for we are told that "by reading the secret purpose of the traitor's heart, Christ gave to Judas the final convincing evidence of His divinity" (DA655). This the ordinary man cannot do, for we recognize that "man looks at the outward appearance, but God looks at the heart" (1 Sam. 16:70). "Christ had not ceased to be God when He became a man" (DA663).

Christ read the hearts of His disciples when they were vying for the highest place in His kingdom (DA548). "He had repeatedly read the hearts of men as an open book" (DA593). He read the hearts of the Pharisees when they tried to trip Him up with respect to whether or not it was lawful to pay tribute to Caesar. Here again He read their hearts like an open book (DA602).

◆ *Christ Raised Himself Through His Own Divine Power*

When the Bible indicates that God raised Christ from the grave according to Acts 2:24, where it says: "Whom God hath raised up," it means that God called Him up from the grave, but that Christ came up from the grave under His own divine power. We are told in DA785: "When the voice of the mighty angel was heard at Christ's tomb, saying, 'Thy Father calls Thee', the Saviour came forth from the grave by the life that was in Himself.... In His divinity Christ possessed the power to break the bonds of death." With such a power He could say of His life, "I have power to lay it down, and I have power to take it again" (John 10:18). He also said: "I am the resurrection and the life" (John 11:25). "These words could be spoken only by the Deity" (DA785).

Christ's Purpose In Healing

◆ *Christ Implanted Spiritual Principles When He Healed*

We are told that "The Saviour made each work of healing an occasion for implanting divine principles in mind and soul" (MH20). To Christ spiritual healing was more important than physical healing. In fact He considered PHYSICAL SICKNESS to be a result of SPIRITUAL WEAKNESS. For this reason physical healing is to be a result of spiritual healing, a result of FAITH. The healing of the body is to be an evidence of the power that affected a change of heart. We must realize that the violation of God's natural laws is also a sin, and in order for Christ to heal us, we must confess our sins and forsake them.

The healing principles that Christ used are the principles which His followers are to adopt. "First meet the temporal necessities of the needy and relieve their physical wants and sufferings, and you will then find an open avenue to the heart where you may plant the good seeds of virtue and religion" (WM 118).

◆ *Christ Wants To Eliminate Sin From The Life*

"Every sin is an offense to God and is to be confessed to Him through Christ" (MH229). With Christ "deliverance from sin and the healing of disease were linked together" (MH111). There was no great virtue in healing a man physically, if he was not taught the spiritual principles that gave him the knowledge of how to eliminate the bad habits that made him sick in the first place. Otherwise, he would merely continue those habits and get sick again because of them. In the healing process, Christ ministered to both soul and body. The gospel which He taught was a message of spiritual life and physical restoration. "It was BY HIS WORD that Jesus healed disease and cast out demons" (GW250). Also His touch made disease flee (MH38) In Him there is healing balm for every disease, restoring power for every infirmity (CH210).

◆ *Sin Is A Spiritual Disease*

Since sin, a spiritual disease, is the basis of physical disease, the healing of the spiritual nature has priority over the healing of the physical nature. The spiritual nature could in large part solve the problems of the physical nature. Christ's prescription of "come unto me, all ye that labor, and are heavy laden, and I will give you rest" (Matt. 11:28), is a prescription for the healing of physical, mental, and spiritual ills. Though men have brought suffering upon themselves by their own wrongdoing, He regards them with pity (MH115). As in the case of the paralytic, before Christ healed a person, the Holy Spirit had usually touched their heart, and had convicted them of their spiritual condition (MH73). For this reason such an individual was ready to be relieved from the burden of sin, and was ready to receive the assurance of forgiveness. Jesus healed him when he repented of his sins, and believed in the power of Christ to make him whole. Indifference to the health of the body is INTEMPERANCE, and that is also a sin which will affect our spirituality (CD43).

Christ told the ones He healed to "SIN NO MORE." In this He taught that SICKNESS is the RESULT OF SIN. However, sickness was not always the result of the sick person's sin. Sickness could be the result of a weakness within the family that was inherited by the individual sick person. It could have been a sin within previous generations back to the third and fourth generation. The individual sick person might have been ignorant of such weakness. If He had known of it he might have been more careful in his eating, drinking and working habits in order to keep himself in health.

One should not assume that once Christ has healed us, that we have no longer a need to restrict our diet. Temperance is the order of the day for every day, lest the same disease through the same bad habits will come upon us again to bring the same bad results. "God demands that the appetite be cleansed and that self-denial be practiced regarding those things which are not good" (9T153).

◆ *Christ Uses His Representatives The Holy Spirit And Angels To Heal*

The Bible throughout makes use of the principle of REPRESENTATIVE or SUBSTITUTIONARY PRESENCE. This means that whenever an agent of Christ is performing an act, or represents Him in any way, it is the same as if Christ Himself were performing the act. John 13:20 says "Verily, verily, I say unto you, he that receiveth whomsoever I send receiveth me; and he that receiveth me receiveth Him that sent me." In Matthew 25:40 Christ says, "Inasmuch as ye have done it unto one of the least of these my brethren, ye have done it unto me." We are told that "The Lord Jesus acts through the HOLY SPIRIT; for it is His representative" (MYP55). The ANGELS are also Christ's representative, for He communicates with man through them (SR51), works through human minds by means of them (7T167), and brings healing to man with their help (6T308). Since the angels are called "ministering spirits" (Hebr. 1:14), they may also be designated as the representatives of the Holy Spirit.

◆ *The Holy Spirit Inspired The Testimonies As Well As The Bible*

The same Spirit that inspired the books of the Bible inspired the Testimonies, which are called the TESTIMONIES of his SPIRIT. The Testimonies are just as inspired as is the Bible, and we must place the same degree of faith upon them. "In ancient times God spoke to men by the mouth of prophets and apostles. In these days He speaks to them by the testimonies of His Spirit. There was never a time when God instructed His people more earnestly than He instructs them now concerning His will and the course that He would have them pursue.

"The Holy Ghost is the author of the Scriptures and of the Spirit of Prophecy" (3SM30). Its purpose is to call attention to the light already given in the Bible (2T660). The Testimonies would not have been needed if God's people had faithfully studied and obeyed the Bible (2T605). God has not given us any additional light to take the place of the Bible

(3SM29). Therefore, it is NOT to be put AHEAD of the BIBLE (Ev. 256), NOT to be an ADDITION to the BIBLE (4T246), NOT to give NEW LIGHT (LS198), but to be a LESSER LIGHT leading to the GREATER LIGHT of the Bible, because little heed had been given to the Bible (CM125). The Testimonies are a lesser light only in the sense that a book of the Bible is a lesser light as compared to the whole Bible. They NEVER CONTRADICT the Bible (3SM32), for there are no degrees of Inspiration, and MRS. WHITE was NOT THE ORIGINATOR of the Testimonies (3SM50). The Bible was written for all people of all times. The Testimonies were given to a special people for a special time.

◆ *The Testimonies Magnify Principles Of Bible Truth For The End-Time*

The Testimonies were given to be a magnification of the principles of Bible truth specifically for the end-time, for the same reason that Christ came to magnify the law and make it honorable in His time (Isa 42:21). A magnification never brings us something new that wasn't there before, but it allows us to see more clearly what was there all the time. In these last days when perilous times shall come, God's people need this enlightened counsel in order to bring them through the terrors of these last-day events. These writings will instruct us as long as time shall last (3SM76), and "All who BELIEVE that the Lord has spoken through sister White, and has given her a MESSAGE, will be SAFE FROM the many DELUSIONS that will come in these last days" (3SM84). We are told that "Those Seventh-day Adventists who take their stand under Satan's banner will first GIVE UP THEIR FAITH in the warnings and reproofs contained in the TESTIMONIES OF GOD'S SPIRIT" (3SM84).

◆ *Testimony Statements Are Scientifically Sound*

When it comes to the Spirit of Prophecy statements of science and specifically in the field of health, such statements have been shown by scientists to be SCIENTIFICALLY UP TO DATE. No reason has ever been found to change any of the scientific statements given us in the Testimonies. In the past many statements by scientists had to be modified and changed. We shall endeavor to give many ideas in which science has corroborated the statements in the Spirit of Prophecy, and to show that they lend themselves to a rational belief in their inspiration. They have not become outdated, but are in many ways still somewhat ahead of modern science in the field of health and nutrition. In accepting them we can be assured of their HARMONY WITH NATURAL LAW. If we want to believe, we will find sufficient evidence of the truthfulness of these statements. God gives us evidence "which must be carefully investigated with a HUMBLE MIND and a TEACHABLE SPIRIT, and all should decide from the WEIGHT OF EVIDENCE. Those who desire to doubt will have plenty of room. God does not propose to remove all OCCASION FOR UNBELIEF. He gives SUFFICIENT EVIDENCE for the candid mind to believe; but he who turns from the weight of the evidence because there are a few things which he cannot make plain to his finite understanding will be left in the cold, chilling atmosphere of unbelief and questioning doubts, and will make shipwreck of faith " (5T676–7).

Christ's Use Of Remedies

◆ *Christ's Used Simple Natural Remedies*

We should understand that "God does not heal the sick without the aid of the means of healing which lie within the reach of man, or when men refuse to be benefited by the SIMPLE REMEDIES that God has provided in pure air and water" (2SM286). "There is a great work to be done in relieving the sufferings of humanity by the use of NATURAL AGENCIES that God has provided, and in teaching how to PREVENT DISEASE by the regulation of appetites and passions" (MH206).

"Christ made use of the simple agencies of nature. While He did NOT give COUNTENANCE to DRUG MEDICATION, He sanctioned the use of simple and natural remedies" (DA824). He taught that HEALTH is the REWARD of OBEDIENCE to the LAWS of GOD. He Himself was an "example of what God designed all humanity to be through obedience to His laws" (MH51). "For the sick we should use the REMEDIES which GOD has PROVIDED in NATURE, and we should point them to Him who alone can restore" (DA824). If Christ used the agencies of nature while here on earth, then we should use them, for He is our example.

Christ works to heal through His representative the Holy Spirit, and we are told that "the influence of the HOLY SPIRIT of GOD is the VERY BEST MEDICINE that can be received by a sick man or woman. Heaven is all health; and the more deeply the heavenly influences are realized, the more sure will be the recovery of the believing invalid" (MM12). "Christ, through the Holy Spirit, comes as a healing power to those who cease to do evil and learn to do well" (CH406). "PHYSICAL DISEASE, however malignant and deep-seated, is HEALED by the POWER of CHRIST" (DA471), He came to DESTROY the WORKS of the DEVIL (1 Jo. 3:8), for "He is the mighty healer of the sin-sick soul"(CH202).

◆ *Christ's Medicines Are In Nature*

Christ Himself has placed in nature the medicines for our use in case of illness. These are therefore the very best medicines that we have available to us. Nothing can be better than the medicines that Christ provides. Since they are His assigned remedies, He places a special blessing only upon the remedies which He has made available to us (CD25). In order for us to benefit from them, we should all have a knowledge of them, and how to apply them (CD301). Hezekiah was asked to take a lump of FIGS and lay it for a plaster upon the boil, and he would recover. (Isa 38:21). On one occasion Christ asked a blind man, whose eyes He had anointed with CLAY, to wash his eyes in the pool of Siloam, and he received his sight (Jo. 9:7). Here Christ used two natural substances with which to heal a man — clay and water. When Christ hung on the cross, He was presented with a stupefying potion of VINEGAR as a pain killer. When He had tasted it He refused it, for "He would receive NOTHING that would BECLOUD HIS MIND" We are told that to do so would have given SATAN an ADVANTAGE (DA746).

"The THINGS OF NATURE are God's blessings, provided to give health to the BODY, MIND and SOUL. They are given to the well to keep them well, and to the sick to make them well" (CD169). This means that the natural remedies which Christ has ordained for our benefit will both HEAL disease as well as PREVENT disease. They are capable of being used when we are well, as well as when we are ill. This is because they are all nonpoisonous remedies "The God of nature directs the human agent to USE NATURAL REMEDIES NOW" (2SM287). We are admonished to "employ every facility for the restoration of health, taking every advantage possible, working in HARMONY with NATURAL LAWS" (2SM286).

◆ *Christ's Remedies Cleanse the System*

We are told that Christ's remedies cleanse the system (2SM289), which means that they are hygienic. They are not substances that pollute the system. But it is Satan who "has tempted man to introduce into the system that which weakens the human machinery clogging and destroying the fine arrangements of God. The DRUGS administered to the sick do not restore, but DESTROY. DRUGS NEVER CURE. Instead they place in the system seeds which bear a very bitter harvest. Our Saviour is the restorer of the moral image of God in man. He has supplied in the natural world remedies for the ills of man, that His followers may have life and that they may have it more abundantly. We can with safety discard the concoctions which man has used in the past. The Lord has provided ANTIDOTES FOR DISEASE IN THE SIMPLE PLANTS, and these can be used by faith, with NO DENIAL OF FAITH; for by using the blessings provided by God for our benefit we are cooperating with Him. We can use water, and sunshine, and the herbs which He has caused to grow, in healing maladies brought on by indiscretions or accident. We do not manifest a lack of faith when we ask God to bless HIS REMEDIES" (2SM289).

The use of drugs ignores the cause and TREATS the EFFECTS, SUPPRESSES the SYMPTOMS, LOWERS the FEVER, STOPS the PAIN, but at the same time causes CHRONIC DISEASE to develop. One must pay the price for interfering with the WISDOM OF THE BODY. This price is paid with HEART DISEASE, ARTHRITIS, CANCER, and other DEGENERATIVE DISEASES. CHRONIC DISEASE is a more serious problem than ACUTE DISEASE.

◆ *Disease Is Healed By The Cleansing Action Of Christ's Remedies*

The natural remedies for disease are both God's remedies as well as Christ's remedies, and the elimination of disease is brought about by their cleansing action. The DIVINE PHILOSOPHY of health says that disease is an effort by nature to free the system of POISONOUS IMPURITIES. The HEALING PROCESS is therefore A CLEANSING PROCESS (CH60–1). If the impurities of the body are not allowed to escape, they are taken back into the BLOOD and are forced upon the INTERNAL ORGANS (HL143). This causes a diseased condition in the body, the blood becomes impure (3T70), and sickness is the result (3T490). Perfect cleanliness is necessary to freedom from disease, hence, EVERY FORM OF UNCLEANNESS TENDS TOWARD DISEASE (MH276).

◆ *Poisonous Impurities Cause Disease*

We are told that those who are not in health have IMPURITIES IN THE BLOOD (3T490). Many times these impurities are caused by OVEREATING, by having more food in the system than the body can handle. They may be leftover fragments from incompleted digestive processes; they may also be remnants from improper foods, refined products, and harsh chemical additives. Toxic wastes become stored throughout the body, in glands, in cellular spaces, and circulate throughout the bloodstream. They tend to cling together and create barriers that prevent the free movement of your limbs as well as free muscular activity. What then happens is that the vital powers are exhausted in throwing off the excess food, the LIVER becomes burdened and unable to throw off the impurities in the blood, and sickness is the result (3T490). Sometimes not keeping the home clean is the cause of disease. Hence, "PERFECT CLEANLINESS, plenty of SUNLIGHT, careful attention to SANITATION in every detail of the home life, are essential to freedom from disease and to the cheerfulness and vigor of the inmates of the home" (MH276).

Also "the studied habit of shunning the AIR and avoiding EXERCISE closes the pores—making it impossible to throw off impurities through that channel. The burden of labor is thrown upon the LIVER, LUNGS, KIDNEYS etc., and these internal organs are compelled to do the work of the SKIN" (2T524). "The reason that FEVERS prevail in families exposing the attendants is because the sickroom is not kept free from poisonous infection by cleanliness and proper ventilation" (HL213).

◆ *When We Violate God's Laws Of Health*

Since violating the laws of health means violating the laws of God, such violation can be nullified as follows: "When I violate the laws God has established in my being, I am to REPENT AND REFORM, and place myself in the most favorable condition under doctors God has provided — PURE AIR, PURE WATER, and the HEALING, PRECIOUS SUNLIGHT" (CD302). "Let those who are sick do all in their power, by correct practice in eating, drinking, and dressing, and by taking judicious exercise, secure the recovery of health" (CD303). They must all COOPERATE with GOD in restoring their health. "GOD WILL NOT DO WHAT HE HAS ASKED US TO DO" (MM226).

◆ *It Is No Denial Of Faith To Use Christ's Remedies*

"The Lord has provided antidotes for diseases in SIMPLE PLANTS, and these can be used by faith, with no denial of faith; for by using the blessings provided by God we are cooperating with Him. He can use WATER and SUNSHINE and the HERBS which He has caused to grow in HEALING MALADIES brought on by indiscretion or accident. We do not manifest a lack of faith when we ask God to bless His remedies. True faith will thank God for the knowledge of how to use these precious blessings in a way which will restore mental and physical vigor" (2SM288–9).

We are admonished that instruction in the principles of health and healthful living is to be part of the work of every gospel worker (CH40). When we are ill, we are not denying our faith if we use those HYGIENIC METHODS which are available to us to ALLEVIATE PAIN and to AID NATURE in her work of RESTORATION. It is no denial of faith for the sick who request PRAYER FOR HEALING, to COOPERATE WITH GOD, and place themselves in the condition most favorable to recovery. The idea that NO REMEDIES should be used for the sick the Spirit of Prophecy calls an ERROR, because of the fact that God does not heal the sick without the aid of the means of healing which lie within our reach. (2SM286). We are told that thousands need instruction concerning these SIMPLE HYGIENIC METHODS (CH389).

◆ *The True Science Of Healing*

"Those whose minds and bodies are diseased are to behold in CHRIST THE RESTORER. 'Because I live', He says, 'ye shall live also'(Jo. 14:19). This is the life we are to present to the sick, telling them that if they have faith in Christ as the Restorer, if they cooperate with Him, obeying the laws of health, and striving to perfect holiness in His fear, He will IMPART to them HIS LIFE. When we present Christ to them in this way, we are IMPARTING A POWER, a strength, that is of value; for it comes from above. This is the TRUE SCIENCE OF HEALING for body and soul" (MH244). "Christ has empowered His church to do the same work that He did during His ministry. Today He is the same compassionate physician that He was while on this earth. We should let the afflicted understand that IN HIM there is HEALING BALM for every DISEASE, RESTORING POWER for every INFIRMITY" (CH529).

Bible Examples Of Health Principles Applied And Misapplied

◆ *Adam And Eve*

We are told that with Adam and Eve INTEMPERATE DESIRE resulted in the loss of Eden, and that TEMPERANCE IN ALL THINGS has more to do with our restoration to Eden than men realize (CD43). They fell because of the indulgence of appetite, and our only hope of regaining Eden is through the firm denial of appetite and passion. Such a denial will preserve mental and moral vigor, and will enable us to bring our inclinations under the control of our powers of reason, so that we will be able to distinguish between right and wrong, the sacred and the common. Eve was beguiled by the serpent to eat of the fruit of the only tree of which God had forbidden them to eat, or even touch it, lest they die (Gen. 3:3).

Eve had everything to make her happy. She was surrounded by fruit of every variety. Yet the fruit of the forbidden tree appeared more desirable to her than the fruit of all the other trees in the garden of which she could eat freely. She was INTEMPERATE IN HER DESIRES. She ate, and through her influence, her husband ate also, and a CURSE rested upon them both. The EARTH also was CURSED because of their sin. Since that time appetite has controlled reason in the human family because it also has been beguiled by Satan to violate God's laws of health. Disease has been steadily increasing, and the cause has been followed by the effect. (CD145)

◆ *A Lesson From Israel's Failure*

God gave His word to ancient Israel that if they would obey His laws, He would keep them from all of the disease which He had brought upon the Egyptians. Whenever God makes a promise to a people, it is always conditional. Whenever He makes a promise to Himself, it is unconditional. So the promise to Israel was made on the condition of obedience. But Israel did not abide by the conditions. Instead of studying the principles of health, they responded to their appetites and passions, and did not choose to follow the Creator's plan. As a result they brought upon themselves diseases of various kinds by their own wrong habits. People very seldom give the correct reason for their troubles. They seldom accredit them to the true cause — their own wrong course of action. They have often believed that God had caused them, when they themselves were responsible for them. (CD121).

Many articles of food were forbidden to the Israelites by God. But the things forbidden were unwholesome. This was to teach the lesson that the use of INJURIOUS FOODS IS DEFILING THE BODY TEMPLE, and that which defiles the body tends to defile the soul. Because of their murmurings they were given the flesh food they had gotten used to in Egypt, but their demand became a curse to them, for their gluttony produced a plague, from which thousands of them died. "Had the Israelites obeyed the instruction they received, and profited by their advantages, they would have been the WORLD'S OBJECT LESSON of health and prosperity. If as a people they had lived according to God's plan, they would have been preserved from the diseases that afflicted other nations. Above any other people they would have possessed physical strength and vigor of intellect (CD27).

◆ *Daniel And His Companions*

Daniel and his friends were brought into king Nebuchadnezzar's palace in order to partake of the king's meat and wine. But the swine's flesh placed before them was declared unclean by the law of Moses. Daniel decided to stand firm in not defiling himself with the king's food, and he placed his request for simple food of PULSE with Melzar, the officer in charge. Pulse, according to Josephus, consisted of SPROUTED BEANS. Like many in our day, Melzar thought that such a simple abstemious diet would produce pale and sickly individuals who would be deficient in muscular strength. At Daniel's request the matter was to be decided by a ten days trial. At the end of the trial, Daniel and his companions exhibited a marked superiority in personal appearance, physical activity, and mental vigor over those who had indulged their appetite. As a result they were permitted to continue their diet during the whole course of their training. This is an example of the triumph of principle over the temptation to indulge the appetite. It shows that a strict compliance with the requirements of God is beneficial to the health of body and mind. (CD31–2)

◆ *The Experience Of Nadab And Abihu*

Nadab and Abihu were the sons of Aaron. They partook freely of wine which God forbade because it had an influence to becloud the intellect. They nevertheless ministered in the office of the priesthood. The priests who burned incense before the Lord were required to use the fire of God's kindling, which burned day and night and was never extinguished. No sacrifice was acceptable to God which was not seasoned with divine fire, which represented the communication between God and man. The incense kindled by the holy fire was to arise before God mingled with prayers which represented an emblem of the mediation of Christ.

Instead of the holy fire Aaron's sons used the common fire which God did not accept, and He consumed them because of their disregard of His directions. We are told that if they had been in full command of their reasoning faculties they would have discerned the difference between the common and sacred fire. The gratification of appetite debased their faculties and so beclouded their intellect that their power of discernment was gone. We may ask whether an individual is responsible for the results that follow his use of a substance which beclouds his intellect, and limits the full use of his mental faculties. The answer that is given us is that when they put the cup to their lips they made themselves RESPONSIBLE FOR ALL THEIR ACTS committed while under the influence of wine. An individual becomes responsible for any injury sustained when he barters away his reasoning faculties and lets appetite control him. As a result, the indulgence of appetite cost them their lives. (Te 43–4). We are told that the use of wine among the Israelites was one of the causes that finally resulted in their captivity (Te52).

◆ *Other Examples*

✓ ADAM—"Adam fell by indulgence of appetite. Christ began His ministry by conquering appetite" (CD54). "That long fast in the wilderness was to be a lesson to fallen man for all time. Christ was not overcome by the strong temptations of the enemy, and this is encouragement for every soul who is struggling against temptation. All who would live godly lives may overcome as Christ overcame, by the blood of the Lamb, and the word of their testimony. THAT LONG FAST OF THE SAVIOUR STRENGTHENED HIM TO ENDURE. He gave evidence to man that He would begin the work of overcoming just where the ruin began—on the point of appetite. When Christ was most fiercely beset by temptation, He ate nothing" (CD186). "For our sake He exercised a self-control stronger than hunger or death" (CD185).

✓ ESAU—"Esau lusted for a favorite dish, and sacrificed his birthright to gratify appetite" (CD148).

✓ SODOM AND GOMORRAH—"The gratification of unnatural appetite led to the sins that caused the destruction of Sodom and Gomorrah. God ascribes the fall of Babylon to her gluttony and drunkenness. Indulgence of appetite and passion was the foundation of all their sins" (CD147).

✓ JOHN THE BAPTIST—We are told that the diet of John the Baptist was purely vegetable, composed of locusts and wild honey. His diet was a rebuke to the indulgence of appetite and the gluttony that everywhere prevailed. His was a message of temperance in all things. Since his diet was vegetable, it means that the locusts were not grasshoppers, but the pods of the locust tree, or carob pods. (CD71)

✓ PAUL—"Paul was a health reformer. Said he, 'I keep under my body, and bring it into subjection; lest that by any means, when I have preached to others, I myself should be a castaway'. He felt that a responsibility rested upon him to preserve all his powers in their strength, that he might use them to the glory of God. If Paul was in danger from intemperance, we are in greater danger, because we do not feel and realize as he did the necessity of glorifying God in our bodies and spirits, which are His. Overeating is the sin of this age" (CD133).

SATAN, THE ORIGINATOR OF DISEASE

Satan The Destroyer

◆ *He Destroys The Good And The Evil*

We are told that "sickness, suffering, and death, are the work of an antagonistic power. Satan is the destroyer; God is the restorer" (CH168). "SATAN IS THE ORIGINATOR OF DISEASE" (HL60). Satan is called the destroyer because he destroys both good and evil. He destroys the good as far as God allows because of his enmity against the law of God, and against God's servants who keep His law. He destroys evil persons who have given themselves into his hands, because he doesn't want them to get the chance to be converted and be saved in God's kingdom. "Satan has control of all whom God does not especially guard. He will favor and prosper some, in order to further his own designs; and he will bring trouble upon others and lead men to believe that it is God who is afflicting them" (CH460). In this way he is leading men to look upon disease as from God (5T193).

◆ *God Allows Satan To Destroy*

The history of Job is to show us that SUFFERING IS INFLICTED BY SATAN, and is overruled by God for purposes of mercy (DA471). In Job's case Satan destroyed that which was good. In the case of the destruction of Jerusalem he destroyed that which was evil. He destroyed his own kind. We are told, "Then God withdrew His protection from them and removed His restraining power from Satan and his angels, and the nation was left to the control of the leader she had chosen" (GC28). If God had told Satan exactly what he could do to Job, then God would have been directly responsible for the consequences. The direct responsibility for Job's family and property was Satan's. He planned it and carried out the plan. However, God recognized his indirect responsibility in allowing Satan to do this by giving Job an even greater family and greater property in the end.

◆ *God Destroys Only Evil Doers*

Satan destroys because that is part of his nature. God also destroys, but that is not a part of His nature. That is why it is called, "HIS STRANGE ACT" (Isa 28:21). In the Old Testament God many times executed the wages of sin upon evil doers directly and immediately. The flood is a case in point. He didn't have to wait until the end of the world before He destroyed the wicked people in Noah's day by a flood. He says, "I kill and make alive. I wound and I heal" (Deut. 32:39). God does all of these things directly and indirectly. He does them directly through the agency of His angels. He does them indirectly when He allows Satan and his angels to destroy within limits, as well as when men, tempted by Satan, exercise their freedom of choice to destroy themselves. Such is the case when smoking causes a fatal disease, or when drinking causes a fatal accident. These fatalities happen when men are disobedient to God's laws of health which were ordained as laws of life (Rom. 7:10).

We are told that "A single angel destroyed all the first-born of the Egyptians, and filled the land with mourning. When David offended against God by numbering the people, one angel caused that terrible destruction by which his sin was punished. The same destructive power exercised by HOLY ANGELS when God commands, will be exercised by EVIL ANGELS when He permits" (GC614). When people commit sin, Satan has an indirect responsibility in their sin, because he tempted them to commit it. But the individual sinner has a direct responsibility in his own sin, because there was power available to him to help him overcome the temptation, but he chose not to utilize that power. He exercised his God-given freedom in the wrong direction. God may indirectly take the blame because He gave them their freedom of choice. But He doesn't take the responsibility for their action. If He took the direct responsibility for their action, then He could not in the end destroy the unrepentant sinner.

Satan Has Corrupted God's Creation

◆ Satan's Influence Has Weakened The Human Race

The physical condition of the human race has been growing weaker and weaker because of his influence. We are told: "The present enfeebled condition of the human family was presented before me. Every generation has been growing weaker, and disease of every form afflicts the race" (1T304). "Satan has the power of disease and death, and he has been learning how to annoy and enfeeble the race" (EW184). "He can bring disease and disaster until populous cities are reduced to ruin and desolation. He imparts to the air a deadly taint, and thousands perish by the pestilence. These visitations are to become more frequent and disastrous" (GC589). "Thousands of poor mortals with deformed sickly bodies, shattered nerves, and gloomy minds are dragging out a miserable existence. Satan's power upon the human family increases. If the Lord should not soon come and destroy his power, the earth would erelong be depopulated" (CH18). We are told that "If Adam, at his creation, had not been endowed with twenty times as much vital force as men now have, the race, with their present habits of living in violation of natural law, would have become extinct" (3T138).

◆ He Has Corrupted Wholesome Fruits And Grains

Specifically, Satan's corruption of the earth took the form of taking the fruit of the vine, wheat, and other things which were given by God as food and converted them into POISONS which would ruin man's physical, mental, and moral powers, and so overcome the senses that Satan would have full control. "God did not mean that man should have this knowledge. They are using the poisonous productions that SATAN himself has PLANTED to take the place of the tree of life, whose LEAVES ARE FOR THE HEALING OF THE NATIONS. Under the influence of liquor, men would be led to commit crimes of all kinds. Through perverted appetite the world would be made corrupt. By leading men to drink alcohol, Satan would cause them to descend lower and lower in the scale…. This APPETITE, which has no foundation in nature, has destroyed its millions" (Te12). Under its influence men have become DEMONS (Te36).

◆ Satan Has The Power To Modify God's Creation

Satan's agents claim to cure disease by ELECTRICITY, MAGNETISM, and SYMPATHETIC REMEDIES (5T193). He also has the power to cause sickness (2SM53), and for this reason sickness should not be attributed to God (MM297). We understand that Satan has no power to create or to give life, which is the prerogative of God alone (PP264; 5T697). But he apparently has the power to work with living material already in existence so as to modify its nature. He has the power to modify germs so as to produce disease and death (EW184; GC589), and in a limited manner he has power to perform miracles of healing (5T589). We are told that GOD "NEVER MADE A THORN OR A THISTLE. These are Satan's work, the result of DEGENERATION, introduced by him among the precious things" (6T186). However, when God cursed the earth because of Adam's sin, it brought forth thorns and thistles (Gen. 3:17, 18). This means that when God cursed the earth He allowed Satan to corrupt some life forms so as to produce degenerate life forms. He corrupted not only plant and animal life but human life also. We are told that "Every species of animal which God had created were preserved in the ark. The confused species which God did not create, which were the result of AMALGAMATION, were destroyed by the flood. Since the flood there has been amalgamation of man and beast, as may be seen in the almost endless varieties of species of animal, and in certain races of men" (3SpG75).

The process of amalgamation refers to the modern term of HYBRIDIZATION, or of the intermingling of two more or less diverse varieties of plant or animal life by means of genetic material. It means that animals were intermingled with related animals but not with man. The process of amalgamation we are told "defaced the image of God and caused confusion everywhere" (3SpG64)

◆ The Threefold Curse

Because of this confusion, God did not allow the earth to carry out the purpose which He had originally designed for it. The curse which He placed upon the earth was placed upon ALL CREATION. We are to read in it the LAW OF CONDEMNATION. The Lord's curse is upon MAN, upon BEAST, upon the FISH in the sea.

The FIRST curse was pronounced upon the POSTERITY of Adam and upon the EARTH because of disobedience. The SECOND curse came upon the GROUND after Cain slew his brother Abel. The THIRD most dreadful curse from God, came upon the earth at the FLOOD. The sin of man has brought the sure result,— decay, deformity, and death. As the transgression becomes almost universal, the curse will be permitted to become as broad and as deep as the transgression. (1BC1085).

◆ *Satan Has Power To Produce Poisonous Plants*

When Satan was allowed by means of God's curse, to produce THORNS and THISTLES he also produced degenerate harmful plants of all kinds, many of which exist today as poisonous plants. He no doubt was allowed to produce them from some of the nonpoisonous helpful plants which God had created, by modifying their seeds. We are told that "Christ never planted the SEEDS of DEATH in the system. Satan planted these seeds when he tempted Adam to eat of the tree of knowledge which meant disobedience to God. Not one NOXIOUS PLANT was placed in the Lord's great garden, but after Adam and Eve sinned, POISONOUS HERBS sprang up. In the parable of the sower the question was asked the master, 'didst thou not sow good seed in thy field? from whence then hath it tares?' The master answered, 'An ENEMY hath done this' (Matt. 13:27, 28). All tares are sown by the EVIL ONE. Every noxious herb is of his sowing, and by his ingenious methods of amalgamation, he has corrupted the earth with TARES" (2SM288).

◆ *Satan's Power To Produce Disease, Death, And Healing*

Satan has a degree of power over a person's body, who, if he indicates his willingness to subject himself to such power, can be HEALED AS WELL AS MADE SICK. We are told that "Satan will work in these latter days through his evil agencies to make it appear that he is the great healer and benefactor of the race. 'Men under the influence of EVIL SPIRITS will work MIRACLES. They will make people sick by casting their SPELL upon them, and will then remove the spell, leading others to say that those who were sick have been miraculously healed. This Satan has done again and again.'" (CH461).

◆ *Satan Will Perform Miracles Of Healing*

Before the close of time Satan will perform actual MIRACLES as far as God will allow him to do so (5T698), but he cannot control the mind or the will unless they are yielded to his control (DA125; GC510). He makes sin attractive by the covering of light which he draws over it (Te16). "HEALING THE DISEASES of the people, and professing to present a new and more exalted system of religious faith" (GC589). Evil angels "are constantly seeking access to us, and against whose attacks we have, in our own strength, no method of defense. If permitted, they can DISTRACT OUR MINDS, DISORDER AND TORMENT OUR BODIES, DESTROY OUR POSSESSIONS AND OUR LIVES. Their only delight is in misery and destruction" (GC517)

◆ *h. Satan Will Counterfeit Faith Healing*

Many will be deceived to receive these wonders of Satan as coming from God. "By departing from the plain precepts and commandments of God, and giving heed to fables, the minds of many are preparing to receive these lying wonders. We must all now seek to arm ourselves for the contest in which we must soon engage. Faith in God's word, prayerfully studied and practically applied, will be our shield from Satan's power and will bring us off conquerors through the blood of Christ" (1T302).

Pharaoh's magicians in Egypt counterfeited the miracles performed by Aaron, of turning the rod into a serpent: "Moses, by the power of God, had changed the rod to a living serpent. Satan, through the magicians, counterfeited this miracle. He could not produce living serpents, for he has not the power to give life. This power belongs to God alone. But all that Satan could do he did—he produced a COUNTERFEIT. By his power, working through the magicians, he caused the rod to ASSUME the appearance of serpents." (5T697). "So far as his power extends, he will perform ACTUAL MIRACLES" (5T698). Rev. 13:14 says: "And deceiveth them that dwell on the earth by the means of those miracles which he had power to do" not merely those which he pretends to do. He "will work miracles of all kinds, to deceive, if possible, the very elect" (9T16). "Satan has control of all whom God does not especially guard" (CH460). "Through

SPIRITUALISM, Satan appears as a benefactor of the race, healing the diseases of the people, and professing to present a new and more exalted system of religious faith; but at the same time he works as a destroyer" (CH460).

"The mother, watching by the sickbed of her child, exclaims, 'I can do no more! Is there no physician who has power to restore my child!' She is told of the wonderful cures performed by some CLAIRVOYANT or MAGNETIC HEALER, and she trusts her dear one to his charge; placing it as verily in the hand of Satan as if he were standing by her side. In many instances the future life of the child is controlled by a satanic power, which it seems impossible to break" (Ev. 606).

◆ *Appetite Is Satan's Strongest Weapon*

"Satan comes to man as he came to Christ, with his overpowering temptations to indulge appetite" (CD153). Adam and Eve were first tempted in the garden of Eden on the point of appetite. Christ was tempted by Satan in the wilderness first on the point of appetite. He began the work of overcoming where Adam's and Eve's failure originated. They failed the test, but Christ passed the test successfully. In doing so, Christ had to show that by the denial of appetite man could overcome this temptation of Satan. In human nature Christ fasted and prayed and overcame the temptation. That long fast was to be a lesson to fallen man for all time. "For our sake He exercised a self-control stronger than hunger or death" (CD185). His victory made it possible for every member of the human family to resist the temptations of appetite, and to overcome as He overcame.

◆ *Indulgence Of Appetite—The Foundation Of Sin*

"In our own strength it is impossible for us to deny the clamors of our fallen nature. Through this channel Satan will bring temptation upon us. Christ knew that the enemy would come to every human being, to take advantage of hereditary weakness, and by his false insinuations to ensnare all whose trust is not in God" (CD152). "Entire cities have been blotted from the face of the earth because of the debasing crimes and revolting iniquity that made them a blot upon the universe. INDULGENCE OF APPETITE was the FOUNDATION of all their sins" (CD153).

◆ *Appetite Will Prove The Ruin Of Thousands*

It takes a lot of self-control in order to resist the temptations of Satan, and we are told that those without self-control are the DUPES OF SATAN (Te34), and are helpless to resist him. The reason is that under these circumstances they cannot distinguish between right and wrong. Christ "knew that appetite would be man's idol and would stand directly in the way of salvation" (Te20). He also showed how strong the power of appetite was upon man. We are therefore told that "the controlling power of appetite will prove the ruin of thousands, when, if they had conquered on this point they would have had moral power to gain the victory over every other temptation of Satan. He deceives man in transgressing the laws of nature in eating and drinking. But those who are slaves to appetite will fail of PERFECTING CHRISTIAN CHARACTER" (Te21-2). While we can receive all of the help we need, WE MUST FOR OURSELVES, INDIVIDUALLY EXERT EVERY EFFORT TO OVERCOME. "As we near the close of time, Satan's temptations to indulge appetite will be more powerful and more difficult to overcome" (3T491).

Diet has much to do with the disposition to enter into temptation and commit sin, If we are determined to overcome God will help us and will give us strength to resist every temptation (CD485). Appetite is one of the strongest temptations that we have to meet. If we are to overcome as Christ overcame, we must restrict our appetites and passions and place them under the control of ENLIGHTENED CONSCIENCE (Te21). But if we depart from God's directions, we are placing ourselves under the control of Satan (Te123).

"Those who choose to be presumptuous, saying, 'The Lord has healed me, and I need not restrict my diet; I can eat and drink as I please', will erelong need, in body and soul, the restoring power of God. Because the Lord has graciously healed you, you must not think you can link yourself up with the self-indulgent practices of the world. Do as Christ commanded after His work of healing,—'GO AND SIN NO MORE' Appetite must not be your god" (CD25).

Christ's Warning To Us

"Our Saviour warned His disciples that just prior to His second coming a state of things would exist very similar to that which preceded the flood. Eating and drinking would be carried to excess, and the world would be given up to pleasure. This state of things does exist at the present time. The world is largely given up to the indulgence of appetite; and the disposition to follow worldly customs will bring us into bondage to perverted habits,— habits that will make us more and more like the doomed inhabitants of Sodom. I have wondered that the inhabitants of the earth were not destroyed, like the people of Sodom and Gomorrah. I see reason enough for the present state of degeneracy and mortality in the world. Blind passion controls reason, and every high consideration is, with many, sacrificed to lust.

"We have the example of ancient Israel and the warning for us not to do as they did. Their history of unbelief and rebellion is left on record as a special warning that we should not follow their example of murmuring at God's requirements. How can we pass on so indifferently, choosing our own course, following the sight of our own eyes, and departing further and further from God, as did the Hebrews? God cannot do great things for His people because of their hardness of heart and sinful unbelief" (3T172).

"To keep the body in a healthy condition, in order that all parts of the living machinery may act harmoniously, should be the STUDY OF OUR LIFE. The children of God cannot glorify Him with sickly bodies and dwarfed minds. Those who indulge in any species of intemperance either in eating or drinking, waste their physical energies and weaken moral power"(CD17–18)

PRAYER AND HEALING

Conditions Of Answered Prayer

◆ *Prayer Should Be Carefully Considered*

We are told that "Prayer should not be entered into without careful consideration" (MH227). It must be based upon true faith and not upon presumption. Presumption means claiming the promises of God without endeavoring to meet their requirements. Many individuals bring sickness upon themselves by wrong habits of living, dressing, and working, which is not according to God's natural laws. They want most of all to receive bodily healing, and God is ready and willing to give it to them, for He says, "Beloved, I wish above all things that thou mayest prosper and be in health, even as thy soul prospereth" (3 Jo. 2). But sickness has a great spiritual side, and that is that the sick person must be willing to give up his sinful physical habits so that God can release His spiritual power to heal. This is one limitation to prayer healing which the individual must adjust to. God does not heal just anybody under any circumstances. God does not heal so that the individual can go back to his old bad habits and get sick all over again for the same reasons. He must give up his perverted appetite and unhealthful practices. The Holy Spirit "will renew every organ of the body, that God's servants may work acceptably and successfully. VITALITY increases under the influence of the Spirit's action" (MM12). "The Lord will remove infirmities in answer to prayer" (MM242).

◆ *Sins Must Be Confessed*

"To those who desire prayer for their restoration to health, it should be made plain that the violation of God's law, either natural or spiritual, is sin, and that in order for them to receive His blessing, sin must be CONFESSED and FORSAKEN" (MH228).

The individual who asks for healing must exercise faith without presumption in order to meet the requirements for healing. If his own sins caused his sickness, he must endeavor to change his ways, his lifestyle, in order to make healing effective. He must cease to do evil and learn to do good. The guilty conscience must be aroused to confession. Sin must be confessed and forsaken, for every sin is an offense to God.

Otherwise, if healed he would continue in the same sins of heedless transgression of nature's law. Often "Sin has brought many of them where they are—to a state of feebleness of mind and debility of body. Shall prayer be offered to the God of heaven for His healing to come upon them then and there, without specifying any conditions? I say, No, decidedly no. What then shall be done? Present their cases before Him who knows every individual name" (CH373). Sins that are of a private nature should be confessed only to God, unless the individual is impressed by the Holy Spirit to confess them to a human being. "Who forgiveth all thine iniquities; who healeth all thy diseases" (Ps. 103:3).

◆ *Sins Must Be Forsaken*

When a person has been healed through prayer, he cannot presumptuously say, "'The Lord has healed me, and I need not restrict my diet; I can eat and drink as I please', will erelong need, in body and soul, the restoring power of God. Because the Lord has graciously healed you, you must not think you can link yourself up with the self-indulgent practices of the world. Do as Christ commanded after His work of healing,—'go and sin no more'" (CD25). We are told that if all the sick were healed by prayer, there would then be very few who would improve their opportunities to become acquainted with the right way of eating, drinking, and dressing (MM260). Hence, what is wrong with the so-called "miracle" healings of television evangelists is that people are not asked to change their lifestyles so as to keep themselves from disease in the future. Christ no doubt instructed the ones He healed in the avoidance of the sinful practices which caused their disease in the first place.

Al. Wolfsen, an Adventist herbalist, tells a personal experience of a woman who was healed of cancer through prayer. After the healing she said that now she could live any way she wanted to because she was healed. Al reminded her that now she had a responsibility to God to live according to His principles of life. She said that if she can't live the way she wanted to she might as well be dead. At that point the cancer returned in its full fury, and without an inclination to repent, eight months later she died of the same disease from which God had healed her earlier.

◆ *We Are Not Denying Faith When We Apply God's Remedies*

It is not a denial of faith to use those remedies against disease which God has provided for us in nature to help us alleviate pain, and to help nature in her work of eliminating poisonous substances from the system. We are told that nature will want some help in doing this. "We are not denying faith when we cooperate with God by placing ourselves in a condition most favorable to the healing process" (MH232). The things which God has not approved do not place us in a position where God can apply His miraculous power to heal. He will then allow nature to take its course. If we have overpowered nature through our bad habits, God will then not perform a miracle to avoid the obvious results.

Not all Are Healed

◆ *We Must Have Faith In God's Response*

"God knows the end from the beginning. He is acquainted with the hearts of all men. He reads every secret of the soul. He knows whether those for whom prayer is offered would or would not be able to endure the trials that would come upon them should they live. He knows whether their lives would be a blessing or a curse to themselves and to the world. This is one reason why, while presenting our petitions with earnestness, we should pray for the sick only in one way which is, 'Lord, if it be in accordance with Thy will, for Thy glory and the good of the one who is sick, heal the sufferer, we pray. Not our will but thine be done' (2SM345–6). 'The sick will be healed when we have faith to come to God in the right way' (MM16) If requested the elders of the church can be called to pray for the sick. In this case we are told that 'They shall lay hands on the sick and they shall recover' (Mark 16:18). 'God is too wise and too good to answer our prayers always at just the time and in just the manner we desire' (MH230) In Christ there is healing balm for every disease, restoring power for every infirmity, and 'the prayer of faith shall save the sick' (Jam. 5:15)."

◆ *When Prayers Are Not Answered*

When some person's prayers are not answered, the fault does not lie with God but with the person. While they may be professing godliness, they do not bear fruit to the glory of God; their works are not what they should be. They are living in neglect of positive duties. Unless this is changed in the life, God cannot answer their prayers for healing according to His glory. Mrs. White states, "I saw that the reason why God did not hear the prayers of His servants for the sick among us more fully was, that He could not be glorified in so doing while they were violating the laws of health" (CD25–26). "Sick persons cannot be healed while knowingly committing sin" (SD297). All that can be done in praying for the sick is to earnestly importune God in their behalf, and in perfect confidence rest the matter in His hands. We should acknowledge our acceptance of His will, and should not pray that He concede to ours. "It is not always safe to ask for UNCONDITIONAL HEALING" (CH375)

"It is labor lost to teach people to look to God as a healer of their infirmities, unless they are TAUGHT also to lay aside UNHEALTHFUL PRACTICES. In order to receive His blessing in answer to prayer, they must cease to do evil and learn to do well" (MH227).

◆ *God Does Not Hear The Prayer Of The Unrepentant Sinner*

When we pray for a sick person who has not confessed all of his sins, God will not hear our prayer in his behalf. The sick still may have something in his life that he hasn't repented of, for we are told that "if we regard iniquity in our heart the Lord will not hear us" (Ps. 66:18). A prayer is more efficacious, or brings better results if it is expressed by a person who is dedicated to God and His work, a man of faith. As the sick person has purified his heart in order to receive the benefit of prayer, so also the intercessor in prayer must be a person who is pure in heart if the expected results are to be achieved. Mrs. White gives an example where a sick sister who feared God was immediately healed of consumption when both she and a minister prayed earnestly for her healing. She arose and prepared supper, a thing she had not done in ten years. Because of her life she was healed, for the minister was said to be a vile and corrupt person. (2SM347).

When we pray for a sick person, and we have not confessed all of our sins to God, He will not hear our prayer in the sick person's behalf. Prayer will not be efficacious unless sins are repented of. We are told that "Fasting and prayer will accomplish nothing while the heart is estranged from God by a wrong course of action. The promise of God to us is on CONDITION OF OBEDIENCE, compliance with all his requirements" (CH377). That is why the Bible says in Jam. 5:16, "Confess your faults one to another and pray one for another, that ye may be healed. The effectual fervent prayer of a righteous man availeth much." If the person who prays is righteous, there is a greater likelihood for his prayer to be answered according to the way it is given, but God is nevertheless the final arbiter of the desires expressed in the prayer.

◆ *The Healing Must Glorify God*

Jam. 5:14, 15 says, "Is any sick among you? let him call for the elders of the church; and let them pray over him, anointing him with oil in the name of the Lord: and the prayer of faith shall save the sick, and the Lord shall raise him up; and if he have committed sins, they shall be forgiven him." "Many have expected that God would heal their sickness simply because they have asked Him to do so. But God does not regard the prayers of some because their faith was not made perfect by works. God will not work a miracle to keep those from sickness who have no care for themselves, but are continually violating the laws of health, and make no effort to PREVENT DISEASE.

"When we do all on our part to have health, then we may expect that the blessed results will follow, and we can ask God in faith to bless our efforts for the preservation of health. He will then answer our prayer, if His name can be glorified thereby. Those who will gratify their appetite, and then suffer because of their intemperance, and take DRUGS to relieve them, may be assured that God will not interpose to save health and life which is so recklessly periled. The cause has produced the effect. Many, as their last resort, follow the directions in the word of God, and request the prayers of the elders of the church for the restoration to health. God does not see fit to answer prayers in behalf of such, for He knows that if they should be restored to health, they would again sacrifice it upon the altar of unhealthy appetite" (CD26)

In order for an individual to be healed, God must be glorified through his healing. In some cases God did not hear the prayers of His servants for the sick, because He could not be glorified in raising them to health because they were violating the laws of health. "Many persons bring disease upon themselves by their self-indulgence. They have not lived in accordance with natural law or the principles of strict purity. Others have discarded the laws of health in their habits of eating and drinking, dressing, or working. If God were to work a miracle in restoring these persons to health, He would be ENCOURAGING SIN" (MH227). "Faith and good works go hand in hand in relieving the afflicted among us, and in fitting them to glorify God here, and to be saved at the coming of Christ" (CD26)

◆ *We Should Not Urge God To Heal.*

We should not urge upon God that He heal any specific person, for we might be urging a recovery without submission to His will on the part of the sick. "But to press our petitions without a submissive spirit is not right; our prayers must take the form, not of command, but of INTERCESSION" (MH230). "We do not know whether the blessing we desire will be best or not. Therefore our prayers should include this thought, 'Lord, thou knowest every secret of the soul. Thou art acquainted with these persons. Jesus, their advocate, gave His life for them. His love for them is greater than ours can possibly be. If, therefore, it is for thy glory and the good of the afflicted ones, we ask, in the name of Jesus, that they may be restored to health. If it be not Thy will that they may be restored, we ask that thy grace may comfort and Thy presence sustain them in their sufferings" (MH229).

God Responds To Prayer According To His Will

◆ *No Answer May Mean Wait*

It is often better that the Lord does not answer our prayers for the sick in the manner that we desire, God does more and better for us than to answer our prayers in the manner that we might desire. He knows that other solutions are even better than the one which our finite mind might suggest. When we ask God for special healing we are asking Him for a miracle to be performed, which goes beyond the gradual healing by means of the laws of health. If this is what we are asking for, then we must have a worthy individual for God to perform such a miracle upon.

Sometimes God answers our prayer for the sick to be restored in the manner in which we asked it only because we were too insistent to have this person restored. He restored him accordingly, and a short time later He laid this person to rest. In cases of this type God answered our prayer positively as well as fulfilling His own plan a short time later.

There are some who remember God only on their DEATH BED, and if they were to be restored to life and health, they would continue to forget God afterward. Their restoration would not be a blessing to themselves nor to God. They would then have been restored to a life of disobedience which finally leads to eternal death. Mrs. White asks the question as to how she can present people to the Lord for healing when they have made the subject of health reform a matter of jest by using TEA, COFFEE, SPICES, AND FLESH MEAT.

◆ *Natural Methods Bring Supernatural Results*

We are told that "those who seek healing by prayer should not neglect to make use of the remedial agencies within their reach" (MH231). "Nature is God's physician" (MH263). God desires to heal especially when His natural methods of healing have been previously applied. Just because we pray for the sick does not mean that we should stop using God's remedies as an assistance for his condition. God's miracles often do not look like miracles. They often look like nature taking its natural course. When we pray for the sick we also work for them, and by working for them we are God's assistants in His endeavor to heal. We are cooperating with God when we use His remedies. "NATURAL MEANS, used in accordance with God's will, bring about SUPERNATURAL RESULTS. We ask for a miracle and the Lord directs the mind to some simple remedy" (2SM346). God asks us to do for ourselves what we can do for ourselves, and what we can do for ourselves He doesn't do for us. In doing this we are working out our own salvation as a patient, as well as an intercessor for the patient. We are told to work out our own salvation with fear and trembling (Phil. 2:12).

◆ *God Makes Us Responsible For The Methods Used*

If His methods have not been used, God may not answer our prayers in a special way, and will simply allow the laws of nature to take their natural course. The individual may continue to live if his vitality overcomes the disease, or he may die without miraculous intervention if the disease overcomes him. If we allow doctors to use harmful and poisonous methods which God does not approve of, He will allow these methods to take their natural course toward unnatural results, which in all likelihood will be more negative than positive. We must remember that God makes us responsible for the methods that are applied to us in sickness, and not the doctor directly. He may make the doctors responsible for themselves for the methods which they are using, but He makes us responsible for the methods which we allow the doctor to apply to us, as long as we are in the condition to make such a decision.

◆ *The Healed One Is Under Renewed Obligation To God*

When one has been healed through prayer, the healed one is under renewed obligation to God to live according to His will. The LEASE ON LIFE that God has given is to be used to honor Him to a greater degree than ever before. By restoring the sick one to health, God has seen a blessing which this person can still be to Him, to the benefit of His name, and to others. Besides being prayed for and finally healed, this person must also be educated to live better after he is restored to health. He should then become a health reformer and change his life completely around, for faith must be made perfect in works. "It is labor lost to teach people to look to God as a healer of their infirmities, unless they are taught also to lay aside UNHEALTHFUL PRACTICES. In order to receive His blessing in answer to prayer, they must cease to do evil and learn to do well" (MH227)

◆ *Pray Without Ceasing*

We are admonished to keep on praying even if we don't receive an immediate answer to our prayer. "Ask and it shall be given you" (Luke 11:9). A delay in the answer to prayer is for our special benefit. It is for God to determine if our faith is strong enough to wait upon the Lord for guidance, direction, and answers. Faith strengthens as we exercise it, and maintain it in time. "God answers prayer for those who place themselves in the channel of His blessings" (MH256). If God does not decide to heal immediately, He may want to determine if we in faith are continuing to apply His remedies. If we are wishing and hoping for a quick answer to our prayer for healing, and time lingers, our faith may grow dim, and we may be tempted to use fast acting poisonous substances which God does not approve of. Nature's processes of healing are deliberate, and to the impatient patient they will appear slow. But a slow process will test our faith more than a doubtful quick fix.

◆ *Blessed Are The Dead Which Die In The Lord From Henceforth*

Those who die in the Lord are blessed, and their works do follow them (Rev. 14:13). They are blessed because they have blessed God and others by their works. In this sense whether the sick live or die, they are the Lord's. They have the privilege of resting from their labor. They have done their part in spreading the gospel, and have lived the life that counts for God. They have influenced others toward the good, and have brought other souls into God's kingdom. They have their reward which will be given them when the Lifegiver calls them home. "Some died in the days of Christ and in the days of the apostles because the Lord knew just what was best for them" (MM17). We must remember that God looks upon DEATH AS A SLEEP, and not the very serious matter which we consider it to be. To be sure, our righteous life honors Him much more than our premature death. However, death is of less consequence than the salvation of souls (2T549)

◆ *Deathbed Repentance Is Not Always Genuine*

When Mrs. White was on a boat trip from Portland to Boston a violent storm came up and they were in great peril. Many were confessing their sins and were crying to God for mercy. One of the passengers had solemnly promised that if she were preserved, she would be a Christian. When they all reached land, this lady said: "Glory to God, I am glad to step on land again." When Mrs. White reminded her of her vow a few hours back, she turned from her with a sneer. This experience reminded Mrs. White of the matter of DEATHBED REPENTANCE. Some people serve themselves and Satan all their lives, and then when sickness comes upon them, they manifest some sorrow for sin. But when they recover, they turn out to be as rebellious as ever. What would be God's response under these circumstances? Proverbs 1:27, 28 give us the answer: "When your fear cometh as desolation, and your destruction cometh as a whirlwind; when distress and anguish cometh upon you. Then shall they call upon Me, but I will not answer; they shall seek me early, but they shall not find Me" (1T81–82).

THE DIVINE SCIENCE OF HEALTH AND HEALING

Disease As A Cleansing Crisis

◆ *A Crisis In Toxemia*

In general hygienists would say that disease is a CLEANSING CRISIS. It is an evidence that the body has found more resistance than it can handle in its attempt to keep itself in health. Basically, they would say that there is only one cause for disease, and that is TOXEMIA, or the gradual poisoning of the body from within and without, besides mechanical damage which might have occurred. During such a time the body has reduced its less vital functions, in order to apply its resources to the emergency at hand, of cleaning toxic matter from the system, and healing damaged tissue. This has increased to such an extent as to become a hindrance and a danger to life. This process can also be observed in ANIMALS that are sick. Under these circumstances they STOP EATING in order to rally all of their energies toward the process of healing. All HEALING therefore becomes SELF-HEALING, or of making the body whole again.

Without toxemia, there can hardly be any disease. The waste products of metabolism are toxic, and the reason that we are not poisoned by them is because they are being removed from the system almost as soon as they are produced. When the body is enervated such a process is slowed down, and can be almost stopped, and we then have the basic conditions for disease. Every so-called disease is a CRISIS in TOXEMIA or SELF-POISONING. This has occurred because toxins have accumulated in the blood above the toleration level. Any treatment which obstructs this effort at elimination confuses nature in her self-healing, house-cleaning, effort. It is said that CANCER, TUBERCULOSIS, BRIGHT'S DISEASE, and all chronic diseases were once innocent colds which were "ameliorated" several times, until the body was enervated, and in an enervated state the body does not react strongly against poisons, but tolerates them to a greater and greater extend, thereby weakening itself further.

Heredity

◆ *Physical Weaknesses Are Transmitted*

Physical, mental, and emotional weaknesses are inherited by the children from their parents. We are told that "as a rule, every intemperate man who rears children transmits his INCLINATIONS AND EVIL TENDENCIES to his offspring; he gives them disease from his own inflamed and corrupted blood" (4T30). "Many have inherited disease and are great sufferers because of the wrong habits of their parents, and yet they pursue the same wrong course in regard to themselves and their children which was pursued toward them" (1T488). Such hereditary evils are passed on even to the third and fourth generation. "MENTAL INABILITY, PHYSICAL WEAKNESS, DISORDERED NERVES, and UNNATURAL CRAVINGS are transmitted as a legacy from parents to children" (Te56). "Our ancestors have bequeathed to us customs and appetites which are filling the world with disease" (CH49). If left to themselves, children are inclined to act toward the weakened tendencies more strongly than toward the stronger tendencies because their inclination toward them agree more strongly with their unregenerate nature.

◆ *Christians Not To Follow Customs Of The World*

Good habits are almost as easy to learn as bad habits, if we practice good habits to begin with. They may take a little more effort, but they are well worth learning. In the endeavor to learn good habits, our environment may or may not be conducive to such habits. This means that we cannot always copy or imitate that which others are doing. Here is where sound principles come in. In all of our habits of life we must follow sound principles, and not merely good actions on the part of others. In this regard the habits and customs of the world may go contrary to sound principles. For this reason we are admonished that "Christians should not follow the customs and practices of the world" (CH50). The

◆ Good Habits Start with The Mother

We are told that the well-being of "the child will be affected by the habits of the mother. Her appetites and passions are to be controlled by principle…. If before the birth of her child she is SELF-INDULGENT, if she is SELFISH, IMPATIENT, and EXACTING, these traits will be reflected in the disposition of the child. Thus many children have received as a birthright almost unconquerable tendencies to evil. But if the mother unswervingly adheres to right principles, if she is TEMPERATE and SELF-DENYING, if she is KIND, GENTLE, and UNSELFISH, she may give her child these same precious traits of character" (CD217). So we find that the reform must begin with the mother before the birth of her children (CD225), for "the appetites of the mother are transmitted to the children" (Te292). In general parents transmit to their children by means of acquired habits. the tastes and tempers that were allowed to develop in their own characters (5T325). Because of these bequeathed customs and appetites, the world is being filled with disease (CH49).

◆ Children Inherit Tendencies To Sin But Not Sin Itself

"Children inherit inclinations to wrong, but they also have many lovely traits of character." (RH 1-24-1907). Also "men are born with the propensity to disobedience" (5BC1128). It is evil INCLINATIONS that are received by heredity, but not evil acts (4T30). Children before birth have not broken any of the commandments, for Rom. 9:11 says that children before birth haven't done any good nor evil. For this reason they cannot be born as sinners, for sin is the transgression of the law (1 Jo. 3:4). The reason for this is that "Adam's nature, depraved by sin, lessened man's strength to resist evil" (PP61) It is for this reason that "parents transmit evil tendencies to their children" (MYP237). What we can say is that children are born SINFUL, with tendencies and propensities to evil. However, they are not sinners until they have acted upon these tendencies and have committed unlawful acts.

◆ Guilt Is Not Inherited But Acquired

In PP61 it says that "The sin of our first parents brought GUILT and SORROW into the world." But since children only inherit inclinations to wrong and not wrong itself, this statement means that sin brought guilt not in the INHERITED SENSE, but in the ACQUIRED SENSE. It brought guilt in the sense that children PARTICIPATE in the sins of their parents and thereby make themselves guilty also. Children must repeat the sins of their parents for them to become guilty. Ez. 18:20 says: "The son shall not bear the iniquity of the father, neither shall the father bear the iniquity of the son." However, "It is inevitable that the children should suffer from the consequences of parental wrongdoing, but they are not punished for the parents guilt, except as they participate in their sins. It is usually the case, however, that children walk in the steps of their parents" (PP306). "By INHERITANCE AND EXAMPLE the sons become partakers of the father's sin. Wrong tendencies, perverted appetites, and debased morals, as well as physical disease and degeneracy, are transmitted as a legacy from father to son, to the third and fourth generation" (PP306). By "inheritance" is here meant the inheritance of tendencies to certain types of acts, and not the inheritance of formed habits.

◆ Evil Inclinations Are Acquired By Heredity

"Many suffer in consequence of the transgression of their parents. While they are not responsible for what their parents have done, it is nevertheless their duty to ascertain what are and what are not violations of the laws of health. They should avoid the wrong habits of their parents, and by correct living, place themselves in better conditions" (MH234). "Because of Adam's sin our natures are fallen"(SC62), and because of our fallen natures "without the transforming process which can come alone through divine power, the original propensities to sin are left in the heart in all their strength to forge new chains to impose a slavery that can never be broken by human power"(Ev. 192). Evil inclinations are received by heredity (4T30), and there is no need to retain one sinful propensity (7BC943). It is up to enlightened intellect to control animal propensities (MYP237), which represent our natural desires to do wrong.

In the process of adjusting to nutritional intake,

especially children need to learn that they EAT TO LIVE AND NOT LIVE TO EAT. In this matter also they must learn to develop the right and good habits. Any unhealthful habit will produce an unhealthful condition in the system, and we are told that habits which are contrary to the laws of nature are constantly warring against the soul (Te61). We are also told that if our physical habits are not right our mental and moral powers cannot be strong, for great sympathy exists between the physical and the moral (Te13). "Satan leads the human family to indulge in habits which destroy themselves and one another, for by this means he is robbing God of the service due Him" (Te14).

Accidents

When a person has been in an accident of any kind, and a part of the body has gotten hurt, the whole body has gotten hurt because it has been put in a WEAKENED CONDITION. Such weakened condition can contribute to the starting of a disease in the specific part that was hurt, for disease generally starts in the weakest part of the body. The body will immediately begin to repair the damage done, and in good time the body will attain to its normal functioning again. However, if the body is otherwise not in good condition, and there exists a condition of impurities within it, such a condition will limit the speed of restoration, and it will allow germs and viruses to settle there so as to prolong the healing process, and perhaps produce another disease state.

Germs And Infections

◆ *Germs Are Generally Harmless*

We have been taught that disease is caused by the invasion of GERMS, VIRUSES, and other MICROORGANISMS. We deal with such an invasion by attacking these so-called "enemies" with poisonous substances so as to destroy them. In this process we also harm the body by means of the poisonous substances which we have introduced into it. In reality, these invaders do not cause disease, but we do. Their contribution to the process of disease is only by way of our invitation. Just like ants do not come into our homes unless they can smell food therein, so germs do not come into our body in excessive numbers, unless we contain the food or soil for their multiplication. In order to eliminate them, we don't really have to focus on killing them outright, we merely have to focus on eliminating the internal physical environment which nutritionally feeds them. Changing our HABITS, DIETS, LIFESTYLE, INTERNAL and EXTERNAL ENVIRONMENT, can change the chemistry of our body so that germs cannot survive in it and are thereby eliminated.

There are more beneficial germs than there are harmful germs in the world. There are nitrogen-fixing bacteria that help man in the development of his food. There are bacteria in the intestines of man which produce B-vitamins therein. There are bacteria which help to develop lactic acid in milk products. Bacteria are indispensable for the fertility of our fields. The benign bacteria in our bodies fight the malignant ones and thereby preserve our health. They are vital to our digestive processes. As long ago as 1954 it was pointed out to us that YOGURT would help protect us from the bacteria causing DYSENTERY, TYPHOID, PNEUMONIA, AND NUMEROUS OTHER DISEASES. Yogurt develops in our intestines an overabundance of beneficial bacteria which destroy the harmful bacteria. The friendly bacteria in the colon are AEROBIC, that is, they flourish in high oxygen environments, and thrive in the presence of hydrogen peroxide (H_2O_2), which has an extra oxygen atom as compared to water (H_2O). Harmful bacteria, on the other hand, are mostly ANAEROBIC, and therefore cannot survive in the presence of OXYGEN OR H_2O_2. HENCE, H_2O_2 works its magic on a number of health problems by increasing the oxygen levels of the tissues.

◆ *The Beneficial Effects Of Germs*
- ✓ ACIDIFY THE COLON—They do so by developing LACTIC and ACETIC ACIDS. Such acidic environment inhibits the growth of undesirable bacteria.
- ✓ THEY NORMALIZE BOWEL MOVEMENTS — They can also stop the opposite problem of DIARRHEA.
- ✓ IMPROVE THE IMMUNE SYSTEM—By stimulating the formation of antibodies, which might be considered to be a natural form of VACCINATION.

- ✓ HELP TO FORM VITAMIN K—This vitamin aids in the CLOTTING OF BLOOD and the formation of NEW BONE.

- ✓ HELP TO PRODUCE LACTASE—This enzyme is necessary for the digestion of MILK. Without it milk allergies are produced.

- ✓ NEUTRALIZE CANCER COMPOUNDS—They may be produced by other organisms or found in food.

- ✓ REGULATE CHOLESTEROL LEVELS—Much of the cholesterol produced in the liver is converted to BILE ACIDS which are used to digest fats. With LOW FIBER DIETS, the bile acids are broken down into toxic substances which slow down the process of converting CHOLESTEROL into bile acids, and cholesterol begins to accumulate in the blood stream. A high fiber diet changes the bacteria in the colon to FRIENDLY BACTERIA which do not break down the bile acids and thereby allow more cholesterol to be excreted, and more bile acids to be retained.

- ✓ REGULATE HORMONE LEVELS—When the BACTERIAL FLORA is out of balance, a large part of the ESTROGEN circulating in the blood is not deactivated by the liver as it normally is, and then put into the GALLBLADDER with the bile, and reactivated by the friendly bacteria. It is then lost in the stool. The remaining low estrogen level can then produce OSTEOPOROSIS, PMS, MENSTRUAL CRAMPS, and MIGRAINE HEADACHES. Taking antibiotics also decreases the estrogen level by killing off the friendly bacteria in the bowels.

- ✓ ELIMINATE GAS AND BAD BREATH—When the bad bacteria take over in the colon, they frequently cause HALITOSIS or BAD BREATH, as well as foul smelling gas in the colon. YOGURT will under these circumstances be a lot better than breath mints.

◆ *Germs Are The Results Of Disease Conditions*

In his book *The Health Secrets Of A Naturopathic Doctor*, M.O. Garten says; "Germs do not cause Disease. The germs are the results of disease." Germs of all kinds are always in our bodies, but when kept under control by the advantageous conditions of the body, they are not harmful to us. But if we permit our bodies to undergo changes of degeneration, the rapidly propagating germs could become dangerous. It is said that flies do not create garbage, or the filthy conditions in which they breed, and that mosquitoes do not create the stagnant pool. In the same manner germs do not create the conditions of impurity in our body which represent fertile soil for their propagation. Germs and viruses are symptomatic factors in the production of disease. The IMPURE CONDITIONS within the body are the PRIMARY CAUSES of disease. Germs are the SECONDARY CAUSE.

◆ *Bacteria Find Their Soil And Food In Dead Matter*

Whenever the body is not properly cleansed both internally and externally, bacteria multiply. Bacteria find their soil and food mainly in dead matter. They are SCAVENGERS who break up and decompose the trash in our system just as they do in soil. For example, if we take raw milk and add it to a culture of BACILLUS BULGARICUS, the culture will die before it sours the milk. But if we first pasteurize or boil the milk, cool it to about 100 to 110 degrees, and then add the bacterial culture, we will have YOGURT in 6 to 8 hours. This shows us that the culture could not act on fresh milk, but only after some essential substance had been destroyed by heat, the milk became ready soil for bacteria which could then quickly multiply in it. In this case, however, the lactic acid which developed was beneficial to the body. We should realize that our lifestyles rather than bacteria are the cause of most of our diseases. Waging war against bacteria is like waging war against ourselves, since many bacteria normally exist in balance with ourselves, and only contribute to our disease processes as a result of our own imbalances. In reaction to ANTIBIOTICS, bacteria become stronger, develop a resistance against them, and finally evolve into new strains that we can't even identify, much less fight against.

◆ *Bacteria Themselves Produce Toxins*

Bacteria themselves give off poisonous substances, some of which are among the most poisonous substances known. The symptoms and morbidity they produce are due to these toxins. They give off poisons while they live, and dissolve into poisonous matter when they die. They add poisons to the poisons already in the system, of which the body has not yet been cleansed. When the impurities of the body are cleansed from it, the fertile soil for bacteria is eliminated, and the multiplication of bacteria is greatly restricted to a level where they cannot produce the symptoms of disease. The IMPURITIES of the body themselves lower the RESISTANCE of the body.

Bacteria are credited with a lot of diseases such as TUBERCULOSIS, SYPHILIS, TOXIC SHOCK, etc. They can also contaminate our food, thereby causing severe food poisoning. VIRUSES are responsible for everything from INFLUENZA to POLIO, RABIES, AIDS, and some types of CANCER. They threaten what stands between you and them, your IMMUNE SYSTEM, which is like a police force in your body, which is constantly on patrol, fighting any and all unwelcome invaders. The condition of the immune system determines the outcome of the fight.

◆ *Bacteria Can Change Their Nature*

In 1914 Dr. Rosenow, America's foremost bacteriologist, verified the conclusions of French scientist Bechamp that there exist no specific bacteria. One kind of bacteria was changed to another kind and back again by altering conditions of FOOD and TEMPERATURE of the ENVIRONMENT. Deadly bacteria were converted to harmless ones and vice versa. As early as 1897 Dr. Lemke observed that the dietary change from MEAT to BREAD, FRUITS, and VEGETABLES resulted in complete alteration in the intestinal bacteria, and in the disappearance of poisonous substances caused in the breakdown of protein by bacteria. Dr. Metnikoff of Russia found that the inhabitants of Bulgaria reached the greatest age and remained free of aches and pains even in their old age. The cause was determined to be the LACTIC ACID as found in YOGURT, SOUR MILK, and SAUERKRAUT. The good bacteria counteracted the effect of putrefaction and left lactic acid as their end-product. They also manufactured nine vitamins in the intestines, among them vitamin K and the B-COMPLEX vitamins.

◆ *Chemical Destruction Of Germs Is Harmful To The Body*

Munich professor Baumgaertle declared in 1954 that the chemotherapeutic treatment of many infectious diseases created drastic harm to the patients. The treatment destroyed the intestinal flora, which led to serious symptoms of vitamin deficiencies and to more dangerous intestinal infections. Dr. Gosselin of Dartmouth said that modern medicines are capable of doing a great deal of good, and an almost equal amount of harm. ANTIBIOTICS, while destroying the specific germs of primary infection also destroy the vitamin producing bacteria. After the first antibiotics were introduced in 1935 and 1936, hospitals throughout the nation found to their dismay that bacteria which had hitherto given little trouble began to take a toll of patients' lives. The villain was STAPHYLOCOCCUS AUREUS, a bacterium which had formerly been held in check by aseptic methods. New strains of staph germs developed that were resistant to all treatments. By the middle of the 50's the new infection had reached epidemic proportions. In Texas one epidemic took 22 lives. The result was traced to the destruction of a large number of the intestinal flora by the antibiotics.

When a cow gets a shot of PENICILLIN, the beneficial bacteria which help to make sour milk are destroyed, and the milk often does not clabber. A guinea pig can be killed with one shot of penicillin, because it is more dependent on the intestinal B-vitamins than we are.

If ANTIBIOTICS are given too frequently one's immune system becomes suppressed. Under these circumstances fewer natural antibodies are produced, and the body's WHITE BLOOD CELLS are less active in attacking bacteria that have been treated with antibiotics. Such suppression of the immune system explains why even minor infections re-occur over and over again, thereby needing multiple courses of treatments.

Furthermore, the bacteria frequently exposed to antibiotics change their nature or mutate, and become immune to the antibiotics effect, and many people die because the new strain of bacteria is difficult to destroy. To avoid this we should make sure that through the use of cultured foods like YOGURT, our intestines are supplied with plenty of beneficial bacteria which destroy the harmful bacteria.

◆ Germs And The Spirit Of Prophecy

Does the Spirit of Prophecy mention the role of germs as the causative factors in disease? At times it does, but in general not. Then what does it emphasize as the main cause of disease? Basically, it emphasizes that the lack of external and internal CLEANLINESS causes disease. "A neglect of cleanliness induces disease" (CD63).

During the 6th and 7th centuries the LEPROSY began to spread all over Europe, until it reached its peak during the 13th and 14th centuries. People were more afraid of it than they are of cancer today. In the 14th century also the BLACK PLAGUE swept over Europe and took the life of one person out of four, or an estimated total of 60 million people. The physicians were helpless. Finally leadership was taken over by the church which took as its guiding principle the principle of CONTAGION. The procedures came from Lev. 13:46. "All the days wherein the plague shall be in him he shall be defiled; he is unclean: he shall dwell alone; without the camp his habitation be." Both the Black Plague and the leprosy were brought under control by this means.

During the Black Plague the herb ANGELICA was also used by some. It was reported that those who kept a piece of ANGELICA ROOT in their mouth all day were preserved from the plague. Angelica root contains VALERIAN, MALIC and ANGELIC ACIDS.

Since the people of the Middle Ages didn't as yet live up to all of God's principles of health, there were other serious diseases which continued to decimate them. Diseases such as DYSENTERY, CHOLERA, and TYPHOID FEVER continued to take a heavy toll up to the 18th century. This happened because the hygienic conditions even in the great cities were quite primitive. It was a rule for refuse to be dumped out into the streets which were unpaved and filthy. It was a heyday for flies as they bred in the filth and spread intestinal diseases that killed millions.

◆ How A Biologic Doctor Treats Disease

A biologic doctor looks at the matter of disease from the standpoint of the WHOLE PERSON. He reasons that in the case of sickness it is the whole person who is sick, and hence, it is the whole person who must be treated, even though the disease may be localized in one part of the body.

1. The first principle of the art of healing is that the treatment must DO NO HARM to the patient. This principle is perhaps more commonly violated than any other. It is therefore not rational to concentrate on destroying the harmful bacteria, if at the same time we destroy the helpful beneficial bacteria.

2. The second principle is that of IMPROVING THE BODY'S OWN RESISTANCE against disease by the elimination of all hindrances, such as impurities, to its recovery.

3. The third principle is that the treatment must work in harmony with the natural principles of the body and not against them, by BUILDING UP THE BODY'S OWN DEFENSES IN THE IMMUNE SYSTEM.

Nutritional Causes

◆ Overeating

Most people eat far more than they should, more than they need, and more than their system requires. We are told that "as a people, with all our profession of health reform, we eat too much. Indulgence of appetite is the greatest cause of physical and mental debility, and lies at the foundation of a large share of the feebleness which is apparent everywhere" (CD135). We are more liable to eat too much if we eat fast than if we EAT SLOWLY. One reason for this is the fact that if we eat fast the bodily appestat mechanism, which tells us when we are full, often does not quite catch up with our eating, and doesn't tell us that we are full until after we have already imbibed too much. This is not as likely to occur when we eat more slowly.

Dr. Vogel of Switzerland says that half of the people of Switzerland are ill because they are overfed. The VARIETY OF THINGS available to satisfy their palates IS TOO GREAT.

When we eat too much we are first of all wasting food, and are injuring the whole system. We defile God's temple, weaken our natural powers, clog the living machinery, and hinder it in its work (CD131). We are also told that "nearly all members of the human family eat more than the system requires. This excess decays and becomes a putrid mass" (CD132). "Overeating is the sin of this age" (CD133). God places the sin of GLUTTONY in the same category with DRUNKENNESS. It is the greatest cause of physical and mental debility (CD135). It causes FORGETFULNESS and LOSS of MEMORY. "A clogged stomach means a clogged brain" (CD137).

The remedy is first of all to EAT AS LITTLE as you can and NOT AS MUCH as you can. Eat only TWO or THREE KINDS of food at each meal; eat no more than is required to SATISFY HUNGER; eat proper COMBINATIONS of food; If possible eat only TWO MEALS A DAY rather than three, and remember that "excessive indulgence in EATING, DRINKING, SLEEPING, or SEEING. is sin" (CD140–42). If this is done we will be more clearly able to discern the difference between the sacred and the common, and be better able to maintain our physical, mental, and moral health.

◆ *Improper Diet*

The more we get away from the food which God gave to Adam and Eve, the more we move toward a disease-producing diet. The food which God created in its natural interrelationships, we have artificialized by extracting from them the things which we think are important, and thereby eliminating the COMPLEMENTARY SUBSTANCES which are just as important to our health. We should never consider the idea that it doesn't matter much what we eat (CD196). We are told that "poor food cannot be converted into good blood" (CD199), and that diseases caused by an impoverished diet are difficult to cure (MH321). Foods that have been chemically altered, that have been extracted from whole foods as the essential substances usually lack the vitamins and minerals of their natural relationships, and therefore create a liability toward disease in the individual who partakes of them. Every time a natural substance is removed from a food, the natural balance is disturbed. Also every time a chemical is added to the food, the natural balance is disturbed. Butter is taken from cream, bran is taken from wheat, sugar is extracted from sugar cane with all of the vitamins and minerals left behind. Hippocrates said: "Leave your chemicals in the chemist's pot if you can't cure your patient with food."

◆ *The Customs Of Society Not Our Guide*

We are told that we cannot be guided by the customs of society. "The disease and sufferings that everywhere prevail are largely due to POPULAR ERRORS IN REGARD TO DIET" (CD127). APPETITE IS NOT ALWAYS A SAFE GUIDE as to what is good for us to eat, because through wrong habits of eating the appetite might have become perverted. "Our artificial civilization is encouraging evils destructive of sound principles. Custom and fashion are at war with nature. The practices they enjoin, and the indulgences they foster, are steadily lessening both physical and mental strength, and bringing upon the race an intolerable burden" (Te247). "It is possible for one to spoil his spiritual experience by an ill-use of the stomach" (CD126). An improper diet increases the animal passions (CD244), and leads to unnatural cravings, which can lead to strong drinks, and disordered nerves (Ed203). Once correct tastes are acquired we will realize that foods which we formerly regarded as harmless were laying the foundation for disease.

Sinful Habits

◆ *We Should Reason From Cause To Effect*

In everything that we do that affects our health, we are admonished to gain as much knowledge as possible. When we apply such knowledge correctly with respect to cause and effect, our health would be ensured. Whatever we sow we shall also reap. This is a constant law of life. We are told that "the Lord has made it a part of his plan that man's reaping shall be in accordance with his sowing" (HL18). "Sickness and premature death do not come without a cause" (HL53). The body's attempt at the restoration of its health is a normal biological process. Its success at SELF-HEALING depends upon the removal of the CAUSE of its ills. The body will CURE ITSELF when the cause is removed. There is actually no cure outside of the correction of cause.

◆ *Appetite Has Controlled Reason*

We have been told that to an alarming extent. APPETITE has controlled man's reason. Worldly people often give liberal amounts of money to a cause in which the inducement toward the gratification of appetite is a major appeal. However,

Christians should take their appeal on the right side to endeavor to reform these fashionable health and soul destroying customs. A depraved appetite craves those things which are the most injurious to health (2SM417–18). We are told that "the first thing to be done is to ascertain the true character of the sickness, and then go to work intelligently to remove the cause. If the harmonious working of the system has become unbalanced by overwork, overeating, or other irregularities, do not endeavor to adjust the difficulties by adding a burden of poisonous medicines." (MH235).

THE CAUSES OF DISEASE

The Definition Of Disease

◆ *Violation Of Natural Law—Standpoint Of Individual Action.*

"Disease is the penalty of nature's violated laws" (CH347). When Christ said, "Sin no more, lest a worse thing come unto thee" (Jo. 5:14), He taught that disease is the result of violating God's laws, both natural and spiritual (CH31). "There is sickness everywhere, and much of it might be prevented by attention to the laws of health" (CH389). "Thousands need to be educated patiently, kindly, tenderly, but decidedly, that of their complaints are created by their own course of action" (MM225). "Sickness is the result of transgression" (CH37).

✓ CH347—"DISEASE, the penalty of nature's violated law."

✓ CH37—"It is a sin to be sick, for all sickness is the result of transgression."

✓ CH202—"The burden of SIN, with its unrest and unsatisfied desires, lies at the very foundation of a large share of the maladies the sinner suffers."

✓ 2SM411—"Man has disregarded the laws of his being, and disease has been steadily increasing. The cause has been followed by the effect.... he has gratified TASTE at the expense of HEALTH.

✓ CD121—"The human family have brought upon themselves diseases of various forms by their own WRONG HABITS. Wrong habits in eating and drinking lead to errors in THOUGHT and ACTION" (CD62).

✓ 2SM465—"As a result of WRONG HABITS in parents, disease and imbecility have been transmitted to their offspring."

✓ MH127—Disease is an effort of nature to free the system from conditions that result from a violation of the laws of health.

◆ *Impurities Within The System—Standpoint Of Body Condition*

✓ Dr. J.H. Tilden—"Disease is the body's effort at expelling TOXINS"

✓ Kuhne—"Disease is the presence of FOREIGN MATTER in the system."

◆ *The Body's Effort At Correcting Unhealthful Conditions*

✓ MH235—Disease is nature's effort to correct UNHEALTHFUL CONDITIONS.

✓ 2SM287—Disease is nature's attempt at SELF-HEALING. "Disease is an effort of nature to free the system from conditions that result from a violation of the laws of health. In case of sickness, the cause must be ascertained. Unhealthful conditions should be changed, wrong habits corrected. Then nature is to be assisted in her effort to EXPEL IMPURITIES and to re-establish right conditions within the system" (MH127). Disease is usually SELF-CAUSED, and health is also largely SELF-CAUSED. Disease is nature's effort to correct unhealthful conditions (MH235). In allowing the disease to take hold, the body is acting in its own best interest, for purification and cleansing are a prerequisite for the return to high level functioning. The reconstruction of cells and tissues that have suffered damage is necessary to the resumption of normal function. The broken down tissue is toxic. In a healthy body this toxic material is eliminated from the blood as fast as it develops.

The organism manufactures all the substances it needs, along with its proper nutrition. Hence, is it scientific to be always developing new chemicals to replace what the body once made but cannot make anymore? Or is it more scientific to find out why the body stopped making what it is supposed to make? It selects out of what we eat and drink those substances which it wants and needs and can use. It rejects those substances which are incompatible with body chemistry. The body has a 100 different organs that perform a 1000 different functions all at the same time with precision. They manufacture all the chemicals one needs, all the CORTISONE, ADRENALINE, and PEPSIN out of the food we eat, the fluids we drink, and the air we breathe, if we don't put obstructions in its way. Since prescribed MEDICINES SUPPRESS SYMPTOMS, they are exactly what one must avoid to get well.

The speediest way to gain health is to stimulate the eliminating organs to eliminate poisonous substances, and to avoid poisonous substances. This can be accomplished by means of exercise, bathing, water-drinking, elimination etc. At such a time nature deprives us of our normal appetite. If we dig our spur into a tired horse it will start running faster, but we cannot say that the spur gave it new energy. It merely stimulated it to expend its reserve energy more quickly. It is the same with STIMULANTS. They impart a false feeling of strength, and the same is true with DRUGS.

Ehret says that disease is nature's healing eliminating process. Dr. Herbert M. Shelton said that "Diseases are eliminative or purification crises wherein the body devotes itself intensely to rejecting toxic matters from the vital domain. The body is purging itself of matters that are destroying cells or tissue; it is freeing itself of toxic matter that is ANTIVITAL in character, to the extent that it interferes with normal life processes."

◆ *The Body's Effort to Free The System*

Tests have revealed that nearly all processed foods are contaminated with organic toxins from molds, insects, animal excrement, metallic compounds from herbicides, insecticides, and unassimilable chemicals. These are substances which hinder the process of bodily assimilation, and at the same time clog the body with substances which it cannot utilize.

The process of metabolism consists of digestion, assimilation, as well as the use of vitamins and minerals required for efficient bodily functioning. This process of metabolism also results in the production of waste products which are not needed by the body, and which would harm it if retained. The body must also eliminate those substances which were in our food, water, and air which are non-nutritive, and not assimilable, and which are not essential to the efficient functioning of all body processes. A pure body is not subject to disease, for all diseases are basically body disabling processes. Illnesses are generally crises in the elimination of substances which hinder the process of maintaining healthy functions.

◆ *Evidences Of An Impure Body*

Some of the evidences of a polluted body are COLDS, FEVERS, ACHES, PAINS where no injury has been sustained, CONSTANT FATIGUE, HEADACHES, SINUS PROBLEMS, EXCESSIVE MUCUS, PSORIASIS, PIMPLES, BOILS, RASHES, etc. The body will cleanse itself if we allow it a chance to do so. Such a special cleansing will begin when we stop eating solid foods and take in only water and fluids. These will lighten the digestive load and allow the body to direct its attention to the hindrances to its proper functioning.

◆ *Internal And External Cleansing*

While external cleansing represents the elimination of poisonous substances through and from the skin as one of the eliminative organs, the more important of these is internal cleansing. If such a process ceased we would all die in a very short time of self-poisoning. It is the function of our "drainage system" to prevent the poisons of our metabolic wastes from taking our life.

Normally the body is self-cleansing and self-purifying, and it operates as such every minute of our lives. The LUNGS eliminate largely gaseous wastes into the air; the KIDNEYS expel poisonous wastes through the medium of water; the LIVER excretes wastes and poisons through both kidneys and bowels; The COLON disposes of indigestible wastes and food eaten in excess of digestive capacity; the SKIN excretes wastes in gaseous and liquid form, and forms boils, pimples, sores, etc. when other organs of elimination are overloaded. The MUCOUS MEMBRANES are our "internal skin," where elimination proceeds on the basis of mucus discharges as an emergency "safety valve" outlet for extraordinary detoxification.

A thorough physiological rest, such as FASTING, represents a universal step which allows the body the opportunity to detoxify. Fasting is the abstention from everything except water, or other fluids, pure air, and sunshine. Under these conditions expenditures of nerve energy are greatly reduced, stresses are discontinued, and emotional drains are avoided. The body is freed from the burdens of activity and food digestion, and can devote its energies to cleansing, bodily repair, and healing.

In women an extraordinary form of elimination is menstruation, which is a periodic discharge of blood, mucus, and mucosal tissue. Such a process is really not a normal process in very healthy women. In them menstruation does not occur. The healthier the person, the less pronounced the flow, and the shorter its duration. Nature does not impose blood letting as a part of her plan. Many women who have adopted a very healthy regimen have found the cessation of bloody menstruation to be a by-product.

✓ SELF-HEALING CRISIS—It is not the superficial symptoms which are being suppressed. When a healing crisis occurs, the body is rejecting old accumulated wastes and toxins. This is nature's way of keeping the body clean and healthy.

✓ STUDY HEALTH—The proper way to study disease is to STUDY HEALTH. When we know what a condition ought to be, then we can easily see to what condition the system needs to return. Then we need to study every influence that is either favorable or unfavorable to the continuance of health. Any influence that lowers NERVE ENERGY can become disease-producing.

✓ DISEASE IS NOT ITS OWN CAUSE—Disease does not cause itself. It has an antecedent cause. Conditions precede it which influence the body toward disease. If we say that a lack of nerve energy or ENERVATION is the cause of disease, then we must ask as to where the enervation came from. Then we can put the blame on POISONOUS SUBSTANCES which were either generated by the body itself, or which were introduced from without. Enervation checks SECRETION and EXCRETION, resulting in a general or systemic poisoning of the body. Checked excretion causes a retention of metabolic waste to accumulate in the fluids and tissues of the body. It results in impaired digestion and impaired nutrition. There are waste products of METABOLISM which are toxic to the system. They are self-generated. They can poison us if we let them, but the reason they are not poisoning us is because they are eliminated from the body soon after they are produced.

External poisons, which are taken in from the air, water, mouth, or skin can poison us if their quantity is more than the body can quickly eliminate. If the body is not in good order, then there is a checking of the eliminative processes, and more poisons are retained within the system, and disease is more easily produced. Thus poisonous substances, and largely SELF-GENERATED POISONOUS SUBSTANCES, become the basic cause of disease.

Dr. R.T. Trall said: "It has always been one of the most difficult practical problems in the world how to present NEW TRUTHS so as not to offend OLD ERRORS; for persons are very apt to regard arguments directed against their opinions as attacks upon their persons; and many there are who mistake their own ingrained PREJUDICES for established PRINCIPLES."

◆ *Lack Of Harmonious Action—Standpoint of Body Workings*

"The BRAIN is the organ and instrument of the mind, and controls the whole body. In order for the other parts of the system to be healthy, the brain must be healthy. And in order for the brain to be healthy, the BLOOD must be pure. If by correct habits of eating and drinking the blood is kept pure, the BODY will be properly nourished.

"It is the lack of harmonious action in the human organism that brings disease. The imagination may control the other parts of the body to their injury. All parts of the system must work harmoniously. The different parts of the body, especially those remote from the heart, should receive a free circulation of blood. The limbs act as an important part, and should receive proper attention" (MM291).

AMERICAN HERITAGE DICTIONARY—"An abnormal condition of an organism or part, especially as a consequence of infection, inherent weakness, or environmental stress, that impairs normal physiological functioning.

◆ *Chemical Shortage—Standpoint Of Nutritional Needs*

Every disease is a sign of a chemical shortage in the body.

✓ HEREDITY and ENVIRONMENT—are two major contributors to all illness. Environment refers to all the chemicals in our life and surroundings which have an effect on us. Heredity represents inherited weaknesses which are constant forces within the body which tend to lead it toward disease.

✓ HIPPOCRATES—said that we will never understand disease until we know our FOOD. He taught that sickness is the result of the type of LIFE we lead, of man's own making, the end-result of a longtime abuse in the form of poor living habits, faulty nutrition, and other health destroying environmental factors. People live on excuses. They blame GOD, NATURE, PEOPLE, and the ENVIRONMENT, but never THEMSELVES. They could achieve HEALTH BY THEMSELVES, if they would straighten out their lives, and live the life that emphasizes God's Nature and its healing and maintaining powers.

◆ *Stages Of Disease*

✓ ACUTE LEVEL—Waste is eliminated in the form of CATARRH, PHLEGM, MUCUS, FOREIGN MATTER, or TOXINS. When the body is doing this it is called a "cleansing process." In most cases this cleansing process should never be interfered with. Here the body is ready, willing, and able to perform its own cure, in its own way. Here is the best opportunity we have to cooperate with nature.

✓ SUBACUTE LEVEL—develops when we use DRUGS as a suppressive measure to drive CATARRHAL DISCHARGES back into the body. The condition which then exists represents the beginning of disease. When this stage is suppressed with drugs, it produces PAIN, FEVER, ACHES, and DISCOMFORT. Pain and discomfort are warning signs for us to do something beneficial for the condition. The HEALING CRISIS—which then has arrived is an acute reaction that comes when the body still has the energy to throw off toxic materials.

✓ CHRONIC STAGE—healing agents are forced to take a back seat. Nature is being overpowered by DRUGS, polluted air and water, and junk foods. Vitality is decreasing and CHRONIC DISEASE comes upon us. Chronic diseases are made. We eat and drink them into existence. This DISEASE CRISIS—which then has arrived is a reaction resulting from the dominance of disease conditions over the healing forces of the organism.

✓ DEGENERATIVE STAGE—represents the almost total loss of function of an organ or tissue. Here the body is too weak for organs to be strengthened. Reversal here can take place only under the most intense methods of body cleansing. We have earned the consequences that go along with our SELF-DESTRUCTIVE HABITS, which we were unwilling to change.

Find The Basic Cause Of Disease In Order To Heal Disease

Medical science is generally based upon the idea that there is an ENTITY called disease which is caused by outside influences, and that such disease can be expelled and eliminated when the right drug is found for it. But such disease is tackled without any clear UNDERSTANDING of its CAUSE. Hence, what is tackled is the EFFECT of the disease, for in most cases the real cause is said to be unknown. Searching for the cause of disease therefore becomes a matter of treating the EFFECT of the disease and not the CAUSE. We are here reasoning from effect to cause and not from cause to effect. But an effect is not the cause, and treating an effect is not treating the cause. The effects of disease are the SYMPTOMS of disease, and to treat the symptoms of disease is not treating the disease. The cause of disease can be followed by a chain of symptoms of disease, any one of which is often given as the "cause" of the disease, because they do follow one another in a cause-effect manner. The basic cause, however, has not as yet been determined, but it must be found in order to completely eliminate the disease.

If a headache is caused by blood pressure in the

brain, the headache is the effect of the pressure, which is the cause of the headache, but the pressure is also an effect of a cause which causes it. In this case the BASIC CAUSE has not as yet been determined, and therefore both the headache and the pressure are symptoms of the basic cause which could be impurities in the system. We may be able to reduce or eliminate the pressure with drugs, but this is merely ameliorating a symptom. The basic cause is thereby not affected. Disease is damaged health, and the proper way to study disease is to STUDY HEALTH, and every influence which is favorable or unfavorable to its maintenance. Disease will not occur unless we cause it, and we cause it if we live contrary to the principles of life and the laws of health.

Germs As The Cause Of Disease

◆ *The Germ Theory Of Disease*

Louis Pasteur, the famous French chemist, developed the GERM THEORY OF DISEASE which says that microbes enter the body and cause disease therein. Drugs and vaccines are used to destroy these germs to prevent them from doing damage to the body. But Pasteur denounced his own theory on his deathbed by saying: "Bernard is right. The microbe is nothing. The environment is all-important."

Claude Bernard, a French physiologist. claimed that the seeds of disease—the germs or microbes—would not grow and cause disease, unless the environment was favorable to their multiplication.

Antoine Bechamp, also a contemporary of Pasteur, emphasized that pathogenic microorganisms are a secondary manifestation of a state of toxicity in the body. He believed that there exists no specific bacteria. One kind of bacteria is changed into another kind and back again by altering the environmental conditions of food and temperature which will change deadly bacteria into harmless ones and vice versa. It is the condition of the host that determines the behavior of the germs.

Dr. Ray Rife proved in his laboratory that by altering the environment, he could change harmless bacteria into deadly ones. He classified all pathogenic bacteria into 10 groups, and showed that any organism within this group could be readily changed to any other organism within the ten groups depending upon the medium with which it is fed and grown. For example, by changing the medium as little as two parts per million by volume, he could change BACILLUS COLI within 36 hours to BACILLUS TYPHOSIS. He thereby altered disease states by altering the environment. Bacteria and viruses become dangerous only when the body's natural balance is disturbed. Dr. Rene Dubois named the COMMON COLD and BASILLARY DYSENTERY as two diseases that experiments had found practically impossible to communicate by contact alone, but which are easily contracted when the internal balance has been disturbed. He then warned that the ANTIBIOTICS, in curing one illness leave the person far more susceptible to others. Instead of being wiped out by antibiotics, bacteria have the ability often to simply change themselves into a different specie that is not harmed by antibiotics, and which brings us new and hitherto unknown diseases.

Blind acceptance of Pasteur's theories lies behind modern medicines inability to cope with DEGENERATIVE DISEASES. So long as modern medicine treats the disease rather than the patient, and attempts to cure rather than prevent diseases, it will continue to fail. It is the ill health that causes the bacteria which then go on to cause the specific disease determined by the form they have taken.

◆ *Germs Are Always In The Human Body*

If we think that germs are the cause of disease, then we can use drugs to kill them, but in this process we will do harm to the body in other ways. In most cases, an overabundance of germs cannot live in a healthy body. The IMMUNE SYSTEM will destroy their effectiveness. Disease germs are at all times in the human body, but they are kept in check by a well-functioning immune system. Germs thrive and multiply themselves because there is something in the body for them to feed on. That is why we have to take care of the body first. We have to keep well. We must be clean and well within first, and then we will not be affected by germs from without.

◆ *Germs Are The Body's Scavengers*

Germs play a most important part in the workings of the body. It is in breaking down dead organic matter that germs are employed by nature. They are agents of disintegration of refuse or toxic matter. Germs decompose the trash in our system. Germs are parts of the results of disease, not its cause. They are helpers brought there by nature to rid the body of disease. They will disappear when the body's toxic matter has been disposed of. Research has shown that germs can change their size and shape, and become the size of a virus. The BACTERIAL FORM does not produce CANCER, but the VIRAL FORM does.

◆ *Germs Thrive In Conditions Of Low Vitality*

Killing the germs ignores the real cause of disease. If a transfer of cold germs from one person to another person causes a cold in the second person, it is because these germs find fertile soil in the form of toxic matter in the second person in which to propagate. No one who is clean and healthy inside can be affected, or become the victim of germ infection. People in ordinary health contain in their bodies the same germs that are claimed to be the cause of those infectious diseases. The predisposing factors are a LOWERED VITALITY, and a body clogged with IMPURITIES.

A Natural Treatment Maintains Body Energies

When a child develops an ACUTE DISEASE of any kind, we should allow it to run its natural course. The mother must not become impatient and lose faith in the natural treatment. It may take a week or more to cure a COMMON COLD, or an attack of BRONCHITIS, or from 2 to 8 weeks to cure a case of WHOOPING COUGH. The child should not be forced to eat, but should be given vegetable and fruit juices, possibly every 2 or 3 hours. The child's energy should be directed toward the elimination of impurities, and not so much toward the process of digesting food. Giving them lots of food takes energy away from the ELIMINATIVE and HEALING process. To suppress nasal mucus with drugs drives it back into the tissues, and maintains their impure conditions. A MILK FORMULA represents synthetic food for the child, and it may cause diabetic tendencies in later years. We are told: "He causeth the GRASS to grow for the cattle, and HERB for the service of man; that he may bring forth food out of the earth" (Ps. 104:14).

Why We Should Maintain Our Health

"God requires the body to be rendered a LIVING SACRIFICE to Him, not a dead or dying sacrifice.... All should be very careful to preserve the body in the best condition of health, that they may render to God PERFECT SERVICE and do their duty in the FAMILY and in SOCIETY" (CD21). True health begins with an AWARENESS OF SELF, to discover how we function. True healing begins with discovering why we are sick. The body is a complex interactive organism of various actions and functions. One organ affects another. One activity affects another. Whenever one part is hurt the whole body sympathizes. External stimuli interact with internal stimuli to affect the organism's actions. We must respond harmoniously with external BENEFICIAL factors so as to give a harmonious response which assists the organism's functions and which will maintain it in health. Maybe we should act as though we already have every disease, take the steps to cure these diseases, and by taking these steps we are preventing them.

Disease Never Comes Without A Cause

◆ *Violating The Laws Of Health*

"Disease never comes without a cause. The way is prepared and disease invited, by disregard of the laws of health. Many suffer in consequence of the transgression of their parents. While they are not responsible for what their parents have done, it is nevertheless their duty to ascertain what are and what are not violations of the laws of health. They should avoid the wrong habits of their parents, and by correct living, place themselves in better conditions. The greater number, however, suffer because of their own course of action.... But God is not responsible for the suffering that follows disregard of natural law"(CD122).

◆ *The Cause Represents A Chain Of Events*

The cause of disease always represents a chain of events made up of many different links. Every link is a necessary part of the chain. We can give as the cause of the disease any one of the different links. We often use the link which is the most convenient, which places the blame on some external agent, and which therefore casts the least amount of reflection upon the individual himself. So we can say that the disease to which we have succumbed was due to our lack of resistance, or we can say that it was due to germs. Since germs are always present, the first initiative has to be given to our lack of resistance, and with such a helpful start, the germs are taking over, can multiply, give off toxins, and therewith poison the whole system into more disease.

◆ *For Health Our Lifestyle Must Be Changed*

"In case of sickness, the cause should be ascertained. UNHEALTHFUL CONDITIONS should be changed, WRONG HABITS corrected. Then NATURE is to be assisted in her effort to expel IMPURITIES and to establish right conditions in the system" (MH127).

"If we are sick, we impose a weary tax upon our friends, and unfit ourselves for discharging our duties to our families and to our neighbors. And when premature death is the result of our violation of nature's law, we bring sorrow and suffering to others; we deprive our neighbors of the help we ought to render them in living; we rob our families of the comfort and help we might render them, and rob God of the service He claims of us to advance His glory. Then are we not in the worst sense transgressors of God's law" (CD21)?

◆ *Our Own Bad Habits Create Our Suffering*

Most people "suffer because of their own wrong course of action. They disregard the principles of health by their habits of EATING, DRINKING, DRESSING, and WORKING. Their transgression of nature's laws produces the sure results; and when sickness comes upon them, many do not credit their suffering to the true cause, but murmur against God because of their affliction.... If the harmonious working of the system has become unbalanced by OVERWORK, OVEREATING, or other IRREGULARITIES, do not adjust the difficulties by adding a burden of POISONOUS MEDICINES" (MH234–235)

Any crime against the body—such as SMOKING, DRINKING ALCOHOLIC BEVERAGES, COFFEE, TEA, EATING FRIED, REFINED, or PROCESSED FOODS, or trying to TOLERATE THE CHEMICALS in food, or even in the ENVIRONMENT—PREVENTS the body from DEFENDING itself, from FIGHTING its battle, and from WINNING the battle and HEALING itself.

◆ *Nature Bears Long Abuse*

"Nature bears abuse as long as she can without resisting; then she arouses and makes a mighty effort to rid herself of the encumbrances and evil treatment she has suffered. Then come HEADACHE, CHILLS, FEVERS, NERVOUSNESS, PARALYSIS, and other EVILS too numerous to mention" (CD125).

Drugs Thwart The Body's Effort At Healing

◆ *Nature Must Fight Both Drugs And Disease*

As civilization has advanced many new diseases have developed. UNNATURAL LIFESTYLES lower vitality and favor the accumulation of waste matter and poisons. SULFUR and COAL TAR MEDICINES suppress skin eruptions, just as ANTIHISTAMINES, ANTIPYRETICS, and PAIN RELIEVERS suppress COLD SYMPTOMS. Drugs suppress disease, and the suppression of disease causes more disease in the future.(MM225). KIDNEY TRANSPLANT PATIENTS who receive drugs to suppress the immune system's ability to reject a new kidney, have a higher rate of CANCER as a result than would be expected. DRUGS act against the body by OPPOSING its SELF-HEALING WORK. The body has to relinquish work in order to deal with the newly created threat of the drugs. This thwarts nature's effort at cleansing and healing. Nature has to reduce her battle against disease in order to combat the poisons that have been introduced into the body in the form of DRUGS. The disease is still in the system, and so is an ADDED BURDEN of POISONS. Nature's well-meant effort at healing has been well-nigh defeated. The tissues are then so loaded with waste material, that the body can no longer react to them with ACUTE responses. The CHRONIC conditions of the body proceed further in the direction of the INCURABLE STAGE, and try to eliminate these waste materials by means of SKIN ERUPTIONS and ULCERS in various parts of the body.

◆ *Medicine Adds to The Poisons*

Instead of allowing poisons to be eliminated from the system, medicine adds to the poisons by means of drugs and serums of all kinds, and forces the poisons farther back into the system to create other diseases or new forms of diseases that may be more serious. It actually contributes to the increase of disease in two ways: First, by making people believe that diseases have been cured when they have been forced beneath the surface, and secondly, by changing simple ACUTE diseases such as COLDS, DIARRHEA, or SKIN ERUPTIONS into CHRONIC diseases which are more persistent and harder to eradicate from the system, such as RHEUMATISM, BRONCHITIS, ASTHMA, DIABETES, KIDNEY DISEASE, HEART DISEASE, and CANCER. Chronic disease does not follow immediately upon the suppression of acute diseases. It is the continued SUPPRESSION of ACUTE DISEASES which leads ultimately to chronic disease. One will pay a price for interfering with the God-given wisdom of the body.

Medical science, as currently practiced with drugs causes bodily ENERVATION. As such it builds disease rather than correcting or ameliorating man's sufferings. Even drugs used to relieve pain wind up by causing greater pain, and even destroying the body itself. Drugs used to relieve cough in pneumonia sometimes prove fatal. Removing the stones from a gallbladder does not remove the cause of the stones. As a result more stones will form.

Modern Medicine Looks For External Causes

◆ *Modern Medicine Adds To Disease*

Modern medicine tends to look for the CAUSES or ETIOLOGICAL AGENTS of disease OUTSIDE of the body. Hence, it therefore tends to think that the CURE of disease must also come from outside the body. So it searches for BETTER DRUGS, more REFINED SURGICAL TECHNIQUES, and more effective methods of CHEMOTHERAPY and RADIATION. It attempts to "cure" disease by means of the administration of poisonous drugs and vaccines, thereby adding to the diseases instead of eliminating them. It DAMAGES NORMAL CELLS as well as TUMOR CELLS, SUPPRESSES BONE MARROW FUNCTION, and KILLS OFF WHITE BLOOD CELLS as well as RED BLOOD CELLS. Common side effects are NAUSEA, VOMITING, and HAIR LOSS. It uses the method of TRIAL and ERROR, because it has no fundamental PHILOSOPHY based upon the fundamental bodily processes.

◆ *Medicine Is Concerned With Pathology*

Orthodox medicine looks upon disease as something that happens to man quite by ACCIDENT, BAD LUCK, or CHANCE. It is something that enters the body from without, such as germs or microbes, and has to be fought against and defeated. It exonerates man from all blame, to pity himself at the mercy of unknown forces. Men actuated by the highest motives—for the alleviation of the suffering of mankind—are by virtue of the METHODS they employ, directly instrumental in actually causing disease to be far more widespread and prevalent than it needs to be. Modern medicine is concerned with PATHOLOGY, and not really with health. The treatment of disease is not the same as the maintenance of health.

◆ *Natural Methods Help Body Heal Itself*

On the other hand, NATURAL METHODS recognize the power of the body to heal itself, and place outside reliance only upon those substances which can help the body HEAL ITSELF. The HEALING comes automatically from the elimination of toxic obstructions to further and enhance the healing process. These toxic obstructions have produced the symptoms of disease, and their elimination removes the causes of disease. The NATURAL METHOD has no harmful SIDE EFFECTS, no LONG TERM ADVERSE EFFECTS, no TIME-BOMB effects. NATUROPATHY believes that disease EMANATES FROM WITHIN the body, is SELF-GENERATED as a result of errors of living, and is nature's attempt at SELF-HEALING. Albert Schweitzer said: "Each patient carries his own doctor inside him. We are at our best when we give this doctor a chance to work"

◆ *Medicine Suppresses Symptoms*

A symptom by itself reveals little about the underlying cause. The symptom of a stalled car can have dozens of causes. Hence, there are probably a hundred or more causes for a HEADACHE. If only the symptom is relieved by suppressing it, we have done nothing to get rid of the cause of the disease. To remove enlarged TONSILS and ADENOIDS is not to get rid of the underlying causes of the trouble; to relieve a headache by taking aspirin is not to remove the cause of the headache. A drug relieves only the pain effect of the disease. To take vitamin B_6 for a migraine headache relieves the pain effect, but it does so by healing the immediate cause of the headache, since vitamin B_6 is a healing substance also.

A Hurt Organ Means A Hurt Body

A patient is never just sick in one part of the body. If an organ is affected, so is the rest of the body or the whole organism. This means that it is better to pay attention to healing the body as a whole, and in so doing we are healing what needs to be healed in any part of the body. The healing of the whole body is emphasized, for whenever you assist the body in healing itself, it will heal itself totally. The healing forces always extend themselves all over the body and endeavor to correct that which needs to be corrected.

Vaccinations

Mrs. White hadn't been given any light from God on the matter of vaccinations. As a result, whenever the matter of vaccination came up she would go along with the prevailing custom. However, vaccination is not a natural way of preventing disease. It is an accepted social method for controlling disease as a mass medium method. It is similar to putting chlorine in the water supply which can prevent an epidemic, but it is not a health measure for individuals who drink such water.

It is said that a SMALLPOX VACCINE used by the World Health Organization triggered a virus, now identified as the AIDS VIRUS. It was widespread in Africa but harmless at the time. It was changed into a deadly killer virus by its interaction with the smallpox vaccine. The search is now on for a drug that would suppress the aids virus and knock out the symptoms of the disease. The great danger here is that suppression of the AIDS virus could develop another virus with even more deadly results of a different kind of plague. We need to realize that suppressive drugs are part of the problem, not part of the solution.

THE PREVENTION OF DISEASE

It Is Better To Prevent Than To Cure Disease

◆ *Learning What To Do To Stay Healthy*

We must KNOW, THINK, and ACT prevention. No one can do this for us. A DOCTOR can treat your angina, but we must learn how to stop our arteries from clogging up. An ORTHOPEDIST can fix a fractured hip, but we can prevent the bones from becoming brittle and breakable. A NEUROLOGIST can diagnose a stroke once a person becomes paralyzed, but we must acquire the knowledge to help us to keep the stroke from happening. A SURGEON can remove a cancerous breast, or bowel, or lung, or thyroid, but we must take those steps necessary to reduce the likelihood of such diseases happening.

We have been told that "it is far better to prevent disease than to know how to treat it when contracted" (MH128). God wants us to apply the principles of health to our lives daily in order to prevent disease and maintain our health. He wants us to make use of his God-given "doctors," or natural energies, such as the SUN, AIR, and WATER, etc., to keep us from disease. He wants us to work for our health, instead of doing nothing in this regard, and let sickness creep up on us and surprise us. It is not enough for us to pray to God to keep us healthy.

◆ *God Will Not Work A Miracle For The Intemperate.*

"Many have expected that God would keep them from sickness merely because they have asked Him to do so. But God did not regard their prayers, because their FAITH was not make perfect by WORKS. God will not work a MIRACLE to keep those from sickness who have no care for themselves, but are continually violating the laws of health, and make no efforts to PREVENT DISEASE. When we do all on our part to have health, then we may expect that the blessed results will follow, and we can ask God in faith to bless our efforts for the preservation of health. He will then answer our prayer, if His name can be glorified thereby.... God will not work in a miraculous manner to preserve the health of persons who are taking a sure course to make themselves sick, by their careless inattention to the laws of health" (CH59).

◆ *God Will Keep Us From Disease Only With Our Help*

"A great amount of suffering might be saved if all would labor to prevent disease, by strictly obeying the laws of health. Strict habits of cleanliness should be observed." (CH61). "Those who will gratify their appetite, and then suffer because of their intemperance, and take DRUGS to relieve them, may be assured that God will not interpose to save health and life which is so recklessly periled. The cause has produced the effect." (CD26). God will keep us from disease when we keep ourselves from disease. The person who does what he can to prevent disease exists on a higher level than the doctor who knows how to help heal disease after it has been contracted. The doctor helps us get over our disease, and then we say what a wonderful man he is, when we could do even better by our intelligent application of God's health principles which keep us from getting a disease in the first place. But there is no human being who gives us credit for keeping ourselves in health. We should recognize again that "A great amount of suffering might be saved if all would labor to prevent disease by strictly obeying the laws of health" (2SM460).

◆ *How Disease Is Prevented*

"God desires suffering human beings to be taught how to avoid sickness by the practice of correct habits of EATING, DRINKING, and DRESSING.... they need to be taught the divine laws given by Christ for the good of all mankind. This is the work that is to be done in our Sanitariums" (CH221). If we cannot properly teach ourselves, then we can find teachers who can teach us the principles of prevention. "Disease is prevented by PURE WATER, AIR, and DIET" (1T491). but those who ignore pure air and water, we are told, cannot be free from disease (MM226). Mrs White was asked many times what one should do to preserve health. Her answer was, "Cease to transgress the laws of your being; cease to gratify a depraved appetite; eat simple food; dress healthfully, which will require modest simplicity; work healthfully; and you will not be sick" (CH37). "An ounce of prevention is worth a pound of cure" (2SM291). We should also remember that there is a big difference between PREVENTION and CURE, and this difference has not been emphasized enough. (MM221).

Physicians Are To Be Instructors In Health

◆ *Physicians Must Instruct Patients In Regard To Prevention*

"The first labors of a physician should be to educate the sick and suffering in the very course they should pursue to PREVENT DISEASE" (2SM282). "In the providence of God, many of the sick are to be given the opportunity of separating for a time from harmful associations and surroundings and of placing themselves in institutions where they may receive health-restoring treatments and wise instruction from Christian nurses and physicians" (CH470). It is to be the work of the physician to enlighten his patients as to the nature and causes of their maladies, and to teach them how to avoid disease. Such a physician may have a difficult task, but if he is conscientious he will talk of the ruinous effects of self-indulgence in eating, drinking and dressing, of the overtaxation of the vital forces that have brought the patients to where they are. He will instruct the patients how to form correct habits, and to aid nature in her work of restoration by a wise use of her remedies (CH451–2).

◆ *We Must Assist The Immune System*

The term "doctor" means teacher. This means that one of the important functions of the doctor is to teach the patients the best ways of avoiding disease. Overcoming disease has been the function of medicine ever since its beginnings. This has in the past been effected through many external agents. Recently however, more and more attention has been given to the conquering of disease through the INTERNAL POWER OF THE BODY ITSELF. Emphasis has been placed upon the power of the IMMUNE SYSTEM to control and eliminate disease. Many notorious diseases are caused directly or indirectly by a weakened immune system, the body's own defense against disease. Diseases such as AIDS, CANCER, EPSTEIN-BARR, and CANDIDIASIS imply a weakened immune system as an intermediate cause of the disease. The immune system can counter almost any invasion of foreign bodies if it is strong enough. Almost anything that we engage in that is harmful to the body is harmful to the immune system. Examples are STRESS, TOXINS, BAD DIET, LIFESTYLE, LACK OF SLEEP, DRUGS, ETC.

◆ *Prevention Of Disease Through Proper Diet*

Studies have shown that some of the strongest supporters of the immune system are HEALING HERBS. However, they cannot do the job alone. The proper lifestyle habits must be engaged in order to help the whole process to succeed. Disease can be prevented by eating a diet of the natural foods which God gave to Adam and Eve in the garden of Eden. Such a diet should not contain any artificial chemicals which do not belong in the body, which cannot be assimilated, which do not give energy, which do not stimulate natural growth, which do not have preservatives added to them, to which poisonous substances are not attached. Chemicals do keep food from decaying and give it longer shelf life. But those chemicals that preserve food do not generally preserve the human body. They are generally a cause of its deterioration. They generally harm the body's effort to maintain its health. We are told that "The proper diet of God's people should consist of food made from materials God has provided" (7T125), and we also "prevent sickness by the regulation of appetite and passions" (CH206)

Dr. Jean Mayer of Harvard, said: "The main diseases we deal with, and the main causes of death are influenced by NUTRITION—and they are more easily prevented than cured."

◆ *Prevention Through Right Habits Of Eating*

Every disease of mankind springs in whole or in part from wrong habits of eating. Most diseases have their origins in substances which we put into our bodies. We put unacceptable, unassimilable, impure, and toxic substances into our system which can gradually poison us out of existence. What affects one organ affects every organ. Each organ contributes to the well-being of every other organ. Dr. Spies said: "If we only knew enough all diseases could be prevented and could be cured through proper nutrition." Another doctor said: "The only sickness which exists in the body is TOXICITY. Healthy cells nourished properly, are immune to attack." No known disease can penetrate the strength of a healthy body. A LOW PROTEIN, LOW STARCH, LOW FAT, HIGH ENZYME, HIGH VITAMIN, HIGHLY ALKALINE, and HIGH MINERAL DIET is the KEY. No disease can exist when the bloodstream is clean, and the cells are well nourished.

A study has shown that anyone can restore health by way of detoxification and rebuilding healthy cells so that the BODY CAN HEAL ITSELF. Sickness is a failure to understand the balance of the body, mind, and spirit which creates well-being. A HEALTHY DIET and a CLEAN COLON are most important in maintaining health and preventing disease. The human bloodstream is a closed circuit. God made it so. Everything that goes into the blood in a natural way must pass through the intricate natural filters which keep out dangerous substances. The doctor with the HYPODERMIC NEEDLE bypasses these protective filters and subverts the defenses, while setting up weak spots for ill health to start.

THE USE OF DRUGS

DRUGS AND THE SPIRIT OF PROPHECY

Poisonous Substances

◆ *The Term 'Medicine' Should Be Reserved For Nonpoisonous Substances*

The Spirit of Prophecy is replete with warnings regarding the harmful effects of poisonous drugs. The expression "poisonous drugs" is not used simply because there may also exist nonpoisonous drugs, but because all drugs in their very nature are poisonous substances. One author states that "all drugs are poisons, and all poisons are drugs." A pharmacy took it upon itself to test the toxicity of 10,000 drugs. Out of the 10,000 drugs they found 3 that were nonpoisonous. Hence, we may say with confidence that all drugs are poisonous to a greater or lesser degree. While Webster gives us practically the same definition for a "drug" as for "medicine," as substances used for the prevention and cure of disease, it is clear that a definite distinction must be made between these terms.

Strictly speaking, the term "medicine" should be reserved for those substances which are OBJECTIVELY HEALING SUBSTANCES, and not for those which are SUBJECTIVELY used as such. A substance used as a healing substance may not be a healing substance. That drugs are not healing substances has been made perfectly clear to us when the Spirit of Prophecy tells us that "DRUGS NEVER CURE" (2SM451). Because of the light that has been given us we must reject a part of Webster's definition and say that drugs are not objectively healing substances. They are merely used as such. Objectively speaking, the term "MEDICINE" should be reserved for HEALING SUBSTANCES, and the two terms should not be confused so as to create confusion and misinformation.

The healing substances which we have been given through the Spirit of Prophecy are called HERBS. They must be called objective healing substances because God has created them for us as such. They actually have healing power within the body because they have been given us to cleanse the system of impurities which process definitely aids the healing process. When the Spirit of Prophecy tells us that "drugs never cure," this information could be given us only by the Mind of Omnipotence. This means that God was not only referring to the drugs used in Mrs. White's day, but to drugs used in all times present, past, and future. God did not limit Himself to any specific time for he did not want us to take into the body temple poisons which would tend to destroy it. He foresaw the multitudinous chemicals which would be developed and applied as medicines without their being healing substances. This means that we should not use any of these substances because they do not heal but destroy.

◆ *The Poisonous Nature Of Drugs*

Drugs are poisonous chemical substances used by doctors to bring about a change in a disease condition. They are chemicals which are not normally found in the body, and as foreign to the body, the body regards them usually as enemies to be eliminated as fast as possible. Medical science is based upon the FALSE PREMISE that disease is caused by extraneous outside influences, and that such an affliction may be cured by drugs. All of these "therapeutic" substances are then administered without a clear understanding of the cause of the affliction. It is believed that the entity called DISEASE can be expelled when the right drug is found and applied.

Chemicals which are not normal to the body can harm the body in many ways. Drugs as poisons have a poisonous effect upon body cells and functions. This also means that a substance which is not poisonous should not be called a drug, even though it may have a drug effect in excessive quantity. For example, the Bible says that honey is good (Prov. 24:13), but it also says that much honey is not good (Prov. 25:27). It is no accident that the words "poison" and "potion" come from the same root, and that the Greek word "pharmakon," which we find rooted in our word "pharmacy," originally meant both a healing substance and a deadly one.

The basic truth about all drugs is that if they are improperly used, or even if properly used, they are poisons without qualification, producing unwanted reactions ranging from temporary NAUSEA to DEATH. A POISON is a substance which has the tendency to threaten the life of the organism which partakes of it. THEY may seem to have a beneficial effect for a time (4SG135), they may produce temporarily favorable results (MM224), but they are nevertheless a CURSE upon mankind (4SG133), because they merely change the FORM and LOCATION of the disease (MH126), but do not cure the disease. "In nature's effort to expel the drug from the system, intense suffering is sometimes caused the patient, and the disease which the drug was given to cure, may disappear, but only to reappear in a new form, such as SKIN DISEASES, ULCERS, PAINFUL DISEASED JOINTS, and sometimes in a more dangerous and deadly form" (2SM451). Some experts estimate that one hospital patient in ten is in the hospital as a result of REACTIONS TO DRUGS prescribed by their doctors. The doctors rationalize such effects by saying that from the standpoint of the risk factors involved, that the beneficial effects outweigh the harmful effects for most patients most of the time. This is a rationalization upon which a lot of doubt can be placed, for LONG-RANGE EFFECT OF DRUGS can hardly ever be ascertained, so that drug-taking is a matter of faith in the drug and in the doctor who prescribes it. All drugs injure and enervate the body, suppress or suspend the restorative processes, and prolong the disease, if they do not prevent recovery altogether.

◆ *Most Diseases Are Self-limiting*

We say that most diseases are SELF-LIMITING, which means that the patient, with a little extra rest, with or without treatment, will sooner or later get well. Hence, it is impossible to say whether or not the patient recovered because of the treatment, or in spite of it. Dr. John Forbes said: "Some patients get well with the aid of medicines; more without it; and still more in spite of it." Even more puzzling is what is called the "PLACEBO EFFECT." The word "placebo" means "to please," and refers to any substance that is given to the patient to benefit him by pleasing him, even if the substance doesn't have any medicinal value. Sometimes the psychological value of giving the patient something that makes him feel better, and as a result get better by relieving ANXIETY, TENSION, PAIN, is a direct illustration of the great effect which the mind has upon the body.

◆ *Harmful In Health And In Disease*

A poisonous substance will react as a poisonous substance chemically in the same manner whether a person is ill or well. This means that if a substance is harmful to a person in health, then it is also harmful to the body when ill. Hygienists point out that it is indeed a strange "science" which teaches that substances which make us sick when we are well, should be taken when we are sick to make us well. A PERSON CANNOT BE POISONED INTO HEALTH. Poisons add disease problems instead of solving disease problems. They are obviously less harmful in smaller amounts than in larger amounts, in lesser concentrations than in greater concentrations. It is therefore a mistake to think that diseases can be overcome by agencies that are poisonous to the body. Nevertheless, the MATERIA MEDICA of the doctors says in the preface: "If it is not POISON, it is not good for MEDICINE." In contrast we should be saying: "If it is poison, it is not good for health." Oliver Wendell Holmes, himself a medical doctor, recognized the effect which drugs have upon the body when he said: "I firmly believe that, if the whole materia medica could be sunk to the bottom of the sea, it would be all the better for mankind and all the worse for the fishes."

◆ *Drugs Are Inimical To Life*

When it comes to drugs, we find that they are harmful in any amount, because they are poisons by their very nature. A small quantity may not have any noticeable effect or reaction that can be observed, but we cannot therefore say that it is good because we cannot see or feel any bad reaction, or notice any harmful effect. The Spirit of Prophesy has given us the PRINCIPLES to live by under these circumstances. It first of all tells us that God's method of healing is "healing without drugs" (MM225), that drugs "Imperil life and health" (MM14), that they "increase rather than decrease evils" (MM222), that they are "health-destroying inventions" (2SM279), that "they derange the system generally" (2SM281), that "they are worse than the disease for which they are given" (2SM443), that they are the "seeds of death" (MM229), that they "kill but never cure" (2SM289), that "thousands are killed by drugs" (MM57), and that "they have resulted in more harm than good" (Loma Linda Messages 62).

We are told that we are CONTRADICTING THE LIGHT which God has given us when we use drugs (MM27, 228), that they are an offense to God (MM229), that we should use HERBS in the place of drugs (2SM288), and that thousands would recover health if they discarded drugs and lived healthfully (MM229).

When the Spirit of Prophecy tells us that "we should employ every facility for the restoration of health" (MH231), it certainly does not mean drugs, for it adds that we should work in harmony with natural law, and it was indicated that drugs work contrary to natural law (MM223). These statements categorically dismiss all DRUGS AS NON-HEALING LIFE-ENDANGERING SUBSTANCES. In response to the statement that drugs never cure, Adventist doctors have said that the drugs that are used today are different from the drugs that were used in Mrs. White's day. This is no doubt true, since 4000 or more new drugs are put on the market every year. However, we must look at this situation from the standpoint of the way God sees it. We cannot claim that God did not foresee the development of new drugs. If this were true then those Spirit of Prophecy statements have no relevancy for us today. But they were written for our benefit to be relevant till the end of time (MMxiii). God made His statement about the use of drugs an ABSOLUTE STATEMENT by the use of the word "NEVER."

◆ *Drugs Do Not Cure Disease*

Drugs contain no nutrients. They have no intelligence for creating new cells or to repair damaged tissue. They are not corrective. No tissue can use drugs nutritionally, but only nutrition can restore damaged tissue. They do not supply materials for the manufacture of AMINO ACIDS or PROTEINS, or substances needed by the body in the performance of its bodily functions. They cannot remove TOXIC MATTER from the system, for they themselves represent toxic matter. They combine chemically with cells and vital fluids so as to interfere with their functions by depriving them of OXYGEN and NUTRIENTS. They can produce harmful GENETIC CHANGES, and often reduce the BODY'S RESISTANCE to disease. They can have a TIME-BOMB EFFECT in that they produce disease conditions that arise years after their use as CHRONIC and DEGENERATIVE diseases. They also have "no power to cure."

Drugs may suspend the vital activity of the body so that symptoms disappear, but they do not remove the cause of disease. They may kill germs, and sometimes patients too, but they do not eliminate the bodily condition which allows germs to thrive and grow in the body. If they do not remove the cause of disease, they do not cure the disease. If they do not enable us to avoid the cause of disease, then they do not prevent disease. They are not factors out of which good health is built. They do not heal because they do positive harm to the body. THERE IS NO CURE WITHOUT THE REMOVAL OF CAUSE.

◆ *Restorative Power Is In Nature Only*

Healing is nature's prerogative. We are told that "people need to be taught that drugs do not CURE disease. It is true that they sometimes afford present relief, and the patient appears to recover as the result of their use; this is because nature has sufficient VITAL FORCE to expel the poison and to correct the conditions that caused the disease. Health is recovered IN SPITE OF the drug. But in most cases the drug only changes the FORM and LOCATION of the disease. Often the effect of the drug seems to be overcome for a time, but the results remain in the system, and work great harm at some later period. By the use of poisonous drugs, many bring upon themselves lifelong illness, and many lives are lost that might be saved by the use of NATURAL METHODS OF HEALING" (CH89). "Poisonous drugs.... destroy the power of the patient to help himself" (2SM281).

◆ *Drugs Radically Alter Body Processes*

Drugs are poisonous substances which are either derived from poisonous plants, or are manufactured synthetically in the laboratory. They do not change their nature regardless of what type of environment they are in. As chemicals they will react indifferently with everything that they are capable of reacting with. They work by radically altering body processes adversely. No drug is free of potentially DANGEROUS SIDE EFFECTS. As one doctor put it: "Every drug upsets some function of the body—that is how it works." PENICILLIN affects body processes even though it is intended only to kill bacteria. One doctor said that the PILL is supposed to affect only one hormone system, but instead it affects 50 hormone systems. SIDE EFFECTS reduce the quality of life and the sense of well-being. They often decrease potassium levels, cause cramps in the legs, heart arrhythmias, and increase the likelihood of cardiovascular mortality.

CHEMICAL ACTIONS are the only actions of which drugs are capable. If ASPIRIN is taken the effect may be the ACCELERATION OF THE HEARTBEAT which is the action of the body; the EROSION OF THE STOMACH WALL is the chemical action of the SALICYLIC ACID; the damage to the KIDNEYS represents a chemical action. When DIGITALIS is taken there is a change in HEART ACTION, which is the action of the body. The MYOCARDIAL ACTION which may follow, is the result of chemical action. The VOMITING that follows the taking of a drug, the PURGING that follows the taking of a LAXATIVE, the SWEATING that follows the taking of a DIAPHORETIC, are all reactions of the body for purposes of expelling the poisons before they combine chemically with the tissues. We are DECEIVED by these actions because we tend to ascribe the actions of the body to the actions of the drugs. They are in reality all DEFENSIVE, REMEDIAL, and ELIMINATIVE actions of the body.

These DEFENSIVE actions of the body exact a toll of its VITALITY. Some bodies do not react to the influence of the drug taken. If this is the case it means that the vitality of the body is exhausted, and its condition is near death. No matter how powerful the drug is, the more powerful it is, the more it devitalizes the body's resources. It is impossible to produce a reaction in a body whose vitality has been exhausted. When drugs are taken regularly over a period of time, they gradually lose their effect, and larger and larger doses are needed to have the same original effect. The loss of effect of these drugs is the result of the loss of, or weakening of, the defensive power of the body to defend itself against the poisonous onslaught. The drugs, however, have done nothing to remove the cause of the disease.

◆ *Chemical Actions Are Non-rational Actions*

Chemical action is not rational action as far as the chemical's relationship to the body is concerned. A substance which is HARMFUL to the body in HEALTH is also HARMFUL to the body in DISEASE. The same amount of poison given by a doctor will have the same effect as if given by a layman, or if taken by the person himself. The poisonous nature of a substance is not changed by a change in the person who is administering it. Poisons are not capable of being assimilated by the body, and therefore the body cannot direct and control their use as it does with HERBS, FOOD NUTRIENTS, or VITAMINS. As soon as a drug is taken, the powers and the wisdom of the body are devoted to eliminating it. In their chemical action, drugs may permanently damage the body. They form chemical combinations contrary to the needs of the body economy. Hence, they interfere with or destroy VITAL PROCESSES, so as to threaten the existence of the body in whole or in part. They are substances which bear no beneficial or health-promoting relationship to the needs of the human organism. They are not compatible with it, and are not adapted to it. The doctor who administers drugs to suppress a FEVER or other symptoms, is actually stopping vital, restorative and reparative body processes. Drugs do not have any restorative action. They are not selective because they are NON-RATIONAL.

DRUGS form chemical unions that PARALYZE NERVES, DESTROY CELLS, and SUSPEND VITAL ACTION, thereby causing the SYMPTOMS of disease to disappear. The person so treated is actually sicker than he was before, even though for the time being he may be feeling better. Drugs goad the body into activities which exhaust an already exhausted body even more, resulting in his being even worse off than he was before. All HEALING that takes place after the administration of drugs does so IN SPITE of the drugs, and not because of them. The rest in bed did most to allow the body to restore itself to health.

◆ *Drugs Relieve The Symptoms Of Disease*

Drugs do not cure disease, but they do alleviate

many of the SYMPTOMS of disease. They also often make the evidence of a disease to disappear. They submerge or SUPPRESS the disease so that one does not notice an inward or outward effect of the disease. The individual may feel better without being cured of the disease. ALL DRUGS MASK SYMPTOMS, and they mask symptoms of even fatal diseases. Giving poisonous drugs amounts to HARMFUL INTERFERENCE with the healing processes of the body. Giving HERB TEAS as well as FRUIT and VEGETABLE JUICES does not represent an interference with the healing processes of the body, because these substances are adapted to the natural body processes, and help the system cleanse itself of impurities. They therefore advance the healing processes of the body. To eliminate the symptoms of the disease is not to cure the disease. It is merely to eliminate the superficial evidences of the disease. Generally, when the elimination of the symptoms of a disease is emphasized, the LAWS OF NATURE ARE BYPASSED as not being powerful enough to alleviate the disease situation.

◆ *Drugs Reduce Vitality*

The body has been working to cleanse the tissues of impurities in the healing process. Now its attention is called to the elimination of the poison that has just been introduced. The sick person's body is already at a point of low vitality. Its remaining vitality is now directed at the greater enemy which has been introduced, and the symptoms of the cleansing and purification process disappear. The fact that fevers and other symptoms of disease disappear indicates the further loss of vitality. The body is not able to fight on both fronts, and it therefore withdraws from the eliminative and remedial process that has caused the symptoms in the first place. The body has now been placed in double jeopardy in now having to overcome a double dose of poisonous substances.

◆ *Drugs Interfere With Nutrition*

✓ ANTACIDS THAT CONTAIN ALUMINUM—reduce the absorption of FLUORIDE and PHOSPHOROUS in the body as well as the amount of CALCIUM, by increasing the amount of calcium lost in the urine.

✓ ANTACIDS WITH MAGNESIUM—lower the absorption of PHOSPHOROUS in the body by increasing the amount of phosphorous lost in the urine

✓ ANTACIDS WITH SODIUM-BICARBONATE — result in BLOATING due to water retention and SODIUM retention.

✓ ASPIRIN—interferes with levels of FOLIC ACID and ASCORBIC ACID in the blood, and causes a deficiency of IRON.

✓ CORTICOSTEROIDS—inhibit the absorption of PHOSPHOROUS and CALCIUM, and raise the body's need for other vitamins, such as VITAMIN D, ASCORBIC ACID, and FOLIC ACID.

✓ LAXATIVES—interfere with the absorption of CALCIUM in the body

✓ MINERAL OIL—interferes with the absorption of VITAMINS A, D, and E.

✓ PENICILLIN — reduces the amount of POTASSIUM in the body by increasing the amount of potassium in the urine

✓ TETRACYCLINES—inhibit the absorption of minerals such as IRON, CALCIUM, MAGNESIUM, and ZINC.

◆ *"Cures" Don't Last*

So-called "drug cures" pass away in a very short time. New drugs are continuously developed because the "old" drugs were found not to do what they were expected to do, simply because they were NOT HEALING SUBSTANCES that could eliminate disease. That is why a French physician said to one of his patients: "Here, take this while it is still a remedy." People are often "cured" repeatedly, for the "cures" do not stick. The wound of a nail in the foot cannot be cured without removing the nail, and a drunk man cannot be made sober while he continues to drink. Some years ago it was estimated that the medical profession had 130,000 remedies for 407 diseases. With so many "remedies," why should anyone ever remain sick or die of disease? Hosea 4:6 says: "My people are destroyed for lack of knowledge." IGNORANCE leads people to ignore causes and to rely upon remedies.

Drugs Themselves Cause Disease And Death

Drugs as poisons do not in any way harmonize with body processes. To the body they are foreign substances, and the body itself reacts to them as unwelcome substances that hinder rather than help the body. They make conditions worse rather than better, and destroy the life which Christ came to restore (2SM288). They represent a disease themselves, by producing a disease of a different kind (2SM448).

We are furthermore told that "thousands have gone down to the grave by the use of poisonous drugs, who might have been restored to health by simple methods of treatments" (MM227), and that therefore "drugging should be FOREVER ABANDONED, for while it does not cure any malady, it ENFEEBLES THE SYSTEM, making it more susceptible to disease" (CD83). "MORE DEATHS HAVE BEEN CAUSED BY DRUG-TAKING THAN FROM ALL OTHER CAUSES COMBINED. If there was in the land one physician in the place of thousands, a vast amount of PREMATURE MORTALITY would be prevented. Multitudes of physicians, multitudes of drugs, have cursed the inhabitants of the earth, and have carried thousands and tens of thousands to untimely graves" (2SM450).

The Results Of Taking Drugs

◆ *They Harm The Immune System*

Dr. Moss of the University of Rochester said that DIGITALIS, one of the oldest and widely used heart drugs, increases the risk of sudden death in people who have survived a heart attack. They often die later of sudden heart rhythm disorder within 60 seconds. However, it has been determined that digitalis is neutralized in the body by VITAMIN E. In the case of BROAD SPECTRUM ANTIBIOTICS, the person using them often develops severe DIARRHEA. This is the result of upsetting the INTESTINAL FLORA. The SULFA DRUGS have caused serious LIVER involvements, and have also caused inflammatory disease of the ARTERIES, with symptoms similar to blood poisoning and other SYSTEMIC INFECTIONS. Patients treated with HYDRALIZINE, which has been used extensively in the treatment of HIGH BLOOD PRESSURE, have shown symptoms resembling RHEUMATOID ARTHRITIS, with PAIN at the JOINTS and MUSCLES. Patients receiving CORTISONE, ACTH and other STEROID therapy are in serious danger of death from ADRENAL EXHAUSTION when exposed to new stresses such as SURGERY, ACCIDENTS, BURNS, and even CHILDBIRTH. All known CANCER DRUGS not only act against CANCER CELLS, but also suppress the IMMUNE SYSTEM. They can do more harm than good by destroying what limited capacity the patient's system has to protect itself.

"Young men who are sent to Ann Arbor to obtain an education which they think will exalt them as supreme in their treatment of disease by drugs, will find that it will result in the loss of life rather than restoration to health and strength. These mixtures place a double taxation upon nature, and in the effort to throw off the poisons they contain, thousands of persons lose their lives. We must LEAVE DRUGS ENTIRELY ALONE, for in using them we introduce an ENEMY into the system" (Letter 67, 1899)

◆ *They Mask Symptoms*

There are reports of people having been driven to SUICIDE as a result of having taken TRANQUILIZERS. They tend to mask symptoms that the doctor could find helpful in diagnosing the patient's problem. There is no specific antidote for many of the tranquilizing drugs, and many of them have proven fatal when given in seemingly small doses. The common drug ASPIRIN is rapidly absorbed and circulates in the blood stream as SODIUM SALICYLATE. A moderate dose of aspirin can cause a more RAPID HEARTBEAT, a rise in BLOOD PRESSURE, PERSPIRATION, FULLNESS in the HEAD, RINGING in the EARS, DEAFNESS, IMPAIRMENT of VISION, and a slight fall in BODY TEMPERATURE. Larger doses may cause DELIRIUM, DISTURBED RESPIRATION, a FALL in BLOOD PRESSURE, ALBUMIN in the URINE, HEMORRHAGING, VOMITING of BLOOD, and IRRITATION of the GASTRIC MUCUS.

◆ *The Remedy Is Worse Than The Disease*

In a conclusive test at the Mayo Clinic, 2114 patients, who were treated for ARTHRITIS with aspirin-type medications, were found to have 4 times as many ULCERS as other patients. The Spirit of Prophecy tells us that "Everywhere you may go you will see DEFORMITY, DISEASE, and IMBECILITY, which in very many cases can be traced directly back to the DRUG POISONS, administered by the hand of the doctor, as a remedy of some of life's ills. The so-called REMEDY has fearfully proved itself to the patient, by stern suffering experience, to be far worse than the disease for which the drug was taken." "There are more who die from the use of drugs than all those who would have died of disease, had nature been left to do her own work" (2SM452). Drugs have INCREASED THE DEGENERATION OF THE RACE (2SM442).

Drugs Produce Side-Effects

Drugs being poisons, produce what are called SIDE-EFFECTS. It is easy to see why this should be so because side-effects are a result of the POISONOUS EFFECTS of drugs on body processes. They represent the body's strong reaction against being mistreated. It has been estimated that about 4 million people a year are poisoned so severely by their physicians as to be hospitalized. Some side-effects are due to the destruction of the body's beneficial germs, of which there are at least as many as there are of the harmful germs. One doctor said: "If you swallow an antibiotic you may kill off a large number of your necessary intestinal flora. Many of the dangerous side-effects of antibiotics are the result of just this phenomenon." He continues by saying: "If an antibiotic cures your pneumonia, and leaves you with an incurable liver condition, it has done you more harm than good. In the past 10–15 years, drugs, like insecticides, have been made progressively more and more potent. This means that they have become potentially more and MORE DANGEROUS TO THE PATIENT also."

If you have been given a drug that produces a noticeable side-effect, another drug is given to take care of that side-effect. But the second drug has side-effects of its own also, and how is that to be taken care of? On the other hand, if there is an absence of clinical symptoms after taking a drug, this does not mean that no side-effects have been caused by the drug. They just simply haven't been felt. This fact leads one to the conclusion that drugs should not be taken as a MATTER OF PRINCIPLE, for no one can ever know how many adverse side-effects there may be. Drugs in the body are treated as foreign objects which the liver endeavors to detoxify. White blood cells engulf them in an endeavor to protect the body from them. So instead of enhancing our natural defenses, drugs tend to weaken them, and to open the door to more disease. "Drug medication gives nature two burdens to bear, in the place of one. She has two serious difficulties to overcome, in the place of one" (MM223).

Drugs Should Not Be Called Medicines

The term "medicine" is defined as a healing substance. It is a term which therefore should not be applied to substances which are non-healing. The Spirit of Prophesy makes a distinction between poisonous and nonpoisonous plants, as well as poisonous and nonpoisonous substances used for healing purposes. In order not to cause confusion we cannot use the term MEDICINE for both types of substances, but must by way of definition distinguish between them. The term DRUG being a non-healing substance, should therefore not be considered to be a healing substance. The confusion comes when the term "medicine" is applied to both types of substances. The term "medicine" should be applied only to a healing substance, and not indiscriminately to whatever the doctor gives you with the intention of healing you. The intention on the part of the doctor that the drug heal does, however, not make the drug heal. This is what it means in the minds of most people. To apply the term "medicine" to a drug represents a deception in terminology and definition. Furthermore, natural nonpoisonous herbs or food substances should not be called drugs. Vitamins should be considered as food substances and not as drugs, even though some of them may have a drugging effect if taken in excessive quantities. To apply the term "medicine" to all substances used for the purpose of healing is a cover-up. It makes the patient believe that he is getting a healing substance when he is actually getting a NON-HEALING HARMFUL SUBSTANCE. If the doctor had an absolute degree of integrity, he would say to his patient: "I want to give you this poison to make you well, and if that doesn't do the job I have an even stronger poison for you to use." Under these circumstances very few patients would take the so-called "medicine" prescribed for them.

Doctors often speak of the new drugs that have been developed. But why should a new substance always be a drug if it is designed for healing purposes? Why shouldn't we be able to say that a new plant has been discovered which has such and such healing properties? When the Bible says: "A merry heart doeth good like a medicine" (Prov. 17:22), it did not mean drugs, but rather nonpoisonous plant substances which the Lord has created to grow in the field as nature's healing agents.

Present Benefit And Future Harm

Not even the statement that drugs relieve present suffering, which is often true, may be a good enough reason for using them. Under these circumstances what the doctor is doing is to emphasize a present short-term benefit in place of a future harm (2SM281), and the sum total of the two effects turns out to be on the harmful side, which means that DRUGS DO MORE HARM THAN GOOD. A present good is turned into a greater future harm. We are told that when health is recovered, it is RECOVERED IN SPITE OF THE DRUGS TAKEN and not because of them (CH89). It is because nature had enough vital force to overcome the poison, and to correct the condition that caused the disease in the first place.

When the Spirit of Prophesy tells us that "Christ's remedies cleanse the system" (2SM289), it indicates to us that it isn't germs that are the major cause of disease, but rather that it is IMPURITIES of every kind, including drugs, that are a major cause of disease. It means impurities produced within the body as well as impurities introduced from without. A drug takes away the symptoms of a disease by changing the form and location of the disease, and such a change is falsely labeled as healing. The poison is distributed to other parts of the body and produces great harm there at some future time. This cause and effect relationship doctors are usually not aware of, and they consider a later illness simply as a new illness, without recognizing it as an effect of possibly some previous drug treatment. That is why drug treatment should be abandoned as a matter of principle, because man isn't wise enough to discern a present treatment's future effects.

Satan Temps Us To Take Poisons

We are told that "Christ never planted the seeds of death in the system. Satan planted these seeds when he tempted Adam to eat of the tree of knowledge which meant disobedience to God. Not one noxious plant was placed in the Lord's great garden, but after Adam and Eve sinned, poisonous herbs sprang up.... All tares are sown by the evil one. Every noxious herb is of his sowing, and by his ingenious methods of amalgamation, he has corrupted the earth with tares. Then shall physicians continue to resort to drugs, which leave a deadly evil in the system, destroying that life which Christ came to restore? Christ's remedies cleanse the system. But SATAN HAS TEMPTED MAN to introduce into the system that which weakens the human machinery, clogging and destroying the fine, beautiful arrangements of God. The drugs administered to the sick do not restore, but destroy. DRUGS NEVER CURE. Instead, they place in the system seeds which bear a very bitter harvest" (2SM288–9).

Let us remember that if the doctor is not using God's method of healing he is using Satan's method of healing, and there is no in-between. If a mixture of the two methods is used, the matter becomes more insidious, for then it tends to blur the great distinction between the two methods, and it makes the patient think that Satan's drug method is on a par with God's natural herbal method. Drugs are used because "It is easier to use drugs than to use natural remedies" (Te85).

The Plant Origin Of Drugs

God created all of the nonpoisonous plants. Satan, by his ingenious methods of amalgamation or hybridization was allowed by God to modify some of the existing plants, which God had created, in order to produce poisonous plants or tares. Usually, drugs that come directly from plants come from poisonous plants. Some of the drugs may come from nonpoisonous plants, but they become poisonous substances when they are processed and refined. For example, MOLDS are poisonous substances to the body. Penicillin, having been produced from a poisonous substance, is also a poisonous substance. This is attested to by the fact that every year about 300 persons die from adverse reactions to penicillin injections. God does not want a single person to die from the medicine he is taking. That is why he admonishes us to use nonpoisonous harmless herbs which have the property of assisting the individual toward health without harming him.

When the Spirit of Prophecy speaks of HERBS, it does not imply that the pharmaceutical industry should process and refine them until they are no longer recognizable as herbs. God means for us to use the natural product just AS HE HAS CREATED IT without any tampering by man so as to change a harmless substance into a powerful harmful drug. It is not merely what chemicals are in a plant that is important, but rather it is the synergistic effect of all the substances working together in the way that God has put them together that brings the desired result. Man cannot chemically fractionate a plant, take one substance out of it, and expect that one substance to work with the same beneficial effect as the natural whole plant. With plants we must apply the principle that the whole is greater than the sum of its parts. The chemicals of a plant produced separately in the laboratory and then combined artificially will not produce the same effect as the natural product. We cannot combine substances the way God can.

OUR PERSONAL RESPONSIBILITY REGARDING DRUGS

We Should Accept God's Light On Drugs

Our first duty to God is to accept the light which he has given us on the matter of drugs. We would be doing this not only to please God, but to do that which favors our greatest welfare. Mrs. White says: "I have been pained when many students have been encouraged to go where they would receive an education in the use of drugs. The light I have received on the subject of drugs is altogether different from the use made of them at these schools or at the sanitariums. We must become enlightened on these subjects.... drugs are to be discarded and RATIONAL METHODS of TREATMENT followed.... By observing these rules many who have been given up by the physicians may be restored to health" (MM228).

"After seeing so much harm done by the administering of drugs, I cannot use them and cannot testify in their favor. I must be true to the light given me by the Lord" (2SM293). The patient who relies on drugs feels no RESPONSIBILITY for his recovery, does not understand his capacity for helping himself to health, places negligible trust in the laws which rule his physical being, and is thus led to place his responsibility for his own health in the hands of another. We should remember that principles don't change. The nature of their application may be modified according to circumstances. This means that the principles which were presented to God's people in the early days of Mrs. White's ministry are as valid today as they were then. God's principles do not change, for God doesn't change. That is why Mrs. White wrote: "I have been shown that the principles that were given us in the early days of the message are as important and should be regarded just as conscientiously today as they were then" (9T158).

Parents Sin Against Themselves And Their Children

We are told that "If those who take drugs were alone the sufferers, then the evil would not be as great. But parents not only sin against themselves in swallowing drug poisons, but they sin against their children. The vitiated state of their blood, the poison distributed throughout their system, the broken constitution, and various drug diseases, as a result of drug poisons, are transmitted to their offspring, and left them as a wretched inheritance, which is another great cause of the degeneracy of the race." They also "sin against their intelligence and endanger their whole afterlife" (2SM290). One reason why parents are tempted to use them is because "it is easier to employ drugs than to use natural remedies. Many parents substitute drugs for judicious nursing" (Te85).

We Should Use Herbs Instead Of Drugs

We are told that "There are simple herbs that can be used for the recovery of the sick, whose effect upon the system is very different from that of those drugs that poison the blood and endanger life" (2SM288). "God has caused to grow out of the ground herbs for the use of man, and if we understand the nature of these roots and herbs, and make a right use of them, there would not be a necessity of running to the doctor so frequently, and people would be in much better health than they are today. I believe in calling upon the Great Physician when we have used the remedies I have mentioned" (2SM297).

"There are simple HERBS and ROOTS that every family may use for themselves and need not call a physician any sooner than they would call a lawyer" (2SM279). "There are herbs that are HARMLESS, the use of which will tide over many apparently SERIOUS DIFFICULTIES" (2SM291). "The Lord has given some simple herbs of the field that at times are beneficial; and if every family were educated in how to use these herbs in case of sickness, much suffering might be prevented and no doctor need be called. The old-fashioned, simple herbs, used intelligently, would have recovered many sick who have died under drug medication" (2SM294).

"Our Savior is the restorer of the moral image of God in man. He has supplied in the natural world remedies for the ills of man, that his followers may have life and may have it more abundantly. We can with safety discard the concoctions which man has used in the past. The Lord has provided ANTIDOTES FOR DISEASE in simple plants, and these can be used by faith, with no denial of faith; for by using the blessings provided by God for our benefit we are COOPERATING WITH HIM. We can use water and sunshine and the herbs which he has caused to grow for healing maladies brought on by indiscretion or accident" (MS 65, 1899).

We Should Live Healthfully

We are to make use of all of the healthful agencies which God has placed within our reach, and we should eliminate all of the substances that we know are harmful to the health of the body. When the Spirit of Prophecy told us that "we should employ every facility for the restoration of health, it certainly did not mean drugs, for she added that we should work in harmony with natural law, and drugs work contrary to natural law" (MM223). If we know what is right to do under the circumstances, then we should do it. We should not become victims of our own ignorance. When we have done what we ought to do, then we can expect that GOD'S BLESSINGS will follow. We are told that "If the sick and suffering will only do as well as they know in regard to living out the principles of health reform perseveringly, then they will in NINE CASES OUT OF TEN recover from their ailments" (2SM288). "Thousands need to be educated patiently, kindly, tenderly, but decidedly, that NINE TENTHS of their complaints are created by their own course of action" (MM225)

We Should Heal Without Drugs

◆ *Taking Drugs Is Our Responsibility*

One of the first things we should do is to have confidence in God's remedies which he has placed in nature, which have the power to OVERCOME EVEN THE MOST DIFFICULT DISEASES. This fact has been demonstrated many times. Some may feel that herbs are not powerful enough to heal a serious disease, but if God placed them there for that purpose, then they can do whatever needs to be done. We are told to "avoid the use of drugs, and carefully observe the laws of health. If you regard your life, you should eat plain food, prepared in the simplest manner, and take more physical exercise. Each member of the family needs the benefits of HEALTH REFORM. But DRUGGING SHOULD BE FOREVER ABANDONED; for while it does not cure any malady, it enfeebles the system, making it more susceptible to disease." (CD82). The responsibility for taking drugs is ours, not the doctor's. We are told that "we are not excusable if through ignorance we destroy Gods building by taking into our stomachs poisonous drugs under a variety of names we do not understand. It is our DUTY TO REFUSE ALL SUCH PRESCRIPTIONS" (2SM283). Disease can be successfully treated without drugs (Ev535).

◆ *Should Not Be Taken To Relieve Present Suffering*

Sometimes we may feel that under circumstances of great pain in an affliction, that drugs are the proper remedy to relieve the pain. But even this is questionable, for even herbs have the ability to reduce pain. We are told that "God's servants should not administer medicines which they know will leave behind INJURIOUS EFFECTS upon the system, even if they do RELIEVE PRESENT

SUFFERING" (2SM281), and the reason given is that they will derange the system and destroy the power of the patient to HELP HIMSELF. "The sick themselves, if they would be patient, (meaning undergoing pain without complaint), diet and suffer a little, and give nature time to rally, would RECOVER MUCH SOONER without the use of any medicine" (2SM452).

Naturopaths have seen many patients, who by doing away with drugs or chemical medicines, have overcome the disease for which these drugs were taken. They have seen people get rid of DIABETES by taking away the INSULIN. They have seen many patients get a good night's rest after doing away with the TRANQUILIZERS. Doctors who have been taught no other way fear to leave the patient without those medicines, so that they have never seen the comparison between their drugs and natural medicines. The naturopath uses natural medicines without fear and produces many expected results.

Drugs And Emergencies

The use of some drugs in cases of emergency is not denied by the Spirit of Prophecy. Emergencies do not represent cases of gradual healing from disease. When an emergency occurs we must do the best that we can with the material immediately available. Mrs. White herself, when she was on board of ship crossing the ocean, became ill and partook of a cup of tea as a medicine. She did not want people to think, however, that she used Chinese or Java tea as a drink. The tea that she drank every day was RED CLOVER TEA. The same held true for coffee. At another time she drank a cup of very strong coffee as a medicine with a raw egg broken into it when she had become ill (2SM302).

While in Australia Mrs. White was told of the sickness and death of the son of a brother who had been a missionary in the islands. He was afflicted with MALARIA, and his father was advised to give him QUININE, but he did not give it to the boy because of the counsel given in the testimonies to avoid the use of quinine. Thereafter the son died. When the father later asked Mrs. White if he would have sinned if he had given the boy quinine to check the malaria when the prospect was that he would die without it, she said: "No, we are to do the best that we can" (2SM282). The general statement which Mrs. White made about quinine is given in 4SGa139, where she says: "MERCURY, CALOMEL, and QUININE have brought their amount of wretchedness, which the day of God alone will fully reveal."

One can contract MALARIA from a blood transfusion if the donor was infected and was unaware of it. This is possible because it can take as long as a year after being bitten by the mosquito before symptoms appear.

An Indian woman who had a reputation as a healer told two men suffering from malaria to sprinkle common table salt inside their shoes and to wear thin white socks. This they did and in one week's time their malaria symptoms disappeared and never returned. Al. Wolfsen, an Adventist herbalist and missionary to the South Seas, cured malaria among the natives with a hot steam bath while the patient was beginning to chill and before the fever started. If done properly, he says, there will be no more malaria unless a malaria mosquito bites again. If one is too late with the heat, then try it again at the next chill.

Substances Which Counteract Poisonous effects

✓ VITAMIN C—Large doses of vitamin C up to 10 gm will neutralize poisons
✓ VITAMIN B COMPLEX—is especially needed after treatment with ANTIBIOTICS
✓ LECITHIN—2 to 3 tablespoons a day. All of these three substances protect against the harmful effects of drugs, and prevent damage to the liver and other organs.

HOW MEDICAL WORKERS SHOULD RELATE TO DRUGS

They Should Understand The Needs Of The Human Body

◆ *Drugs Injure The Whole System*

In order for us to aid nature properly, we must know how nature works. Only in this way can we assist her in her work. Only with such understanding can we intelligently cooperate with her in her work of healing, for ONLY NATURE HEALS. Without such knowledge we are more likely to hinder her than help her. The human organism represents a delicate machinery. Poisonous substances can destroy it and thereby do more harm than good. "Every pernicious drug placed in the human stomach, whether by prescription of physicians or by man himself, doing violence to the human organism, injures the whole machinery" (2SM280). "The physician who depends upon drug medication in his practice, shows that he does not understand the delicate machinery of the human organism. He is introducing into the system a SEED CROP that will never lose its destroying properties throughout the lifetime. I tell you this because I dare not withhold it. Christ paid too much for man's redemption to have his body so ruthlessly treated as it has been by drug medication" (2SM284)

◆ *The Physician Is Not Helping Patients By Using Drugs*

The physician should not claim that he is helping patients by giving them drugs, and NATURE wants none of such help as many claim that they have given her (MM223). "Nature will want some assistance to bring things to their proper condition, which may be found in the simplest remedies" (MM223). "But if the physician encourages a MEAT-EATING DIET to his invalid patients, then he will make a necessity for the use of drugs" (MM222). The physicians "prescribe drugs to cure disease which is the result of indulging unnatural appetites, and two evils are produced in the place of removing one" (MM225). "DRUG MEDICATION IS TO BE DISCARDED. On this point the conscience of the physician must ever be kept tender and true and clean. The inclination to use poisonous drugs, which kill if they do not cure, needs to be guarded against. Matters have been laid open before me in reference to the use of drugs. Many have been treated with drugs and the result has been DEATH. Our physicians, by practicing drug medication, have lost many cases that need not have died if they had left their drugs out of the sickroom" (MM227). It is seldom that a doctor investigates the tests to which a drug treatment has been subjected before he uses it on his patients.

The Physician Should Use Rational Methods

The function of hygienic practices is to RESPECT THE LAWS OF LIFE, base them upon the fundamental principles of physiology, and upon the built-in powers of nature. Hygienic methods strike at the cause of the trouble and endeavor to correct the underlying conditions which cause the symptoms. We are told that "in the work of healing let the physician work intelligently, NOT WITH DRUGS, but by following rational methods. Then let them by the prayer of faith draw upon the power of God to stay the progress of disease." (MM29). By rational methods is meant that "the patients must not be given ALCOHOL, TEA, COFFEE, or DRUGS; for these always leave traces of evil behind them. By observing these rules, many who have been given up by the physicians may be restored to health" (Te88). It is also not rational to give drugs for a disease which is not known or understood. "Very many lives have been sacrificed by physicians administering drugs for unknown diseases" (2SM452).

THE ATTITUDE OF OUR INSTITUTIONS TOWARD DRUGS

Mrs. White's Light Regarding Our Sanitariums

Mrs. White states regarding our SANITARIUMS that "As to drugs being used in our institutions, it is CONTRARY TO THE LIGHT which the Lord has been pleased to give. The drugging business has done more harm to our world and killed more than it has helped or cured. The light was first given to me why institutions should be established, that is, SANITARIUMS were to reform the medical practices of PHYSICIANS" (MM27). "Years ago the Lord revealed to me that institutions should be established for treating the sick without drugs" (MM229). "Institutions for the care of the sick are to be established where men and women may be placed under the care of God-fearing medical missionaries and be treated without drugs" (CH212). "Man is God's property, and the ruin that has been made of the living habitation, the suffering caused by the SEEDS OF DEATH sown in the human system, are an offense to God" (MM229). "It would have been better if from the first, all drugs had been kept out of our SANITARIUMS, and use had been made of such simple remedies as are found in PURE WATER, PURE AIR, SUNLIGHT, and some SIMPLE HERBS growing in the field. These would be just as efficacious as the drugs used under mysterious names, and concocted by human science. And they would leave no injurious effects in the system" (2SM291), for drugs "POISON THE CURRENT OF THE BLOOD" (CD303). "A simple diet and the entire absence of drugs, leaving nature free to recuperate the wasted energies of the body, would make our sanitariums far more effectual in restoring the sick to health" (CD303).

Health Reform Should Be Taught

We are told that "facilities should be provided at Loma Linda that the necessary instruction in medical lines may be given by instructors who fear the Lord and who are in harmony with his plans for the treatment of the sick" (MM62). "We must have medical instructors who will teach the science of healing without the use of drugs. We are to prepare a company of workers who will follow Christ's methods. I have been instructed that here (at Loma Linda) we should have a school conducted on the principles of the ancient SCHOOLS OF THE PROPHETS" (MM75). She was further shown that by Loma Linda "a solemn and sacred work was to be done. The teachings of HEALTH REFORM were to stand out clearly and brightly that all the youth in attendance might learn to practice them. ALL OUR EDUCATORS SHOULD BE STRICT HEALTH REFORMERS" (MM63).

How Nature Responds To Drugs

Whatever substances a patient is given in order to aid him in his restoration to health must be in harmony with the laws of his being. Drugs do not in any way harmonize with nature's laws and principles. They limit, restrict, and counteract natural processes, and therefore act contrary to them. When a patient recovers his health, he recovers it in spite of the drugs which hindered it and lengthened his recovery time (MH126). In such recovery honor is often given to the doctor and to the drug for the restoration of health. But there was no restorative power in the drug, it was all nature's doing. The drug actually hindered nature in the recovery process, but nature had sufficient vitality to overcome the hindrance (4SGa133). The general response of nature is to try to expel the drug from the system as quickly as possible (MH126). Nature will respond positively only to God's physicians of PURE AIR, PURE WATER, PROPER EXERCISE, AND A CLEAR CONSCIENCE.

Drugs Militate Against Patients Recovery

A recent study of a group of men in the age range from 35 to 57 who were in the category of HIGH BLOOD PRESSURE, and who received medication for their ailment, determined that they were DYING SOONER than men who received no drugs. It was further found that the more drugs were used by individuals, the higher was the rate of death. It is said that 10% of the 30 million people admitted to hospitals are there because of adverse drug reactions. One large hospital attributed 25% of its in-house deaths to adverse drug reactions.

GOD'S ATTITUDE TOWARD DRUGS

GOD WANTS US TO USE HIS NATURAL REMEDIES, the natural herbs which He Himself has created for our healing in the place of drugs (2SM287). He wants us to FOREVER ABANDON DRUGGING (CD83). He APPROVES and BLESSES ONLY HIS OWN REMEDIES (2SM287). The lack of approval and blessing in the taking of drugs implies that He will not in a special way intercede to restore a person to health who has disregarded His remedies. It means that He will not necessarily in a special way interpose the health and life of drug users. He will not in a special way answer their prayers, nor the prayers of the elders in their behalf, for He knows that they would repeat the same mistakes and would use the same wrong methods if He worked a miracle in their behalf. (2SM464) Under these circumstances, if their restoration is nevertheless brought about, it will be due to the vitality which still remained in their system (Te84). He will not supply a neglect that is due to IGNORANCE when knowledge was available (MM226). HE BLAMES GOD'S PEOPLE themselves when they take drugs (Te88). God wants us to call upon Him for help if we use His remedies (2SM289), and he pledges Himself to keep our bodies in good condition if we use His methods and means (MM221).

GOD'S DOCTORS FOR THE RESTORATION TO HEALTH

GOD'S TRUE REMEDIES

The Simple Agencies Of Nature

We are told that "there are many ways of practicing the healing art, but there is only ONE WAY THAT HEAVEN APPROVES. God's remedies are the SIMPLE AGENCIES OF NATURE that will not tax or debilitate the system through their powerful properties. PURE AIR and WATER, CLEANLINESS, a PROPER DIET, and a firm TRUST IN GOD are remedies for want of which thousands are dying; yet these remedies are going out of date because their skillful use requires work that the people do not appreciate." (CH323).

They are also called GOD'S DOCTORS. "FRESH AIR, EXERCISE, PURE WATER, and CLEAN, SWEET PREMISES are within the reach of all with but little expense; but DRUGS are EXPENSIVE, both in outlay of means and in the effect produced upon the system" (2SM287). God told Adam and Eve, "I have given you every HERB bearing seed, which is upon the face of all the earth, and every tree, in the which is the fruit of a tree yielding seed; to you it shall be for meat" (Gen. 1:29). Modern students of natural methods of healing have found that not only are the plants of the field good medicine, but that also the fruits and vegetables can be used for healing purposes. That is why some of them have written books entitled *Food Is Your Best Medicine*. God's specific MEDICINES are the HERBS OF THE FIELD, the nonpoisonous plants which He has allowed to grow upon the whole earth, so that everyone can avail himself of them. God does not want us to rely wholly on PRAYER in order to get well. It is good for us to have a part in our own restoration. It helps us to cooperate with God in this process. It will remind us of what we did to get sick, and of the great amount of energy that is expended in order to get well again. The chances are that we have probably "earned" our sickness, and we will thereby obtain a knowledge of what not to do in the future in order to avoid all of this pain and suffering. We must make the best use of the means which the Lord in His goodness has provided for us in our necessities. A knowledge of God's principles of health will allow us to prevent sickness in the future.

The methods and means which God has ordained for the healing of the body all HARMONIZE with all of the functions of the body. From the foundation of the world He has established remedies in nature which are available to everyone. This means that all of the available REMEDIES for disease are already in existence, and we should not have to look for new remedies of man's invention as something superior to that which God has ordained. The 8 doctors which He has established are "PURE AIR, SUNLIGHT, ABSTEMIOUSNESS, REST, EXERCISE, PROPER DIET, the USE of WATER, TRUST in DIVINE POWER,— these are the TRUE REMEDIES" (MH127).

We Must Know And Understand God's Remedies

We are told that "Every person should have knowledge of nature's remedial agencies and how to apply them. Health does not depend on CHANCE. It is the result of OBEDIENCE TO LAW" (MH127, 128). If in the 8 remedies for disease we replace the word "diet" with the word "nutrition," then the acronym that can be formed from these first letters is NEWSTART. Tom Kopko gives us the acronym GOD'S PLAN, which can be formed from the first letters of the following phrases: GOLDEN SUNSHINE, OPEN AIR, DAILY EXERCISE, SIMPLE TRUST IN GOD, PROPER REST, LOTS of WATER, ALWAYS TEMPERATE, and NUTRITION. "Through the agencies of nature, God is working day by day, hour by hour, moment by moment, to keep us alive, to build up and restore us. When any part of the body sustains injury, a healing process is at once begun; nature's agencies are set at work to restore soundness. But the power working through these agencies is the power of God. All life-giving power is from him. When one recover from disease it is God who restores him" (CH168).

God's Natural Methods Are Superior To Man's Method

◆ *God's Remedies Cleanse The System*

Many may question the idea as to whether these simple natural remedies are as effective as the powerful drugs which are generally dispensed by modern day physicians. First of all, God's methods will help cure disease, when drugs will not cure any disease. Secondly, God's methods will help cleanse the system when drugs will pollute the system. Thirdly, God's methods will cure diseases which cannot be cured in any other way. We are told that with God's methods "many who have been given up by physicians may be restored to health" (Te88). With God there are NO INCURABLE DISEASES. It is obvious why this should be so. Since drugs are poisons which do not cure any disease, they can only make a patient worse on that account. Except for his strong recuperative powers, he would naturally get worse and be finally given up by the doctor. The lack of the healing power of drugs also leads the doctor to perform MORE OPERATIONS. Since a diseased organ cannot be healed otherwise, it is finally determined that it must be taken out in order to save the patient's life. It is for this reason that hygienists say that 90% of all operations are unnecessary, in that the problem could be alleviated by other more natural means, by "the wise use of heaven's remedies."

"Christ never planted the SEEDS OF DEATH in the system. Satan planted these seeds when he tempted Adam to eat of the tree of knowledge which meant disobedience to God. Not one noxious plant was placed in the Lord's great garden, but after Adam and Eve sinned, POISONOUS HERBS sprang up. In the parable of the sower the question was asked the master, 'Didst not thou sow good seed in thy field? from whence then hath it tares?' The master answered, 'An enemy hath done this' (Matt. 13: 27, 28). All tares are sown by the evil one. Every noxious herb is of his sowing, and by his ingenious methods of amalgamation, he has corrupted the earth with tares.

"Then shall physicians continue to resort to drugs, which leave a deadly evil in the system, destroying that life which Christ came to restore? Christ's remedies CLEANSE the system. But SATAN HAS TEMPTED MAN to introduce into the system that which weakens the human machinery, clogging and destroying the fine, beautiful arrangements of God. The drugs administered to the sick do not restore, but destroy. DRUGS NEVER CURE. Instead they place in the system seeds which bear a very bitter harvest" (2SM288–9).

◆ *Nature's Processes Are Gradual*

When we study the natural process of healing, we find that it often does not proceed as fast as we would like to have it go. When we are sick we are in a hurry to get well. Patients are often impatient, and that strong desire to get well often leads us to adopt methods which appear to get us over our difficulty faster, but which have many effects which are harmful to us in the future. We are told that "The use of NATURAL REMEDIES requires an amount of care and effort that many are not willing to give. Nature's process of healing and upbuilding is gradual, and to the impatient it seems slow. The surrender of hurtful INDULGENCES requires SACRIFICE. But in the end it will be found that nature, untrammeled, does her work wisely and well. Those who persevere in obedience to her laws will reap the reward of health of body and health of mind" (MH127).

◆ *Natural Remedies Require More Skill*

"God's remedies will not tax or debilitate the system through their powerful properties. PURE AIR and WATER, CLEANLINESS, a PROPER DIET, PURITY of LIFE, and a firm TRUST IN GOD, are remedies for the want of which thousands are dying, yet these remedies are going out of date because their skillful use requires work that the people do not appreciate. Fresh air, exercise, pure water, and clean, sweet premises, are within the reach of all with but little expense; but DRUGS are EXPENSIVE, both in the outlay of means, and in the effect produced upon the system." (CH323).

Even though it takes more work to apply the natural remedies, we are admonished to minister to the sick with these remedies, and to teach them how to regain health and avoid disease (CH397). We are told that "If the sick and suffering will do only as well as they know in regard to living out the principles of HEALTH REFORM perseveringly, then they will in 9 cases out of 10 recover from their ailments" (MM224).

◆ *The Sick Must Have Confidence In Nature's Remedies*

The sick cannot be healed very effectively unless they have confidence in and believe in the natural remedies which God has provided. Physicians often prescribe drugs to cure a disease which is the result of INDULGING UNNATURAL APPETITES, and TWO EVILS ARE PRODUCED in the place of removing one. Thousands need to be educated patiently, kindly, tenderly, but decidedly that of their complaints are created by their own course of action. Also the obstructions to health must be removed, and opportunity must be given for nature to exert her healing forces, which she will surely do, if every abuse is removed and she is given a fair chance. We are told that many lives could be saved by natural methods of healing that would be lost by other methods (MH126–7). If nature had been left left to herself, and with the help of PURE AIR and PURE WATER, a speedy cure could have been effected in many cases.

If a healing agent is a naturally occurring BOTANICAL, it cannot be patented, and a drug company cannot control the rights to it. Hence, it cannot make the profits it might want to get from it. It then labels such products as "unproven," even though other countries have plenty of documentation supporting their effectiveness.

THE IMPORTANCE OF EXERCISE

Adam And Eve In Eden

Man's organic structure is made for movement and exercise. Adam and Eve were created to be useful and not idle. They were given the work of tending trees and bushes in the Garden of Eden. Such labor was to call into exercise the wonderful organs of the body. Their happiness was bound up with their labor. "Useful occupation was appointed them as a blessing to STRENGTHEN the BODY, to EXPAND the MIND, and to DEVELOP CHARACTER" (Ed21). The physical powers were to be kept in health by EXERCISE so as to also maintain and strengthen the spiritual powers.

It Is Necessary For Good Health

Sufficient exercise is an imperative for good health for two reasons. One is that it will tone up your muscles, improve digestion and general metabolism, keep the eliminative organs doing their work effectively, and contribute to better circulation and better function of all of the organs and glands. Secondly, it will increase and improve tissue oxygenation. THE ULTIMATE CAUSE OF ALL DISEASE AND PREMATURE AGING IS A LACK OF OXYGEN IN THE CELLS. Vigorous daily exercise will keep all of your cells and tissues well oxygenated, and in the peak of their efficiency.

We are told that "action is a law of our being" (MH237). It is impossible to maintain good health without it. All the organs of our organism depend upon it. The KIDNEYS, LIVER and MUSCLES are strengthened by it (2T533), and the SKIN and LUNGS are kept in a healthy condition through it (MH238). Exercise stimulates the ADRENAL HORMONES which are ANTIDEPRESSANTS. This develops what is called a "high," which is similar to the feeling which people get who are "high" on drugs. Such a "high" is due to the hormone NOREPINEPHRIN which is released by the adrenal glands. It is said to produce euphoric emotions. Exercise increases CHEST EXPANSION and OXYGEN intake; it increases LUNG CAPACITY, and thereby assures greater RESISTANCE to DISEASE; It is necessary for MUSCULAR DEVELOPMENT; it is essential for GROWTH and DEVELOPMENT of all organs; it encourages SKIN ACTIVITY, PERSPIRATION, and increases the ELIMINATION of WASTE PRODUCTS from the system. Dr. Kellogg has said: "All food that enters the mouth must leave the rectum within 16 hours, otherwise, damaging putrifaction begins."

Regular exercise is the single most important thing you can do for yourself if you want to live a long and healthy life. It can give you the equivalent of 10 years rejuvenation. The exercises which men prefer in their order of preference are: 1. fishing, 2. swimming, 3. weightlifting. The exercises which women prefer are: 1. swimming, 2. bicycling, 3. aerobic dance. A perfect exercise is the one that you stay with. Exercise is also a vital component of beauty, because it helps to NOURISH YOUR SKIN from the inside and enhance the entire cardiovascular system which in turn aids BLOOD FLOW to the skin which increases the skin's supply of NUTRIENTS, OXYGEN, and increases VITALITY and a RADIANT APPEARANCE. The most important factor which is likely to initiate a person's physical activity is his physician's recommendation.

It Quickens The Circulation Of The Blood

The quickened circulation of the blood through exercise invigorates every organ of the body. It is said to AID DIGESTION, PREVENT DISEASE, helps in the RECOVERY OF HEALTH, gives TONE to the Muscles, and keeps the SKIN in a healthy condition. It increases the flow of OXYGEN to all the ORGANS, which promotes the CLEANSING of the BLOOD by stimulating PERSPIRATION. It BURNS CALORIES, STRENGTHENS the IMMUNE system, REDUCES STRESS, LOWERS SERUM CHOLESTEROL, TONES the NERVOUS SYSTEM, DECREASES MUSCULAR FATIGUE, and gives a sense of WELL-BEING by releasing ENDORPHINS which reduce PAIN, and give the individual a sense of WELL-BEING. With regular exercise the heart can pump blood with LESS EFFORT, and the HEART ATTACK RISK is reduced by 20%. Much of the work of pushing the blood back to the heart is done by the CALF MUSCLES which squeeze the deep veins and force blood upward against gravity. That is why WALKING is often called the SECOND HEART.

Exercise In The Open Air

We need most of all to exercise where there is plenty of fresh air and pure OXYGEN. We are told that "Exercise in the open air should be prescribed as a LIFE-GIVING NECESSITY" (MH265). This is called AEROBIC exercise, and as one type of such exercise "there is nothing better than the CULTIVATION of the SOIL" (MH265). "Outdoor exercise combined with hygienic treatment, will work miracles in restoring and invigorating the diseased body, and refreshing the worn and weary mind" (CH171). "It is God's medicine for the restoration of health" (CH166). "The tiller of the soil finds in his labor all the movements that were ever practiced in the GYMNASIUM" (FE73). It is suggested that one wait at least two hours after eating before exercising, otherwise BLOOD FLOW to the STOMACH is decreased and food will digest more slowly. However, light exercise or a short walk after meals is beneficial (CD104). We are also advised that we should not eat after excessive exercise when one is exhausted or heated (MH306).

Sufficient exercise is imperative for good health for two reasons: 1. It will tone up your MUSCLES, improve DIGESTION and general METABOLISM, keep your ELIMINATIVE ORGANS doing their work effectively, and in general contribute to the better CIRCULATION and better function of all your organs and glands. 2. It will increase and improve your TISSUE OXYGENATION. Vigorous daily exercise will keep all your cells and tissues well oxygenated, and in the peak of their efficiency.

Exercise Eliminates Impurities From The System

◆ *The Skin Is Greatly Activated through Exercise*

Since we are told that the life is in the blood (Lev. 17:1), it means that the blood brings life to all parts of the organism. In order to have perfect health, we must have PERFECT CIRCULATION of the blood (MH293). Exercise also helps in the elimination of the body's BY-PRODUCTS of METABOLISM which may be impurities which are to be eliminated from the body. One of the organs that is greatly activated through exercise is the SKIN. We are told that through the process of sweating the skin can eliminate as much as 30% of all of the impurities that are generated. This takes a heavy burden from the other organs of elimination. For this reason the skin is referred to as ONE OF THE BODY'S ORGANS OF ELIMINATION.

◆ *The Benefit Of Massage.*

✓ IMPURITIES—We are told that "IMPURITIES are constantly thrown off from the body through the skin. Its millions of pores are quickly clogged unless kept clean by frequent bathing, and the impurities which should pass off through the skin become an additional burden to the other eliminative organs" (MH276). Leading medical men believe that 90% of all diseases are due to faulty elimination which allows poisons to remain in the body. A WARM BATH after a workout will UNTENSE your MUSCLES.

✓ ELIMINATES LACTIC ACID—A MASSAGE is effective after a workout, for it helps eliminate metabolic waste products, like LACTIC ACID, which develops in the muscles, of which an excess can clog the muscles. The body must drain this residue or convert it into sugar for storage. If lactic acid is left in the muscles, it forms tiny crystals that can cause pain and cramping. Lactic acid is formed in YOGURT when bacteria break down the milk sugar LACTOSE. Lactic acid is also developed in the muscles through exercise and exertion. When too much is developed, the muscles feel tired or have a burning sensation. But when you eat lactic acid it is broken down into sugar and used for energy, and therefore does not accumulate in the bloodstream or muscles.

✓ STIMULATES THE CIRCULATION—Massage increases blood flow to an area, helps RELAX MUSCLES, improves PERFORMANCE, and prevents INJURY. This is also what a DRY BRUSH MASSAGE does after a bath. It STIMULATES THE CIRCULATION and brings blood to the surface, keeps SKIN clean from DEAD CELLS and IMPURITIES, and it opens the PORES. The best time for it is after a cold shower in the morning and before going to bed.

Exercise reduces the risk of heart disease because it speeds up the removal of TRIGLYCERIDES from the bloodstream, says new research from Rockefeller University. Triglycerides flood the bloodstream after a meal and deposit part of their unneeded fatty load onto the walls of the arteries and thereby set the stage for a heart attack. The exercise reduces the risk of CORONARY HEART DISEASE.

✓ IMPROVES RECOVERY RATE—Massaging the soft tissues and muscles speeds up the release of the fluid toxins. It also gives an improved recovery rate, that is, it speeds up the ability of the muscles to perform normally after exertion and rest. For example: 5 minutes of rest after doing 50 push-ups produces a 20% recovery, which means that the subject can manage another 10 push-ups. But if the 50 push-ups are followed by 5 minutes of massage, the subject is able to do from 37 to 50 more push-up, or up to a 100% recovery.

✓ RELIEVES PAIN—A massage can relieve STIFFNESS, PAIN, NUMBNESS, and help reduce some SWELLING in sprains and fractures. It can stimulate DIGESTION, TONE MUSCLES, and relieve CONSTIPATION. Dilates the BLOOD VESSELS, relaxes SPASMS, and increases the NUTRITION of the TISSUES. Various massage techniques are good for HEADACHES, NERVOUS UPSET, and INSOMNIA.

✓ HELPS BABIES' MENTAL DEVELOPMENT—Dr. Field of Miami Medical School found that babies who are massaged showed signs of faster neurological development, and become more active and responsive than other babies. He found that slow strokes on a baby's back and legs helps it to relax, while light strokes on its face, belly or feet tend to stimulate. Dr. Wacks of Purdue University found that babies which are held more in the first six months of life were likely to have an advantage in mental development over babies held less.

◆ *The Skin As An Eliminative Organ*

It is estimated that of body impurities are excreted through the SKIN. If the skin becomes inactive and its pores are clogged with millions of dead cells, the impurities will remain in the body and may cause AUTOINTOXICATION therein. Over one pound of waste products is discharged through the skin every day. A Dutch physician by the name of SYLVIUS once said: " of all diseases can be cured by SWEATING."

Exercise And Disease

◆ Inactivity A Cause Of Disease

One of the basic causes of disease is the poisonous substances which are produced by the process of metabolism, and which are not readily eliminated from the body. We are told that "IMPURITIES are not expelled as they should be if the circulation had been quickened by vigorous exercise" (MH238). For this reason "inactivity is a fruitful cause of disease" (MH238). In many sickness cases, where it can be applied, it is BETTER THAN MEDICINE (MH240), for there are many sick people who will never get well without exercise (3T76). "Morning exercise, in walking in the free invigorating air of heaven is the surest safeguard against COLDS, COUGHS, CONGESTIONS of the BRAIN and LUNGS.... and a hundred other diseases" (HL903).

◆ Exercise Reduces Blood Pressure

Dr. Fahim found low levels of NEUROTRANSMITTERS in inactive animals, and higher levels in animals that had exercised regularly. Neurotransmitters such as NOREPINEPHRIN, SEROTONIN, and DOPAMINE, help the brain communicate with muscles and nerves. They tend to alleviate depression because they are thought to be low in depressed people. Lack of COORDINATION is a sign of low levels of neurotransmitters. Regular aerobic exercise, however, can restore their levels in about 5 months. Regular exercise can reduce BLOOD PRESSURE by 4 or 5 points by forcing blood into capillaries which were previously closed. OVERWEIGHT people tend to eat less when they exercise. Non-insulin dependent diabetes can be controlled and prevented through diet and exercise, especially with caloric restriction without drugs. It helps the pancreas by boosting its tolerance of carbohydrate foods, burning more food and thereby controlling weight. It also eases the need for insulin by lowering the blood sugar level.

◆ It Prevents Even Cancer

Exercise also speeds up the removal of TRIGLYCERIDES from the bloodstream, lowers the risk of ARTERY BLOCKAGES, and reduces the risk of heart disease. In normal hearts, muscle fibers are never injured by physical strain. Endurance exercises are best for heart development. A number of studies have shown that higher levels of fitness and exercise are correlated with lower rates of colon and breast cancer. Regular exercise increases the body's production of tissue PLASMINOGEN ACTIVATOR, a protein that helps dissolve blood clots that block arteries feeding the heart. Exercise helps those people who suffer from demineralization called OSTEOPOROSIS. It has been said that regular running from 3 to 5 miles a day can PREVENT CANCER because of the great amount of OXYGEN that is brought into the cells. It also eliminates cancer because exercise raises the body temperature, and a HIGH TEMPERATURE inhibits cancer growth. That is why a FEVER THERAPY has the beneficial effect of reducing and eliminating cancer growth. AEROBIC EXERCISE can actually decrease JOINT PAIN in people with ARTHRITIS, and has entirely eliminated arthritis in some people. In spite of this fact, arthritis patients are often advised to curtail physical activity.

A Harvard study in 1985 of 5400 women, all college graduates, showed that those who participated in SPORTS while in college had lower incidence of cancer than did their classmates who did not participate in sports.

Females who train in ballet, swimming, or running before puberty are more likely to begin menstruating at a later date, and have longer intermittent menstrual cycles than other girls.

◆ It Increases White Blood Cell Count

Exercise helps your infection fighting abilities by increasing the infection fighting WHITE BLOOD CELLS. Science has found out that exercise prevents HEART DISEASE, prevents strokes, prevents HIGH BLOOD PRESSURE, and prevents some forms of CANCER. SWIMMING is a non-weight-bearing sport. It is great for the JOINTS, especially for people with ANKLE, SHOULDER, or BACK PROBLEMS. It doesn't put any STRESS on the joints. Hence, it is great for anybody with arthritis. It is the standard exercise for older people who find it difficult to jog or walk. Studies show that you can get into good shape by swimming only twice a week for 15 minutes at a time. It means swimming about 25 yards every minute.

Go Out Of Your Way To Exercise

It has been shown that 75% of the people who exercise in the morning stick with it. Only 25% of the people who exercise in the evening stick with it. It is suggested that you go out of your way to exercise. Park half a mile from work and walk the rest of the way. Get off the bus two stops before your regular stop and walk the rest of the way. Walk the stairs even though there is an elevator in the building. Stair climbing requires as much energy as running, but it places only about the same amount of stress on the joints as walking. Also take a hiking vacation.

Exercise For Brain Workers

The brain is invigorated and relieved of weariness through exercise. When you exercise, the brain produces low levels of NATURAL OPIATES that actually improve your mental outlook. During exercise the mind is diverted from self to paying attention to those events and activities going on around us, and a greater degree of mental health is achieved thereby. It is often true that brain workers such as STUDENTS, TEACHERS, and MINISTERS do not get enough exercise. They often suffer from illness as a result of severe mental taxation, unrelieved by physical exercise. What they need is a more active life. Strictly temperate habits combined with proper exercise, would ensure both mental and physical vigor (MH238). They must become extra conscious of the need for exercise. Under these circumstances some GAIN WEIGHT because the SYSTEM is CLOGGED. Others becomes LEAN, FEEBLE, and WEAK, because their VITAL POWERS are EXHAUSTED, throwing off the excess food; the liver becomes burdened and is unable to throw off the impurities in the blood, and sickness is the result (CH572). The MIND is intimately connected with the BODY; suffers by its infirmities; is debilitated by its under-use, and is made much more efficient by its perfection. For this reason PHYSICAL EDUCATION is a necessary part of MENTAL EDUCATION.

The Results Of Inactivity

"The tendency of the misuse of all of our organs is toward decay and death" (MH237). "IDLENESS is the cause of many diseases" (CH166). Those individuals who do not exercise are not giving their lungs the FOOD they need which is PURE FRESH AIR. It is therefore impossible for the blood to be vitalized (CH173). "By neglecting to take physical exercise, by overworking mind and body, we UNBALANCE the NERVOUS SYSTEM. Those who thus shorten their lives by disregarding nature's laws are guilty of robbery toward God" (CH41). It is not exercise that kills people, but the diseases which so often come from a lack of exercise. The heart only functions well when demands are made upon it.

The lack of exercise has a depressing effect upon the whole organism. The BOWELS are ill-affected, DIGESTION is hindered, slowed down, or incompletely performed, and DYSPEPSIA or INDIGESTION develops, the MUSCLES are weakened, The MENTAL and MORAL POWERS are enfeebled, and the GENERAL HEALTH is affected adversely. "More people die for want of exercise than through overfatigue; very many more rust out than wear out" (2T525). "Neither study nor violent exercise should be engaged in immediately after a full meal. When mind or body is taxed heavily, the process of digestion is hindered" (HL576).

Exercise Increases Bone Mass

Medical researchers of Washington University studied exercising and non-exercising women ages 55 to 70. In 9 months the non-exercising women lost 1% of their bone mineral content. After 17 months of workouts the exercisers had increased their mineral content an average of 6.2%, a significant gain. 13 months after they stopped exercising, the exercisers bone mineral content had dropped 4.8%, which was still better than when they started. Hence, as indicated in another experiment also, exercise was shown to be one of the best ways to prevent age-related bone loss. By age 70 a sedentary woman has lost up to 30% of her total bone mass. By age 65, 25% of women have OSTEOPOROSIS. The bones become brittle and break spontaneously. Bones lose small amounts of calcium during the hours you lie asleep each night. Our bodies interpret LACK OF MOBILITY as a signal that CALCIUM is no longer needed. Tennis players and baseball pitchers increase the bone mass in the dominant arm.

It suggests that the strength of bones is definitely increased by exercise. WALKING also increases bone strength. A lack of exercise begins the process of thinning the bones.

Exercise Under Normal Conditions

For the average person in reasonably good condition, exercising 20 minutes a day is sufficient to maintain physical fitness. Your basic METABOLIC RATE slows down from 2 to 3% every decade after age 19, and it is said that a lower metabolic rate tends to increase the lifespan. Under normal conditions the circumference of your waist should not be larger than the circumference of your expanded chest. If you carry HAND WEIGHTS while walking, you can burn more calories per mile than you would while running. But they increase your blood pressure somewhat, so that they are not recommended for those with high blood pressure. A one mile walk uses up about 100 calories. Running for an hour at 10 miles per hour uses up 900 calories. Exercising just hour per day will keep you burning calories at a faster pace all day long. With moderate exercise a person can achieve the MAXIMAL OXYGEN VOLUME of a person 15 years younger. With a high degree of regular exercise the oxygen volume of a person 40 years younger can be achieved. Those people who exercise feel better about themselves than those who don't. It improves their SELF-IMAGE as well as their MENTAL SHARPNESS. For CALORIES NEEDED: Multiply your ideal weight by 10 if you are sedentary; by 17 if very active; 150 x 10 = 1500 cal. ; or by 17, 150 x 17 = 2250 cal.

Exercise And Aging

◆ *Exercise Makes You Live Longer*

With exercise you are never too old to grow young, for it will make you FEEL BETTER, LOOK YOUNGER, and LIVE LONGER. It can give you the equivalent of 10 years rejuvenation. A study of men between the ages of 35 and 74 who exercised regularly showed that they could expect to live an hour or two longer for every hour they exercised. The DEATH RISK is reduced by 50% if a person walks from 25 to 30 miles a week. Another study found that ATHLETIC STUDENTS have a longer life span than NON-ATHLETIC STUDENTS. It compensates for bodily decline by increasing HEART OUTPUT, LUNG CAPACITY, and BLOOD VOLUME. HARD WORK is the secret of staying young. The heart is a muscle that improves with work. It will produce a BETTER MEMORY, BETTER REASONING, and QUICKER REACTIONS.

◆ *Swimming, The Anti-aging Formula*

Higher levels of physical fitness appear to DELAY MORTALITY due to lowered rates of CARDIO-VASCULAR disease. Dr. Kraus believes that aging MUSCLES deprived of exercise, go through a progressive SHORTENING. They actually go through a progressive shortening the longer they are neglected. Scientists have found that they can actually predict how long a person may live by measuring the strength of his lungs VITAL LUNG CAPACITY. They say that SWIMMING stops the deterioration of lung capacity, or restores what age and disuse have taken away. Dr. Hutinger says that SWIMMING is the closest thing to an ANTI-AGING FORMULA.

The Miracle Of Walking

◆ *Walking Is Better Than Medicine*

One of the simplest, natural, inexpensive, controlled, and stressless exercise is walking. We are told that "there is no exercise that can take the place of walking. By it the circulation of the blood is greatly improved" (CH200). "When weather permits, all who can possibly do so ought to walk in the open air every day, summer and winter" (2T529). From the health standpoint one cannot think of a better exercise which is equal to swimming. "Walking in all cases where it is possible, is the best remedy for diseased bodies, because in this exercise all of the organs of the body are brought into use" (CH200). Walking stimulates thought by increasing the brain's supply of oxygen, and elevates one's spirit through the release of natural mood-elevating chemicals called ENDORPHINS. Walking is BETTER THAN MEDICINE, for we are told that "a walk, even in winter, would be more beneficial to health than all the medicine the doctor may prescribe" (CH53). It is the prescription without a medicine and the weight control without a diet.

A doctor examined an elderly man's left knee that hurt, and he said that that was to be expected. It is just a part of growing older. The patient replied that his right knee was just as old, but that it didn't hurt.

A woman from Louisiana walked to work for two years, and went from a size 16 to a size 10 dress, but she never went on a diet. Everyone wanted to know what kind of diet she was on. They could not believe that walking could do that.

A woman from Washington state was on blood pressure pills for 10 years and completely eliminated them by walking. She lost weight, reduced her salt intake, ate a low-fat high fiber diet, and ate garlic.

◆ *Walking Improves The Immune System*

"Walking is preferable to riding or driving, for it brings more of the muscles into exercise. The lungs are brought into healthy action, since it is impossible to walk briskly without inflating them" (MH240). A Loma Linda study of 50 women showed that walking improved the immune system, as well as the infectious illness rate. The more you walk the more you will maintain the circulation in your legs, the less PAIN you have, and the more you feel like walking. "When pain is felt in certain muscles after walking, or other exercise, it is caused by the effort of nature to give life and vigor to those parts that have become partially lifeless through inaction. Nature is awakening them to life" (CH200).

◆ *Walking—A Natural Body Healer*

Walking acts as a natural BRONCHO-DILATOR, releases CHEST CONGESTIONS, and helps the body expel TOXIC WASTES, and improves your BREATHING CAPACITY. If you experience SHORTNESS of BREATH, this is nature's indication that your body needs more oxygen. If you slow your breathing and concentrate on exhaling, you will restore oxygen to your system more rapidly.

Walking Is Everybody's Opportunity

Walking is the TRANQUILIZER without a pill; It is the COSMETIC not sold in a drugstore; it is the THERAPY without a psychoanalyst; it is the FOUNTAIN of YOUTH that can extend your lifespan; it is the VACATION that doesn't cost a cent; it is the EXERCISE that needs no gym; it is the GYM that needs no equipment; it requires no LESSON from the pros; it requires no EXPENDITURE beyond the price of an extra pair of shoes a year. It can take away ANGER and ANXIETY, solve a PROBLEM, and untangle PHYSICAL and PSYCHOLOGICAL KNOTS. It can be engaged INDIVIDUALLY or in GROUPS. Its TIME is anytime; its place is anyplace; and it fits into anybody's and everybody's SCHEDULE.

Walking stairs gives us 10 times the amount of work required in walking on the level. You will get more exercise out of your walking if you walk faster. Maintain the fastest pace that is natural for you. It is better to take longer strides, because it puts less weight on the feet and makes less work for the muscles. A good average pace is 3 miles per hour with an average number of 106 steps per minute.

Walking is Good Medicine

◆ *Making Use Of The Second Heart*

Walking is the best of all exercises according to physical fitness experts. Here they harmonize with the Spirit of Prophecy statements on the subject. It prevents HEART and CIRCULATORY disorders. It is the NON-DIETING DIET, the NON-EXERCISING EXERCISE that keeps the pounds under control. It is a remedy for RESPIRATORY disorders. It is an aid to SLEEP. It constitutes a SECOND HEART. The diaphragm, the calves, the thighs, the abdomen, and the muscles all help in the circulation of the blood. It lowers BLOOD PRESSURE, the PULSE RATE, and sustains the HEART MUSCLES in a healthy tone. At a time when men's hearts are failing them for fear, it is especially to be recommended.

◆ *A Stress Reliever*

Dr. Selye subjected 10 rats to stresses of LIGHT, NOISE, and ELECTRIC SHOCKS. In one month all had died. Then he took 10 rats and subjected them to the same stresses, but also gave them exercise on a treadmill. After a month they were all well and thriving. The conclusion: Exercise allows the body to make use of its RESTORATIVE POWERS. When Dr. Thomas Cureton put Billy Graham on an exercise program that included swimming, rowing, skiing, and jogging, the exercise that was first on his list was WALKING.

What Nature Lovers Say About Walking

✓ TREVELYAN—said: "I have two good doctors, my right leg and my left leg." SIGMUND FREUD said: "Only clever man invents short cuts to save work, and thereby deprives himself of the activity that can keep him healthy. Only clever man goes to excesses of ease and comfort that may do him harm." JOHN RUSKIN rose at 6 a.m., walked 6 miles, and worked 6 hours every day. WORDSWORTH at the age of 20 walked 350 miles, during a European holiday. When a traveler asked Wordsworth's assistant to show him her master's study, she answered: "Here is his library, but his study is out of doors."

✓ LINCOLN—used to walk to the top of a hillside outside of Springfield, Ill. He found that thoughts came to him as they never could when people and problems were crowding in upon him.

✓ ROBERT LOUIS STEPHENSEN—said that of all possible moods, the one in which a man takes to the open road is the best.

✓ EMERSON—said: "You do well when taking a walk that you take a dog along. A dog is a true pedestrian, who enters thoroughly into the spirit of the enterprise, contentedly sniffing adventure, and who looks upon every field and woods as a new world to be explored." He also said that walking has the best gymnastic value for the mind, and that one will never break down in a speech on a day on which one has walked 12 miles.

✓ THOREAU—said that he could not preserve his health and spirits, unless he spent at least 4 hours a day sauntering through the woods and over the hills and fields, free from all worldly entanglements. The word "SAUNTERING" is derived from people who in the Middle Ages asked for charity under the pretense of going to the Holy Land. They were called "Sainte Terre" in French. When children saw them they would exclaim "There goes a saint-terrer, a saunterer or holy-lander."

✓ JOHN BURROUGHS—a naturalist, said that the American has yet to learn the capability of amusement in a low key. He has nothing to invest in a walk; it is too slow, too cheap. We crave the astounding, the exciting, the far away, and do not know the highways of the gods when we see them.

✓ THOMAS JEFFERSON—said: "The sovereign invigorator of the body is exercise, and of all exercises walking is the best."

✓ HIPPOCRATES—called walking "man's best medicine."

✓ INTELLECTUALS—such as POETS, COMPOSERS, PAINTERS, and PHILOSOPHERS have always gone walking in order to think, to experience, and to dream. Pleasure asked: "Shall I walk or shall I ride?"; "walk," Joy replied.

THE NEED FOR AIR

Air Is A Life Necessity

Air is an important natural healing agent. Life in the open air is God's medicine for the restoration of life. It can restore the sick by natural means (MM233–4). We should encourage every patient to live out of doors, for nature will heal maladies both physical and spiritual. (MM232). The body requires fresh air, and it is even more important than MEDICINE, and more important than FOOD (CH55).

◆ *Air Purifies The Blood*

Without food we can live for months; without water we can live for days, but without air we can live only for a few minutes. "We are more dependent upon the air we breathe than upon the food we eat" (CH173). Fresh air purifies the blood and electrifies the whole body (MH385). The purpose of breathing is to supply the body's need for OXYGEN, and to eliminate CARBON DIOXIDE from the body. The blood flows through the lungs and gives off carbon dioxide from the cells. When in physical effort the amount of carbon dioxide is increased, the amount of oxygen intake is increased through breathing. Any increase in the oxygen content of the blood will decrease the breathing movement. Besides the LUNGS, the SKIN is also a breathing organ. If all the pores of the skin were closed, such as in the case of a burn over most of the body, a person would suffocate in a short time. A young girl died after her body was covered with aluminum paint to make her look like an angel.

◆ *Air Is Food For The Lungs*

In order for the lungs to be healthy, they need a constant supply of fresh air (MH274). Air is the food that God provides for the lungs (2T533). They are "constantly throwing off impurities, and the need to be constantly supplied with fresh air. Impure air does not afford the necessary supply of oxygen, and the blood passes to the brain and other organs without being vitalized. It is close confinement indoors that makes many women pale and feeble. They breathe the same air over and over, until it becomes laden with poisonous matter thrown off through the lungs and pores; and impurities are thus conveyed back to the blood" MH274).

There are other ways by which we obtain a reduced oxygen supply. The chlorination of our DRINKING WATER removes oxygen from it. The COOKING of food as well as the over-processing of our food lowers their oxygen content. Also the extensive use of ANTIBIOTICS destroys the beneficial oxygen-producing bacteria in the intestinal tract.

Air For The Sick

◆ *Air Is More Important Than Medicine*

We are told that "Air is an important natural healing agent. Life in the open air is good for body and mind. It is God's medicine for the restoration of health. PURE AIR, GOOD WATER, SUNSHINE, BEAUTIFUL SURROUNDINGS—these are His means for restoring the sick to health in natural ways" (MM233). "The pure air, the glad sunshine, the beautiful flowers and trees, the orchards and vineyards, and outdoor exercise amid these surroundings are health-giving—the elixir of life" (7T76). "Fresh air will prove far more essential to sick persons than medicine, and is far more essential to them than their food. They will do better and will recover sooner, when deprived of food than when deprived of fresh air" (CH55).

◆ *Fresh Air Conquers Disease*

Some people have felt that night air isn't good for them, but we are told that "night air is not injurious to health. The only air we have to breathe at night is night air. If we refuse to breathe night air, we must stop breathing. Many are suffering disease because of lack of night air" (2T528). Also FEVER cases require lots of fresh air. "Thousands have died for want of pure water and pure air who might have lived" (CH55). During the Spanish-American war and World War I, those of the sick and wounded who were moved outdoors into tents as overflow patients improved much more rapidly than those who were cared for in the hospital wards. During the 1919 flu epidemic, the hospital in Eureka, California was overflowing with patients. The head doctor called the army which gave them tents, cots, and blankets. The overflow patients were moved into the tents in which there was no heat, excepts that hot water bottles were used to keep the feet warm. It was found that no patients in the tents, with the fresh air they were getting, were dying. However, numbers of patients in the hospital were dying. When this was realized, the heat in the hospital was turned down and the windows were raised. The patients had to put on heavy underwear, but their death rate went down.

◆ *Oxygen Destroys Bacteria*

We are told that "if pure air is ever necessary, it is when any part of the system, as the lungs or stomach, is diseased" (CH53). "Many who have died of CONSUMPTION (tuberculosis), might have lived if they had breathed more pure air. Fresh outdoor air is as healing as medicine and leaves no injurious aftereffects" (2SM291). "Work performed in the open air is TENFOLD more beneficial to health than indoor labor" (FE73). Oxygen has been shown to destroy a wide variety of bacteria. It thereby strengthens the immune system. It also increases the number of LYMPHOCYTES which help to destroy bacteria. Extra oxygen is required by the white blood cells that eat germs, because when they engulf bacteria they produce certain poisons with the oxygen which destroys the germs.

Some of our most common diseases can be said to be directly related to OXYGEN STARVATION. Diseases such as ASTHMA, EMPHYSEMA, and diseases of the LUNGS are increasing greatly due to smoking as well as due to the pollution of the air in metropolitan areas. Vitamins such as NIACIN (B$_3$) as well as VITAMIN E promote the oxidation of the blood through their dilation of the blood vessels.

Indoor Air

◆ *Indoor Air Enervates The Whole Body*

"The effects produced by living in close, ill-ventilated rooms are these: The system becomes WEAK and UNHEALTHY, the CIRCULATION is DEPRESSED, the BLOOD MOVES SLUGGISHLY through the system because it is not purified and vitalized by the pure, invigorating air of heaven. The MIND becomes depressed and gloomy, while the whole system is enervated; and FEVERS and ACUTE DISEASES are liable to be generated.... The BODY becomes relaxed, the SKIN becomes sallow, DIGESTION is retarded, and the system is peculiarly sensitive to the influence of cold" (1T702).

◆ *The Destruction Of Negative Ions*

In an overheated apartment or room, the air, which to begin with might have been charged with negative ions, has been neutralized and ions eliminated. Overheated air injures health (4SGa152). STOVE HEAT is called injurious, poisonous, and a destroyer of life. It destroys the vitality of the air, and weakens the lungs (2SM305). The reason for this statement can now be clearly understood, because stove heat neutralizes the negative ions, and takes a lot of oxygen out of the air. People living in closed rooms or apartments may be starving for fresh air unless they keep their windows open, lower the temperature, and wear heavier clothing, in order to adjust to those new conditions. A room really should not be heated higher than 68 degrees Fahrenheit, which is too cool to be comfortable unless one puts on more clothing.

After getting up in the morning the bed should be aired out all day to eliminate poisonous effluent that has passed from the pores onto the sheets of the bed. If those sheets are otherwise slept on again, the poisonous effluent could be reabsorbed.

Once a week the bedding should be hung out in the sunshine.

The Great Benefits Of Pure Air

"Only pure air can make PURE BLOOD" (MH293), and since the life is in the blood, only pure air can give us a well-functioning organism. "Air, air, the precious boon of heaven, which all may have, will bless you with its invigorating influence if you will not refuse it entrance. Welcome it, cultivate a love for it, and it will prove a precious soother of the nerves. Air must be in constant circulation to be kept pure. The influence of pure, fresh air is to cause the blood to circulate healthfully through the system. It refreshes the body and tends to render it strong and healthy while at the same time its influence is decidedly felt upon the mind, imparting a degree of composure and serenity. It excites the appetite, and renders the digestion of food more perfect, and induces sound sweet sleep" (1T702). Air conditioning filters most of the dirt particles and allergens from the air, thus making it safer to breathe. "Pure air leaves no injurious effects in the system" (2SM291). Every day we breathe into our lungs about 30 pounds of air.

The Harmful Effects Of Impure Air

◆ *Impure Air Imperils Life*

A lack of fresh air poisons the blood (CH62), causes the system to be enfeebled and diseased, and this is what the Spirit of Prophecy calls a gradual self-murder (1T701). "The air laden with smoke and dust, with poisonous gases, and with germs of disease, is a peril to life" (MH262). "By inhaling impure air the blood is poisoned, the lungs become affected, and the whole system is diseased" (CH62). "Wastes from lungs and pores of the skin make impure air" (4SGa143). Decaying vegetable matter around the house causes poisoned air (2SM52). "Impure air does not afford the necessary supply of oxygen. It is laden with poisonous matter, and if breathed again, the impurities are pushed back into the blood" (MH274).

◆ *Satan Poisons The Atmosphere*

Even "Satan is working in the atmosphere: he is poisoning the atmosphere, and here we are dependent upon God for our lives—our present and eternal life" (2SM52). "He imparts to the air a deadly taint, and thousands perish by the pestilence" (CH451). Scientists have warned that air pollution carries the seeds of disaster, in that it results in a slow breakdown in the nation's health. An increase in LUNG CANCER parallels throughout the world an increase in AIR POLLUTION.

◆ *The Sun Can Change Substances Into Harmful Chemicals*

Air pollution sources are the incomplete combustion of FUELS, the manufacture of CHEMICALS, DUST, VAPORS, FUMES, MISTS, and specifics such as OZONE, SULFUR DIOXIDE, CARBON DIOXIDE. The HYDROCARBONS from car exhausts have been implicated in lung cancer incidence, while sulfur dioxide, released from pulp paper plants, causes ACID RAIN. Acid rain reduces crop production, reduces fish population in lakes, and damages stone structures. Air pollution causes trees to die, paint to blister, and window glass to discolor. It injures livestock and crops, causes respiratory infections, and diseases such as ASTHMA, BRONCHITIS, PULMONARY EMPHYSEMA, and HEART AILMENTS.

We know that the sun can change the chemicals in the air into other harmful chemicals.

◆ *Smog Can Cause Cancer*

SMOG contains cancer causing agents. These agents, when rubbed on the skin of rats, have caused cancer in them. The smog in Los Angeles is due to the growth in population, industry, chemical plants, auto and truck exhaust fumes, and backyard incinerators. It affects the EYES and causes coughing and sneezing, destroys the protective lining of the RESPIRATORY TRACT and can cause DIZZINESS, HEADACHES, and BLURRED VISION. One report determined that workers breathing unfiltered air in smog-filled Los Angeles are 15% less efficient at their jobs than workers who breathe cleansed air. The Metropolitan Life Insurance Company has found that chronic respiratory ailments are 33% more common among holders of its industrial policies, who breathe polluted factory air.

◆ *Incense Burning Can Cause Leukemia In Children*

It has been said that breathing the air in New York City is equivalent to smoking two packs of cigarettes a day. Since cigarette smoke, industrial fumes, drugs, air pollution, and water pollution use up vitamin C rapidly, take extra vitamin C when you are in such an environment, for the vitamin C helps the oxygen to burn up pollutants as well as the poisons produced by bacteria. Researchers at the University of Southern California found that the children of parents who burn INCENSE at home, had a risk of leukemia almost three times that of children whose parents did not burn incense.

The Beneficial Effects Of Negative Ions

◆ *Negative Ions Contribute To Our Feeling Of Well-being*

Whenever sunlight passes through the atmosphere, it charges some of the air molecules and produces IONS usually in the ratio of 4 negative ions to 5 positive ions. An ion is an atomic particle that carries an electric charge, either positive or negative. The NEGATIVE ions are usually the OXYGEN IONS, while the positive ions are usually contributed by CARBON DIOXIDE. Ions are produced by RADIATION, RADIOACTIVITY in the soil, THUNDERSTORMS, and by WATERFALLS when water breaks up into tiny droplets, which produce a lot of negative ions. It is the NEGATIVE IONS which are of great benefit to us, for they contribute to our feeling of well-being and exhilaration, give us more energy and act as NATURAL TRANQUILIZERS without harmful side effects. This is the reason why one breathes so much more easily at a waterfall as well as at the seashore where waves splash onto the beaches and against the rocks.

◆ *Plants Are Nature's Most Prolific Source Of Negative Ions*

A "healthy" ion level of 1000 to 2000 ions per cubic centimeter, a 5 to 4 ratio of positive to negative ions, is found over an open country field on a clear day. There are more ions in the WOODS than in the FIELD; more on a SUNNY day than on a CLOUDY day; and more where the ground has a high RADIOACTIVE content. PLANTS are nature's most prolific source of negative ions for they conduct the negative energy of the earth into the air by ejecting it from the tips of their leaves. We are told that "there are life-giving properties in the BALSAM of the PINE, in the FRAGRANCE of the CEDAR and the FIR, and other TREES also have properties that are HEALTH-RESTORING" (MH264).

One potted plant per 100 square feet of floor space can help clean the air in the average home or office. It is believed that plants absorb pollutants via the process of PHOTOSYNTHESIS. MICROORGANISMS living in potting soil use airborne TOXINS as a source of food. Plant roots keep the system functioning by taking up the wastes produced by those microorganisms. The plant then returns cleaner air to your home.

15 to 20 potted plants of the right variety, such as PHILODENDRONS, SPIDER PLANTS, ALOE VERA, PEACE LILIES, CORN PLANTS, POTTED IVY, SNAKEPLANTS, and FLOWERING BANANAS would do the work of a good high-efficiency air cleaner in purifying the air in a room.

◆ *Electrical Storms Produce Positive Ions*

Positive ions can be produced by various kinds of FRICTION, which tend to knock negative electrons off substances, leaving them positively charged. Hours or days before an ELECTRICAL STORM, the air is overloaded with positive ions from the CLOUDS that move ahead of it. It is these positive ion that cause ANIMALS to be RESTIVE, and INSECTS to explode suddenly, and become a plague instead of just a nuisance. After the storm has passed, the air is cleared of positive ions, and one feels able to breathe more easily again with an overabundance of negative ions. An excess of positive air ions causes an overproduction of the hormone SEROTONIN, which can lead to severe HEADACHES.

Many people get sick whenever the weather changes. Scientists now think that this is because of a fluctuating balance of positive and negative ions in the air. They speculate that electrically charged particles affect BRAIN CHEMISTRY by altering the secretion of CORTISOL, which is the body's natural steroid that prevents inflammation. This may explain why people with painful arthritic joints are especially sensitive to the changes in the weather.

◆ *Heating Systems Remove Negative Ions From The Air*

HEATING and AIR-CONDITIONING SYSTEMS usually REMOVE most of the negative ions from the air, and add positive charges to it. The increase of positive ions produces adverse effects such as HEADACHES, NASAL OBSTRUCTIONS, FATIGUE, DIZZINESS, and HOARSENESS. A cancer journal reported that negatively charged air has an INHIBITORY EFFECT on CANCER GROWTH. CALCIUM LACTATE, when combined with negatively charged air stops cancer growth completely. Alone calcium lactate has little effect on cancer growth. Negatively charged air has DECREASED the RESPIRATION RATE, has LOWERED BLOOD PRESSURE, while positively charged air has just the opposite effect. OUTDOOR AIR has many more negatively charged ions, while INDOOR AIR tends to have more positively charged ions. Hence, spending a lot more time in outdoor air and sunlight is highly beneficial.

What We Can Do To Counter Air Pollution

◆ *Move out Of The Cities*

One basic suggestion which is given us in the Spirit of Prophecy is to move out of the cities and into the country where the air is much more pure. For example, LUNG CANCER RATES are much higher among city dwellers than among country dwellers.

The air in our atmosphere normally contains about 20% oxygen. It has been reported that in many of our polluted cities the oxygen levels have dropped to about 10%. This pollution allows the extra oxygen containing hydrogen peroxide in the rain water to be neutralized before it reaches the earth.

◆ *Vitamins Give Protection*

Countless studies suggest that VITAMIN SUPPLEMENTATION can protect the body against environmental pollution. Vitamins A and E can neutralize many pollutants by retarding cellular damage. They can neutralize indoor levels of NITRIC OXIDE and NITROGEN OXIDE produced by a gas stove. They can neutralize CARBON MONOXIDE, probably the most health-damaging constituent of polluted air. It is contained in car engine exhaust fumes. It interferes with the oxygenation of all cells of your body by preventing oxygen from being absorbed by the lungs. Vitamin A protects the mucus membrane, including the lungs, against damage by OZONE and NITROGEN DIOXIDE in SMOG.

- ✓ OZONE (O_3)—is another pollutant that can menace our health. It is the principal ingredient in SMOG that passes for AIR in many cities. It may cause chronic lung disease by slowly destroying lung cells. But there is a way to fight ozone with VITAMIN E. Dr. Mustafa of the University of California subjected two groups of rats to a week of ozone after giving them two different amounts of vitamin E. One group he gave 11 parts per million (ppm), and the other group 66 ppm. The 11 ppm of vitamin E is about the amount obtained in the average American diet. This group had quite a bit of lung damage indicating that 11 ppm was not enough vitamin E to protect the lungs. The 66 ppm group had little lung damage. It is suggested that everyone should take about 300 IU of vitamin E as a precaution against ozone-caused lung damage.

Dr. Menzel of Duke University obtained similar results with animals. He found that animals exposed to lower levels of ozone run out of body stores of vitamin E in a few weeks, while animals breathing clean air do not. Experiments have also shown that vitamin E along with ZINC and VITAMIN C, can prevent LEAD absorption.

- ✓ CARBON MONOXIDE (CO)—is the most damaging health-destroying pollutant of polluted air. It interferes with the oxygenation of all the cells of the body by preventing oxygen from being absorbed by the lungs. It can cause RESPIRATORY DISORDERS, IRRITABILITY, LOSS OF MEMORY, HEADACHES, SHORTNESS OF BREATH, ANGINA, EMPHYSEMA, ANEMIA, HEART DISEASE and CANCER. A dose of 400 to 600 IU of VITAMIN E will increase tissue oxygenation as well as decrease the body's oxygen need, by preventing the undesirable oxidation of LIPIDS in the blood stream. Also 25,000 IU of vitamin A per day has a specific property against carbon monoxide.

- ✓ LEAD—Lead is present in air, water, and food in increasing amounts. It is one of the most toxic metal contaminants and can be fatal in even small amounts. It has been taken out of gasoline, and out of paints, but it is still in ceramic glazes and in other industrial sources. Lead is a cumulative poison. It can damage the KIDNEYS, LIVER, HEART, and NERVOUS SYSTEM. It can cause PARALYSIS of the EXTREMITIES, BLINDNESS, MENTAL DISTURBANCES, MENTAL RETARDATION, and even INSANITY. Some researchers believe that MULTIPLE SCLEROSIS is caused by lead poisoning. Lead is particularly dangerous to expectant mothers. Children born to lead-poisoned women suffer GROWTH RETARDATION and NERVOUS and MENTAL DISORDERS. It can be neutralized by CALCIUM which helps the body safely excrete it. Vitamin D, C, B, ZINC, and ALGIN, which is made from brown Pacific kelp, have been shown to help excrete lead from the body.

- ✓ MERCURY—Mercury is one of the universally present poisons in our environment. It is a deadly cumulative poison. It can be neutralized with BREWER'S YEAST which contains SELENIUM, a trace mineral that acts as an antidote, helping to destroy mercury in the body. Also vitamins A, C, E and the B-complex neutralize it.

- ✓ DDT—DDT is a cumulative poison, which is stored mainly in the fatty tissues of the body. While its use has been limited here, it is still widely used throughout the world. YOGURT and other SOURED MILK BACTERIA neutralize DDT in the intestines. WHEY POWDER or tablets feed the beneficial bacteria in the intestines, which help to neutralize DDT. Vitamin C is a powerful antitoxin which helps to neutralize all poisons.

- ✓ X-RAYS—X-rays are cumulative, so that even small amounts, such as those emitted by a color TV set, can add to the total amount received from all sources. Overexposure can cause

BIRTH DEFECTS, CANCER, and a later development of LEUKEMIA in a child born of a mother who received abdominal x-rays during pregnancy. It was shown that VITAMIN P, or BIOFLAVONOID, a natural substance closely associated with citrus fruits, reduced the death rate caused by excessive x-ray exposure by 800% in animal tests. PANTOTHENIC ACID, found largely in Brewers yeast, increased the survival rate in animals by 200% when given prior to exposure. Also vitamin C and a lemon peel concentrate allows patients to withstand larger therapeutic doses of x-rays without damage to healthy tissue.

✓ DRUGS—Most drugs interfere with normal enzyme and vitamin action in the body, causing derangement in metabolism and vital body processes. Drugs destroy vitamins and minerals and prevent their absorption. Many drugs damage the LIVER, KIDNEYS and can cause serious diseases such as IMPOTENCE, INFERTILITY, BIRTH DEFECTS, and CANCER. Large doses of vitamin C, up to 10,000 mg should be taken after heavy drug exposure. The B-complex vitamins are needed especially after treatment with antibiotics. Vitamins C and E are of specific value as protective agents against the damaging effects of ASPIRIN. Aspirin is consumed in the U.S. at the rate of over 30 tons a day, has caused many deaths, and millions of injuries. YOGURT and WHEY help to re-establish a new FLORA of beneficial bacteria killed by antibiotics and other drugs.

✓ ENVIRONMENTAL ADJUSTMENTS TO POLLUTION—Too low humidity in the home dries out the mucus membrane, making it more liable to irritation by pollutants, and leading to respiratory troubles. A HUMIDIFIER would be of help here. AIR-CONDITIONING helps to remove dirt and contaminants from the air, including pollen. A NEGATIVE ION GENERATOR, is said to relieve HEADACHES, RESPIRATORY CONDITIONS, speeds up the healing of BURNS and has a good effect on BLOOD PRESSURE. RESPIRATORY MASKS are good to wear whenever one works in a dusty, fumy atmosphere. PROFESSIONAL COOKS have the highest LUNG CANCER rates of all occupations due to large amounts of BENZOPYRENE occurring in the fumes and smoke from frying with grease. Planting TREES helps absorb carbon dioxide and restores oxygen to the air.

✓ RELIEVING A STUFFY NOSE—
- Boil CHAMOMILE flowers or EUCALYPTUS leaves and inhale the steam.
- A pinch of BASIL pushed up your nose brings back the sense of smell.
- Drink LEMON BALM or VERVAIN tea.

WATER

The Blessings Of Pure Water

We are told that "in health and in sickness pure water is one of heaven's choicest blessings. Its proper use promotes health. It is the beverage which God provided to quench the thirst of animals and man. Drunk freely, it helps to supply the necessities of the system, and assists nature to resist disease.... Thousands have died for want of pure water and pure air, who might have lived.... These blessings they need in order to become well. If they would become enlightened, and let medicine alone, and accustom themselves to outdoor exercise, and to air in their houses, summer and winter, and use soft water for drinking and bathing purposes, they would be comparatively well and happy instead of dragging out a miserable existence" (CD419).

Every drop of water is a gift of redeeming love (SD241). Men are indebted to God for it (CS17). It is one of the doctors provided by God (MM230). It helps nature to keep the body well (4SpGa141), and to resist disease, but it must be used wisely. In the East water is called "the gift of God" (DA83). "Water is the best liquid to cleanse the tissues" (Te101). "It helps remove poisons from the system (CH62). It purifies the blood (ML139). Water is used in the body as is. Its primary role is to serve as a transportation system for carrying on the life processes. Food is carried to all parts of the organism by water, the RED CELLS carry the oxygen by water throughout the body, WASTE is carried along on a stream of water, and all of the vital processes take place in a water solution. GORILLAS drink no water at all. Their diet is water sufficient. They get their water and mineral requirements from the food they eat.

Making The Proper Use Of Water

We are admonished to drink freely of water (CD419), for "it is the beverage which God provided to quench the thirst of animals and man"(MH237). It is within the reach of all and is very inexpensive (2SM287). Water plays a role in maintaining body temperature. By evaporation of perspiration the body is cooled. Water acts as a transporting medium for nutrients and all body substances, as well as for waste products. It is part of all body tissues. Almost all foods contain some water. Most foods rarely contain less than 70% water. CORN—70%, APPLES—80%, TOMATOES—95%. The oxidation of these foods in the body also provides water as an end-product. "Water can be used in many ways to relieve suffering. Drafts of clear hot water taken before eating, will never do any harm, but will rather be productive of good" (CD303). "One cannot be free from disease without pure water to drink" (MM226), and a neglect of cleanliness will induce disease (2SM460). The output of water through the lungs and skin is about the same as that voided in the urine.

Most people do not drink enough water, and this is a neglected and little explored factor in STONE FORMATION, which is also a strain on the kidneys. The tendency for a salt to crystallize out of solution is greater the more concentrated the solution is. In the "stone belts" of the world water is scarce and of poor quality, and the climate is hot so that most of the population is in a chronic state of water deprivation. In Israel where there is a high incidence of urinary stone formation, the incidence was reduced by educating the settlers to drink more water.

Water For Maintaining Health

Water has been used for maintaining health as well as for healing purposes since ancient times. People in various part of the world have sought the healing effect of NATURAL WATERS, MINERAL SPRINGS, SEA WATER, and SPRING WATER. HIPPOCRATES, GALEN, and others praised water for its many CURATIVE PROPERTIES. Father Kneipp of Bavaria said, "Water contains great healing power." To this millions who have taken to the waters can testify. Alternating HOT and COLD BATHS stimulate the body functions, and are excellent ways of revitalizing SKIN ACTIVITY and REPAIRING the CIRCULATION. There are SITZ BATHS, FOOT BATHS, SALT WATER BATHS, SULFUR BATHS, and MINERAL BATHS, all of which are highly beneficial. Dr. Henry Lindlahr sums up the value of a WATER CURE as follows: "There is no such thing as a 'Cure-all,' but if there were such a thing, it would be cold water, properly applied"

RAINWATER given to plants has been shown to be more effective than ordinary TAP WATER. It is the HYDROGEN PEROXIDE (H_2O_2) in the rain water which gives off an extra oxygen atom, which is more beneficial to the plants. Farmers have been increasing their crop yields by spraying them with diluted hydrogen peroxide. One can achieve the same beneficial effects with HOUSE PLANTS by adding 1 ounce of 3% hydrogen peroxide, or 16 drops of the 35% solution, to every quart of water one gives the plants.

Types Of Water

◆ *Soft Water—Distilled water*

The water you drink should be pure, soft water, without contaminants such as CHLORINE, FLUORINE or other chemicals that are designed to destroy germs, but are also poisons to the body. Water helps to maintain the electrolytic balance of the body. Only as long as the osmotic pressure exerted by solutes remains in equilibrium is it possible to have good health. Dehydration thickens the blood, and puts a strain upon the heart and arteries. We even need water to breathe. Our LUNGS must be moist in order to take in oxygen and excrete carbon dioxide. We lose a pint of water a day just exhaling.

"SOFT WATER should be used for drinking and bathing" (2SM456). Soft water is found in SPRINGS, RIVERS, and OCEAN. DISTILLED water and SNOW water is also soft water. Soft water is the ideal water for any cleaning work. Dr. Earp-Thomas added a few blades of WHEAT GRASS to fluoridated water. When the water was tested, no trace of fluorine was to be found. The wheat grass turned the fluorine into a harmless calcium-phosphate-fluoride compound. Without minerals, distilled water lightens the load of the kidneys, and actually allows the body to rid itself of built-up mineral deposits it can't use. Such minerals can form KIDNEY STONES, ARTHRITIC SPURRING, JOINT THICKENING, and even ATHEROSCLEROSIS. One of the best things one can do for kidney problems is to switch to DISTILLED WATER. It has been reported that many cases of ULCERATIVE COLITIS have been cured with it.

◆ *Hard Water And The Spirit Of Prophecy*

According to several studies in the areas of the world where water is HARD, meaning that it contains CALCIUM, MAGNESIUM, and other trace elements, the cardiovascular mortality is less than among those people who drink soft water. It has been shown for a long time that calcium and magnesium are good for the heart. Such results seem on the surface to contradict the Spirit of Prophecy statements. The following rationale can probably explain the apparent contradiction.

Magnesium is a trace mineral that is removed when foods are refined. It is found in whole grain flour but not in white flour. It is present in brown rice but not in white rice. Vitamin E is not present in white flour either, and it's deficiency causes heart disease. The B-vitamins are necessary to prevent heart disease, but they are also refined out of our grains. Our excess consumption of SALT also tends to cause heart disease. An average intake of about 120 pounds of REFINED SUGAR per person per year, robs the body of a lot of calcium. The higher the PHOSPHOROUS content of the diet, the less calcium is absorbed. Hence, diets high in refined cereals tend to rob the body of calcium, for cereals contain lots of phosphorous. MILK is also high in phosphorous, so that some of the calcium in milk is canceled out by its high phosphorous content. MEAT has 20 times more phosphorous than calcium. Hence, the excess phosphorous leads to a calcium deficiency, and also leads to heart disease. So when we see heart disease reduced with hard water, we can say that the people are generally deficient in calcium and magnesium, and that the drinking of hard water brings their calcium and magnesium balance closer to normal so as to give them fewer heart attacks. People who have sufficient calcium in their blood may get too much calcium from hard water and may develop HARDENING of the ARTERIES.

The normal white blood corpuscle count is about 6000/ml. When one drinks HARD WATER, this count will increase to up to 12,000/ml, indicating a pathogenic effect. This does not happen when one drinks pure water. It also happens when one eats cooked vegetables, but it does not happen when one eats raw vegetables and fruits. So mineralized water creates PATHOGENESIS by creating LEUKOCYTOSIS, the proliferation of the white corpuscles. Distilled water is pure water.

◆ *Mineral Water*

Mineral waters have been demonstrated in many places to have curative powers.

✓ BALNEOLOGY—is the science of curing and preventing sickness by the use of water. Russian scientists believe that SPAS prevent disease by stimulating the body's own defensive and resistant forces. It is a rather recent science and still incomplete, but it enforces the idea that mineral waters do have curative powers. This is somewhat obvious since disordered mineral metabolism and biochemical derangement are at the root of many diseases. It used to be believed that the body can utilize only ORGANIC minerals, and not the INORGANIC minerals. But scientists have reversed themselves on this point completely. Studies have shown that inorganic minerals are not only well utilized, but that they are of great importance in the maintenance of health. Dr. Schulf of Hungary has demonstrated that mineral water is actually absorbed through the skin during bathing. This is true when bathing in the sea, and the minerals are also absorbed through the inhaled mineral-rich air by the seashore.

✓ MINERAL BATHS—Many scientist have studied their therapeutic value and have concluded that MINERAL BATHS WORK. Since disordered mineral metabolism and biochemical derangements are at the root of many diseases, mineral water allows the minerals to be absorbed through the skin.

- ✓ HYDROTHERAPY—Biological doctors believe that HYDROTHERAPY is far superior to so-called wonder drugs in helping arthritics.
- ✓ NATURE-CURE SPAS—base their therapies on the belief that the body must build its own resistance to diseases. They are based upon the integrity of the body. Their aim is to find the cause of the illness, eliminate it, and the body will heal itself. Only natural remedies are used with emphasis on FASTING, PROPER NUTRITION, NATURAL HERBS, and VITAMINS. The principle that is applied is that within the organism itself lies the essential healing force for overcoming disease.
- ✓ EUROPE'S DOCTORS RECOMMEND SPAS—In Europe millions of people visit the spas on the recommendation of their doctors, take the CURES, and relieve themselves of ACHES and PAINS, OF ARTHRITIS, HIGH BLOOD PRESSURE, DEPRESSION, ECZEMA, DISORDERS of the HEART and BLOOD, RHEUMATISM, SKIN CONDITIONS, DISEASES of OLD AGE, and many other ailments. The doctors of Hungary have discovered that patients taking CORTISONE can do as well without it after taking the spa treatment. Dr. Kellogg's Battle Creek Spa was one of the most famous spas. Some of the European spas have been used for over 2000 years.
- ✓ SPRINGS FOR HEALTH—Of the different types of springs there are a. IODINE springs—which are helpful in HIGH BLOOD PRESSURE, EYE DISEASES, and CIRCULATORY problems; b. SULFUR springs—which are most helpful for RHEUMATIC problems, METABOLIC DISORDERS, and SKIN DISEASES. c. SODIUM CHLORIDE springs—which are helpful in correcting FUNCTIONAL DISORDERS OF THE CIRCULATION and WOMEN'S diseases; d. GLAUBER SALT springs—which promote the production of BILE, bring back the elasticity of the GALL BLADDER, and give help in OBESITY, DIABETES, and GOUT.
- ✓ INORGANIC MINERALS—Contrary to the opinions of some experts, INORGANIC MINERALS in natural waters are effectively absorbed and well utilized in human metabolism. In fact we need both organic and inorganic minerals for optimum health. The people of HUNZA, considered the healthiest people in the world, who never had any hardening of the arteries, kidney stones, tooth decay, arthritis, osteoporosis, or heart disease, have for 2000 years been drinking water so heavily mineralized with LIME and other inorganic minerals that it is milky in appearance.

◆ *Sea Water*

Some doctors believe that of all natural living waters, SEA WATER has the greatest curative power. They suggest that we use every opportunity to spend some time at the seashore. Salty sea water and salty air are stimulating and rejuvenating elixirs. They also suggest that we take one or two teaspoons of sea water each day with our meals, for sea water is one of the best MINERAL SUPPLEMENTS. It contains most of the TRACE MINERALS that have ever been discovered on the earth, and others some of which may have yet to be discovered. To be healthy we need the minerals that are contained in sea water. It has nearly the same composition as HUMAN BLOOD. This is the reason why doctors on battle ships have used sea water for BLOOD TRANSFUSIONS. Studies have been made to show that if a person who is burned over of his body is placed in a bathtub filled with sea water, and the water temperature is slightly above body temperature, and kept there day and night, he will live and grow new skin. A simulated sea water bath can be made at home with COMMON SALT, MAGNESIUM CHLORIDE, and EPSOM SALTS in the ratio of 7:1:1.

A 92 year old man was completely crippled with ARTHRITIS. He had to be lifted out of bed and could not feed or dress himself. On a doctors advice, he was given one teaspoonful of concentrated sea water per day, which was concentrated to 10 times the usual ocean strength. Soon he began to get up every morning without help and began to dress himself and fix his own breakfast.

Water And Disease

"Water is one of God's means for healing the sick" (MM233). "If those who are afflicted would assist nature in her efforts by the use of PURE, SOFT WATER, much suffering would be prevented. But many, instead of doing this, and seeking to remove the poisonous matter from the system, take a more deadly poison into the system, to remove a poison already there" (CH62). Water can put out the fire of a fever (2SM453). "In cases of severe fever, ABSTINENCE FROM FOOD for a short time will lessen the fever, and make the use of water more effectual" (CD190). "Thousands have died with raging fevers consuming them, until the fuel which fed the fever was burned up, the vitals consumed, and have died in the greatest agony, without being permitted to have water to allay their burning thirst" (CD420). Mrs. White was contradicting the principle of Hippocrates on this point when he said: "I have nothing to say in favor of water drinking in acute diseases."

Water treatments save many lives (2SM288), for water overcomes the system's bad conditions (ML139). It is a most powerful remedy (2SM346), and is more effective than drug medications (7T76). Mrs. White successfully used water treatments on her son Willie, who was ill with LUNG FEVER. Of this experience she said: "We continued to look to God in his behalf, and to use water freely upon his head, and a compress constantly upon his lungs, and soon he seemed as rational as ever.... He has not the injurious influence of drugs to recover from. Nature has nobly done her work to rid the system of IMPURITIES" (2SM304–5).

Dr. Hoffman says that if anything in the world can be called a PANACEA, it is pure water. Water purifies the innumerable passages of the human body. It dilutes and dissolves waste material, and carries nutrients to all parts of the organism. Dr. Balbirnic, a British hydropathic surgeon of the last century, used warm water in his treatments. He noticed that CONSUMPTION (TB), like many other diseases, was caused by a lack of OXYGEN in the bloodstream, and could be eliminated by the use of oxygenated water as well as fresh air. Father Kneipp with his "Water Cure," proved its efficacy by healing the ailing of nearly every known disease. Ann Wigmore has found that a HOT BATH, as hot as can be tolerated, relieves HEADACHES, especially MIGRAINE.

Internal And External Applications Of Water

"The external applications of water is one of the easiest and most satisfactory ways of regulating the circulation of the blood. A cold or cool bath is an excellent tonic. WARM BATHS open the PORES, and thus aid in the elimination of IMPURITIES. Both warm and neutral baths soothe the nerves and equalize the circulation.... There are many ways in which water can be applied to relieve pain and to check disease" (MH237). "Water treatments wisely and skillfully given, may be the means of saving many lives" (MM57). We are told, however, that "the use of water can accomplish little if the patient doesn't strictly attend to his DIET also." (CD304).

◆ *Hot And Cold Baths*

We are told that "Persons in health should on no account neglect bathing. They should by all means bathe as often as twice a week.... respiration is more free and easy if bathing is practiced" (CH104). It has been said that 1. COLD SHOWER will stimulate CIRCULATION and increase MUSCLE TONE and NERVE FORCE, 2. will stimulate the GLANDULAR SYSTEM and increase HORMONE PRODUCTION, 3. build RESISTANCE against COLDS and INFECTIONS, 4. help prevent PREMATURE AGING, 5. and will help increase RED BLOOD CELL COUNT. Some doctors claim that a cold shower is mildly electronic in action, and increases the intake of OXYGEN to a remarkable degree. Oxygen is life itself. The more oxygen in your blood and your cells, the better your health. On the other hand a warm or neutral bath (92 degrees), dilates the blood vessels and increases the circulation to the extremities which dissipate heat throughout the body and restore and induce sleep.

◆ *The Finnish Sauna*

The Sauna, or Finnish steam bath, is especially conducive to profuse sweating. The skin, being our largest eliminative organ, sometimes called "the third kidney," is generally considered to eliminate 30% of the body wastes by way of perspiration. It creates a fever temperature to help DESTROY BACTERIA, STIMULATE the GLANDS, ACCELERATE HEALING, and ELIMINATE TOXINS from the body. Water is thrown over hot stones to produce steam which fills the room and raises the temperature. This steam also contains a lot of NEGATIVE IONS which are beneficial to health. Many toxins are thrown out of the body with the perspiration. URIC ACID, a normal compound of urine, is found in large amounts in the perspiration. The chemical analysis of sweat shows that it has almost the same constituents as urine.

The therapeutic properties of the sauna is attributed to 1. the speed up of METABOLIC PROCESSES, 2. the inhibition of the growth of VIRUSES and BACTERIA, 3. The stimulation of the GLANDS to increased activity, 4. The acceleration of the body's HEALING and RESTORATIVE capacity, 5. and the increase of the ELIMINATIVE, DETOXIFYING, and CLEANSING capacity of the SKIN. Many authorities attribute the phenomenal therapeutic properties of the sauna to the Finnish custom of jumping into cold water or snow during bathing. The sudden changes in temperature are known to stimulate the ADRENAL GLANDS, and such effect of the alternate hot and cold bath is likened to a CORTISONE INJECTION.

◆ *The Schlenz-Bath For Incurable Diseases*

The Schlenz-Bath method is an overheating therapy which is designed to heal with heat, or to heal by means of creating an ARTIFICIAL FEVER. The great physician Parmenides said 2000 years ago, "Give me a chance to create a fever, and I will cure any disease." Fever is one of the body's own healing forces created for the purpose of restoring health. The high temperature of a fever speeds up METABOLISM, inhibits the growth of invading BACTERIA, and burns up the impurities of the system. It is a healing measure not only against simple INFECTIONS and COLDS, but also against more serious diseases such as POLIO and CANCER. It is a method which is widely employed in Europe, and particularly by Prof. Werner ZABEL, the leading biological doctor in Germany, who uses it in his clinic in Berchtesgarden, as well as by Drs. ISSELS and LWOFF, the latter being a Nobel Prize winner. They testify to the fact that it does indeed cure so-called "incurable" diseases.

In this method the patient, in a bathtub, must be totally covered with water, including his head, except for his nose, eyes and mouth. Water is slowly run into the bathtub from a temperature of 95 degrees up to 104 degrees Fahrenheit (36 to 40 degrees Centigrade) and even higher, depending upon the patients reactions. The length of the treatment is one hour. The secret of this method is that the body is totally covered by water, there is no heat escaping from the body, and its temperature will rise to match the temperature of the water.

Impure Water

We are told that "the physical surroundings in the cities are often a peril to health. The constant liability to contact with DISEASE, the prevalence of FOUL AIR, IMPURE WATER, IMPURE FOOD, the crowded dark UNHEALTHFUL DWELLINGS, ARE SOME OF THE MANY EVILS TO BE MET" (MH365).

◆ *Contains Harmful Chemicals*

There can be two types of water poisoning: 1. The pollution of drinking water by NATURAL SOURCES or INDUSTRIAL WASTES, and 2. the CHEMICALS that are ADDED to WATER to remove impurities. This is a matter of adding impurities to remove impurities. Industrial chemicals such as MERCURY dumped into lakes are picked up by organisms, and travel up the food chain to FISH, LIVESTOCK, PETS, and PEOPLE. Protecting crops from insect pests risks the poisoning of our drinking water from PESTICIDES seeping through the soil, and accumulating in body tissues where they jeopardize our health. Researchers found that children whose parents use pesticides inside the home have an almost 4 times greater risk of developing childhood leukemia. Agricultural fertilizers such as NITRATES have been found in well water. They have caused poisoning of INFANTS who are especially susceptible to nitrates.

◆ *Causes Disease*

CHLORINATED WATER can cause ALLERGIES, ASTHMA, HIVES, COLITIS, DIABETES, GOUT, KIDNEY STONES, MUSCULAR SCLEROSIS, MUSCULAR DYSTROPHY, and CORONARY THROMBOSIS. A test with chickens showed that after 7 months every chicken fed chlorinated water had developed atherosclerosis, while not a single chicken fed pure water had done so. Japan has a low incidence of heart disease, but when

Japanese move to Hawaii and drink their chlorinated water, they develop atherosclerosis. 75% of American soldiers who were killed in Korea showed evidence of coronary atherosclerosis. The water in Korea was so heavily chlorinated for sanitary reasons that it was almost undrinkable. When chlorine reacts with organic matter in the water, it forms cancer-causing compounds. A study by the National Cancer Institute found that chlorinated drinking water increased the risk of BLADDER CANCER. It was estimated that it might be responsible for of all bladder cancers among non-smokers.

◆ *Destroys Vitamins*

Chlorinated water destroys vitamin E, and a lack of vitamin E will produce heart disease. It also destroys vitamins A, B, and C as well as the amino acid TRYPTOPHANE. DDT and other chlorinated hydrocarbons are "delayed reaction poisons" which are cumulative in the human body' showing up years after they have been ingested. The effect of chlorine is to reduce TYPHOID FEVER and to increase HEART DISEASE. HOUSE PLANTS will not thrive in chlorinated water, nor will guppies live in such water. The story is told of a cow, brought up on pure ranch water, who could not take part in a contest when brought to the city, because it refused to drink chlorinated water.

◆ *Fluorine Increases Cancer Rates*

A scientific study in the 70's showed that cities with FLUORIDATED water supplies had a 5% increase in CANCER RATES. At levels of 1 part per million fluorine has been shown to increase TUMOR GROWTH RATES, and to increase CANCER DEATH RATES by destroying body ENZYMES. In a study of the water in the city of New Orleans, its high cancer rates were traced to drinking water taken from the Mississippi river. Cooking in ALUMINUM COOKWARE with water containing fluorides increases the aluminum concentration by up to a thousand times more than cooking in fluorine-free water. Boiling will eliminate all traces of chlorine from water, but it will not eliminate fluorine, which can be eliminated through the process of distillation.

◆ *Mass Medication With Fluorine*

Fluorine does help strengthen CHILDREN'S TEETH at ages from 9 to 12, but since it is put into the water for everybody to drink, such a process must be considered to be MASS MEDICATION. Furthermore, the type of fluorine compound put into the drinking water is called SODIUM FLUORIDE. It is a by-product of aluminum production. This compound is a highly toxic PROTOPLASMIC POISON which accumulates in the body. On the other hand, the fluorine in natural water is called CALCIUM FLUORIDE, which is a relatively harmless substance, for it is 85 times less toxic than sodium fluoride. Sodium fluoride is more toxic than LEAD, and is just slightly less toxic than ARSENIC. The government gave it a maximum contamination level of 200 times that of lead. Dr. Steyn says that a deficient diet, and not a fluoride deficiency, is the most important cause of dental decay. Fluoridation also causes FLUOROSIS, or the mottling of tooth enamel, MONGOLISM in infants, KIDNEY DAMAGE, and interferes with ENZYME, MINERAL, and VITAMIN functions of the system. Drinking fluoridated water has been directly linked to BONE MALFORMATION as well as to ARTHRITIS.

Fluorine inhibits over 100 different enzymes in the soft tissues of the body. It DISRUPTS HYDROGEN BONDS, BONE MALFORMATION, CALCIUM DEPOSITS, HYPOTHYROIDISM leading to OBESITY problems, GENETIC DAMAGE, BIRTH DEFECTS, ALLERGY, and CANCER. 1 part per million (ppm) fluoride interferes with COLLAGEN METABOLISM. A .4 to .8 ppm in drinking water causes MOTTLED TEETH. According to Dr. Burk, fluoridation alone results in a 5% to 10% increase in the CANCER DEATH RATE. This means that from 10 to 20 thousand people in the U.S. die of cancer each year due to fluoridation. Death from all causes is 5% higher in fluoridated areas than in non-fluoridated areas. Many countries in Europe, such as Sweden, Holland, Germany, Italy, France, Norway, have abandoned fluoridation for lack of sufficient evidence of its benefit or safety. Over 50% of the population in the U.S. drink fluoridated water.

Water And Diet

◆ *Cold Drinks*

We are told that "many make a mistake in drinking cold water with their meals. Taken with meals, water diminishes the flow of the salivary glands, and the colder the water, the greater the injury to the stomach. ICE WATER or ice lemonade, drunk with meals, will arrest digestion until the system has imparted sufficient warmth to the stomach"(CD420).

◆ *Hot Drinks*

HOT DRINKS are debilitating, and besides, those who indulge in their use become slaves to the habit. Food should not be washed down.

◆ *Drinking With Meals*

"NO DRINK is needed WITH MEALS. Eat slowly and allow the saliva to mingle with the food. The more liquid there is taken into the stomach with the meals, the more difficult it is for the food to digest; for the liquid must first be absorbed" (CD420). The stomach must be approximately 100 degrees Fahrenheit before it can start digestion, and cold drinks reduce the stomach's temperature.

◆ *Drinking Between Meals*

Water should be DRUNK BETWEEN MEALS, and not closer than one half hour before and after the meal.

In an average day, a person loses about 80 ounces of water through URINATION, DEFICATION, RESPIRATION, and PERSPIRATION. This is the reason behind the idea that we should drink 8 10-ounce glasses of water a day.

◆ *Vegetarians May Drink Less Water Than Is Recommended*

This water is replaced by drinking liquids. We also get water from food. An apple, for example, is 84% water. This is why someone has suggested that VEGETARIANS don't need to drink quite 8 glasses of water a day, because their food of fresh fruits and vegetables itself contains more water than other foods. Also when food is digested, water is a BY-PRODUCT of the process of DIGESTION. Whenever one's activity increases, water loss also increases, which means that the consumption of liquids should increase also.

Some have suggested that like in the case of eating food which we should eat only when hungry, that we should drink only when thirsty. This may be a debatable suggestion. It is said that people who eat COOKED FOOD require more water than those who eat raw food, in order to hold noxious substances in solution. Persons who use CONDIMENTS develop strong thirsts because condiments are irritants, and much water is required to hold them in solution. People who use lots of fresh fruit and vegetables, and avoid animal products, and starchy foods require less water. Fruits and vegetables themselves average over 85% water.

SUNLIGHT

Sunlight As Healer

Sunlight is essential to health. It is a healer and health maintainer. For this reason we should avail ourselves of every opportunity to get as much sunlight as possible (2SM296). It is health-giving and life-giving (MH264). Another doctor which God has provided for our health is "the HEALING PRECIOUS SUNLIGHT" (2SM287). It is another one of those blessings which "Heaven has provided to make the sick well and to keep in health those who are not sick" (2T535). Sick people are benefited by lying in the SUNSHINE (MH264), which is one of nature's most healing agents (2T527).

"We have often deprived ourself of that which, if properly used, is of inestimable value for the recovery of health. The sunlight may fade the drapery and the carpet, and tarnish the picture frames; but it will bring a healthy glow to the cheeks of the children" (MH275). Houses need sunlight in every room (MH274). Sunshine is DEATH TO ALL DISEASE-PRODUCING AGENCIES, and it is LIFE and HEALTH to all NATURAL FORMS OF LIFE. Since Christ is also the PHYSICAL and SPIRITUAL HEALER, He is called the SUN of RIGHTEOUSNESS (Mal. 4:2).

Sunlight In Health

◆ *Health Benefits*

Christ provided the sunshine to keep the well in health (2T535). Plenty of sunshine is essential to freedom from disease (MH276). Sunshine is valuable in forming strong bones. It is said that sunshine has the same effect upon the body as EXERCISE. They both decrease the RESTING HEART RATE; also the RESPIRATORY RATE; BLOOD SUG-

AR; the amount of LACTIC ACID in the BLOOD following exercise. They also increase ENERGY, STRENGTH, ENDURANCE, TOLERANCE to STRESS, and the ability of the blood to absorb OXYGEN. Sunlight stimulates the THYROID GLAND to increase HORMONE PRODUCTION, which increases the body's BASAL METABOLISM RATE, which in turn burns up more calories. It helps the absorption of GLUCOSE into the cells, and stimulates the body to convert it into GLYCOGEN to be stored.

Humans are also said to be "photosynthetic." Through our skin and eyes we absorb light as directly as plants do. There are SOLAR ENERGY CELLS all over the body, so that METABOLISM in humans is the same as PHOTOSYNTHESIS in plants. The lower on the food chain we eat, the closer our food is to being directly manufactured from light, the closer we are receiving light's full force. The most LIGHT-FILLED FOODS are probably the BLUE-GREEN ALGAE, and ORGANICALLY GROWN fruits and vegetables.

◆ *It Speeds Recoveries*

There has been found a much larger percentage of recoveries in hospital rooms which are exposed to the sun, than in those which are excluded from its rays. Sunlight reduces the SERUM CHOLESTEROL in the blood. When cholesterol is high, it becomes incorporated into the walls of the RED BLOOD CELLS, which reduces their OXYGEN CARRYING CAPACITY. It has been estimated that 50% of the deaths in this country are attributable to diseases of the HEART AND circulatory system, and are largely caused by excessive cholesterol. One study of school children showed that the incidence of DENTAL CAVITIES was much higher during the SCHOOL YEAR, WINTER and SPRING, than during the summer months. This was directly related to the amount of sunlight they were getting. The more sunlight the fewer the cavities.

SUNLIGHT TREATMENTS cause a definite reduction of ARTHRITIS, for they loosen stiff joints. They are also beneficial for the HEALING of WOUNDS. Wounds heal faster and better, and are kept germ free. They speed up the elimination of toxic agents, and help remove DUST from the LUNGS. In some areas in Russia MINERS are given sunlight treatments every day to help remove coal dust from their lungs. It eliminates all types of disease causing agents, including cancer agents. Under normal conditions sunlight WARDS OFF CANCER by increasing the use of OXYGEN in the tissues. It is good for the BONES, COLDS, METABOLIC PROCESSES, and it PROMOTES SLEEP.

◆ *Exposure To Sunlight*

MULTIPLE SHORT EXPOSURES to sunlight are more effective than a single long exposure. Sunshine is nature's STIMULANT and TONIC, INVIGORATOR, and REJUVENATOR. It revitalizes the function of every gland in your body. It strengthens the IMMUNE SYSTEM. It increases lymphocyte production and thereby increases the production of INTERFERON, which is a substance which has the ability to stop the reproduction of VIRUSES. It is effective against the viruses of CARCINOMA, SARCOMA, and LEUKEMIA. SUNBATHING should be done in moderation like everything else. The TAN that protects the body from overexposure must be built gradually. It has been shown that WET SKIN will burn more readily than dry skin. Take a sunbath only if your shadow in the sun is as long as you are tall or longer. That would be the safest time to be out in the sun. The best time to take a SUNBATH is before 11 a.m. and after 3 p.m., when the rays are less strong. Expose the skin up to 15 min. the first day, and 15 min. a day thereafter until a good tan is produced. BLOND and RED-HAIRED people require less sunlight than do BRUNETTES, because light passes more readily through lighter skin. BETA-CAROTENE gives sunlight relief to those individuals who are sensitive to it.

Sunlight And Vitamin D

The body manufactures vitamin D with the aid of sunlight. It is produced in the skin when the sun's rays are absorbed. CHOLESTEROL CONCENTRATION is higher in the human skin than in any other organ. Cholesterol is changed by sunlight to pre-vitamin D, which is changed to vitamin D by the normal heat of the body in a period of from 24 to 48 hours. If you take a water bath right after you have taken a sunbath, the vitamin D potential is nullified. Sunshine on the back is more effective in producing vitamin D than sunshine on the stomach.

Vitamin D is more of a hormone than a vitamin. It is produced from cholesterol just as are other steroid hormones. Vitamin D is necessary for calcium absorption in the intestines. Dr. Goldberg believes that it is the shorter wavelength radiation that causes the formation of vitamin D in the skin, and that it is ALTITUDE rather than LATITUDE that determines their strength. So the higher you live on the mountain side, the more shortwave radiation you receive, the more vitamin D your skin forms, the more calcium your intestines absorb, and the lower your risk of MULTIPLE SCLEROSIS, COLON CANCER, and other diseases.

On the other hand, excessive vitamin D supplementation causes a MAGNESIUM DEFICIENCY in the heart, as well as higher blood cholesterol. We are getting a lot of supplemental vitamin D in DAIRY PRODUCTS, BEVERAGES, SAUCES, BREAKFAST CEREALS, MARGARINE, MACARONI, NOODLES, FARINA, and FLOUR. The vitamin D added to these products is synthetic vitamin D called CALCIFEROL, which is manufactured in the laboratory. It can cause HYPERCALCEMIA, or too much calcium in the blood, caused by being drained from the bones. It leads to weakness of the bones and muscles. The reason for this is that in nature, in FISH LIVER OILS, vitamin D always comes accompanied with VITAMIN A. Such natural vitamin D with vitamin A has never produced hypercalcemia. The synthetic vitamin D has also caused BLOODY URINE.

◆ *Sunburn*

SUNBATHING forces the skin to increase the production of MELANIN, the pigment that gives dark skin its color, and makes lighter skin look "tan." You can get a tan and a sunburn on a cloudy day, for 60 to 80% of the ultraviolet rays will come through. CAROTENE has been shown to be more effective than VITAMIN E in preventing a sunburn. Using a SUNSCREEN LOTION during a sunbath will avoid a sunburn, but it will also keep the skin from producing vitamin D. Remember that a sunburn is a BURN, which represents some damage to the skin. When the skin is reddened by sunlight, a hormone-like substance called PROSTAGLANDIN is produced. It is produced from LINOLEIC ACID which is found in monounsaturated oil, such as OLIVE OIL and CORN OIL. Prostaglandin is a substance which INHIBITS the IMMUNE SYSTEM.

Most sunscreens protect the skin from the sun's ultraviolet-B rays (UV-B). They do not stop the more damaging UV-A rays. A NATURAL SUNSCREEN which protects the skin from both types of rays can be readily made as a 10% solution of powdered vitamin C and water. It does even more than that: It can prevent SKIN CANCER from overexposure to both UV-A and UV-B rays, and it also heals unhealthy skin conditions such as PSORIASIS, ECZEMA, and IMPETIGO at the same time.

Ultraviolet Light (UVL)

◆ *Benefits Of UVL*

✓ REDUCES ILLNESSES—It has been shown that persons who are regularly exposed to ULTRAVIOLET light develop FEWER ILLNESSES. In 1976 Heding found that UVL could inactivate and destroy CANCER PRODUCING VIRUSES. UVL through the eyes is said to stimulate the IMMUNE SYSTEM. In proper amounts UVL acts like a "life-supporting nutrient" that is highly beneficial.

✓ INCREASES OXYGEN IN THE BLOOD—It increases the OXYGEN in the blood as well as its oxygen carrying capacity, increases the discharge of CARBON DIOXIDE, and gives PAIN RELIEF. After an individual is exposed to UVL, the NEUTROPHILS, one type of white blood cells, in his blood are stimulated to EAT GERMS more rapidly.

SELENIUM is a trace mineral which protects cells against HARMFUL OXIDATION in much the same way that rustproofing protects cars. It keeps free radicals from doing damage after they have formed. If plenty of vitamin E is present to keep free radicals from forming, there would be little need of selenium. Where soil is deficient in selenium, farm animals tend to develop WHITE MUSCLE DISEASE, which is a type of MUSCULAR DYSTROPHY. For this reason some researchers believe that MULTIPLE SCLEROSIS in children is due to a lack of vitamin E in their diet. The average intake of selenium in the U.S. is only of the 300 mcg that is required to prevent CANCER.

- ✓ SAND AND SNOW REFLECT LOTS OF UVL—The beach is a good place to get a lot of UVL. You can get a TAN in the shade from UVL which is reflected from objects, for OVERCAST SKIES filter out only about 20% of the UVL. This is particularly true on SAND and near WATER, both of which are efficient reflectors of the sun's rays. Sand reflects almost 7 times as much UVL as does GRASS, but SNOW reflects 5 times as much UVL as does sand.

- ✓ UVL REDUCES COLDS, PULSE RATE, AND BLOOD PRESSURE—A 10 minute irradiation with UVL 1 to 3 times per week resulted in a reduction of COLDS from 30 to 40% in a study of 4000 college students at Cornell University. Bathing under UVL 3 times a week, in moderate doses, will lower PULSE RATE, and BLOOD PRESSURE, and will increase BASAL METABOLISM.

◆ *Lights In The Classroom*

- ✓ FULL-SPECTRUM LIGHTING—Because of the great benefits that UVL gives to people, it has been suggested that UVL should be substituted for standard classroom lights. One study showed that children in the classroom would have less respiratory infection if UVL were to be substituted for standard classroom lights. FULL-SPECTRUM lighting, which is artificial light or light bulbs which imitate all of the wavelengths of the rays that are in sunlight seems to improve the learning progress of children. Chickens raised under full-spectrum lighting do much better than those raised under other forms of artificial lighting. They live twice as long, lay more eggs, are calmer and less aggressive, and produce eggs that are 25% lower in cholesterol.

- ✓ ORDINARY FLUORESCENT LIGHTING—Has been found to be a slight HINDRANCE TO LEARNING. New studies have shown that skin cancer was twice as prevalent among office workers who worked all day under FLUORESCENT LIGHTS than those whose main outdoor activity was sunbathing. Animal studies have shown that fluorescent office lights can cause mutations in cultures of animal cells. A study by Dr. F. Hollwich showed that individuals sitting under non-full spectrum or normal fluorescent lighting showed hormonal stress responses of ACTH and CORTISOL. This did not occur when they were sitting under artificial full-spectrum illumination, showing that sunlight, real or simulated has an effect in reducing STRESS. Both of these hormones also function as GROWTH INHIBITORS, which may account for the observation that persistent STRESS STUNTS BODILY GROWTH in children. In German hospitals and medical facilities, the normal COOL-WHITE FLUORESCENT BULBS are legally banned.

Sunlight And Disease

◆ *Sunlight Destroys Germs*

Exposure to sunlight DESTROYS GERMS, and thereby has the potential of reducing the incidence of disease. Dr. F.M. Rositerrt said: "Sunlight is a powerful healing and remedial agent of skin diseases and malignant diseases. Skin diseases and malignant diseases are much less common among those who spend a large share of their time in the open air. It helps cure TUBERCULOSIS, and regular exposure would prevent this disease." Many serious diseases have been treated successfully with sunlight—RICKETS, NERVOUS DISORDERS, RESPIRATORY DISORDERS, RHEUMATIC and ARTHRITIC CONDITIONS, PSORIASIS, OBESITY, CIRCULATORY DISORDERS, and GLANDULAR INACTIVITY. NUDISTS suffer from HBP only half as often as the national average. Of all races, the NEGRO RACE is the most susceptible to RICKETS, for the darker the skin, the harder it is for sunlight to penetrate.

◆ *Drugs Can Change Sunlight Into A Disease Potentiator*

There is a direct RELATIONSHIP between the DAYS of SUNLIGHT and the FREQUENCY of COLDS. MEDICINAL DRUGS of nearly every variety can turn the RAYS of the SUN into a POTENTIATOR of DISEASE. When they get into our system or on our skins and are exposed to bright sunlight, they can become very TOXIC,

ALLERGENIC, and even CARCINOGENIC. Too much sunshine can change the structure of the DNA, or DEOXYRIBONUCLEIC ACID in cell nuclei, which is the hereditary basis in many organisms, so that these cells will appear foreign to the immune system, and it will attack them. It changes the genetic code, and some cells may turn into cancer cells.

A substance called CAMP depresses the immune system. It builds up in the LYMPHOCYTES and keeps them from destroying cancer cells. COFFEE, TEA, and CHOCOLATE contain, THEOPHYLLINE, and THEOBROMINE which increase the amount of CAMP in the body cells because they block the destruction of CAMP. Sunlight relaxes the nervous system by decreasing the levels of CAMP. This has a sedating effect, which is the reason why many sunbathers fall asleep easily in the sun.

Sunlight And Skin Cancer

◆ *Sunlight Produces Sex Hormones*

When sunlight strikes the skin, it produces SEX HORMONES in the skin. It produces ESTROGEN in FEMALES and TESTOSTERONE in MALES. It also increases ADRENALINE. Adrenaline can stimulate the PINEAL BODY to produce more MELATONIN, which in turn affects the hormone producing glands. When the pineal gland in humans becomes calcified, it cuts down the production of MELATONIN. This stimulates the production of ESTROGEN which may cause an increase in BREAST CANCER.

◆ *UVL On Fatty Tissue Produces Cancer*

Dr. Zane Kime says that it is the FAT in SUNTAN LOTIONS that causes skin cancer. He says that it stimulates the formation of cancer cells. UVL causes oxidation of the cholesterol in the skin which then turns into FREE RADICALS such as CHOLESTEROL ALPHAOXIDE which can cause cancer. A HIGH FAT DIET promotes SKIN CANCER with the aid of UVL, and not the sunshine itself. When polyunsaturated fat is refined, it is changed somewhat in structure into PARTIALLY HYDROGENATED VEGETABLE OIL. It is these refined oils that can cause SKIN CANCER. When more vitamins such as VITAMIN C, E, and BETA CAROTENE are taken, however, which are antioxidants, more of them are delivered to the skin, and their presence decreases the synthesizing of cholesterol alphaoxide, and no cancer is formed.

Excessive sunlight can cause several types of skin cancer. The chemicals in our FOOD and ENVIRONMENT make our skin more sensitive to the damaging effects of sunlight. UVL produces FREE RADICALS in skin cells in the test tube, and they can produce small raised lumps on the skin called ACTINIC KERATOSIS which are pre-cancerous. A mild sunburn decreases the function of circulating LYMPHOCYTES for as long as 24 hours. The SCOTCH and IRISH, who are the lightest complexioned people, have the highest incidence of skin cancer. Beta-carotene is one of the most efficient scavengers of singlet high energy oxygen. VITAMIN E does the same.

◆ *Immune System Depression Can Cause Skin Cancer*

Skin and heart transplants patients have the IMMUNE SYSTEM DEPRESSED so that the body will not reject the donated organ. Such suppression seems to cause more skin cancer in these patients when they are exposed to the sun. When sunlight plays on the skin of people who have used too many DRUGS, the skin reacts with the formation of MOLES, WARTS, and even with low-grade SKIN CANCER.

Sunlight And Aging

◆ *Aging Reduces Vitamin D Production*

Aging impairs the body's ability to produce active forms of vitamin D, which in turn slows down the absorption of calcium through the intestines, resulting in an increased risk of FAULTY BONE MINERALIZATION. Most investigators believe that a high fat diet is the main contributor of aging. The skin of a 70 year old person can produce about the vitamin D of a 20 year old person.

◆ *Vitamin Saturated Skin Will Not Wrinkle*

The sun will WRINKLE the SKIN only if the tissues are not saturated with the necessary vitamins. If the tissues are saturated with VITAMIN C by a diet of fresh fruits and vegetables, it will prevent free radical formation as well as accelerated tissue aging. The vitamins and minerals that prevent free radical formation are abundant in natural foods, but they are largely removed when foods are refined. The natural foods that contain vitamin E give protection from sunlight by preventing FREE RADICAL DAMAGE. Mice on polyunsaturated fat aged faster because they needed more vitamin E to prevent the attack of free radicals, but they got less of vitamin E because it had been refined out. When polyunsaturated oils are used in COOKING where they are heated, they break down into free radical compounds. These combine with oxygen to form PEROXIDES which are TOXINS that damage the cells. When CORN OIL is heated for more than 15 minutes, it can contribute to the development of atherosclerosis.

◆ *Sunscreens And Photosensitivity*

Sunscreens are lotions used to protect the skin from excessive ultraviolet radiation. People who spend a lot of time in the sun with bare skin are wise to put on some sunscreen in order to avoid skin damage from such radiation. Some skins are very sensitive to these rays and therefore need protection. The best sunscreens will contain the B-complex vitamin PARA-AMINOBENZOIC ACID, or PABA for short. People with light skin color and blue or green eyes are inclined to burn easily. They can exceed their sunburn threshold tolerance in 10 or 20 minutes under a noontime summer sun. People with darker skin who rarely burn and readily tan, may not even become red after 45 minutes or so under the same conditions.

PABA protects against the B-rays of UVL. They are the waves that cause sunburn. At the same time PABA permits the A-rays of UVL to travel through the skin. They are the less dangerous tanning rays.

A person who has PHOTOSENSITIVITY, which represents an exaggerated reaction to sunlight, will be helped by sunscreens. With them he may avoid REDNESS, SWELLING, ITCHING, HIVES, SKIN IRRITATION, RASH, AGING SPOTS, WRINKLES, or even SKIN CANCER. DRUGS will cause photosensitivity. Those that are likely to do so are RETIN-A®, THIAZIDE DIURETICS, or "water pills" used in treating high blood pressure, TETRACYCLINE, ANTI-DIABETICS, PSORALENS, ORAL CONTRACEPTIVES ANTI-PSYCHOTICS, ANTI-DEPRESSANTS, ANTIHISTAMINES, ANTI-BACTERIALS, ANTI-CANCER DRUGS, and CORTICOSTEROIDS.

REST

Gods Example Of Rest

After God had created the world in six days He rested on the seventh day from all of the works which he had created and made (Gen. 2:2, 3). He did not necessarily rest because He was tired, but in order to give us an example to show the human organism needs rest after labor. He therefore appointed a day of rest for man. The fourth commandment deals with the seventh day of the week as a special day of rest for the purpose of meditating on the Creator's work of creation. He created us with a need for REST, RELAXATION, and RECUPERATION of our exhausted energies. We will need rest also after every day's work in order to restore the expended energies. "God wants His people to take time for rest" (4BC1144).

Our Need For Rest

◆ *The Heart Beats More Slowly On Saturdays*

REST and SLEEP are some of the essentials of life. Without them we cannot thrive nor exist very long. We cannot withstand sleeplessness for more than a few days. The need for rest was also recognized by Christ when He said to His disciples, "Come ye yourselves apart into a dessert place and rest awhile" (Mark 6:31). They sought rest among the scenes of nature (DA359). He was to give them rest for their soul (Matt. 11:24, 28).

Tests that have been made on body processes have determined that for everybody, regardless of religious belief, the HEART BEATS MORE SLOWLY ON SATURDAY than on any other day of the week. Even if a person has a day off on any other day of the week, the heart still beats more slowly on Saturdays. The heart rests at the end of every beat. The lungs rest after every exhalation. The stomach should have at least 5 hours of rest between meals. The brain is the master control and directing authority for the entire body economy. Most brain functions and their results are carried on beneath the level of consciousness. In sleep the brain regenerates and renews its fund of nerve energy and marshals other vital factors. The body needs only rest. Old people suffer from a deficiency of SEROTONIN, an important neurotransmitter that initiates SLEEP. TRYPTOPHAN, an amino acid, is the substance used by the brain to make serotonin. Tryptophan is contained in relatively large amounts in MILK and BANANAS. This means that hot milk before bedtime really does help you to sleep. Serotonin is manufactured in the brain only when enough vitamin B_6 is present, and it is often found to be abnormally low in HYPERACTIVE CHILDREN.

There is evidence that people who are getting inadequate rest SHORTEN THEIR LIFE span by 8 to 10 years. A simple test which determines whether or not you need more sleep is indicated if you need an alarm clock to get you up in the morning. Another is in evidence when you have a strong physical letdown in the middle of the day.

◆ *Rest before Midnight*

The work of building up the body takes place during the hours of rest. "Proper periods of sleep and rest and an abundance of physical exercise are essential to health of body and mind. We must also rest in bed" (7T247). The more rest we can get in BEFORE MIDNIGHT the better. They are the most valuable hours for rest and body building. If you must work at night, do it early in the morning, but get your sleep before midnight. The soundest sleep is before midnight, and one sleeps more lightly after midnight. The first half of the night's sleep gives us the deepest, most efficient sleep, and is far more beneficial than the second half. If we have extra work to do we should get to bed even earlier than usual, and then get up earlier in the morning to do the work. ONE hour of sleep BEFORE midnight is worth TWO hours of sleep AFTER midnight. Or one hour of phase four sleep, the deepest stage, is worth two hours or more of lighter phases of sleep. One hour of work early in the morning is worth two or more hours before midnight. NOISE disturbs sleep. A TIGHT GARMENT interferes with sleep. An hour's NAP in the afternoon decreases our need of nighttime sleep by about 2 hours. In a study it was shown that men who napped at least 30 minutes a day were 30% less likely to have heart problems as compared to those who did not nap. Those people who FAST require only from 2 to 5 hours of sleep daily. All drugs hurt our sleep. LACK OF EXERCISE tends to cause us to sleep more than we should. The last meal should be 4 to 5 hours before bedtime. ANIMALS rest after eating; humans should too.

◆ *Where And When Rest Is Best*

If we are in a fine state of health, if suspended in fresh air of ideal temperature and humidity, in a weightless condition, in a dark noise-free environment, in a pleasant aromatic atmosphere, without emotional problems, or bodily disturbances, we should get by on about 3 or 4 hours of sleep a day.

The more comfortable our body, the more conducive to sleep. In the house the BEST SLEEP is with an OPEN WINDOW. If you move onto a PORCH, it will improve your sleep even more. If you take your bed UNDER the STARS it is still better. If you sleep on the GROUND, it is still better. If you sleep near WATER, that is better yet, and if you sleep on a PIER above the water, bodily rest and repair is still faster.

The Simmons Mattress Company did some research about how people slept. They found out that people never MOVED in bed, regardless of position, until about MIDNIGHT. After midnight they seemed to move all of the time. People who had to work at night never suffered if they got only 4 or 5 hours of sleep before midnight. Rest should come BEFORE EXERCISE. If one rests first one can do good work when doing physical labor.

◆ *Rest And Disease*

Proper periods of rest are part of an intelligent system of treating disease (1T553). The work of building up the body takes place during the hours of rest. In fact one might say that the biggest part in the recovery from disease is the rest the individual gets while recuperating. Rest invigorates and renews. Tired nerves need rest. James White was such a hard worker, and saw so much work to be done, that he could not afford time for rest (1T519). He believed that it was better to wear out than to rust out, and as a result he died somewhat prematurely at the age of sixty. But these are not the two alternatives given us. Work must be applied in moderation so as to preserve health and extend life.

We are told that "many have made themselves sick by overtaxing their strength. Their exhausted energies compel them to cease labor, and they are brought to a bed of suffering. Rest, freedom from care, light, pure air, pure water, and a spare diet, is all that they need to make them well" (2SM458). Research is hinting that regular relaxation may help avoid infections, because it boosts KILLER CELLS activity. A suggested type II diabetes prescription for the future is: Relax after every meal. This was shown to improve glucose tolerance by 20%. One gets more pleasure out of life in health than in sickness. Weakness and ill health are poor foundations for joy and happiness.

The Best Scientific Principles Of Rest

◆ *Go To Bed Early*

One of the first requirements for sleep is that the nerves should not be disturbed. There should be darkness and quiet. Go to bed early; early sleep is beauty sleep. People who retire late are more fatigued than those who retire early; sleep in a well-ventilated room; maintain a comfortable temperature; practice a few moments of mental and physical quiet before retiring.

◆ *Go To Sleep With An Empty Stomach*

Don't eat before retiring. If one goes to sleep with an empty stomach, one can often get along with six or seven hours of sleep. With a full stomach you would need from 8 to 9 hours. Those who sleep 9 HOURS have a HIGHER MORTALITY rate than those who sleep 7 or 8 hours. During sleep the body is continually at work. It REBUILDS its TISSUES and ALKALINIZES ITSELF; BURNS UP STORED ENERGY; PRODUCES POISONOUS WASTES; and REPAIRS CELLS and TISSUES. BRAIN WORKERS require more sleep than others.

◆ *Take Warm Showers At Night*

Researchers found out that people should do their showering at night with fairly hot water before retiring. The warmer you go to bed the longer you'll sleep. They also found out that adult males who took hot showers before going to sleep had much better REM (rapid eye movement) sleep than did a control group who took hot or cold showers upon arising the next morning.

◆ *Sleep Outdoors If Possible*

The most healthful position in sleep is on the right side, because it avoids pressure upon the heart. Sleep outdoors if possible. One night's sleep outdoors is worth three nights indoors. The best sleep producer is outdoor exercise. With a good day's work and physical exercise, with a clear conscience and untroubled mind, there should be no difficulty in going to sleep. A sufficient amount of rest between exercises is as important as the exercise. children especially need frequent intervals of rest (AH289). Rest should come before extreme fatigue, for it requires 2 to 10 times as long to fully recuperate after thorough fatigue as from the beginning of fatigue.

◆ *Go To Sleep As Soon As You Are Sleepy*

The mind is rested when the topic of thought and concentration is turned to less demanding considerations and diversions. Go to sleep as soon as you feel sleepy, and sleep until you wake up on your own. Sleep should come naturally and should NOT BE INDUCED BY DRUGS. Natural sleep is the most effective form of sleep. As one adapts to the practice of natural living, and reduces the amount of FATIGUE POISON in the body, the need for sleep is reduced.

◆ *Sleep In A Weightless State*

Sleeping apartments should have a circulation of air through them day and night, because the lungs, in order to b e healthy must have pure air (2SM463). Sleeping time is lessened in a WEIGHTLESS STATE such as floating on air or suspended in water. This is due to lack of pressure points. PRESSURE POINTS reduce the circulation of the blood. Weight must be evenly distributed. When pressure points exist, the phase of sleep never becomes deep. The compression forces the brain into a lighter phase of sleep, and shifts the body to another position. When this is the case it takes a greater length of time for the brain to regenerate its fund of nerve energy.

Dr. Jay T. Shurley of the Veterans Administration Hospital in Oklahoma City observed that sleepers who floated on a bed called the "Royalaire Air-Fluidized Bed" with controlled air flow, temperature, and humidity, increased the depth and duration of PHASE FOUR sleep (the deepest and most efficient phase of sleep), and reduced their sleep needs from 8 to 4 hours. The reason was the lack of PRESSURE POINTS. Body weight is evenly distributed, and blood circulation is not restricted. On a normal bed the body shifts 30 to 40 times a night in order to change the pressure points. Hence, in ideal sleep the body will be perfectly quiet, and not move at all. It is SLEEPING LIKE A LOG. It will be free of pressure points. Since the SKIN ALSO BREATHES, it must be able to take in oxygen, and eliminate waste products. The better air circulates around the body, the easier the body will maintain sound sleep. Anything against the skin that prevents AIR CIRCULATION, denies the skin air, and causes its own EFFLUVIA to collect so as to suffocate the area. When we shift during sleep, we sacrifice DEEP SLEEP for a lighter stage of sleep. The ideal sleeping temperature of the air we breathe while asleep is from 65 TO 70°. Body temperature must be maintained. Overheating or excess cooling disturbs sleep.

NASA kept a man WEIGHTLESS IN WATER for 23 of 24 hours a day with a special suit which fed him fresh air continuously. He got by well on a mere 2 hours of sleep a day. Sleepers on WATER BEDS, AIR BEDS, AND HAMMOCKS report that sleep need is satisfied with one or two hours less sleep than on conventional beds.

◆ *Sleep In Health And Disease.*

Recent research reveals that many changes are taking place inside the body—the BLOOD PRESSURE falls, the temperature drops more than 1 degree from its normal afternoon high. When you awake, your body makes the transition by producing a surge of "stimulation" chemicals called CATECHOLAMINES. This causes the heart rate to increase and the blood vessels to constrict, resulting in higher BLOOD PRESSURE and REDUCED BLOOD FLOW to the heart muscle. That is why during the first two hours after getting up people are more likely to suffer a HEART ATTACK or a STROKE. At this time people are also most vulnerable to many other leading causes of death such as CANCER, EMPHYSEMA, ASTHMA, BRONCHITIS, and ISCHEMIC HEART DISEASE.

As a rule, HEALTHY PEOPLE require less sleep and are better able to sleep. Unhealthy people require more sleep and are less able to sleep. Sleep will improve with your health. Sick people have disturbed bodies that generate more pain and sensory phenomena which involve the brain in trying to overcome them through eliminative and restorative activities. The brain needs more nerve energy to regenerate a degenerative condition. Healthy people have only to regenerate that small fund of nerve energy which a wholesome day of life has expended. Sleep need will be less if the conditions of sleep are improved, and it will improve with your improvement of health. Sleep needs only be long enough for the brain to achieve the requisite REGENERATION OF NERVE ENERGY, the building up of energy reserves, the replacement of spent cells, the casting out of spent cells, and the elimination of the by-products of METABOLISM. Sleeping in a cool room lowers the metabolism rate, while sleeping in an overheated room increases it. One rule is: Go to bed and get up every day at the same time. Never sleep late—not even on weekends.

Those who eat COOKED FOODS require more sleep than those who eat RAW FOODS. Meat eating animals require more sleep than vegetarians. Lions and tigers may sleep as much as 20 hours a day. Their bodies have more poisons to eliminate. A 1 hour nap during the afternoon lessens our need of nighttime sleep by about two hours. Fasting institutions have noticed that fasters who are undergoing a thorough physiological rest need only from 2 to 5 hours of sleep daily.

Sleep laboratories have reported that OLDER PEOPLE spend less time in the deeper phases of REM sleep than younger people. SLEEPING PILLS will not offer a good night's sleep, because most sleeping pills will inhibit the REM stage of sleep, and they also depress breathing.

TEMPERANCE, ABSTINENCE, AND FASTING

Temperance In All Things

Temperance means moderation or self-restraint in the indulgence of natural appetites and passions. We are told that "With our first parents, INTEMPERATE DESIRE resulted in the LOSS OF EDEN. Temperance in all things has more to do with our restoration to Eden than men realize" (MH129). "It is impossible for an intemperate man to be a Christian, for his higher powers are brought into slavery to the passions" (CH36). "Our only hope of regaining Eden is through the firm denial of appetite and passions" (3T491). Paul says that "every man that striveth for the mastery is temperate in all things" (1 Cor. 9:25). And he added: "Let your moderation be known unto all men" (Col. 4:5). This means that we should shun that which is harmful, avoid unneeded extremes, and be moderate in the enjoyment of those things which are lawful. Health of BODY, MIND, and SOUL is impossible without temperate living. Whatever we do in our daily habits of life, we should honor God by doing that which is most pleasing to Him, and which maintains our MENTAL, PHYSICAL, and SPIRITUAL POWERS to the highest efficiency. We must do all things to the glory of God (1 Cor. 10:31).

Christ's Example Of Temperance

Christ as well as Adam and Eve experienced the matter of appetite as their first great temptation. "As by the indulgence of appetite Adam fell, so by the denial of appetite Christ must overcome" (CD185). He fasted 40 days for our sake, and in doing so "He exercised a self-control stronger than hunger or death" (CD185). This fast was to be a lesson for man for all time, because Christ was not overcome by Satan's temptations, and neither need we be. "All who would live godly lives may overcome as Christ overcame.... He would begin the work of overcoming just where the ruin began,— on the point of APPETITE. When Christ was the most fiercely beset by temptation, HE ATE NOTHING" (CD186)

Fasting And The Spirit Of Prophecy

◆ *The Best Fasting Is Moderate Eating*

The best fasting is the type of eating, and the type of lifestyle which does not lead to disease, but which continually replenishes, recuperates, and purifies the body as the body is operating, so as to keep it in a high condition of function. Such maintenance will not allow disease to get started in the body, and that is the way God would have it. We are told that "The true fasting which should be recommended to all, is abstinence from every stimulating kind of food, and the proper use of wholesome, simple food, which God has provided in abundance" (CD90). At times we are imitating the worldling with the use of fanciful dishes which will contradict our faith by our works. Our concentration should be less on physical food than on spiritual food so as to enhance our religious experience.

Fasting And Prayer

If we want to obtain the clearest understanding of scriptural passages, the process of fasting and prayer is recommended. In the past "difficult points of present truth have been reached by the earnest efforts of a few who were devoted to the work. Fasting and fervent prayer to God have moved the LORD to unlock His treasuries of truth to their understanding. By this means those facts which immediately concern the salvation of souls will be made so clear that none need err, or walk in darkness. Unless God's people PRACTICE TRUE TEMPERANCE, they cannot be susceptible to the sanctifying influence of the TRUTH" (CD451). Mrs. White says of her past experience along this line, "Often we fasted that we might be better fitted to understand the truth. For certain things fasting and prayer are recommended and appropriate. In the hand of God they are a means of cleansing the heart and promoting a receptive frame of mind" (CD187). "The spirit of true fasting and prayer is the spirit which yields mind, heart, and will to God" (CD189). We are admonished to unite in fasting and prayer for the WISDOM that God has promised to supply liberally. Till the close of time we should set aside DAYS of FASTING and PRAYER, in which prayer is offered and supplicants may not need to abstain from food entirely, but are admonished to eat sparingly of the most simple food (CD188–9).

Fasting As A Remedy For Disease

◆ *The Meaning Of Fasting*

Fasting means the reduction or elimination of food except water, herbal teas, fruit or vegetable juices. It means a minimum intake of food for purposes of resting the organs to restore their maximum strength, and for allowing the body the time for regeneration of bodily functions and the healing of damaged organs and tissues. Fasting allows the body to HEAL ITSELF through the recuperative powers which God has placed within it, because it is then given the opportunity to do so WITHOUT HINDRANCE. Fasting may involve SKIPPING A MEAL OR TWO, or skipping meals for ONE, TWO, or MORE DAYS, according to the need of the constitution. This is especially valuable in CASES OF SICKNESS.

◆ *Fasting — A Self-Healing Process*

The practice of fasting acknowledges the fact that our organism is a self-healing organism. Healing occurs naturally if it is allowed to. Under these circumstances EXCESSIVE FOOD THWARTS the natural ongoing healing process. Forcing a sick person to eat "to keep up his strength" overlooks the fact that the process of digestion itself uses up strength also. Here the limited available strength might be better used for the healing process than for the process of digestion. Fasting is also known to release a HORMONE that stimulates the immune system. Hence, it can speed recovery from FEVER, INFECTION, and other diseases.

The body is always SELF-CORRECTING, SELF-REPAIRING, SELF-RESTORING. You will suffer for every sin that you commit against yourself. Not one transgression is forgotten. All bad practices have bad effects. For example, the body requires far less food than we think it does. With less food we can maintain more health.

When fasting, the body loses about 1 POUND A DAY, and experiments have shown that this is about the amount of food we should eat in order to maintain the body in good condition. Most people eat several times this amount and become sick doing it.

No DEFICIENCY DISEASE ever develops during a fast. People who suffer from deficiency diseases experience improvement during a fast. The number of RED CELLS in ANEMIA PATIENTS increase. Patients with RICKETS experience REMISSIONS, and problematic CALCIUM METABOLISM experiences dramatic IMPROVEMENT. HEARING becomes MORE ACUTE. All the SENSES become more acute, and many people are able to discard their glasses after a fast. Also an increase of KEENNESS of the INTELLECT is experienced. During a fast all the processes of the body continue at a reduced rate with the exception of the PROCESSES of ELIMINATION.

◆ *Fasting — A Cleansing Process*

If food is withheld from the outside, the body begins to feed itself from within, in a process called AUTOLYSIS. The "inner physician" takes over, and whatever is least essential to the body economy is used up first. In this category we find MUCUS, FAT, DISEASED CELLS OR TISSUES, URIC ACID,. CHOLESTEROL, CALCIUM CARBONATE, and other RESIDUES of METABOLISM. They represent IMPURITIES which are substances which hinder the normal operations of the body, and these are metabolized first. Also TUMORS and ABSCESSES are eliminated. Tumors are the body's method of quarantining toxic material. Dr. Trall mentions that abnormal growths possess lower degree of vitality than normal growths, and are therefore easiest to get rid of. The body economy can now accomplish chemical changes so perfectly, that they are unmatched by any other laboratory process, which indicates that dietary reform is best accomplished with temporary food withholding. URIC ACID can actually be transformed into PROTEIN, from where it came. CHOLESTEROL is converted into FAT, and CARBONIC ACID is changed to STARCH or SUGAR. It represents an incredible manifestation of a higher intelligence taking over command.

After the third day of fasting hunger disappears, and all organs are undergoing a well-deserved rest. STARVATION does not take place until all of these nonessential substances are used up and eliminated, and the whole system is cleansed of impurities, which process usually takes up to three weeks. At that point hunger returns, and a sweeter BREATH is in evidence. Hippocrates made the statement that "if a sick person is fed, one feeds the disease. On the other hand, if the sufferer is withheld from food, the disease is fasted out."

◆ *When Is Fasting Beneficial?*

Fasting is of benefit to everyone who maintains

in his body a degree of internal pollution, which is almost everybody. There are signs which can determine that the particular body can benefit from fasting. An easy way to determine that the body is impure involves an abstention from food for from 24 to 36 hours. One should go without food for at least a whole day, and take in water only as the thirst demands. By the end of the first day or day and a half, the TONGUE will be COATED a FROSTY WHITE, which coating cannot be rubbed off no matter how hard you try. Such condition will be accompanied by a strong smelling breath. These symptoms are signs of a toxic overload. COLDS, FEVERS, certain ACHES and PAINS, CHRONIC FATIGUE, HEADACHES, ETC. are some of the evidences of an impure body. A body that is relatively pure will not get a cold.

When fasting, the MUCUS MEMBRANES also become an organ of elimination besides the LUNGS, KIDNEYS, LIVER, COLON, and SKIN. The flow of mucus from the nose during a cold represents an extraordinary elimination of toxic matter and should therefore not be stopped, and especially not with drugs. The mucus membranes are pressed into service as a special outlet by a body that is loaded with toxins beyond toleration levels. It is endeavoring to eliminate its toxins which are causing SINUS PROBLEMS, PSORIASIS, PIMPLES, BOILS, BLACKHEADS, RASHES, FEVER etc. Such processes would not occur if the body were internally clean. In women one of the avenues of special compensatory elimination is the UTERUS. This occurs as MENSTRUATION, the periodic discharge of mucus and blood.

◆ *Fasting — Is The Oldest Medical Therapy*

Fasting is not recognized by official American medicine as a legitimate form of therapy, but it is employed in Europe on a grand scale by reputable medical doctors. There it is used routinely for almost every disease condition. One clinic has supervised the fasts of over 100,000 patients. Dr. Werner Zabel of Germany, has said that "Together with FEVER and OPTIMAL NUTRITION, fasting is man's oldest healing method." It has been a dependable curative measure throughout medical history. It was prescribed by HIPPOCRATES, PARACELSUS, GALEN, and practiced by PLATO and ARISTOTLE to "attain mental and physical efficiency."

The therapeutic values of fasting are well documented by a large number of scientific studies, and those doctors who use it testify to the fact that it not only works, but that it is one of the SAFEST HEALING METHODS there is. Paracelsus said that "Fasting is the greatest remedy, the physician within." Many modern doctors agree with Adolph Mayer that "fasting is the most efficient means of correcting any disease." Dr. Otto Buchinger calls fasting "a royal road to healing." Fasting for serious conditions such as CANCER, TUBERCULOSIS, DIABETES, OR CARDIO-VASCULAR DISORDERS should be carried out under the supervision of a doctor who is trained in this therapy. But otherwise, fasting for a few days, especially JUICE FASTING, can be safely undertaken by anyone.

In a fast the body eliminates, attacks, and disposes of the least necessary tissues first. Waste and poisons are disposed of, then fatty tissue. When this process is completed, hunger returns. If at this time food is not taken in, then starvation begins. The average person can fast for 40 days as did Christ, Moses, Daniel and other patriarchs. Fasting is a CONSTRUCTIVE PROCESS, while STARVATION is a destructive process which begins by attacking the vital organs themselves.

When one takes food away from a sick person, one does not begin to starve the sick person, but rather to starve the disease. Hippocrates said: "The more you feed a diseased body, the worse you make it." In disease we have a LOSS OF DIGESTIVE POWER, and digestive conditions. We derive benefit from our food not in proportion to the amount we eat, but in proportion to the amount we can properly utilize and ASSIMILATE. In a diseased condition food is improperly converted in the body so that it only partially nourishes the patient.

We must understand the proper PHILOSOPHY OF FASTING. It will not only benefit the digestive organs, but it will act on seemingly unrelated conditions such as DEAFNESS, JAUNDICE, COLD in the HEAD, HEADACHES, PARALYSIS, ULCERS, PLEURISY, HBP, ARTHRITIS, TONSILLITIS, and scores of other conditions. The reason for this is because the body is a unity. FASTING effects and benefits every condition in the body.

IN FASTING NATURE ATTENDS TO THE HEALING PROCESS IN THE FASTEST POSSIBLE WAY.

◆ *Fasting Often Better Than Medicine*

We are told that "Intemperate eating is often the cause of sickness, and what nature most needs is to be relieved of the undue burden that has been placed upon her. In many cases of sickness, the very best remedy is for the patient to fast for a meal or two that the overworked organs of digestion may have an opportunity to rest. A FRUIT DIET for a few days has often brought great relief to BRAIN WORKERS. Many times a short period of entire abstinence from food, followed by simple, moderate eating, has led to recovery through nature's own recuperative effort" (CD189). SCHIZOPHRENICS have been restored to mental wholeness through fasting, for schizophrenia is considered to be a disease of PROTEIN IMBALANCE in the brain. Fasting can more than any other method correct deficient conditions. The HEARING becomes more acute, and hearing impairments are sometimes corrected; the TASTE is improved, and food tastes unbelievably better; the sense of SMELL is heightened, and fasters can smell food at great distances; the INTELLECT is made more keen along with a new sense of awareness and understanding.

Throughout a prolonged fast, all of the processes of the body continue at a reduced rate, with the exception of the organs of elimination, which are greatly accelerated. The tongue becomes heavily coated, and there is an unpleasant taste in the mouth, and a bad breath. This is a sign that the body is engaged in the process eliminating toxins from the system. There is a decrease of saliva secretion during the fast. People will be able to recognize the taste of drugs they have taken, even years before, which had remained in the body's fatty tissues. Skin eruptions are sometimes seen as a part of the body's eliminative process. After the second or third day on the fast, people will lose all desire for food. The signal for the return of true hunger is the clearing of the coated tongue, the bad taste in the mouth, and the bad breath. At this time the fast must be broken, else starvation will set in. In most cases, however, the fast is broken before this time arrives. A fast is usually broken with fruit juices, and gradually heavier food is taken as the stomach becomes better able to assimilate it.

◆ *No Nutritional Deficiency During A Fast*

There develops no nutritional deficiency during a fast. The condition of the blood remains normal. The body economy is able to re-synthesize new proteins from the discarded amino acids of dead cells. No new diseases develop during a fast, except for the indications of eliminated toxins by means of the organs of elimination. An Indiana girl was cured of EPILEPSY through a prolonged fast, and had one epileptic convulsion during her fast and never one after that. She experienced severe HEADACHES and WITHDRAWAL SYMPTOMS for several days while the body was correcting the disease condition. DIARRHEA during a fast is rare, and some fasters experience no bowel activity at all. NAUSEA and VOMITING occur in about 10% of the patients, and result in the disposal of the bile from the overworked liver, when reverse peristalsis has caused the bile to back up into the stomach. If the vomiting persists, dehydration may be a threat, and the fast may have to be broken. Not much SLEEP is required while fasting. The expected amount of sleep is usually from 3 to 5 hours during a 24 hour period.

◆ *Self-Denial—The Path To Health*

"The true fasting which should be recommended to all, is abstinence from every stimulating kind of food, and the proper use of wholesome, simple food, which God has provided in abundance" (CD188). "The sick have their lesson to learn. They must be educated to lay aside every wrong practice and cease to indulge perverted appetite. They must be taught to use the provisions which God has given" (MM260, 262).

We are told that "he who is thoroughly converted will abandon every injurious habit and appetite. By total abstinence he will overcome his desire for health-destroying indulgences, — Abstinence from all hurtful food and drink is the fruit of true religion" (CD457). "An ABSTEMIOUS DIET for a month or two would convince many sufferers that the path of self-denial is the path to health" (CD189). We should let our self-denial and our victory over appetite be an example to others of our obedience to

Fasting Helps Us Enjoy Good Food

People who have PERVERTED their TASTE by eating rich and highly spiced foods, often have no taste for simple wholesome food. They have no taste for a diet of FRUITS, PLAIN BREAD, and VEGETABLES. Fasting will help eliminate the craving for foods which excite the taste buds, but which are at the same time harmful to their health. We are told that if persons with a perverted taste "cannot at first enjoy plain food, they SHOULD FAST until they can. The fast will prove to them of greater benefit than medicine, for the abused stomach will find that rest which it has long needed, and REAL HUNGER can be satisfied with a PLAIN DIET. It will take time for the taste to recover from the abuses it has received, and to gain its natural tone. But perseverance in a self-denying course of eating and drinking will soon make plain wholesome food palatable, and it will soon be eaten with greater satisfaction than the epicure enjoys over his rich dainties" (CD190).

Short Fasts Are Recommended

Christ fasted in the wilderness for forty days, and resisted the temptation to take in food. This example was to show us that even in our weakest moment we can with God's help resist the temptations of the devil. He began the work of overcoming on the point of where the evil began, namely with APPETITE. In doing so Christ exercised a SELF-CONTROL stronger than hunger or death (CD185), and we are told that we can all overcome as Christ overcame(CD186). We do not have to repeat such long fasts that Christ, Moses, and Daniel subjected themselves to, but it is short fasts that are recommended. "Fast for a short time and give the stomach a chance to rest. Reduce the feverish state of the system by a careful and understanding APPLICATION OF WATER. These efforts will help nature in her struggles to FREE THE SYSTEM OF IMPURITIES." (CD190).

Whenever we follow the principles of Health Reform, we will not get seriously ill. We may be all worn out at times, and may be subjected to some short-term acute disability which we can clear up through applying the principles of rest and abstinence. If we don't apply these principles under those circumstances our condition may degenerate into a chronic degenerative disease which then can only be cured by means of many weeks of fasting. The Spirit of Prophecy here addresses itself largely to those who are in one way or another endeavoring to follow the principles of HEALTH REFORM, and if they are indisposed they do not have to subject themselves to long periods of fasting.

If the taste buds have been perverted with the eating of the wrong type of food, good food does not then immediately taste good to such a person. What he can do to establish or re-establish a taste for good, wholesome food, is to fast for a few days to allow the digestive organs to readjust themselves so that they will be able to benefit from partaking of good food. We are told that "If they cannot at first enjoy plain food, they should FAST until they can. That fast will prove to them of greater value than medicine, for the abused stomach will find that rest which it has long needed, and real hunger can be satisfied with a plain diet" (CD158). "An abstemious diet for a month or two would convince many sufferers that the path of SELF-DENIAL is the path to health" (CD189).

The Benefits Of Fasting

✓ VITAL ORGANS—It gives them a complete rest.

✓ FOOD—It discontinues the intake of food.

✓ DIGESTION—It empties the digestive tract and disposes of putrefactive material.

✓ ELIMINATION—It allows the organs of elimination to catch up with their work.

✓ SECRETIONS—It establishes normal physiological chemistry

✓ DISEASED TISSUES—it promotes the absorption of diseased tissues.

✓ RESTORATION—It restores a youthful condition to the cells and tissues.

✓ CONSERVATION—It permits the conservation of energy.

✓ ASSIMILATION—It increases the powers of assimilation.

- ✓ MIND—It clears and strengthens the mind.
- ✓ BODILY FUNCTIONS—It improves all bodily functions.

NUTRITION

The Proper Diet

◆ *God's Original Diet*

"In order to know what are the best foods, we must study God's original plan for man's diet. He who created man and who understands his needs appointed Adam his food" (CD81) "And God said, Behold I have given you every herb bearing seed, which is upon the face of all the earth, and every tree, in which is the fruit of a tree yielding seed; to you it shall be for meat" (Gen. 1:29). When Adam and Eve had to leave the garden of Eden and gain their livelihood by tilling the earth, they received permission to eat the "herb of the field" also. (Gen. 3:18). This meant that altogether Adam and Eve were to eat GRAINS, FRUITS, NUTS, and VEGETABLES. "These foods, prepared in as SIMPLE and NATURAL a MANNER as possible, are the most healthful and nourishing. They impart a STRENGTH, a power of ENDURANCE, and a vigor of INTELLECT, that are not afforded by a more complex and stimulating diet" (CD81).

◆ *Flesh Not Part Of Original Diet*

It was in the beginning contrary to God's plan to have the life of any creature taken for food, for there was to be NO DEATH IN EDEN. The food which God originally gave to man was food to which man's biological makeup was adapted. He did not create man's organism to be naturally adapted to MEAT EATING. The organisms of animals who are meat eaters were designed somewhat differently from man's organism. They have sharp teeth, shorter intestines to limit the factor of putrefaction, and much stronger digestive juices.

After the flood God gave man permission to eat animal food, because all of the vegetation had been destroyed by the flood. But He allowed Noah to eat the flesh of the clean animals which he had taken with him into the ark. Nevertheless, we have been told that "animal food was not the most healthful article of food for man" (CD373). The result was that animal food shortened the sinful lives of the post-diluvian people, and "the race began to rapidly decrease in size, and length of years" (CD373). "Of the meats permitted, the eating of the FAT and the BLOOD was strictly forbidden" (CD374).

◆ *God Wants To Bring Us Back To His Original Diet*

In order to purify a people for translation and the second coming of the Lord, God wants to bring His people of today back to the diet which he originally gave to man, and to eliminate entirely the flesh of dead animals from our dietary (CD82). We are told that "if a liking for fruits and grains is encouraged, it will soon be as God in the beginning designed it should be. No meat will be used by His people. If there ever was a time when the diet should be of the most simple kind, it is now" (CD82). We are told that "the food which God gave to Adam in his sinless state is the best food for man's use as he seeks to regain that sinless state" (7T135).

Herbalist Jethro Kloss says in his book *Back To Eden* (p. III), that "God has provided a remedy for every disease that might afflict us. Satan cannot afflict anyone with any disease for which God has provided a remedy. Our Creator foresaw the wretched condition of mankind in these days, and made provision in nature for all the ills of man. If our scientists and medical colleges would put forth the same effort in finding the virtues in the 'true remedies' as found in nature for the use of the human race, then poisonous drugs and chemicals would be eliminated and sickness would be rare indeed. If they would make use of only these remedies that God has given for the 'service of man' it would bring an untold blessing to the world. In these distressing days, the use of a simple natural diet would prevent much suffering and save money. The most important subject for people to study, should be: How can we live our allotted time without suffering? God has surely made this possible."

Food In Natural State Represents Proper Diet

◆ *Adopt A Vegetarian Diet*

Diet is the major influence of health which is entirely under the individual's control. It determines in great measure one's entire well-being. Other influences cannot always be completely controlled.

The grains, fruits, nuts, and vegetables which God gave to Adam and Eve in the beginning, were foods which were to be eaten in their NATURAL STATE. There wasn't any COOKING going on in the garden of Eden. The need of some cooking may have come in later with the use of some root vegetables. If we become intelligent in regard to the use of a proper diet, then we will also be considered sound in BIBLE DOCTRINE (CM133). Our diet may have to change somewhat in the future because of conditions prevailing on the earth, but we should continue to increase in knowledge regarding what a proper diet is. Diet reform should be progressive (MH320). To be sure we should adopt a vegetarian diet (CD81).

It has been discovered that most VEGETARIANS have a MORE ACTIVE IMMUNE SYSTEM. Their WHITE BLOOD CELLS are twice as deadly to TUMORS as those of MEAT EATERS, because it is thought that they have more natural KILLER CELLS among their WHITE CELLS.

◆ *The Unnatural State Of Processed Foods*

One naturopathic scientist applies Matt. 19:6 "What therefore God hath joined together, let no man put asunder" to the principle of natural foods. God has combined the food elements in the best possible way for nourishment. Here the principle applies that "the whole is greater than the sum of its parts." Food that is taken apart, separated, and processed is UNBALANCED, and will therefore not nourish us as much as it should, and it can even be detrimental to our health.

Dr. Josephs Evers points out that today our foods, because of wrong agricultural methods, processing, and chemical additives, contain over 2000 substances to which man is not adapted, and which his system is therefore unable to handle. He specifically points out that the replacement of wholesome whole meal bread by devitalized white bread, and raw milk by pasteurized and homogenized milk, are some of the most serious assaults on man's natural foods.

The rules we live by must be in harmony with our nature in order to contribute to our health. With the harmful substances which are placed in our food we have found a way to deceive ourselves and to ruin ourselves without knowing that we are doing so. We engage in self-injury when we believe that we are engaged in self-enhancement. For the evils of ignorance the remedy is knowledge. For the evils of false ideas the remedy is truth. For the source of truth and knowledge we have divine wisdom as represented in the laws of nature. To follow them is making such wisdom personal. HEALTH is a state of soundness and integrity of the organism, vigor, efficiency of function and the excellency of mental faculties.

◆ *All Elements Of Nutrition Are In A Vegetarian Diet*

In His original diet, God placed all of the elements of nutrition necessary to sustain the life of man (CD92). Since God gave it, it must be the best food that man can eat. It has all the nutritive properties necessary to make good blood. This a flesh diet cannot do (CD322). We must remember that the life is in the blood (Lev. 17:11), and the food we eat determines the condition of the blood. Man was to subsist upon the NATURAL PRODUCTS of the earth (CD380). "Our bodies are built up from the food we eat. There is a constant break down of the tissues of the body; every movement of every organ involves waste, and this waste is repaired from our food. Each organ of the body requires its share of nutrition" (MH295). "Foods in their NATURAL STATE are best adapted to the wants of the system" (CD241). By partaking of natural living foods, we will increase our nutrition on less food. If God gave man no meat to eat as part of his diet, then it must not be essential for his bodily needs. It is therefore "not essential for health or strength, else the Lord made a mistake when he provided food for Adam and Eve before their fall" (CD395).

If man would use only whole, complete, natural, and never refined, fragmented, or processed foods, he would not be concerned about protein, carbohydrates, and fats, because in whole food the body would be getting a proper balance of all essential nutrients.

◆ *Seeds, Nuts, And Grains*

From the standpoint of the order of importance, natural nutritionists consider the seeds, nuts, and grains of first importance in our dietary; the vegetables next; and the fruits after that. They believe that the nutritional value of seeds, nuts and grains is unsurpassed. Even cooked they contain all the important nutrients for human GROWTH, SUSTENANCE of health, and PREVENTION of disease. What makes them of basic importance is the fact that they contain the SEAT OF LIFE itself, the GERM, the REPRODUCTIVE POWER, or the SPARK OF LIFE that assures the perpetuation of life itself.

Seeds, nuts, and grains are excellent sources of proteins, and also the best natural sources of UNSATURATED FATTY ACIDS, without which health cannot be sustained. They are also nature's best source of LECITHIN, the B-COMPLEX VITAMINS, and the best source of VITAMIN E which prevents premature aging. They are also a gold mine of MINERALS, and help increase man's natural RESISTANCE to DISEASE.

◆ *Sprouted Seeds*

The practice of sprouting seeds has been known and applied from earliest times. It is now known that sprouted seeds contain more vitamins than dry seeds. When a seed is given water and warmth, it puts forth a sprout which develops vitamins within it, especially vitamin C, and thereby increases the nutritional value of the seed tremendously. It also improves the protein value in seeds and grains. Some seeds become complete protein food after sprouting, when they did not have complete protein before sprouting. WHOLE OATS will increase their vitamin C content from 11 mg before sprouting to 42 mg after 120 hrs. of sprouting. DRY PEAS will increase the vitamin C content from zero to 86 mg after 96 hrs. 7 parts of THIAMIN become 9 parts in the SPROUTED WHEAT, and it increases all of the other B-vitamins also. Dr. Francis Pottenger says that the sprouts develop into complete proteins, and Dr. Clive McCay says that soybean sprouts are rich in protein, fat, minerals, including calcium, usable iron, and vitamins.

MILLET, BUCKWHEAT, WHEAT, OATS, BARLEY, BROWN RICE, SESAME SEEDS, and BEANS are all wonderful HEALTH FOODS. WHEAT, MUNG BEANS, ALFALFA SEEDS, and SOYBEANS make excellent SPROUTS. SPROUTING increases the nutritional value of these seeds tremendously by creating new VITAMINS. Most of these seeds contain COMPLETE PROTEINS of the highest biological value. The few that do not contain complete proteins will become complete proteins if eaten with other vegetables or with milk. Some grains and legumes which contain only incomplete protein, become complete protein foods after they are sprouted. Josephus said that the PULSE (Dan. 1:16) which Daniel and his companions ate at Nebuchadnezzar's palace was SPROUTED SEEDS. Complete proteins are those which contain all of the ESSENTIAL AMINO ACIDS, which the body cannot supply, and which therefore must be obtained from food. Examples are MILK, COTTAGE CHEESE, ALMONDS, SOYBEANS, PEANUTS, POTATOES, and all LEAFY GREEN VEGETABLES.

◆ *Vegetables*

Vegetables are generally considered the REGENERATORS of the body, while fruits are considered to be the CLEANSERS of the body, although the vegetables have cleansing qualities also. They are not as palatable as fruits, but we are told that they can be made palatable with a little milk or cream (CD322). Since we are made up of what we eat (CD322), we should make sure that the vegetables are fresh, and do not show the slightest sign of decay. We are told that more die of decayed fruit and vegetables which ferment in the stomach and result in blood poisoning, than we have any idea of. (CD309). Most vegetables should be EATEN RAW in the form of SALADS. Some vegetables such as Potatoes, YAMS, SQUASHES, or GREEN BEANS, can also be COOKED, BAKED, or STEAMED.

Vegetables are extremely important sources of vitamins, minerals, and enzymes. They also contain complete proteins of highest quality, which are often of better biological value than those from animal sources. The Proteins of potatoes and leafy green vegetables are of highest biological value. A generous use of GARLIC and ONIONS should be made use of. Many HERBS should be used as replacements for salt and sugar. They will improve the health and turn dishes into delectable foods. It has been said that "food is our best medicine, and vegetables are our best MEDICINAL foods.

◆ *Fruits*

Like vegetables, fruits are excellent sources of minerals, vitamins, and enzymes. They are easily digested, and exert a cleansing effect on the blood and digestive tract. At least 75 to 80% of our diet should consist of natural foods in their uncooked state, and the rest only lightly steamed. Raw foods MAINTAIN HEALTH as well as PREVENT and HEAL DISEASE. We are told that "we should avoid eating fruit with vegetables at the same meal" (CD395), because it causes distress if our digestion is not strong. It will affect our thinking process negatively. It produces acidity of the stomach and impurity of the blood (CD113). "The more we depend upon fresh fruit just as it is plucked from the tree, the greater will be the blessing" (CD96). "It would be well for us to do LESS COOKING, and to eat more fruit in its NATURAL STATE" (CD309). "Eat largely of fruits and vegetables" (CD200). "APPLESAUCE, put up in a glass, is wholesome and palatable…. APPLES are superior to any fruit for a standby that grows" (CD312). Fruit with bread is good for the third meal (CD178). One biologist gave the following definition for a fruit and a vegetable. She said that "Anything that is a FRUIT is a seed and or a seed pod. A VEGETABLE is a root, stem, or leaf." On the basis of this definition peas, beans, and peanuts are fruits because they have a seed and a seed pod.

Hygienic Principles Of Food Intake

◆ *Food Must Be Palatable In Its Natural State.*

This means that it must largely be taken in its raw condition. Many experiments have shown that only a raw food diet will sustain HEALTH at the HIGHEST LEVEL. It can then also reverse disease conditions. Food must be relished in its raw state without destroying its nutritional value through HEAT. Heat tends to disintegrate many natural substances into chemicals that are less nutritional, and may possibly be harmful. Food must be delicious in its raw state to the undepraved taste of healthy human beings.

◆ *Food Must Contain No Harmful Substances*

Food lovers believe that EATING is one of life's greatest pleasures. But if we look at it not only in terms of the present but also in terms of the future, it can become one of life's greatest pain with respect to what a bad diet might cause.

We should not eat food which excites desire for stimulating drink (CD235). Among these are BUTTER and MEAT (CD48). TEA is poisonous to the system, as well as is COFFEE (CD421), and its effect upon the system is even worse than tea. There is NO NOURISHMENT in them. We are told that tea and coffee drinking is a SIN.(CD425). They have the tendency to BECLOUD the INTELLECT and BENUMB the ENERGIES (CD426). The nervous system is EXCITED, temporarily INVIGORATED, and VIVIDNESS of the imagination increased. These temporarily agreeable results make people think that they really need them.

But such a stimulation only means that one is borrowing energy for present use from future resources of strength. The after effects of coffee are MENTAL DEPRESSION, NERVE EXHAUSTION, DECREASE in MUSCULAR POWER, and damage to LIVER and KIDNEY. As great as the stimulation is, so great will also be the letdown afterwards. We are told that the safe course with these things is to TOUCH NOT, TASTE NOT, and HANDLE NOT. The temptation of Satan to indulge in these things is now twice as great as it was several generations ago (CD428). "HEALTH, CHARACTER, and even LIFE, are endangered by the use of these stimulants which excite the exhausted energies to unnatural spasmodic action"(CD429). Anything that the body cannot utilize as food can cause CANCER.

CIDER is a good drink if it is sweet, and used in an unfermented state. But if it has become strong cider through the fermentation process, persons can become just as intoxicated on it than on stronger drinks. We are told that "moderate drinking is the school in which men are receiving an education for the drunkard's career" and that it awakens a taste for stronger drinks. "licentiousness, adultery, and vices of almost every type, are committed as the result of indulging the appetite for wine and cider." (CD433).

"Many articles of food eaten freely by the heathen about them were forbidden to the Israelites. It was no arbitrary distinction that was made. The things forbidden were unwholesome. The fact that they were unclean taught the lesson that the use of INJURIOUS FOODS is DEFILING. That which corrupts the body tends to corrupt the soul. It unfits the user from communion with God, unfits him for high and holy service. (MH280).

◆ *Eat Mostly Natural Raw Food*

The food eaten should be whole, UNPROCESSED, UNREFINED, and be ORGANICALLY GROWN in FERTILE SOIL. It is preferable to have it grown in your own environment, and eaten in their season (CD273). It is an established scientific principle that one's health and longevity are in direct relationship to the NATURALNESS of the foods one eats. Where natives eat a diet of whole, natural, unprocessed, and unrefined foods, they enjoy perfect health, absence of disease, and a long life. When denatured, processed, refined, manmade foods such as white sugar and white flower comes to be used among these natives, disease becomes rampant among them.

Natural foods are foods that are grown in fertile soil, without chemical fertilizers and sprays, and are consumed in their natural state with all the nutrients which God put in them intact, nothing removed and nothing added. WHITE BREAD, for example, is a denatured food from which most vital nutrients have been removed. SUPERMARKET QUALITY EGGS cannot strictly be called natural foods, for they are produced by cooped up chickens without a rooster, and are therefore infertile. They are fed chemicallized commercial mash, hence, such eggs have a lower nutritional value, less vitamins, and more cholesterol than natural eggs. Organically grown fruits and vegetables contain more vitamins, minerals, and enzymes, as has been shown in many tests. Recently researchers reported that ANTI-MALIGNANCY FACTORS are present in organically grown foods. One may say that only natural, whole, unprocessed, and organically grown foods may be said to possess THERAPEUTIC VALUE.

The foods in nature which God wants us to eat are well-balanced in their nutrients. In one sense each NATURAL FOOD is a complete food in and of itself. On their own they do not create disease. Each has its natural complements of proteins, carbohydrates, fats, enzymes, and other food factors, known and unknown. They may differ in their quantitative relationships, but most foods have some of the essential nutrients. For example, when it comes to protein, all fruits together average about 1%. All vegetables average about 2 to 3% protein, with SOYBEANS containing from 35 to 40% protein. POTATOES contain about 2% PROTEIN. The story is told of a lady who could digest no food except potatoes. She lived for years eating only potatoes without getting sick. Potatoes represent a well-balanced food.

◆ *Eat For Physical Need*

Most people eat out of habit instead out of hunger. The body doesn't need food when it is not hungry. At that time not as many enzymes are ready to digest food.

Eating when we are not hungry means eating beyond our physiological need. All such eating is OVEREATING. Money is wasted on such food, for such food is merely stored as fat. That is why so many people are overweight. It becomes the source of poisoning which may lead to more serious diseases. The organism then becomes a depository of fermenting and putrefying matter. When one eats for GRATIFICATION of TASTE without regard to physical need, one makes a garbage receptacle out of the stomach. One's maxim should be, "Take pleasure in what you eat, but don't eat for pleasure." It is said that "up to the age of 20, man can eat as much as he can, up to 40 as much as desired, and after that he should eat as little as possible."

MISSING A MEAL is not at all harmful; in fact, it is positively beneficial. We are told that "there are some who would be benefited more by abstinence from food for a day or two every week than by any amount of treatment or medical advice. To fast one day a week would be of incalculable benefit to them" (CH477). There are benefits in a spare diet (2T61).

We are told that "indulging in eating too frequently, and in too large quantities, overtaxes the digestive organs and produces a feverish state of the system. The blood becomes impure, and then diseases of various kinds occur. A physician is sent for, who prescribes some DRUG WHICH GIVES PRESENT RELIEF but which does not cure the disease. It may change the form of the disease, but the evil is increased TENFOLD. Nature was doing her best to rid the system of an accumulation of impurities, and could she have been left to herself, aided by the common blessings of heaven such as PURE AIR and PURE WATER, a speedy and safe cure would have been effected" (MM281). "Overeating DEBILITATES the stomach, WEAKENS the digestive organs, and brings on DISEASE" (CD101). It has a worse effect upon the system than overworking (CD102). It is a most pernicious violation of the laws of health. It is a sin to be intemperate in the quantity of food eaten, even if the quality is unobjectionable (CH160). We are told to "Teach the little ones that they should eat to live, not live to eat; that appetite must be held in abeyance to the will; and that the will must be governed by calm, INTELLIGENT REASON" (CH113). "It is not the chief end of man to gratify his appetite" (CH116)

◆ *Eat Only Unadulterated Foods*

If at all possible obtain food which has been grown without the aid of chemical fertilizers. It should contain no residues of toxic insecticides, chemical additives or preservatives. Most of the foods sold in supermarkets today contain some chemicals which were added when food was processed or packed. Many of the poisons in fruits and vegetables are SYSTEMIC, which means, that they cannot be washed out, as they penetrate the whole food. Here the solution seems to be to buy only ORGANICALLY GROWN FOOD, or to GROW OUR OWN FOOD. Also avoid canned, processed, preserved, and packaged foods, for they contain the most chemicals. Chemicals used in the process of preserving food, are usually those which have little relationship to food, and are therefore not compatible with the human organism. For this reason, they usually represent poisonous substances to the body. Since in this poisoned world one cannot entirely escape imbibing some poisonous substance, it is advisable for us to use extra vitamins and minerals.

The average American eats 9 lbs. of chemical additives a year including PRESERVATIVES, FLAVORING AGENTS, STABILIZERS, and ARTIFICIAL COLORINGS.

◆ *The Less You Eat, The Less Hungry You Will Feel*

Scientific studies in the U.S. and Russia show that overeating is one of the prime causes of most DEGENERATIVE DISEASES. Food eaten in excess of body needs acts in the system as a POISON. It INTERFERES with proper DIGESTION, causes internal SLUGGISHNESS, GAS, INCOMPLETE ASSIMILATION, and PUTREFACTION. The unbelievable truth seems to be that the less you eat the less hungry you feel, because the FOOD will be more EFFICIENTLY DIGESTED and BETTER UTILIZED. The rule is "EAT AS LITTLE AS YOU CAN, NOT AS MUCH AS YOU CAN."

◆ *Don't Overeat—Excess Weight Shortens Life*

The Italian Luigi Carnaro wrote in 1538 that "he who would eat much must eat little, for by eating less he would live longer, and so be able to eat more." The Framingham Study showed that for every pound of excess weight you gain after age 30, you shorten your life by 6 months. For every pound you gain after 50, you shorten your life by one year. When people ate LOW FAT MEALS, they lost nine pounds every two weeks, although they were eating as much as they wanted. Eating earlier in the day allows you to lose 10 pounds a month without changing calories. You will lose weight if all your daily calories are eaten at BREAKFAST. Eat slowly. It takes several minutes for the stomach to tell the brain that it is full. This will keep you from overeating. According to Baylor College of Medicine eating SOUP can help suppress the appetite. It helps people eat more slowly. Hence, they eat less food and gain less weight. "Overeating, no matter what the quality of the food, CLOGS the LIVING MACHINE and thus hinders it in its work" (CH119). The CAUSES OF OVERWEIGHT are: 1. eating too much; 2. eating the wrong foods; 3. eating late at night; 4. eating between meals; 5. eating empty calories; 6. eating fiberless foods; 7. lack of self-control. Eating just enough to maintain a lean body has proven the following: 1. it extends the LIFE SPAN; 2. it slows down physical deterioration; 3. it retards the process of age-related diseases such as KIDNEY and HEART PROBLEMS.

"Some eat three meals a day, when two would be more conducive to physical and spiritual health" (CD141). We are also told that "EXCESSIVE INDULGENCE in eating, drinking, sleeping, or seeing is SIN " (CD141). "Overeating is the SIN OF THIS AGE" (CD133). A great variety of dishes at a meal also causes overeating (3T563). The BEST RULE is to "take only TWO OR THREE KINDS if simple food, and eat no more than is required to satisfy hunger" (CD139).

OVERWEIGHT PEOPLE are largely cooked food eaters. COOKED, ENZYMELESS FOOD, is FATTENING, whereas the same amount of RAW FOOD is not. Dead cooked food is soil for bacterial fermentation and putrefaction. It has been demonstrated that when people change to a NATURAL LIVING FOOD DIET, they quickly lose their excess weight. Nature sees to it that no excess weight is tolerated.

◆ *Masticate Your Food Thoroughly—Eat Slowly*

It also means that we should EAT SLOWLY. When one eats fast, the APPESTAT of the body, which tells us when we are full, is slow to indicate that fact, and we may be full before we feel that we are. Then we continue to eat and overeat as a result. That is why we are told that "many eat too rapidly" (CD136). One of the more natural ways to slow down eating is to consume more FIBER. Fiber provides mouthfuls that must be chewed thoroughly, and that takes time. The end result will be that you will eat less food than you would if you hurried through your meal. Fiber also requires lots of room in the stomach, and this reduces the appetite and makes you feel full sooner and longer. You are more likely to be satisfied before you eat too much. On a high fiber diet you will also excrete more fat than on a low fiber diet. The bacterial decomposition of the refuse left in the body due to overeating causes toxic substances to be formed, for bacteria give off poisonous substances.

WE MUST NEVER EAT UNTIL WE ARE FULL. We should stop eating before that time arrives. An overeater is also a person who, when he relaxes on Sabbath will fall asleep during the sermon. "Upon the Sabbath, in the house of God, GLUTTONS will sit and sleep under the burning truths of God's word" (CD136). "Nearly all the members of the human family eat more than the system requires" (CD132). This includes also eating too much of GOOD FOOD. On the other hand, it is said that today people with full stomachs are starving from overeating of DEFICIENT FOOD.

Slow eating and thorough mastication are essential. GOOD CHEWING increases the assimilation of nutrients and makes you feel satisfied with a smaller amount of food. "Solid foods requiring mastication will be far better than mush or liquid foods." (FE227). "Fletcherize" your food, and chew every mouthful at least 30 times. Saliva contains digestive enzymes. Hence, well chewed and generously salivated food is practically half-digested before it enters the stomach. Also food should be eaten in a relaxed atmosphere and enjoyed. A peaceful, unhurried, and happy atmosphere around the table will pay good dividends in improved digestion and assimilation of food, and, as a result, in better health. "Soft or LIQUID FOODS are less wholesome than DRY FOODS, which require thorough mastication" (CD514).

◆ *Eat Only When Free from Emotional Stress*

DON'T EAT when in PAIN, ANGRY, FRUSTRATED, UPSET, or FEELING ILL. It means that when we are in a FIGHT or FLIGHT SITUATION, or when the body's reserves are marshaled to save the organism from a threatening situation, then there EXISTS LITTLE DIGESTIVE POWER. When we are sick our energies are used for the HEALING PROCESS. Digestive juices are very limited in quantity or next to nonexistent. Under these circumstances let us not be coaxed into eating by those who mistakenly think that we must eat to keep up our strength.

"If your time to eat is limited, do not bolt your food, but EAT LESS and masticate slowly. The benefit derived from food does not depend so much on the quantity eaten as on its THOROUGH DIGESTION.... Those who are excited, anxious, or in a hurry, would do well not to eat until they have found rest or relief; for the vital powers, already severely taxed, cannot supply the necessary DIGESTIVE FLUIDS" (CD107).

◆ *Do Not Drink Immediately Before, During, Or After Meals*

Water, especially cold water, requires up to 30 minutes to go through the stomach. At the fastest it can leave the stomach in 5 minutes if at the right temperature. Drinking before meals INHIBITS the SECRETION of DIGESTIVE JUICES. "Many make a mistake in drinking cold water with their meals. Taken with meals, water diminishes the flow of the salivary glands; and the colder the water, the greater the injury to the stomach. Ice water or ice lemonade, drunk with meals, will arrest digestion until the system has imparted sufficient warmth to the stomach to enable it to take up its work again. HOT DRINKS are debilitating.... Food should not be washed down; NO DRINK IS NEEDED WITH MEALS.... The more liquid there is taken into the stomach with the meals, the more difficult it is for the food to digest; for the liquid must first be absorbed." (CD420).

◆ *Eat A Good Breakfast*

The omission of BREAKFAST in order to lose weight is no advantage in a weight reduction program. To do so means that you will suffer a significant LOSS of EFFICIENCY, invite the devastating effects of LOW BLOOD SUGAR, and SLOW down your METABOLISM. When you fail to eat breakfast, your blood sugar drops slowly but continuously throughout the morning. The "morning calorie" will burn up quicker than the "evening calorie" because it has all day to be acted upon by the activities of the body.

In a study, those who started their day with a HIGH FIBER cereal ate an average of 90 fewer CALORIES at lunch. Their combined calorie consumption was also lower. Over the span of a year, a high fiber diet could result in a 10 lbs. weight loss.

We are told that "in most cases, TWO MEALS a day are preferable to THREE. Supper when taken at an early hour, interferes with the digestion of the previous meal. When taken later, it is not itself digested before bedtime. Thus the stomach fails of securing proper rest. The sleep is disturbed, the brain and nerves are wearied, the appetite for breakfast is impaired, the whole system is unrefreshed, and is unready for the day's duties" (CD176). If for some a third meal is needed, it should be light, but most people will enjoy better health with two meals a day (CD176). Benjamin Franklin said: "Dine with little, sup with less, do better still; sleep supperless."

As the blood sugar supply dwindles there is less energy and a feeling of lassitude. When the sugar level drops to about 70 mg/%, hunger is experienced and lassitude becomes fatigue. If the blood sugar drops to about 65 mg, a craving for sweets become irresistible. A continued drop develops sheer exhaustion. Then follow HEADACHES, WEAKNESS, SHAKINESS, PALPITATIONS of the HEART, RUBBERY LEGS, and possibly NAUSEA and VOMITING. In one study several subjects actually gained weight during the period they went without breakfast. If you are not hungry for breakfast in the morning, the chances are that you ate too much the night before. Supper should be a very light meal. Then you will be able to eat a good breakfast. Try a little exercise before breakfast to increase your morning appetite This is a good time for you to jog around the block.

The Spirit of Prophecy tells us that "It is the custom of society to take a slight breakfast. But this is not the best way to treat the stomach. At breakfast time the stomach is in a better condition to take care of more food than at the second or third meal of the day. The habit of eating a sparing breakfast and a large dinner is wrong. Make your breakfast correspond more nearly to the heartiest meal of the day" (CD173).

◆ *Eat Food That Agrees With You*

We need good judgment to determine what combination of foods best agrees with us. "It is our duty to act wisely in regard to our habits of eating, to be temperate, and to learn to reason from cause to effect. If we will do our part then the Lord will do His part in preserving our brain-nerve power" (CD492).

It may be that at times good food does not agree with you. The reason may be that you have gotten used to eating unhealthy food, so that the healthy food may taste flat and unappetizing. It may be that you have developed a perverted appetite. It may be that even some good food does not agree with you. Under these circumstances you might want to decide to change the habits of you taste buds, and allow them to undergo a transformation. The way to do this is to FAST for a while so that the taste buds will adjust themselves to more normal, less stimulating food. We are told that "If they cannot at first enjoy plain food, they should fast until they can. That fast will prove to them of greater benefit than medicine, for the abused stomach will find that rest which it has long needed, and real hunger can be satisfied with a plain diet" (CD158).

All good food does not agree with all people. Mrs. White says: "Avoid food which does not agree with you" (CD136). One example of this would be people who do not have enough of the enzyme LACTASE in their system to digest milk. Also "It is important that the food should be prepared with care, that the appetite, when not perverted can relish it" (CD259). Since we do not use condiments to stimulate the taste, we must be adjusted to the taste of natural foods in their natural condition. This we can do only if our taste buds are not deranged through the use of unnatural, artificial, and stimulating types of food.

◆ *Eat Mainly Raw, Living Foods*

At least 75% to 80% of your diet should consist of foods in their natural uncooked state. There are a lot of studies which indicate the SUPERIORITY OF RAW FOODS for the MAINTENANCE OF HEALTH, the PREVENTION of disease, as well as for the HEALING of disease. Cooking destroys much of the nutritional value of most foods. Many vitamins are partly destroyed, minerals are leeched into the boiling water, and all ENZYMES are destroyed at temperatures of over 120° F. It is estimated that the human body requires about 600 various enzymes to maintain proper health, and cooking destroys all of them. Cooking also changes the biochemical structure of PROTEINS, AMINO ACIDS, and FATTY ACIDS, and makes them only partially digestible. It has been demonstrated that you need only one-half the amount of protein in your diet if you eat protein foods raw instead of cooked.

◆ *Eat Only Natural Foods*

Your food should be whole, unprocessed and unrefined. It should be preferably grown in your own environment, and eaten in its season. An established scientific fact is that your HEALTH and LONGEVITY are in direct relationship to the naturalness of the food you eat. Natural foods are foods that are grown in fertile soils without chemical fertilizers and sprays, and are consumed in their natural state, with all the nutrients God put in them intact, nothing removed and nothing added. Organically grown fruits and vegetables contain more VITAMINS, MINERALS, and ENZYMES, than the produce grown on depleted, chemically fertilized soil. Such foods have greater health-building and disease-preventive potential. Recent research has also shown that ANTI-MALIGNANCY FACTORS are present in organically grown foods. Synthetic, denatured, and devitalized foods will not sustain health, but will inevitably bring about a gradual degeneration of normal body functions, which ultimately leads to disease.

◆ *Avoid Foods That Have Been Processed, Blended, Mixed, Or Tampered With.*

Almost all food sold at supermarkets contains some chemicals, either used in food producing, or added during food processing or packing. Many of the poisons in fruits or vegetables are systemic, that is, they cannot be washed out or peeled out, as they penetrate all of the fruit. The only solution is for you to grow your own food, or buy the certified organically grown food. If possible, avoid the eating of all processed and packaged foods, which contain the most chemicals. Since in our poisoned world it is almost impossible for us not to get some poisons into our systems, it would be wise for us to learn about the vitamins and minerals and PROTECTIVE FOODS such as BREWER'S YEAST, KELP, WHEAT GERM, and FISH LIVER OILS, which will neutralize the poisons in our system.

◆ *Eat Only When Really Hungry*

Nature has provided a built-in mechanism within your brain which will tell you unmistakably when you should eat or drink. You should eat when you are hungry, and drink when you are thirsty. Contrariwise, you should never eat when you are not hungry, and some say that you should not drink when you are not thirsty, but this is debatable. Your requirements for food and drink are unique, different from those of everybody else. But you can not go wrong if you follow your hunger and thirst signals. Food eaten without appetite will do you no good. It may harm you by overburdening the digestive organs with unwanted material and create INDIGESTION, GAS, and other disturbances.

◆ *Do Not Mix Too Many Foods At The Same Meal*

There is a lot of evidence to the effect that the fewer foods you mix at the same meal, the better your digestion and assimilation will be. Every food, every fruit or vegetable, requires a different enzyme system, and too many at one meal result in less effective digestion. "There should not be a great variety at any one meal, for this encourages

OVEREATING, and causes INDIGESTION." We are told that "the habit of overeating or eating too many kinds of food at one meal frequently causes DYSPEPSIA" (CD139). Do not make a battleground out of your stomach. "All mixed and complicated foods are injurious to the health of human beings. Dumb animals would never eat such a mixture as is often placed in the human stomach" (CD113). "There is intemperance in eating and in the many varieties of food taken at one meal. In the preparation of food there are unhealthful mixtures which ferment in the stomach and cause great distress." (MM225).

We do not need to try to get every important nutrient in at every meal. The principle here is to try to get them in with the meals that we eat during ONE WHOLE DAY. Even this is not an absolute necessity, for the body maintains reserves of nutrients which allow us to extend the full complement of nutrients over more than one day.

The simpler the foods you eat, the less complex is the digestive task. The less complex the digestive task, the more efficiently does the digestive function proceed.

◆ *Do Not Eat Raw Fruits And Raw Vegetables At The Same Meal*

Fruits and vegetables taken at one meal produce ACIDITY of the stomach; then impurity of the blood results. Raw fruits and raw vegetables require totally different ENZYME COMBINATIONS for their effective digestion. Such combination will only result in poor digestion and gas. It would be advisable to make one meal of the day a FRUIT MEAL, with possibly YOGURT, RAW SEEDS, and NUTS, and another meal a VEGETABLE MEAL. The exception to the rule are THE ACID CITRUS FRUITS, PINEAPPLE, PAPAYA, and AVOCADO, all of these fruits can be eaten with vegetables. We are told that "it is not well to eat fruit and vegetables at the same meal. If the digestion is feeble, the use of both will often cause distress, and inability to put forth mental effort. It is better to have the fruit at one meal, and the vegetables at another. The meals should be varied. The same dishes prepared in the same way, should not appear on the table meal after meal and day after day. The meals are eaten with greater relish, and the system is better nourished, when the food is varied" (CD112).

◆ *If Possible Eat Protein Foods First*

Proteins require a generous amount of HYDROCHLORIC ACID (HCL) in your stomach. Your stomach secretes only a limited amount of HCL, for it is not needed for the digestion of CARBOHYDRATES. If you eat the carbohydrates foods first, then you are diluting the hydrochloric acid for the protein foods, and these foods will remain largely undigested. Hence eat the protein foods first on an empty stomach. Those who have tried it say that it works. It works even with the bad effects of eating beans. If fruit juice sours in your stomach, it is usually a sign that you have a deficiency of hydrochloric acid.

◆ *Practice Systematic Undereating*

SYSTEMATIC UNDEREATING may be the number 1 health and longevity secret. On the other hand, OVEREATING of even good food is one of the main causes of disease and premature AGING. Studies of CENTENARIANS have shown that all of them are moderate eaters. You never saw, and never will see, an obese centenarian. Studies have shown that overeating is one of the prime causes of most degenerative diseases. Food eaten in excess of actual body needs acts in the system as a POISON. It is especially dangerous for older people, who are less active and have a slowed down metabolism.

Undereating extends the lifespan, delays sexual maturity, and influences hormonal and immunological systems in ways that extend life.

The Cooking Of Food

◆ *Cooking And The Spirit Of Prophecy*

"For want of knowledge and skill in regard to cooking, many a wife and mother daily sets before her family ill-prepared food, which is steadily and surely impairing the digestive organs, and making a poor quality of blood; the result is frequent attacks of inflammatory disease, and sometimes DEATH. We can have a variety of good, wholesome food, cooked in a healthful manner, so it will be palatable to all. It is of vital importance to know how to cook. Poor cooking produces DISEASE and BAD TEMPERS; the system becomes deranged and heavenly things cannot be discerned. There is more RELIGION in GOOD COOKING than you have any idea of. Scanty, ill-cooked food depraves the blood by weakening the blood-making organs. deranges the system and brings on disease, with its accompaniment of irritable nerves and bad tempers. The victims of poor cookery are numbered by thousands and tens of thousands. Over many graves might be written: 'Died because of poor cooking' 'Died of an abused stomach' (CD256–7). "In reality, cooking.... is a science in value above all other sciences"(CD251). "Before children take lessons on the organ or the piano they should be given lessons in cooking. The work of learning to cook need not exclude music, but to learn music is of less importance than to learn how to prepare food that is wholesome and appetizing.(CD263). Often HEALTH REFORM is made HEALTH DEFORM by the unpalatable preparation of food" (CD263).

◆ *Bread Making*

"For use in bread making, the superfine white flour is not the best. Its use is neither healthful nor economical. Fine-flour bread is lacking in nutritive elements to be found in bread made from the whole wheat. It is a frequent cause of constipation and other unhealthful condition. The use of SODA or BAKING-POWDER in bread-making is harmful and unnecessary. Soda causes inflammation of the stomach, and often POISONS the ENTIRE SYSTEM.... In the making of raised or yeast bread MILK should not be used in place of WATER. The use of milk is an additional expense, and it makes the bread much less wholesome.... Bread should be light and sweet. Not the least taint of sourness should be tolerated. The loaves should be small and so thoroughly baked that, so far as possible, the yeast germs shall be destroyed." (MH300–1). "It takes thought and care to make good bread; but there is more RELIGION in a loaf of good bread than many think." (MH302).

Sourness in bread is due to the incomplete drying of the bread which allows the moisture in it to react with other substances. On the other hand, SOURDOUGH BREAD is produced due to the enzymatic action on the grain whereby valuable LACTIC ACID develops, which is a health-promoting and disease preventing factor as demonstrated by Dr. Johannes Kuhl and others. Also the fermentation makes certain nutrients in grains more easily available for assimilation in the intestinal tract. This is particularly true in the case of ZINC, MANGANESE, and other trace minerals. RYE is the most suitable grain for making sourdough bread.

◆ *No Food Is Made More Nutritious By Heating It*

There was no cooking in the Garden of Eden. Food was eaten raw in the manner in which God had created it, and after all, who knew better how to serve up food that was fitted to man's organism. There was no fire used in the Garden of Eden, for there Adam and Eve ate only fruits, nuts, seeds and grains. The vegetables were eaten later on after they had to leave the Garden. There were some vegetables which could be softened through heat after the discovery of FIRE was made. Since that time we may say that fire in connection with cooking has been more of a detriment than a blessing to man. Cooked food is an inferior food, for some vital elements such as VITAMINS, MINERALS, and ENZYMES are destroyed during the cooking process. It is said that NO FOOD IS EVER MADE MORE NUTRITIOUS BY HEATING IT. Cooked foods are foods that are more dead than alive. "Dead foods sooner make dead people."

◆ *Cooking Destroys Food Value*

Cooking destroys food from the moment that heat is applied. The more cooking foods receive the more they are destroyed. Cooking modifies the chemistry of food toward non-food, until food is disorganized, made unusable, made less palatable and more poisonous until only poisonous ashes are left. Heat changes the nature of nutrients so that they are not assimilated as well by the body. The less time food is cooked the more nutritious it is. Steamed SPINACH loses 50% of its vitamin C. Only 40 to 60% of the vitamins remain in vegetables cooked by the conventional method on the stove. In some cases one can get close to 100% nutrient retention with a MICROWAVE oven. The IRON in food becomes inorganic as a result of cooking and therefore less assimilable. The same is true with CALCIUM and other minerals which our body requires. Uncooked foods are foods that are living, that are raw. Only in these living foods exist the vital principle of life on which we can thrive to the maximum extent. Only through them can we truly achieve our biological potential.

Cooking destroys the vitamins, and one author says that vitamins are turned into gases, the gases which you can smell when you smell the food. They are escaping as you are smelling them. We like to smell the food as it is boiling, the bread as it is baking, but they represent a part of the vitamins which you are losing as nutrients. They are evaporated vitamins. This does not happen when you eat raw food.

One study has shown that CANCER CELLS from a human body will thrive on cooked food, but they were unable to thrive on the same kind of food when it was raw. One author says that all bodily disease originates in the colon, because the colon is the dumping ground for the waste material from the digestive organs. Heating food destroys the enzymes which are absolutely necessary for proper digestion. This means that much of the modern food that is eaten is not properly digested because of the lack of ENZYMES in the food. Cooked food saturates the blood with waste and foreign matter. Dr. Otto Warburg demonstrated that poisons in the system interfere with the enzyme system which carries OXYGEN to the cells.

◆ *Cooked Food Considered As Enemy Substance By Body*

The WHITE BLOOD CORPUSCLES are the body's first line of defense against toxic or harmful substances. The normal white corpuscle count of the blood is about 6,000 per cubic centimeter (ccm). When this count doubles, triples, or goes up four or five times, this is indicative of a pathological condition. Dr. Kouchakoff of Switzerland conducted over 300 experiments with cooked and processed foods, foods that are not natural to the human dietary. Foods cooked at temperatures from 120° to 190° F, which destroys all enzymes, caused LEUKOCYTOSIS in his subjects. Leukocytosis is a term applied to an abnormally high white blood corpuscle count. Within a short time after food had been cooked at this temperature range, his subjects' white corpuscle count TRIPLED. But foods eaten in this temperature range by his subjects did not cause leukocytosis if certain types of raw foods were added to the meal. But, if the food was cooked at temperatures higher than 190°, no amount of raw food would offset the pathological effects of the cooked food, and leukocytosis always occurred. The fact that the body treats cooked and processed food as antagonistic to it, should be a sufficient message to us to limit cooked and processed foods in our diet.

◆ *Pulse Rate Reflects Body Condition*

When unwelcome foods enter the body, our pulse rate may shoot up as high as 100 pulses per minute. A normal pulse for a healthy person is in the 40 to 60 range, with some outstanding athletes having pulses in the low 30's. Cooked food eaters have a normal pulse rate of about 72 per minute. Such pulse is symptomatic of a somewhat pathological condition. The heart is stimulated to greater effort to faster circulate the blood to rid the system of pathogenic matters. Dr. Claunch who wrote the book *Exploding the Germ Theory*, proved that just as garbage conditions are favorable to the fly, so it is with bacteria. Unless we provide the soil, bacteria are harmless. He says that there are nearly 700,000 species of animal life, and everyone of these species except man, live exclusively on natural, uncooked, organic food. No other animal except man eats devitalized food. It is no surprise therefore that man is the only species in the entire animal kingdom that is sick, with the exception of some domestic animals that have their diet prescribed for them by man.

◆ *Natural Foods Do Not Cause Pathological Effects*

Cooking foods and processing them — REFINING, STERILIZING. PRESERVING, PICKLING, FLAVORING, and COLORING — all devitalize and rob of nutrients. It is clear that living foods that are natural to the human dietary do not cause pathological effects, and if we want to live to the full extent of our life potential, we should change to a 100% living food diet as one of the necessary factors toward achieving this goal. Hygienists advise us to eat at least 75% natural foods, and the rest only lightly steamed, as in Chinese food.

◆ *Heat Destroys Living Force In Food*

Heat applied to food destroys their LIVING FORCE, the ENZYMES and AUXONES. Enzymes speed up reactions and induce chemical changes without being changed themselves. Auxones also promote growth in plant cells and tissues. They are absolutely indispensable to human well-being. Although a healthy person synthesizes within himself with the aid of intestinal bacteria 1,000 enzymes and co-enzymes, co-enzymes being called VITAMINS, he still requires those enzymes inherent in natural foods.

◆ *Heat Makes Food Less Digestible*

The Max Planck institute For Nutritional Research determined that one needs only the amount of protein in the diet if one eats protein foods RAW instead of COOKED.

Cooking coagulates proteins which are broken down into URIC, HIPPURIC, SULFURIC, and PHOSPHORIC ACIDS. They become unwelcome in the system. It deaminizes essential and nonessential amino acids, which means that the amino acid chains are broken down and rendered largely indigestible. It destroys hormones. It caramelizes sugars, and they become, in effect, a sweet syrup not easily assimilated by the body. It breaks up natural fats and makes them completely indigestible and poisonous, and it coats other food particles and renders them indigestible too. Especially poisonous is ACROLEIN, which is formed as a result of cooking fats. It renders minerals inorganic, alters or destroys flavors, and also destroys the co-enzymes or vitamins. Not only are nutritive factors destroyed by heat, but those substances destroyed, and altered become toxic and harmful to the body. The frying pan can become a very deadly weapon. POLYUNSATURATED FATS are highly susceptible to oxidation and the generation of free radicals. Cooking changes PROTEINS into a form that deposits FREE RADICALS in your system. FOOD RULE; "Either keep it hot or keep it cool." THAW FOOD in the refrigerator, not in the kitchen. "Food grows mold when it grows old."

Cooking renders food less digestible and of less utility to the body economy. RAW CABBAGE, for example, is digested in about 2 hours. Cook it and it requires about 4 hours in the digestive tract. Cooked foods are often appropriated by the body in unassimilable forms. This stimulates the body to extraordinary eliminative efforts which can exhaust our nerve energy.

◆ *Natural Food Gives More Nutrition With Less Food*

By eating raw natural foods, you INCREASE your NUTRITIONAL INTAKE on LESS FOOD. You require less food, and you put less toxic material into your system. Once you get used to natural foods you will enjoy their taste, and you will not have to use CONDIMENTS with which to deceive your taste buds. ALL EXCITANTS to the taste PERVERT our taste. They deprave our taste. They make acceptable to the palate foods that are hurtful to us. Foods worthy of the human dietary can be relished in their natural living state without cooking, sauces, seasonings, or condiments. Not only do you eat less, but foods in their natural state COST LESS.

◆ *Cooked Foods Are Disease-causing*

Dr. Pottenger experimented with feeding cooked and natural food to two groups of cats. Control groups fed exclusively on cooked foods suffered MENTAL DERANGEMENT, DECREASED SEXUAL ABILITIES, DEVELOPMENT of MENSTRUATION in the FEMALES, ARTHRITIS, HEART TROUBLES, HOMOSEXUALITY, GENERAL SICKLINESS, and a SHORTENED LIFE. Test groups fed on the very same foods in their natural state enjoyed superb vigor and health. Experiments on calves have demonstrated that calves cannot live on their own MOTHER'S MILK, if the milk has been subjected to the heat of pasteurization. Calves died within one to two months from diseases born of MALNUTRITION and SYSTEMIC POISONING.

◆ *Cooked Foods Spoil Readily*

If we eat cooked food, or what may be called dead organic matter, bacteria have a Roman holiday. Starches and sugars ferment quickly, and the body becomes a vinegar and alcohol factory, especially when we eat incompatible combinations. INDIGESTION then means that most of the food will be acted upon by bacteria and not by digestive juices. BACTERIA cannot exist on living cells. They are a very weak form of life. They are scavengers. Their soil is dead organic material. They are responsible for the SYNTHESIS of VITAMIN B_{12} within our and animal bodies. Cooked foods spoil inside and outside the body quite readily, whereas natural foods are slow to lose their vital qualities to become soil for bacteria. Bacteria breakup and decompose the trash in our systems just as they do in soils. Bacterial action renders usable some waste matters that would ordinarily be expelled. They are essential to our lives and without them our existence would not be possible.

Let us illustrate again the heating of food such as in making yogurt from raw milk. If we take the raw milk and add a culture of BACILLUS BULGARICUS, the culture dies before it sours the milk. But if we first PASTEURIZE or BOIL the milk, or render it dead and then cool it to about 100° or 110° F, and add the bacterial culture, keeping it at this temperature, we will have yogurt in about 6 to 8 hours. Note that the bacterial culture could not act on milk in a fresh state, whereas in a dead state the milk readily became soil for bacterial proliferation. The by-products of bacterial action are ACID EXCRETA, VINEGARS, ALCOHOLS, AMMONIAS, etc., all death dealing to bacteria and man alike.

◆ *Cooked Food Causes Constipation*

Cooked foods are to a great extent responsible for bowel irregularity or CONSTIPATION. The majority of Americans suffer this unnatural, abnormal and unnecessary affliction. The nerves controlling peristalsis are perpetually intoxicated, and will eventually be completely destroyed. Cooked fats are especially deadly to the heart, even if the fats are obtained from vegetable sources. They are also suspected of being CARCINOGENIC, but it has been shown that a NATURAL FOOD DIET corrects cases diagnosed as cancer.

◆ *Being overweight — A Symptom Of Cooked Food*

✓ FAT CELLS INCREASE AS YOU GAIN WEIGHT—The removal of salt and sugar from baby food has taken place because of mounting scientific evidence that early exposure to these substances may contribute to the problems of obesity and hypertension. Infants show no preference for salt in food. This was added for the benefit of the mother.

The diseases of OVERWEIGHT and OBESITY, which are heart ailments, high blood pressure, peptic ulcers, diabetes, gall bladder ailments, cirrhosis of the liver, and poor circulation, are largely symptoms of cooked food eaters. If they would revert to a diet of fruits, nuts, and vegetables, they would speedily lose their excess baggage. Many people are pot-bellied. This is mostly retained wastes, and many individuals have lost 50 to 60 pounds upon a lengthy FAST. The FAT CELLS of the body increase in number as you gain weight, but when you lose weight, the fat cells do not decrease in number; they simply grow smaller. After obesity, therefore, a person will have a constant struggle against gaining weight, because the number of fat cells cannot be reduced.

✓ FAT CELLS DON'T DECREASE WITH LOSS OF WEIGHT—Statistics show that if a child is obese before the age of two, he will likely be obese in adulthood, because he has already an increased number of FAT CELLS. These fat cells will remain with him the rest of his life. It is more difficult for an obese adult to lose weight if he was obese before the age of two, which means that he has more fat cells than normal. 99% of obesity is directly related to overeating. Obese adults have a higher than normal DEATH RATE for their age group. The risk of death correlates almost directly with how much a person is overweight.

✓ OBESITY DECREASES LONGEVITY AND INCREASES CANCER—In 1935 C.M. McCay showed that feeding rats a low protein diet yielded lean animals that lived much longer than animals fed a high protein diet. Also in humans obesity decreases LONGEVITY, and increases CANCER DEVELOPMENT. Hence, caloric restriction has the greatest influence on cancer development as determined by experimental studies. POST-MENOPAUSAL women produce a lot more of the female hormone ESTRONE. This production is directly related to the size of the fat cells, for estrone is manufactured in them.

✓ OBESE PERSONS USUALLY CONSUME MORE FAT IN THEIR DIET—People who are obese usually consume more fat in their diet, which is a major risk factor for the development of BREAST and COLON CANCER. If food intake is reduced, lower amounts of PROLACTIN and ESTROGEN are produced, thereby producing a lower risk of cancer development. Diets high in fat also depress a person's resistance to TUBERCULOSIS, MALARIA, and PNEUMONIA. Obesity also interferes with the action of INSULIN. Hence, obese persons have a 2 to 3 times higher risk of developing DIABETES.

◆ *Cooked Food And Menstruation*

In nature animals do not menstruate. Man domesticates his animals and feeds them an unnatural diet, and his pet dogs therefore menstruate. Wild dogs do not. During menstruation the womb becomes an eliminative organ, while the other eliminative organs are overloaded. Females of pristine peoples and apes do not menstruate when they ovulate. In civilization menstruation accompanies ovulation in more than 99% of our women. Healthy women living in healthy circumstances do not menstruate. It is suspected that cooked foods are the main cause of the unhealthful condition that brings on this monthly affliction.

FEMALE ATHLETES experience bloody menstruation little or not at all. Women who go through a lengthy fast often have only a little mucus discharge instead of a bloody flow. Observers have been amazed to discover that in many TRIBAL SOCIETIES, whose members live close to nature, very few women have bloody menstruation, and that even among these the flow is exceptionally light. Many women who have adopted a completely HEALTHY LIFESTYLE have been surprised to find the cessation of bloody menstruation to be a by-product.

The Acid-Alkaline Balance

◆ *Foods Can Be Divided Into Acid And Alkaline Foods*

When we talk about certain foods, such a LEMONS, ORANGES, STRAWBERRIES, CHERRIES etc. as being ACID FOODS, we do not necessarily mean that they are acid-forming in the body. They can be alkaline in reaction in the body after they are eaten, provided that the alkaline reserve in the body is high enough to convert the acid. However, in the process of being converted to an alkaline, these strongly acid foods do draw upon the alkaline reserves of the body. Therefore, persons suffering from ACIDOSIS should not eat these strongly acid fruits. They could increase the acidosis. Those foods which have a lot of STARCH, PROTEIN, and FATS in them, such as BEANS, NUTS, EGGS, and CHEESE, are the real acid-forming foods.

◆ *Both Extreme Conditions Are Harmful*

It is good for us to remember that how we COOK and how we EAT a certain food may have a lot to do with whether or not it is an acid or alkaline-forming food. For example, a mealy baked potato is alkaline in reaction if it is CHEWED WELL, and if the SKINS are eaten. If it is washed down or swallowed whole, the digestion then is not complete, and it is acid-forming. Similarly, fried, greasy potatoes are acid-forming. It is just as bad for the body to become TOO ALKALINE as TOO ACID. Hence, we should not necessarily leave off all acid foods. ALKALOSIS is often the result of an excessive intake of ALKALINE DRUGS such as SODIUM BICARBONATE for the treatment of gastric or peptic ulcers. Alkalosis may cause calcium to build up in the body such as in the case of BONE or HEEL SPURS. The organs of elimination are supposed to normally handle a certain amount of acid-forming foods, which are considered to be the body-building foods. If the BLOOD becomes too alkaline, one can suffer from LOW BLOOD PRESSURE, POOR CIRCULATION, COLD FEET AND HANDS, ANEMIA, EMACIATION, NEURASTHENIA, LACK OF PEP, ENERGY, AND AMBITION. If the blood becomes too acid, one may suffer from SKIN ERUPTIONS, PYORRHEA, TOXEMIA, HIGH BLOOD PRESSURE, NEURITIS, RHEUMATISM, INSOMNIA, NERVOUSNESS, BAD TEMPER, and numerous other disorders. To treat acidosis, start with small amounts of CITRUS FRUITS and gradually add larger amounts.

◆ *Disease Conditions Are More Often Acid Conditions*

In living we produce body acids, and by eating we supply food-alkali. We are built up of foods that have both alkali-forming and acid-forming elements. We must maintain normal alkalinity of the blood, or else we will develop disease. If the body is lacking in alkali, it will be kept from neutralizing some of the poisonous organic and mineral acids. A HEALTHY DIET is predominantly ALKALINE in effect, while an UNHEALTHY DIET is predominantly ACID in effect.

The tendency seems to be for people to err on the side of acidity. ACIDOSIS, or OVER-ACIDITY in the body tissues is one of the basic causes especially of the ARTHRITIC and RHEUMATIC diseases. All foods are oxidized or "burned" in the body. This process is more commonly called "digestion." The ash or residue which results from the burning of food is either NEUTRAL, ACID, or ALKALINE, depending upon the mineral composition of the foods. The acid ash results when there is a depletion of the alkali reserves. It is important that there is a proper balance between acid and alkali foods in the diet. The natural ratio in a normally healthy body is approximately 4:1, or four parts of alkaline to one part of acid or an 80% to 20% ratio. When such a ratio is maintained, the body has a strong resistance against disease. In the healing process, the more alkaline elements are in the diet, the faster will be the recovery. ALKALIES NEUTRALIZE THE ACIDS. Therefore, it is important that the patient's diet includes a lot of alkaline foods to offset any effect of the acid foods, and still leave a safety margin of alkalinity.

◆ *Acid And Alkaline Foods*

A healthy body keeps large alkaline reserves which are used to meet emergencies of the sort when too many acid foods have been eaten. But such reserves can be depleted. When the alkaline-acid ratio drops to 3:1, health can be seriously affected. For optimum health and greatest resistance to disease, it is important that the diet be slightly OVER-ALKALINE. The ALKALI-FORMING FOODS are practically all fruits and vegetables, with the top three being FIGS, SOYBEANS, and LIMA BEANS. THE ACID-FORMING FOODS, besides all meats are: EGGS, ALL GRAINS and BREADS except MILLET and BUCKWHEAT, RICE, ALL NUTS except ALMONDS and BRAZIL NUTS, and LENTILS. SPROUTED SEEDS, and GRAINS become more alkaline in the process of sprouting, and VEGETABLE BROTH is an extremely alkalizing drink. NEUTRAL FOODS—are Milk and unheated VEGETABLE OILS. Acid—forming foods thicken the blood and put a strain on the arteries and heart.

◆ *How Our Blood Becomes Acid*

When large amounts of SUGAR, either simple or complex, are taken in, they are absorbed quickly. The GLUCOSE derived from them increases in the body cells, causing an imbalance of OXYGEN, which causes incomplete oxidation. This incomplete oxidation produces many organic acids such as LACTIC ACID, PYRO-RACEMIC ACID, BUTYRIC ACID, and ACETIC ACID, thereby producing an acid condition in the body or ACIDOSIS. For this reason SUGARY FOODS have a tendency to cause acidosis. Black sugar such as MOLASSES, is less acid-forming, because it is a less processed sugar. It contains alkaline-forming minerals and vitamins which aid the combustion of glucose. JUNK FOOD which is high in sugar, high in refined white flour, white rice, cocoa, chocolate, and caffeine products, has a very acid reaction in the body, which means that we are headed for trouble if we eat such food. It is the tendency for acid-forming foods to be MUCUS-FORMING foods. The more ALKALINE the diet, the easier the body will be able to cleanse itself and remove toxins from the system.

◆ *The Acidity and Alkalinity Of Urine*

According to Dr. James F. Balch dietary aspects of acid—base balance are less important than metabolic defects, but can still influence the acidity or alkalinity of the body, and hence that of the URINE. For example:

✓ A RABBIT—has a diet consisting mainly of green and other vegetables. It therefore normally excretes an alkaline urine.

✓ A DOG—which is carnivorous and omnivorous, excretes an acid urine.

✓ VEGETARIAN HUMANS—usually excrete a neutral or slightly alkaline urine.

✓ OMNIVOROUS HUMANS—excrete a slightly acid urine

✓ HEAVY MEAT EATERS—excrete a more acid urine. This is due to the fact that protein is high in sulfur, which the body converts to SULFURIC ACID before excretion in the urine. The high PHOSPHORUS content of meat ends up as phosphoric acid, which also contributes to the acidity of the urine, which can develop into BLADDER CANCER.

◆ *Dietary Acids*

DIETARY ACIDS are organic acids present in FRUITS, VEGETABLES, and YOGURT. Contrary to popular belief they do not produce acidosis, and are in fact alkaline-forming. Examples of such acids in the diet are the following:

- ✓ CITRIC ACID—is oxidized by the body in its normal energy-production cycle. It is contained in CITRUS FRUITS, PINEAPPLES, TOMATOES, and most SUMMER FRUITS.
- ✓ MALIC ACID—is oxidized by the body in its normal energy-production cycle. It is contained in APPLES, PLUMS, and TOMATOES.
- ✓ BENZOIC ACID—is readily excreted by the kidneys, after combining with the amino acid GLYCINE as HIPPURIC acid.
- ✓ TARTARIC ACID—is hardly absorbed, so that it does not contribute to the acid-base balance of the body. It is found in GRAPES.
- ✓ OXALIC ACID—can combine with calcium to form insoluble CALCIUM OXALATE so that it is not absorbed. However, excess oxalic acid can IMMOBILIZE CALCIUM and other minerals to an extent that may cause a mild deficiency. Any oxalic acid absorbed is readily oxidized by existing metabolic processes. It is contained in STRAWBERRIES, GREEN TOMATOES, RHUBARB, and SPINACH.
- ✓ LACTIC ACID—is metabolized by the same body processes that dispose of lactic acid produced from glucose. It is contained in YOGURT, SOUR MILK, SAUERKRAUT, in certain types of PICKLES, KEFIR, ACIDOPHILUS MILK, and COTTAGE CHEESE. It is a fermented food that promotes good digestion and furnishes the body with enzymes. It is pre-digested, cleanses the blood, and helps with elimination. To make it use sea vegetables, such as KELP, instead of salt. Kelp contains only 18%–20% salt.

The Proper Combining Of Food

◆ *Starchy Foods Digest In An Alkaline Medium*

We are told that "Knowledge in regard to proper food combinations is of great worth, and is to be received as wisdom from God" (CD109). It is a fundamental fact of chemistry that ALKALIES and ACIDS are opposites so that they neutralize each other. It is a fact of physiology that all STARCHY FOODS digest in an AKALINE MEDIUM. The starch-splitting enzyme of the mouth, PTYALIN or SALIVARY AMYLASE, is destroyed by acid, even a mild acid. Therefore, if acids are taken with starches, starch digestion is suspended. If breads or cereals or potatoes are eaten with berries or with citrus fruits, or with other acid foods, the digestion of these starches is delayed.

◆ *Protein Foods Digest In An Acid Medium*

It is a fact of physiology that PROTEINS require an ACID MEDIUM for their digestion in the stomach. When proteins are eaten, acid is secreted to enable the enzyme PEPSIN, to begin the work of protein digestion. It is not possible for both starch digestion and protein digestion to both go on at the same time in the stomach. The rising acidity of the stomach will neutralize the saliva, destroy the salivary amylase, and bring starch digestion to a halt. If no protein is taken with the starch, no acid is poured into the stomach and starch digestion proceeds on schedule. The application of this fact is clear: EAT STARCH FOODS at separate meals from ACID FOODS, or foods requiring acid for their digestion. This means do not eat CEREALS, BREAD, GRAINS, POTATOES, PARSNIPS, SQUASH, BEANS, or other starchy foods with EGGS, CHEESE, NUTS, or other protein foods. Also do not eat the starchy foods with the acid foods of ORANGES, GRAPEFRUIT, PINEAPPLE, and BERRIES. There is enough oxalic acid in SPINACH to delay or suspend starch digestion.

◆ *We Should Not Eat A Great Variety Of Food At One Meal*

Because of the fact that in a great variety of foods, acid and alkali food may be mixed, it is unwise to eat a great variety of food at one meal. We are told that "Many are made sick by the indulgence of their appetite.... So many varieties are introduced into the stomach that FERMENTATION is the result. This condition brings on acute disease, and death frequently follows. The variety of food at one meal causes unpleasantness, and destroys the good which each article, if taken alone, would do to the system.... The habit of overeating, or of eating too many kinds of food at one meal, frequently causes DYSPEPSIA. Serious injury is thus done to the delicate digestive organs. In vain the stomach protests, and appeals to the brain to reason from cause to effect. The excessive amount of food eaten, or the improper combination, does its injurious work. In vain do disagreeable premonitions give warning. Suffering is the consequence. Disease takes the place of health" (CD110–11).

◆ *Acids Will Neutralize Alkalies*

All this means that the combinations of FRUITS and CEREALS for breakfast, SOY PRODUCTS and POTATOES are not compatible. Such combinations are largely responsible for what is called "acid indigestion." The retarded digestion that is caused favors FERMENTATION and PUTREFACTION of the foods eaten.

A very small portion of VINEGAR will diminish the digestion of starch by its inhibiting effect upon the PTYALIN. From this fact it becomes evident that PICKLES which are saturated with vinegar, SALADS on which vinegar has been put, and salad dressings containing vinegar, are unwholesome substances to take into the human digestive tract, especially when taken with starchy foods. Vinegar not only destroys PTYALIN, but it also contains alcohol, which precipitates the PEPSIN of the gastric juice and retards or prevents gastric digestion of proteins. It is no wonder that pickles and vinegar have been found useful in reducing weight, because they cripple the first two stages of digestion. Also APPLE CIDER VINEGAR is unfit for use because it contains two poisonous substances such as ACETIC ACID and ALCOHOL.

Dr. Herbert Shelton summarizes the essential rules of food combining as follows:
✓ Eat acid foods and starchy foods at separate meals. Acids will neutralize the alkaline medium required for starch digestion and the result is FERMENTATION and INDIGESTION.
✓ Eat protein foods and carbohydrate foods at separate meals.
✓ Eat but one kind of protein food at a meal.
✓ Eat protein and acid foods at separate meals. Otherwise there will be some protein foods that are not properly digested. Undigested protein putrefies in bacterial decomposition and produces some potent poisons such as INDOL, SKATOL, PHENOL, PHENYLPROPIONIC and PHENYLACETIC ACIDS, FATTY ACIDS, CARBON DIOXIDE, HYDROGEN, MARSH GAS, HYDROGEN SULFIDE, ETC.
✓ Eat FATS and PROTEINS at separate meals. Some foods, especially nuts, are over 50% fat and require hours for digestion.
✓ Eat FRUITS and PROTEINS at separate meals.
✓ Eat FRUITS and STARCHY FOODS at separate meals. Fruits undergo no digestion in the stomach and are held up if eaten with foods that require digestion in the stomach.
✓ Eat MELONS alone. They combine with almost no food.
✓ Desert the desserts. Eaten on top of meals they lie heavy on the stomach, requiring no digestion there, and FERMENT. Bacteria turn them into alcohols and vinegars and acetic acid. Acetic acid is found in vinegar,

The Digestion Of Food

◆ *Acid Fruits Suspend Starch Digestion*

Even those acids that are valuable as food, such as the acids of PINEAPPLES, GRAPEFRUIT, ORANGES, TANGERINES, LEMONS, LIMES, TOMATOES, APPLES, GRAPES, PEACHES, CHERRIES ETC., destroy the ptyalin of the saliva and arrest the digestion of starch. For this reason such foods should not be eaten at the same meal with POTATOES, BREAD, CEREALS, BEANS, PEAS, ARTICHOKES, CARROTS, CAULIFLOWER, PARSNIPS, and similar foods.

◆ *Acid Fruits also Retard Protein Digestion*

Acids also inhibit the secretion of gastric juice,

hence they suspend or retard protein digestion in the stomach. Thus these fruits should not be eaten with protein foods such as eggs, cheese, nuts etc. BAKING SODA also destroys pepsin, and retards gastric digestion. Many drugs, both acid and alkalies, have been used for reducing weight because they retard digestion. Anything that either inhibits the secretion of the digestive juices, or alters their chemistry, or destroys their enzymes, will retard or suspend the process of digestion. CONDIMENTS of all kinds, because of the irritation of the stomach which they occasion, inhibit stomach digestion. SALT inhibits stomach digestion also. The eating of complex mixtures of food is not seen in nature. Animals not only stay strictly with the foods to which their digestive systems and processes are especially adapted, but they refrain from mixing these indiscriminately.

◆ *Digestion Begins In The Mouth*

All foods are broken up into smaller particles by the process of chewing, and they are thoroughly saturated with SALIVA. Of the chemical part of digestion, only STARCH DIGESTION begins in the mouth. There is no sugar digestion in the mouth. When sugar is eaten, there is a copious flow of saliva, but it contains no ptyalin. If soaked starches are eaten, no saliva is poured out upon these, and ptyalin is not poured out upon meat or fat. The SALIVA of the mouth, which is usually an ALKALINE fluid, contains the enzyme PTYALIN when it acts upon starch, breaking it down into MALTOSE, a disaccharide which is present in malt, malt products, and sprouted seeds, which is further acted upon in the intestine by the enzyme MALTASE and is converted to the monosaccharide or simple sugar DEXTROSE. The starch that escapes digestion in the mouth may be changed to maltose by AMYLASE, a pancreatic secretion in the small intestines. The STOMACH or GASTRIC JUICES contain three enzymes: PEPSIN, which acts upon PROTEINS; LIPASE, which acts upon FATS; and RENNIN, which coagulates MILK. Pepsin will initiate digestion on all kinds of proteins. It acts only in an acid medium and is destroyed by an alkali. Low temperatures, as in the case of cold drinks, retards and even suspends the action of pepsin.

◆ *Sensory Indicators Cause Saliva Flow*

Just as the SIGHT, ODOR, or THOUGHT of food may occasion the flow of SALIVA, so these same factors will occasion the flow of GASTRIC JUICE. The TASTE of food, however, is the most important factor in occasioning a flow of saliva. There is no secretory action, when the substances taken into the mouth cannot be digested. In his experiments with the 'conditioned reflex', Pavlov noted that it is not necessary to take the food into the mouth in order to occasion the flow of gastric juice. The mere TEASING of a dog with savory food will serve the purpose. He found that even the noises or some other action associated with feeding time, will occasion the flow of secretion.

HERBS ARE GOD'S MEDICINES

God Gave Man The Herbs Of The Field For Food And Medicine

After He had created man God gave man for food the herbs of the field. This was to be food which would fulfill man's need for sustenance to sustain his life. It was food which was adapted to him, so that the food and the body processes for digesting it were in harmony. He did not give him any food which he could not digest, or which was harmful to his system. "And God said, 'Behold, I have given you every herb bearing seed, which is upon the face of all the earth, and every tree, in the which is the fruit of a tree yielding seed; to you it shall be for meat'."(Gen. 1:29).

God has allowed herbs to grow in the earth which have MEDICINAL PROPERTIES. For the stricken one to use these does not contradict God's healing power. In fact His healing power is combined with these herbs to bring about a successful result. "There are herbs that are harmless, the use of which will tide over many apparently SERIOUS DIFFICULTIES" (2SM291). "God has caused to grow out of the ground HERBS for the use of man, and if we understand the nature of these roots and herbs, and make the right use of them, there would not be a necessity of running for the doctor so frequently, and people would be in much better health than they are today" (MM231). "The use of certain herbs that the Lord has made to grow for the good of man is in harmony with the exercise of FAITH" (MS 31, 1888). Before modern drugs were developed physicians used herbs. The Song of Solomon in 4:14 mentions SPIKENARD, SAFFRON, CALAMUS, CINNAMON, FRANKINCENSE, MYRRH, ALOES, and chief SPICES. The Israelites used bitter herbs with the eating of the paschal lamb (Song of Solomon 4:14).

God created His medicine for man so that it would be easily obtainable. He placed it right under man's feet, in the plants that grow all around him. God has established His laws of healing so that they would be valid forever. Man cannot improve upon them, nor develop any medicine that is better than what God has produced.

Herbal medicine is practiced throughout most of the world. In the Orient and Africa it is the primary medicine of the people. It has been largely ignored in the U.S. because drug companies cannot profit from making herbal products which cannot be protected by patent rights. Neither the FDA nor the AMA will accept herbal research done in other countries. Herbs are allowed to be sold in this country only as FOOD SUPPLEMENTS. As such, claims cannot be made for their effectiveness in treating disease. Drug companies are not interested in botanicals except to synthesize their potent factors into new chemical compounds which can be subjected to control and patented.

God Gave Man No Flesh Food In The Beginning

God gave man in his original diet FRUITS, GRAINS, NUTS, and VEGETABLES. They were prepared for man because they were best for his constitution. They were to be prepared as simply as possible and were to be eaten in as natural manner as possible. They were of such a nature as to be healthful and nourishing; to give strength and the power of endurance, and a vigor of intellect that were not to be obtained from a more complex and simulating diet (MH296). After the flood, because of the destruction of vegetation, God allowed man to eat of the animals, but only those which He considered "clean" animals. Besides this, the eating of FAT and BLOOD was strictly forbidden. Furthermore, it had the effect of shortening man's life. "Flesh was never the best food; but its use is now doubly objectionable, since disease in animals is so rapidly increasing" (CD384). Meat is a stimulating kind of food which is not best for the body, nor for calm consideration of that which is truth. It is a diet that tends to develop us toward ANIMALISM.

God Is Endeavoring To Lead Us Back To His Original Diet

Since meat was never the best diet for man, because he was not created as a meat eater, but rather as a vegetarian, today, God wants us to return to His original diet of the herbs of the field. Such a diet is also designed to purify our lives physically, mentally, and spiritually in preparation for Christ's second coming. We are told that "among those who are waiting for the coming of the Lord, meat eating will eventually be done away; flesh will cease to form a part of their diet." (CD380). He wants us to continue to subsist on the natural products of the earth. These natural products have now been somewhat polluted with chemicals in their preparation, and with the use of chemical fertilizers, that we find it difficult to eat anything that is pure anymore, but we must nevertheless do the best that we can.

There Are No Incurable Diseases With God

In a broad definition of the term "herbs," we could include fruits and vegetables, as well as the medicinal plants which God has created for our well-being. Many fruits and vegetables today are used as medicines with great success. Rev. 22:2 tells us that "the leaves of the tree were for the healing of the nations." The leaves of the tree were to be medicine which would keep God's children from disease and in health. Ps. 104:14 says: "He causeth the grass to grow for the cattle, and herb for the service of man; that he may bring forth food out of the earth." We are to believe that God has a remedy for every disease, and that with him and the medicines which he has created there are NO INCURABLE DISEASES.

Herbs Of The Bible

✓ BALM OF GILEAD—The term "herb" or "herbs" is mentioned 37 times in the Bible, and there are many specific herbs mentioned. Jer. 8:22 says: "Is there no balm in Gilead; is there no physician there? Why then is not the health of the daughter of my people recovered?" The Balm of Gilead is a small tree native to Arabia. By making incisions in the tree a resinous substance is obtained which is still used today in Arabia and other Asiatic countries. When it first flows out of the tree, the liquid is white, but it later turns into a golden yellow color which has the consistency of honey. It has a strong turpentine like odor. The buds are rich in SALICIN, a glucoside that decomposes into SALICYLIC ACID through oxidation in the human system. It reduces CONGESTION, FEVER, INFLAMMATION, and PAIN. The buds of the tree are used as medicine for disorders of the LUNGS, such as COUGHS and CHEST CONGESTION, STOMACH, and KIDNEYS. They are also used as an ointment for the PAIN of ARTHRITIS, RHEUMATISM, GOUT, and MUSCLE SORENESS.

The Balm of Gilead contains RESINS, VOLATILE OILS, and SALICIN, a chemical relative of aspirin.

✓ FIGS—2 Kings 20:7 says: "And Isaiah said, Take a lump of figs. And they took it and laid it on the boil, and he recovered." Here Hezekiah was healed with a lump of figs, and 15 years were added to his life. Among the Hebrews the FIG TREE was associated with the VINE as a symbol of PEACE and PLENTY. The figs are still used as medicine in many lands throughout the world today. In Bavaria they are cooked in milk for use in treating ULCERATED GUMS. Among the Hindus the milky juice of the trees is given to relieve toothache, while in America the juice is used in the treatment of RINGWORMS and WARTS. Figs heated and cut open are placed on GUM BOILS to draw out the matter. For PULMONARY COMPLAINTS they are boiled in BARLEY WATER.

✓ FRANKINCENSE—Matt. 2:11 says: "and when they had opened their treasures, they presented unto him gifts; GOLD, and FRANKINCENSE, and MYRRH. Frankincense was burned both by the Egyptians and Jews in their religious rites. The odor of incense was believed to center the mind on devotion, produce an elevated mental state, and in some way effected the mind. It cannot be denied that certain odors do cause powerful reactions in people. The aroma of certain foods can start the saliva flowing before the food actually enters the mouth. It is still used today as an INCENSE, and in Egypt the GUM is chewed to sweeten the breath.

- ✓ HYSSOP—Hyssop has been known for centuries for its cleansing and beautifying effect on the skin. David drew an important lesson from the use of hyssop when he said, "Purge me with hyssop, and I shall be clean; wash me and I shall be whiter than snow" (Ps. 51:7). When Christ was hanging on the cross he was given vinegar which had been placed upon hyssop (Jo. 19:29). Hyssop was a SYMBOL of PURIFICATION from SIN. Vinegar was given those who suffered death by the cross, as a drug or a stupefying potion, to deaden the sense of pain. But Christ refused it because he would not take anything that would BECLOUD HIS MIND. To do so would have given Satan an advantage (DA748). "The hyssop used in sprinkling the blood was the symbol of purification, being thus employed in the cleansing of the lepers and those defiled by contact with the dead" (DA277). In the old days the early herbalists used hyssop leaves on fresh wounds to protect them against infections and to promote healing. Doctors thought that this was pure superstition until they discovered that the mold which produces penicillin grows on hyssop leaves.

  Contemporary herbalists use hyssop compresses and poultices for BRUISES, BURNS, and WOUNDS, and an infusion for COLDS, COUGHS, BRONCHITIS, FLATULENCE, INDIGESTION, MENSTRUATION, and even EPILEPTIC SEIZURES. Hyssop inhibits the growth of the HERPES SIMPLEX VIRUS which causes GENITAL HERPES and COLD SORES.

- ✓ MYRRH—Myrrh is one of man's oldest romantic favorites among the botanicals. The Ishmaelites that carried Joseph to Egypt also carried myrrh with them (Gen. 37:25). The Egyptians highly esteemed myrrh, as it was one of the chief ingredients in the process of embalming. During this process all internal organs were removed, except for the heart and the kidneys. Then various ointments such as perfumes, spices, and chemicals were employed. The poorer classes used myrrh as a preservative and salted the body for 70 days. Then they wrapped it in coarse cloth and placed it in the catacombs. The ancient Hebrews used myrrh as a medicine which healed their bodies, as an incense it lifted their spirits, and as a perfume it pleased their hearts. One of the wise men offered myrrh to infant Jesus.(Matt. 2:11).

  Myrrh is a shrub or tree native to countries bordering the red sea. The juice flows naturally from the bark and hardens to form gum myrrh which is used as medicine. One of its uses was as an ingredient in holy oils with which they anointed the tabernacle, the ark, the altar, and the sacred vessels. Esther 2:12 tells us that six of the twelve months devoted to the purification of women were accomplished with oil of myrrh. Myrrh has been used to promote PERISTALSIS, and it became the ALL-PURPOSE AROMATIC for perfumes, funerals, and insect repellents.

  In America in the 19th century it was considered for treatment of "indolent sores and gangrenous ulcers." It contains TANNINS which have an astringent effect on tissues. Today myrrh is considered to be a POWERFUL ANTISEPTIC, and as a medicine for weak stomachs. Outwardly applied, it is used for ulcers and bedsores, and is best mixed with charcoal. When applied to fresh wounds, the tincture increases healing action for sore throats, gums, and mouth ulcers.

- ✓ MYRTLE—Isa 55:13 says, "Instead of the thorn shall come up the fir tree, and instead of the briar shall come up the myrtle tree: and it shall be to the Lord for a name, for an everlasting sign that shall not be cut off." Myrtle signified the promise and bounty of God to the Jews. In ancient times its foliage was formed into wreaths for the adornment of heroes, in the performance of religious rites, and as an emblem of civil authority. In some parts of Greece its evergreen quality was symbolic of immortality. The branches of the myrtle tree were waved during the feast of tabernacles (DA448). It is used as a remedy for rheumatism, internal ulcers, and dysentery. The leaves are used in the making of perfume.

- ✓ SPIKENARD—Spikenard is an aromatic plant. The ancients gathered the roots for use in preparing valuable PERFUMES which were used at celebrated feasts, in the baths of the wealthy, and also as a medicine. It makes a powerful perfume from a plant of the valerian family. Its roots and stems produce the essence which was quite an expensive item of commerce from early times. It was customary for the ointment to be kept in sealed alabaster boxes and brought forth on very special occasions. The pound of spikenard with which Mary anointed the feet of Jesus represented almost a year's wages for a laboring man of the time (8BC1039). It is an excellent BLOOD PURIFIER, good in all skin diseases, pimples, eruptions, coughs, colds, and all chest afflictions

The History Of Herbs

◆ *The Symbols Of Medicine*

The symbol of a STAFF AND TWO SNAKES coiled around it, the symbol of modern medicine, has it origin in the "Greek God of Medicine." This was the title given to AESCULAPIUS, an ancient Greek physician whose healing powers were considered so miraculous, that after his death he was honored to the stature of a god. His statue, which was represented with a staff around which a snake was coiled, was placed in all the temples. The snake is shown with an herb in its mouth. One of the daughters of Aesculapius, HYGEIA, became deified as a "Goddess of Health." From her we receive the word HYGIENE. His other daughter, whose success in using herbal remedies for the cure of diseases won her the title of "Goddess of Medicine." Her name was PANACEA, from which we get the word meaning "cure-all."

The Greek word "phisis," meaning natural constitution, came to signify PHARMACY and SORCERY and in this way those who practiced the healing arts came to be known as "physicians." HIPPOCRATES, who became the father of medicine lived from 460 to 377 B.C. The major part of his treatments were HERBS, DIET, BATHS, FRESH AIR, MASSAGE, REST and QUIET. He made his followers swear that they would give no poisonous remedies to their patients.

◆ *Herbal Medicine Held In Highest Regard*

Herbs have been used as healing agents by every race upon the earth since the time of creation. They somehow learned of the medicinal value of many ROOTS, BARKS, LEAVES, SEEDS, and PLANTS. Such knowledge was handed down from generation to generation. The oldest medical literature such as PAPYRUS EBERS of the 2nd century B.C., and all of the Persian, Roman, Hebrew, Chinese, and Egyptian records show that HERBAL MEDICINE was held in highest regard, and was used extensively to cure practically EVERY ILLNESS KNOWN TO MAN. In Mexico herbal medicine was greatly advanced during the Mayan, Incan, and Aztec cultures, and is still used at the present time. In India, China, Central and South America, Africa, and the Pacific Islands, herbs are still widely used.

◆ *How Herbalists Use Herbs*

Herbalists, instead of destroying directly the germs which play a part in the illness, concentrate on changing the INTERNAL and EXTERNAL ENVIRONMENT of the body. They believe that if you strengthen the organs and cleanse the body there is then nothing left for the germs to feed on. The impurities of the body represent the soil and the food that germs feed on. If the germs are starved out by cleaning the IMPURITIES out of the system, then there is no room for germs to settle anywhere, and disease cannot find a foothold there. Simply wiping out the germs still leaves the impurities, and, secondly, it introduces into the body POISONOUS CHEMICALS. These chemicals generally damage the immune system upon which we rely to help destroy the germs. This weakens the body to the extent that it is less able to defend itself against the disease. When the germs are destroyed, the impurities still remain.

◆ *Herbs Help The Body Help Itself*

The herbalists assist the body in doing what it itself is supposed to do in the healing process. While ALLOPATHS use drugs to eliminate SYMPTOMS, herbalists use herbs to CLEANSE and HEAL the entire body. While lowering blood sugar with drugs eliminates a symptom temporarily, herbalists proceed to use herbs to strengthen, stimulate, and cleanse the pancreas. While the allopathic physician will use the poisonous DIGITALIS drug to stimulate the heart, the herbalist will use instead the nonpoisonous herb of the Lily Of The Valley for the same purpose.

◆ *An Herb Has Many Active Healing Factors In It.*

Herbalists believe that while there may be a single strong factor in herbs that participates in the cleansing process, there are other complementary factors which are necessary to make sure that the effect is beneficial. The active principle is MODIFIED, EXTENDED, or BUFFERED by other ingredients in the herb. To extract only a perceived "active" principle out of an herb is to often change the effect in the direction of a drug, in which case the effect often has side effects. Herbs must be used in the manner in which God has created them for them to do good without harm. The herbalist uses whole plants or whole parts of a plants without taking anything out. This would include all of the concomitant factors. Then the herb doesn't have any SIDE EFFECTS, and it will gently stimulate the body's own self-healing mechanisms. An herb not only supplies active ingredients, but it also supplies vitamins as well as mineral nutrients such as IRON, COPPER, or ZINC, which supplement the active factors and make them more effective.

◆ *The Effects Of Extracts Of Herbs*

The roots of the plant RAUWOLFIA have been used for thousands of years as a SEDATIVE. Mahatma Ghandi used to drink rauwolfia tea as a nightcap. An extract of rauwolfdia is the alkaloid RESERPINE which went largely out of fashion because by itself it caused severe DEPRESSION. The same is true with the drug DIGITALIS of the foxglove plant. Clinicians believe that the whole powdered leaf of the plant is more efficacious than the single isolated GLYCOSIDES extracted from the plant. The sad part about this is that drug companies don't want to know that plain old plants can cure disease. They don't want to know that the herb FEVERFEW will prevent migraines, if they make 2 billion dollars a year off migraines with drugs. Herbs can put them out of business. People can pick their own plants and use them. In nature for every disease there is a cure, and nature knows no incurable diseases.

◆ *Animals Instinctive Use Of Herbs*

Wild and domestic animals use herbs instinctively. The instincts of animals makes use of the natural laws for healing themselves. They know unerringly which herbs will cure what ills. Wild creatures first seek solitude and relaxation, then they rely on the remedies of nature, the medicine in plants, pure air, sunshine, water, and rest: a bear grubbing for FERN ROOTS, a wild turkey eating the leaves of the SPICE BUSH, an animal bitten by a poisonous snake chewing on SNAKEROOT. An animal with fever hunts up a shady place near water, eating nothing, but drinking often until health is recovered. An animal with rheumatism finds a spot in hot sunlight until the disease is baked out. Scientific investigation has confirmed the medicinal value of most of the plants which sick animals select instinctively. Naturalists at a national park in Tanzania, noticed that sick chimpanzees ate the leaves from a bush called ASPILIA. Later scientists discovered that aspilia leaves contain a powerful antibiotic. This suggests another ANIMAL INSTINCT — the use of food as medicine. In his journals THOREAU wrote, "A man may esteem himself happy when that which is his food is also his medicine." Since plants can change inorganic substances into organic substances, when we use plants for food, we are using organic substances which are in harmony with our own physical composition. That is the way God has arranged it.

Herbs purify the bloodstream. Hence, one of the fundamental objectives of the use of herbs is to purify the bloodstream and create a normal functioning of the organs and ductless glands. Herbal doctors contend that their treatment is especially suited to deal with chronic complaints. Since plant medicines, which are the true medicines, are administered in small doses and are slow in effect, this slow process will effect more radical and complete cures than the more rapid methods of allopathic medicine. It is estimated that healing herbs are the primary medicines of two-thirds of the world's population.

◆ *American Doctors Are Making Use Of More Herbal Products*

Modern American medicine is isolationist. Rather than building on the substantial knowledge of the past, or even trying to understand it, it simply throws it out. This is because it lacks the traditions present in European and particularly Oriental societies. That is why most American doctors are unfamiliar with the vast scientific literature demonstrating the safety and effectiveness of HERBS. The typical physician's only exposure to it is the medical journal articles reporting harm from the irresponsible use of healing herbs. But the number of people harmed by herbs is only a very small fraction of the number of people harmed by drugs and other accepted medical procedures. Since most of their knowledge about herbs is negative, they feel skeptical about herbal healing. However, doctors are becoming more knowledgeable about herbs now since specialists have recommended the herb FEVERFEW for preventing MIGRAINES, GINGER for preventing MOTION SICKNESS and NAUSEA. Many cardiologists now recommend GARLIC as being effective in reducing cholesterol. Surgeons now speed the healing of incisions with ALLANTOIN, extracted from the COMFREY herb. Some doctors use a form of LICORICE for ULCERS, as it has been shown to be as effective as the drug CIMETIDINE, and without any side-effects.

Under current FDA regulations, the prohibition against unapproved medical claims includes a ban on warnings about possible side-effects. It is therefore illegal for herb packages to list possible problems, even though such warnings are clearly in the public interest. As a result most healing herbs are sold not as medicines but as FOOD SUPPLEMENTS, which do not require pre-approval, but which also allow no healing claims or warnings about potential risks. Ironically, by forbidding appropriate warnings, the FDA is violating its most important mission: that of protecting the public health. In Germany and Canada steps have been taken to exempt "Folk Medicine" from expensive effectiveness tests, as long as they are shown to be safe, and labeled properly.

Common Herbs Used Today

✓ ALFALFA—Alfalfa was named by the Arabs "the Father of all Foods." It is one of the most studied of plants. It contains many important substances such as SAPONINS, STEROLS, FLAVONOIDS, COUMARINS, ALKALOIDS, ACIDS, VITAMINS, SUGARS, PROTEINS, MINERALS, TRACE ELEMENTS, and other nutrients. It is a BODY CLEANSER, INFECTION FIGHTER, and a NATURAL DEODORIZER. It eliminates RETAINED WATER, and relieves URINARY and BOWEL PROBLEMS. It is one of the most nutritious foods known. Instead of being only a food for livestock, scientists are discovering that it contains substances which are valuable to the health of human beings. It contains vitamins A, B, K, D_1, and U. As a healing agent in PEPTIC ULCERS it is believed that vitamin U shows great promise, as it prevents ulcers in laboratory animals. Vitamin U is also present in CABBAGE. Alfalfa contains 8 known enzymes which are necessary to enable foods to be assimilated in the body. It also has a high protein content of 17%, which is equivalent to meat. In India, a poultice of alfalfa seeds is an effective treatment for BOILS. The fluid from freshly squeezed alfalfa KILLS a wide range of BACTERIA. Alfalfa is one of the most nourishing plants on earth, perhaps because its roots penetrate 10 to 20 feet into the ground. The vitamin K guards us against HEMORRHAGING, and helps our blood to CLOT properly. Alfalfa has a high content of calcium, and is rich in many fatty acids. It is also rich in BETA-CAROTENE, CHLOROPHYLL, and XANTHOPHYLL, which are substances noted for preventing CARDIOVASCULAR COMPLICATIONS and CANCER.

The Chinese use alfalfa as medicine for ULCERS, for strengthening the DIGESTIVE TRACT, and to STIMULATE THE APPETITE. Animal studies show that alfalfa leaves help reduce blood CHOLESTEROL levels and plaque deposits on artery walls. Two studies suggest that alfalfa's digestive enzymes help NEUTRALIZE CARCINOGENS in the intestines, and speed their elimination from the body. French scientists have shown that alfalfa can reduce tissue damage caused by RADIATION THERAPY. It can help to remedy BLEEDING DISORDERS such as OBSTRUCTIVE JAUNDICE or BILIARY FISTULA. Other bleeding disorders result from the use of ARTIFICIAL FORMULAS for feeding newborn children, protracted ANTIBIOTIC THERAPY, PANCREATIC INSUFFICIENCY, CHRONIC DIARRHEA, the use of ANTICOAGULANTS, ASPIRIN, and ANTICONVULSANT DRUGS. Dietary vitamin K can remedy all of these conditions.

✓ ALOE VERA—Aloe vera is called "Nature's Miracle" and the "first aid" plant, for it soothes the pain of almost any MINOR BURN, SCRAPE, SKIN IRRITATION, or POISON IVY. It is one plant that every household should have. It is one of the easiest plants to grow indoors. The fresh juice from the leaves heals wounds by preventing or drawing out infections. It speeds healing time and works best in the open air. It has ANESTHETIC, ANTIBACTERIAL, and TISSUE RESTORATIVE properties. The GEL heals burns from flame, sun, and radiation. It soothes itching and burning. It has been taken internally for stomach disorders. It is effective against many different BACTERIA that can invade a wound. Studies show that it may also kill the "CANDIDA ALBICANS" yeast infection. A pint of the gel taken in small doses several times a day has been used for GASTRIC ULCERS without any side effects. A European study suggests that ALOE VERA reduces blood sugar levels in animals and humans with DIABETES. Aloe vera helps to heal internal tissues damaged by radiation exposure such as X-rays and radiation. It contains CALCIUM, POTASSIUM, SODIUM, MANGANESE, MAGNESIUM, IRON, LECITHIN, and ZINC. The aloe that was used to embalm the body of Christ, according to John 19:39, was probably a closely related specie.

✓ CANCERILLO—Cancerillo is a MILKWEED PLANT growing in the jungles of Costa Rica. It is called "cancerillo" by the natives because they have used it for ages as a remedy for CANCERS, WARTS, and TUMORS in general. A Wisconsin team of scientists found an active ingredient in cancerillo that destroys human cancer cells in the test tube, called CALOTROPIN. It had been known for a long time, but they didn't know that it could destroy cancer cells.

✓ CHAMOMILE—Chamomile is a favorite of women and children in Europe and in some parts of the U.S., and is part of the daily diet of many of these people. It is one of the best herbs to keep handy for EMERGENCIES. It is the best-known European "CURE-ALL." Its most firmly established property is its anti-inflammatory effect. It is a soothing SEDATIVE with no harmful effects. It is useful for small babies and children for colds, stomach trouble, colitis, and eczema. Its effects are ANTI-ULCER, ANTI-BACTERIAL, ANTI-TUMOR or ANTI-CANCER. The active principles of chamomile include ESSENTIAL OILS, FLAVONOIDS, GLYCOSIDES, and a very important ETHER. Many divergent cultures have used chamomile for very similar TONIC purposes down through the centuries. It is useful for small babies and children for COLDS, STOMACH TROUBLE, COLITIS, a GARGLE, for inducing SLEEP, and externally for ECZEMA and INFLAMMATION.

Chamomile was used anciently to cure HEADACHES, and illnesses affecting the liver, kidneys, and bladder. It was used to cure FEVER which plagued the ancient civilization. It has a relaxing action on the smooth muscle lining of the digestive tract thereby halting stomach and menstrual CRAMPS. It has an analgesic action on inflamed tissues, and heals CANKER SORES in the mouth. It is also used for GALLSTONES. It contains TRYPTOPHAN, an amino acid which is necessary for the production of vitamin B_3 or niacin.

In an experiment two groups of animals were fed a chemical known to cause ulcers. Those given chamomile developed significant fewer ulcers, and recovered more quickly. Research shows that chamomile is a TRANQUILIZER, for it depresses the central nervous system, and it is a mild SEDATIVE. The tea can be used for MUSCULAR SPASMS, and to relieve PAIN and SWELLING caused by arthritis or an injury. It is beneficial in cases of ANXIETY. Constituents of chamomile, such as the FLAVONES, have smooth muscle relaxing activity, thereby aiding digestion and promoting relaxation. It is also recommended that one add a handful of chamomile flowers to the HOT BATH. In other animal studies chamomile relieved arthritis joint INFLAMMATION. It prevents wound INFECTIONS, and reduces the time it takes for wounds to heal. It kills the yeast fungi CANDIDA ALBICANS that causes vaginal infections, as well as the STAPHYLOCOCCUS bacteria. It prevents infections by stimulating the immune system's infection fighting white blood cells, the macrophages, and the B-lymphocytes. A lady in a village in Europe was known as the "Herb Lady." A man from a neighboring village was brought to her suffering from a severe case of DROPSY, representing an accumulation of fluids in the body, so that he could only sleep sitting up for fear of suffocating. The Herb Lady knew immediately that he was unable to pass urine. She gave him a glassful of CHAMOMILE TEA mornings and evenings, and soon he was able to pass an unbelievable quantity of urine, a fact which he confirmed. After 8 days of this treatment, he was completely cured. It has also been found that a RAW POTATO POULTICE applied and left on all night will help reduce the swelling of dropsy.

✓ CHAPARRAL-CREOSOTE BUSH—The creosote bush is an olive green bush which grows in blistering hot dry desert regions of the southwest. The Indians of the region considered it to be a CURE-ALL and used chaparral for treating BRUISES, TUMORS, STOMACH AILMENTS, and PULMONARY and THROAT COMPLAINTS. It is made from the leaves of the bush as one of the most successful treatments for ARTHRITIS and RHEUMATISM. Some tribes used it as poultices for relieving bodily ACHES and PAINS. Others used it for MUSCULAR ACHES and for SWOLLEN JOINTS. Mexicans called it the governess of the body because it cured so many ailments.

It is one of nature's best ANTIBIOTIC, both internally and externally. It is good for treating BACTERIAL, VIRAL, and PARASITIC infections. It is a bitter herb, and is usually mixed with other herbs.

It has an ANTI-TUMOR effect. One man who refused surgery by University of Utah physicians for MALIGNANT MELANOMA, a most serious SKIN CANCER, told them that he intended to treat himself with chaparral tea. The doctors were greatly surprised when 8 months later he returned with a marked regression of his cancer. Al. Wolfsen, an Adventist herbalist, tells the story of his friend who had stomach cancer. One night his friend had a dream and an angel appeared to him in the dream and told him to go out into the dessert, find the CREOSOTE BUSH, take the leaves and make a tea from it and drink it every day. With it he eliminated his stomach cancer.

Chaparral contains an anti-cancer acid which helps in the treatment of tumors and leukemias. Scientists claim that it extends and even doubles the average life span of laboratory animals. In general it is also an excellent BLOOD CLEANSER. It also prevents the formation of FREE RADICALS, and is therefore believed to not only stop certain kinds of CANCER, but to also retard PREMATURE AGING.

✓ CINNAMON—Cinnamon is a powerful antiseptic, a GERM KILLER. It kills many decay and disease-producing bacteria, fungi, and viruses. It is a common ingredient in folk remedies for COLDS, FLATULENCE, NAUSEA, and VOMITING. It suppresses completely the ESCHERICHIA COLI bacteria, the cause of many urinary tract infections, as well as CANDIDA ALBICANS, the fungus responsible for vaginal yeast infections. It contains the natural anesthetic oil EUGENOL, which helps relieve the pain of cuts and bruises. It helps break down fats in the digestive system. Japanese researchers report that cinnamon helps reduce BLOOD PRESSURE. It makes an excellent mouthwash, clears up athletes foot, and prevents CANCER induced by chemicals in food.

✓ COMFREY—Comfrey is one of the most valuable of herbs known to botanic medicine. It has been used for centuries with success as a WOUND HEALER and BONE KNITTER. It was therefore called "knit bone" and "Boneset" by country folk. It contains the valuable healing agent ALLANTOIN, a cell proliferant found in the leaves and roots. It has dissolved ulcers in various parts of the body. Even in ancient times it had been used to heal ULCEROUS LEG WOUNDS, BROKEN BONES, and especially LEG FRACTURES. It speeds up the formation of new bone cells. It also contains CHOLINE, a constituent of LECITHIN and other phospholipids. It helps promote the secretion of PEPSIN and is a general aid to digestion. It has a strong effect on the CENTRAL NERVOUS SYSTEM, and should be taken only in small amounts. There are 20 varieties, some of which are cultivated for fodder. It is also used for an injured PERIOSTEUM, the connective tissue covering the bones. It has a beneficial effect on all parts of the body, being an overall TONIC.

It is essential in normal fat and carbohydrate metabolism. It is highly esteemed as a remedy in all PULMONARY COMPLAINTS, HEMOPTYSIS or HEMORRHAGE of the LUNGS, and CONSUMPTION or TUBERCULOSIS. It reduces all kinds of INFLAMMATORY SWELLING if used as a fomentation. It helps people with ECZEMA, and other skin troubles, DIGESTIVE DISORDERS, RHEUMATISM, BOILS, ULCERS, as well as ASTHMA. It is an effective ANTACID which helps stomach ulcers to disappear due to the therapeutic agent ALLANTOIN. It is highly recommended as a BLOOD PURIFIER. It is one of the herbs that contains VITAMIN B_{12}.

In case of PAIN, pulped comfrey root can be applied to the painful parts and the pain will gradually disappear. In cream form comfrey is a beauty treatment for the SKIN. With wheat germ oil and honey, it makes an excellent healing paste. Comfrey was banned in several countries because it created tumors in test animals. The reason for this was that the ALKALOIDS which it contains were extracted out of the plant and given to the animals. This did not happen when the whole plant was used.

A woman who heard of comfrey being called a miracle herb, put several big leaves through a juicer, diluted them, put the pulp on some gauze, and used this poultice one a day on her husbands VARICOSE ULCERS on his legs. In 6 weeks the ulcers were all gone. A young woman was in an auto accident and fractured her right hip. The surgeon found it necessary to insert a pin in her hip. After having forgotten about the pin and having neglected any physical check-up, she developed a bone infection that caused great pain, and she hurried to the doctor. The doctor removed the pin and gave injections of a strong antibiotic for the infection, and pain pills for the pain that had developed. However, the bone failed to heal and the pain continued. Then a neighbor prepared a warm poultice of Comfrey root and applied it to the infected joint. She said that it was almost a miracle how her PAIN DISAPPEARED OVERNIGHT. The next day she was able to move around freely without pain.

✓ DANDELION—Dandelion is the weed under our feet which represents a very effective medicine for many purposes. In the dandelion both the LEAVES and the ROOTS are used as medicine. The word means "lion's tooth" according to the appearance of the leaves. The root is a classic European remedy for LIVER DISEASES such as HEPATITIS, CIRRHOSIS, JAUNDICE, and TOXICITY in general. It has a high INSULIN content and thereby aids people with DIABETES MELLITUS. The tea will reduce FEVER in the childhood diseases of MEASLES, MUMPS, and CHICKENPOX. It represents a wonder purifying agent as it contain a good assortment of alkaline salts such as SODIUM, POTASSIUM, and CALCIUM that are needed for purifying the blood. It stimulates the flow of BILE, which helps us digest fats, and also prevents GALLSTONES. Because of its high content of minerals, it is used to treat ANEMIA. It will increase the flow of URINE, and is a good medicine in KIDNEY formulas.

The leaves are also an effective DIURETIC due to their content of POTASH or POTASSIUM CARBONATE. Diuretics usually deplete the body of potassium. However, in the case of dandelions less potassium is lost than with other diuretics because the herb itself has a high potassium content. For potassium eat bananas and lots of fresh vegetables. Dandelions are also used for DYSPEPSIA, KIDNEY TROUBLE, SPLEEN, PANCREAS, and act as a mild LAXATIVE in conditions of chronic constipation. They promote a healthy CIRCULATION, strengthen weak ARTERIES, and cleanse the SKIN of blemishes. It is one of the best herbs for building the BLOOD and curing anemic conditions. It is also useful for CORNS, ACNE, and BLISTERS. The juice of the stem can be applied to WARTS, and it will dry them up in a few days. The inside part of a ripe banana peel is also said to eliminate warts with repeated applications.

When the dandelions first appear, the young leaves can be eaten and used like spinach in salads. They furnish a rich source of vitamins A and C. The inhabitants of the Island of Minorca in the Mediterranean subsisted for quite a while on dandelion roots after their harvest had been entirely destroyed by locusts. One cup of dandelions contains 2000 international units of vitamin A, and also some vitamin C, both of which are antioxidants. Antioxidants help prevent the cell damage that scientists believe eventually causes cancer. Dandelion leaves and roots are believed to be CANCER PREVENTATIVE substances.

Dandelion has a particularly beneficial effect on the liver and is a superior BLOOD CLEANSER and DETOXIFIER. A EUROPEAN HEALTH SPA known for its cures of liver complaints, regularly serves Dandelion greens as well as conventional salads to all patients. Authoritative herbologists recommend that DIABETICS eat up to 10 fresh Dandelion stems daily, gathered when the plant is in bloom. For CHRONIC INFLAMMATION of the LIVER 5 or 6 stems per day bring quick relief. The pains of GOUT, RHEUMATISM, and SWOLLEN GLANDS disappear when the fresh stems are chewed for a period of time which should be from 2 weeks to a month. JAUNDICE and disorders of the SPLEEN yield to the Dandelion also.

✓ ECHINACEA/CONEFLOWER—Echinacea root is a major ANTI-INFLAMMATORY, ANTI-BACTERIAL, ANTI-VIRAL, ANTI-FUNGAL, ANTI-PROTOZOAN, as well as an IMMUNE stimulant in the botanical kingdom. It boosts the white blood cells ability to destroy pathogens. It is one of the BEST BLOOD PURIFIERS. Dr. E. Alstat of Oregon calls it "The best herb for blood and lymph purification." Native American tribes had long been using it for SNAKEBITES. It neutralizes acid conditions of the BLOOD. It is good for BLOOD POISONING, CARBUNCLES, all PUS diseases, ABSCESSES of the teeth, GANGRENE, all LYMPH SWELLINGS, enlargement and weakness of the PROSTATE GLAND. It is thought to confer non-specific immunity to disease. A substance called CAFFEIC ACID GLYCOSIDE, reacts with other substances in the body to facilitate the WOUND-HEALING process. It is a valuable alternative to all ANTIBIOTICS, and assists in removing BACTERIA, GERMS, and CARCINOGENIC SUBSTANCES from the body.

It is used to cure a wide variety of ailments such as RHEUMATISM, STREPTOCOCCUS INFECTION, BEE STINGS, POISONOUS SNAKE BITES, DYSPEPSIA, TUMORS, SYPHILIS, ECZEMA, AND HEMORRHOIDS. It greatly increases the production of infection fighting T-cells up to 30% more than immune boosting drugs. Researchers have successfully treated RHEUMATOID ARTHRITIS with an echinacea preparation. So far it also shows promising ANTI-CANCER ACTIVITY against LEUKEMIA and some animal tumors. It was the Plain's Indians primary medicine. They used it for wounds, insect bites, snakebites, coughs, rabies, smallpox, measles, mumps, and muscle and joint pains.

In a German study 203 women with YEAST INFECTIONS caused by the fungus CANDIDA ALBICANS were treated with either an anti-fungal cream, or the cream plus echinacea. The echinacea group received the herb either by injection or by mouth. After 6 months, 60% of the women treated with the cream only, had experienced recurrence, but among those treated also with echinacea only 16% had experienced recurrence.

Recent research has discovered the mechanism by which Echinacea prevents infection. HYALURONIC ACID (HA) is the substance that maintains the integrity of the cells, and thereby forms an effective barrier against infection. There is an enzyme that attacks HA and its integrity by a process which is not fully understood as yet. When this happens, pathogenic bacteria such as STAPH and STREP penetrate the tissues and make you sick. A similar mechanism is thought to take place in RHEUMATISM, TUMOR FORMATION, and at the beginnings of MALIGNANCY. Echinacea has the ability to prevent the dissolution of HA.

✓ ELDER—The gypsies regard the elder as one of the "healingest trees on earth." Sebastian Kneipp of Worishofen, Bavaria, a renowned herbalist, said that "the elder is excellent for PURIFYING the BLOOD when the tea is taken daily one hour before breakfast." He also said that man "should use his intelligence to discover and bring to light the treasures graciously hidden by God in nature as a means of healing the ills of this human life." ELDERBERRY TEA has been employed for generations as a folk remedy for such conditions as COLDS, COUGHS, INFLUENZA, and promoting SWEATING. It was only in recent years that science discovered that elderberries contain VIBURNIC ACID which induces perspiration, and is helpful in cases of RESPIRATORY AILMENTS. Its leaves, flowers, bark, and berries, have all been used for healing throughout history. The leaves are a traditional English remedy for HEMORRHOIDS.

✓ FENUGREEK—Fenugreek, meaning "Greek Hay," has been used to cure almost everything under the sun. It has been used as a folk remedy for DIABETES, ANEMIA, RICKETS, GOUT, as a FEBRIFUGE or FEVER REDUCER. Applied externally, fenugreek poultices have been said to soothe BOILS, WOUNDS, and ULCERS. The seed contains up to 30% MUCILAGE which makes a good poultice, and which is also responsible for its value as a LAXATIVE. It also contains LECITHIN, LIPOTROPICS (fat attractors), and SAPONIN, which is why it reduces blood cholesterol and fatty accumulations. It is also an aid in curing ULCERS and other STOMACH problems. Many have used it successfully for DIVERTICULOSIS. It reduces cholesterol in dogs, and also reduces blood sugar levels in animals, but neither has as yet been determined in humans.

Fenugreek is useful for all mucus conditions of the lungs. One lady who had COLITIS did so well on fenugreek tea that she told a friend, who also had colitis to try it. She also got good results. A 71 year old man who had colitis went to a health food store where they recommended FENULIN tablets, a preparation of fenugreek seeds. In two weeks he was amazed at the results. It is the first time he felt well in many months.

✓ FO-TI-TIENG—Fo-Ti-Tieng, called "the elixir of life," is a Chinese herb which gained its popularity due to the fact that the renowned Chinese herbalist, professor Li Chung Yun, who lived to be 256 years of age, used the herb daily. He lived from 1677 to 1933. His age was officially recorded by the Chinese government and confirmed by investigators of Chang-Tu University. He had outlived 23 wives and was living with the 24th at the time of his death. At the age of 200 those who saw him declared that he did not appear older than 52, and that he stood straight and strong and had his own natural hair and teeth.

Fo-Ti-Tieng is often compared to goldenseal and chamomile, and its properties are also compared to those of ginseng. In studies with humans it has been found that Fo-Ti-Tieng lowers blood CHOLESTEROL levels, reduces HYPERTENSION, reduces the incidence of coronary HEART DISEASE. It has ANTI-TOXIC, ANTI-SWELLING, and TRANQUILIZING properties. It is used by the Chinese for LIVER and SPLEEN weakness, VERTIGO, SCROFULA, FEVER, INSOMNIA, and CANCER.

✓ GINGER—Ginger is an excellent herb for the RESPIRATORY SYSTEM. It is good for fighting off COLDS and FLU. It relieves HEADACHES and other ACHES and PAINS. It helps to clear SORE THROATS. it is very effective as a cleansing agent for the BOWELS, KIDNEYS, and SKIN. Ginger and CAPSICUM work together against BRONCHIAL CONGESTION and STUFFY NOSES. Ginger is known for RELIEVING GAS, FLATULENCE, INDIGESTION, STOMACH PAIN, and NAUSEA. It contains an enzyme called ZINGIBAIN, which helps relieve INFLAMMATION. It stimulates production of AMYLASE, an enzyme in saliva which breaks down starches. It also increases PERISTALSIS to facilitate digestion. As an ANTI-NAUSEA agent, it is more effective than the drug DRAMAMINE. When DRAMAMINE was compared with ginger root in MOTION SICKNESS, ginger was found to be far more effective. But the dramamine also caused side effects of DROWSINESS, DIZZINESS, and dried the membranes of MOUTH, NOSE, and THROAT. A warm Ginger FOOTBATH is said to invigorate the whole body, and a piece of cotton soaked in Ginger oil is a common treatment for an EARACHE.

In tests it was effective in reducing or eliminating MORNING SICKNESS in over 75% of the cases studied. The women took from 3 to 8 capsules before getting out of bed in the morning, and took one capsule at a time until any NAUSEA they felt upon waking was gone. Throughout the day they took from 3 to 5 capsules at the slightest hint of nausea, and then relaxed until the nausea went away.

Besides eliminating nausea, ginger also eliminates DIZZINESS. Those who took it for nausea were surprised to have their dizziness disappear also when they were previously unable to leave their homes, or ride in a car or train, and there are no harmful side effects. It is also good for SEASICKNESS and POST-SURGERY NAUSEA. Unlike drugs, it does not produce any side-effects, nor even drowsiness.

35 arthritis patients experienced a REDUCTION IN PAIN after taking ginger for 3 months. Ginger also has an anti-inflammatory effect. For arthritis take tsp(teaspoon) of powdered ginger 3 times a day.

✓ GINKGO BILOBA—Ginkgo is one of the oldest of trees in the world. It is native to the Far East. The Chinese used an extract of the fruit to ward off TUBERCULOSIS, BRONCHIAL CONGESTION and KIDNEY INFECTIONS, and an extract of the leaves to treat DEPRESSION, TOXIC SHOCK, and CIRCULATORY AILMENTS. It has been shown to DILATE ARTERIES, VEINS, and CAPILLARIES, thereby increasing peripheral circulation, as well as blood flow to the brain. For this reason gingko may have potential for treating SENILITY, including ALZHEIMER'S disease, SHORT-TERM MEMORY LOSS, RINGING IN THE EAR or TINNITIS. Tinnitis is caused by drugs and medicines which poison the bloodstream such as QUININE, SALICYLATES, ASPIRIN, ANTIBIOTICS, and SLEEPING PILLS. Its extracts are regularly prescribed in Europe and Asia for improving MENTAL FUNCTIONS.

Ginkgo is effective in a broad range of infirmities associated with AGING, such as HEARING LOSS, MEMORY LOSS, STROKE, VERTIGO, and VISION LOSS. It INCREASES BLOOD FLOW to the BRAIN, PREVENTS STROKE, IMPROVES MEMORY and the MENTAL PROCESSES. It improves BLOOD FLOW to the HEART, and prevents formation of BLOOD CLOTS. 40 mg of ginkgo 3 times a day improved INTERMITTENT CLAUDICATION (pain in calf muscles). It is a powerful ANTIOXIDANT and FREE RADICAL SCAVENGER, which means that it may have anti-cancer effects.

Ginkgo acts against FREE RADICALS, and helps to dilate the blood vessels which produces a reduction in BLOOD PRESSURE. It prevents blood clots by reducing the tendency of blood cells to stick together. This reduces the tendency toward CORONARY THROMBOSIS, as well as helping in the recovery from STROKES and HEART ATTACKS. RINGING IN THE EAR as well as VERTIGO or dizziness have been successfully treated with Ginkgo. It is also a most effective treatment for MIGRAINE. DIABETICS who suffer from insufficient circulation are greatly benefited, and it also helps to reduce the INSULIN requirements. By improving the circulation it increases the oxygen supply to the heart and other organs, and slows down age-related diseases to the EYES, such as MACULAR DEGENERATION.

✓ GINSENG—Ginseng, meaning "man plant," is the most famous of all Asian medicinal plants. In the Orient it is called the "King of the Herbs." It stimulates the entire body energy to overcome STRESS, FATIGUE, and WEAKNESS. It is especially stimulating for MENTAL FATIGUE, for it stimulates the BRAIN CELLS. There is Chinese, Siberian, and American ginseng. They are all used for their adaptogenic properties. An ADAPTOGEN is a substance which has the ability to increase an organism's resistance to adverse influences. It has a NORMALIZING action, reducing excesses and stimulating deficient states. It is an herb which the Chinese say the sick take to recover their health, while the healthy use it to resist disease and make themselves stronger. They consider it a PANACEA for all diseases. According to the Chinese, ginseng is the most potent of all CORDIALS, STIMULANTS, TONICS, STOMACHICS, CARDIACS, FEBRIFUGES, and will best renovate and invigorate failing bodily energies. It has a positive effect upon the CARDIOVASCULAR SYSTEM, and without the side effects of many drugs. Other studies report that Ginseng prevents HEART DISEASE, and protects cells from RADIATION DAMAGE. It is best known for its ANTI-FATIGUE and ENERGY-GIVING properties. It stimulates the immune system. Its occasional use, it is said, will add a decade to human life. The root is used faithfully as a disease preventative by means of sucking the juice of the root, or by preparing it as a tea.

The rejuvenating action of ginseng on the sex glands is due to certain RADIOACTIVE substances which it absorbs from the soil. These radioactive substances are beneficial rather than harmful, because they are of organic origin, and not of inorganic origin such as strontium 90 and other inorganic fallout products. They emit a phosphorescent glow at night, called MITOGENETIC RADIATIONS. Garlic and onions were found to emit the same radiations as ginseng, which radiations seemed to have a rejuvenating effect, as discovered by the Russian scientist Gurwitch. Hunters shoot arrows at them at night, for they are hard to spot in the daytime, and then find them and dig them up in the morning.

Ginseng overcomes diseases naturally by

building up the general vitality, and especially by strengthening the ENDOCRINE glands, which control all basic physiological processes. It also strengthens the HEART, the NERVOUS SYSTEM, and increases the HORMONES. Koreans give it to race horses to increase physical endurance. Mice have survived endurance tests up to 70% longer than unboosted mice. In tests telegraph operators improved their performances after taking Siberian ginseng, by making fewer mistakes. Rats treated with ginseng and then exposed to prolonged radiation lived twice as long as expected. In both rats and humans, it seemed to moderate the effects of a high cholesterol diet.

Studies show that ginseng increases STAMINA and ENDURANCE, decreases the time to do COGNITIVE TASKS, and reduces the making of ERRORS. Russian researchers gave factory workers 4 mg of ginseng a day. Compared with workers who did not receive the herb, the ginseng users lost significantly fewer workdays due to colds, flu, tonsillitis, bronchitis, and sinus infections. According to a study of 11,000 people in East Germany and Russia, if you consume 500 mg of Siberian ginseng every day, then you would have 24 hrs of protection against any VIRAL INFECTION known to man today. Siberian ginseng contains only male hormones. In general what ginseng accomplishes are the following:

☞ It stimulates the immune system of both animals and humans

☞ It increases the white blood cells

☞ It spurs the production of interferon, the body's virus fighter

☞ It reduces LDL cholesterol, and increases HDL cholesterol, the good kind

☞ It has an anti-clotting effect which reduces heart attacks

☞ It reduces blood sugar levels

☞ It protects the liver from poisonous substances such as drugs and alcohol

☞ It prevents damage to healthy cells in radiation treatments

☞ It lengthens the lives of cancer patients by as much as four years

✓ GOLDENSEAL—It is largely known for its ANTIMICROBIAL activity which is produced by a substance called BERBERINE, which increases secretions of bile from the liver, thereby improving digestion. It is active against FUNGI, PROTOZOA, and BACTERIA, specifically STREP, STAPH, E. COLI, SALMONELLA, CHOLERAC, SHIGELLA, TRICHOMONAS, GONORRHEA, SYPHILLUS, and CANDIDA.

Many herbalists consider goldenseal one of the best herbs available in North America. It is considered to be very effective as a bitter CURE-ALL type of herb. Like Ginseng, Goldenseal is used for treating the adrenal glands in cases of STRESS, ANXIETY, NERVOUSNESS, ASTHMA, and ALLERGIC REACTIONS. It was used by the Cherokees as a remedy for SORE MOUTH, INFLAMED EYES, SKIN DISEASES, and as a BITTER TONIC in STOMACH and LIVER DISORDERS. An Indian folk healer called Goldenseal one of the "kings of diseases of the MUCOUS MEMBRANE unsurpassed by any other known remedy." In addition Jethro Kloss cites the use of Goldenseal for MORNING SICKNESS, ECZEMA, INDIGESTION, AND GENERAL DEBILITY of the system. It corrects problems of the mucus membrane, and is used as an ANTIBIOTIC to disinfect wounds, and to promote their rapid healing. It reduces yeast infections. It increases the WHITE BLOOD CELLS, thereby boosting the immune system. It was shown to be more effective against CHOLERA than the antibiotic CHLOROMYCETIN. Cholera is transmitted by food and water contaminated by EXCREMENT. It causes a toxic protein to attach itself to cells that line the intestinal tract, resulting in a kind of DIARRHEA.

A 4 year old child fell sick with a serious INFECTION. The parents were told at the hospital that the recovery would take 3 weeks or more. At home a friend suggested that they try goldenseal. They mixed teaspoon into some applesauce and gave it to the child. By the following morning the infection was completely gone.

One lady received instant relief from SHINGLES with goldenseal. She dissolved some of the herb in water and applied it to the infected area several times a day and before going to bed. This worked after a doctor's lotion had failed. The shingles started drying up almost immediately, and were gone in two weeks.

✓ GOTU KOLA—Gotu Kola is said to contain REJUVENATING properties similar to those of fo-ti-tieng and ginseng. Medicinally, it is a DIURETIC AND STIMULANT to the KIDNEYS and BLADDER, as well as a BLOOD PURIFIER. It was always known in India as a longevity plant. It is claimed that it will increase the vitality of 70 and 80 year old people to that of 40. The leaves have an energizing effect on the cells of the brain and are classified as a BRAIN FOOD. It is not related to the cola nut, and it does not contain any caffeine. It has shown its value in MENTAL TROUBLES, BLOOD PRESSURE, ABSCESSES, RHEUMATISM, SWELLINGS, BRUISES, and FEVER REDUCTION. The claim for it by the Sinhalese people of Ceylon is that "Two leaves a day will keep old age away."

It is used in India to treat FADING MEMORY, BRAIN FATIGUE, DEPRESSION, EXHAUSTION, STUTTERING, and other CHRONIC NERVOUS DISORDERS. In 1852 a Dr. Boileau, who had been afflicted for many years with the leprosy, experimented with Gotu Kola and cured himself of the LEPROSY. Herb formulas which have Gotu Kola in them will benefit AGE SPOTS, AGING, HIGH BLOOD PRESSURE, MENOPAUSE, HOT FLASHES, PROSTATE PROBLEMS, and IMPOTENCE.

✓ HAWTHORN—Scientists have discovered that heart disease is our leading cause of death. Yet hawthorn has been virtually ignored in the U.S. while it is widely used in Europe as a treatment for heart diseases. We must say that if it works in Europe it will work here too, for we all belong to the same human race. It is classed as a CARDIAC, TONIC, ANTISPASMODIC AND SEDATIVE. Its activity prevents CHOLESTEROL DEPOSITS in the arterial walls, reduces SERUM CHOLESTEROL, dilates CORONARY VESSELS, increases force of contraction of the HEART MUSCLE, and regulates some CARDIAC RHYTHM disturbances. Its active ingredients are TANNIN and SABONIN. It is a remedy for CIRCULATORY TROUBLE, CONGESTION of the MEDULLA OBLONGATA, HIGH BLOOD PRESSURE, INSOMNIA, ANXIETY, IRRITABILITY, and FATTY DEGENERATION. It is probably the finest HEART TONIC ever discovered. It is extremely rich in vitamin C, and has great value in case of ANGINA. It is not poisonous like DIGITALIS, and is perfectly safe without any poisonous side-effects. It regulates BLOOD PRESSURE and reduces it if it is too high, by dilating peripheral blood vessels. It slows heart action without having any depressant effect.

One herbalist says that hawthorn is one of the best tonic remedies for the heart and may be used safely in the long-term treatment for HEART WEAKNESS or FAILURE, PALPITATIONS, ANGINA PECTORIS, and CONGESTIVE HEART FAILURE. It increases OXYGEN UTILIZATION by the heart. According to legend, Christ's crown of thorns was believed to be made of hawthorn. Therefore, the berries were thought to possess miraculous healing power. It is effective when patients don't respond to digitalis. Hawthorn FLAVONOIDS also have a strong COLLAGEN stabilizing action, which is the primary tissue found in skin, bones, ligaments, and cartilage. By stabilizing these tissues, they are made stronger and more resistant to inflammatory conditions.

✓ KELP—Besides its iodine content, kelp is known today for its use as a protector from RADIATION, HEART DISEASE, AND TOXIC HEAVY METALS. It contains as a trace element IODINE, which is essential to the proper functioning of the thyroid gland, which manufactures the hormone THYROXIN. A lack of iodine causes goiter. It also helps prevent BREAST CANCER. It also produces less HEART DISEASE, less RESPIRATORY DISEASE, less RHEUMATISM and ARTHRITIS, less HIGH BLOOD PRESSURE, less THYROID DEFICIENCY, less GASTRO-INTESTINAL AILMENTS, and less INFECTIOUS DISEASE. In Japan, where seaweed is used as a food, abnormalities of the thyroid are non-existent. In the 1860's physicians observed that people taking a lot of iodine for reasons other than an iodine deficiency, seemed to lose weight more easily. The iodine stimulated their thyroid which boosted their metabolism, and they burned calories faster.

Dr. William Kountz studied 288 LOW THYROID PATIENTS with elevated BLOOD CHOLESTEROL, averaging 67 years of age.

He gave THYROID SUPPLEMENTS to half of this group and none to the other half, the controls. After 5 years, he found the fatality rate of the controls twice that of the patients on the thyroid hormone.

For this reason kelp gained a reputation as a treatment for OBESITY, which it retains to this day. Before iodized salt was introduced more kelp was used. But today iodine deficiency is almost unheard of in developed countries. To function normally, the body needs only 150 micrograms a day, which can easily be supplied by iodized salt. Kelp can be used as a salt substitute in powdered form, and as a seasoning. One will get only one seventh as much salt as with using the ordinary salt shaker. Kelp has a beneficial effect on the reproductive organs, the PROSTATE, UTERUS, TESTES, and OVARIES. It is also an arterial cleansing agent, and gives tone to the walls of the blood vessels. Studies have shown that women are more prone to overweight than men—especially in the menopausal stage. It is also during this stage that THYROID DISFUNCTION is most evident. Thyroid dysfunction caused by lack of iodine includes SLUGGISHNESS, OVERWEIGHT, and GOITER. Iodized salt is not recommended here because one should not add extra salt to the diet. Too much salt in the diet draws potassium out of the cells. Then sodium enters drawing in water which is retained. Cells become waterlogged, and the person appears overweight. This is where GARLIC and KELP come in. These are the richest sources of iodine for the thyroid. They are also rich in POTASSIUM, which pulls out the salt and releases the excess fluid. Garlic and kelp will make the excess pounds melt away.

The SODIUM ALGINATE in kelp prevents the absorption of STRONTIUM 90, a by-product of nuclear explosions, by as much as 83%. It accumulates in bone tissue and has been linked to several cancers: bone cancer, leukemia, and Hodgkins disease. The Atomic Energy Commission advocates the use of 3 oz of kelp a week or 2 tablespoons of alginate supplement a day to prevent strontium 90 absorption. This is especially for those who work in a nuclear facility, live near one, or are occupationally exposed to heavy metals, such as barium, cadmium, plutonium, and cesium.

✓ OTHER SEAWEEDS—Seaweeds known under the collective name of ALGAE, are used as both food and medicine. Three kinds are recognized according to color: the BROWN, the RED, and the GREEN. The Japanese refer to seaweed as "Heaven Grass," so great is their regard for its nutritional and medicinal value. Seaweeds are a rich source of minerals and vitamins. Their total mineral content is said to be 20 times higher than land-grown food. They may contain more than 60 minerals, the total complement of what is found in the sea. Seaweeds contain valuable amounts of ZINC. Zinc is a trace mineral which is concentrated in the thyroid, sex organs, liver, and pancreas. An insufficient amount of zinc in the diet can cause STERILITY. Other studies have shown that disorders of the prostate are often traced to a deficiency of zinc. CANCER and LEUKEMIA victims are often found lacking in this mineral. An inadequate supply may also be related to DIABETES, as well as possibly being one of the causes of ATHEROSCLEROSIS.

CARRAGEEN is commonly known as "Irish moss." It resembles the parsley plant. It has remarkable emulsifying properties, and is used in disorders of the KIDNEY and BLADDER. It has prevented PEPTIC ULCERS in laboratory animals. It apparently interferes with the formation of ULCERS by blocking the overaction of pepsin in the stomach. Such tests lend support to the theory that it is not acids but increased secretions of pepsin that causes stomach ulcers. It is considered an excellent substitute for animal GELATIN. The preponderance of alkaline salts in carrageen is of particular value in the diet of convalescents, the aged invalids, and children. It is low in calories and possesses easily assimilated plant phosphorus, calcium, and other valuable elements.

✓ LICORICE—Licorice is one of the oldest and best known remedies for coughs and chest complaints. Clay tablets of Mesopotamia indicate its use as a medicine and elixir of life. King Tut who died in 1344 B.C., was buried with a generous supply of licorice root. In China it was considered by herbalist doctors to be a potent and effective curative agent. It acts mainly on the LIVER in aiding it in discharging the poisons it filters from food. This allows the kidneys to eject these poisons from the blood once they have been released from the liver.

Because of its positive influence on the hormonal system, the Chinese have also used licorice to strengthen the FEMALE REPRODUCTIVE SYSTEM. Licorice contains compounds similar to those found in ginseng, sarsaparilla, cortisone, and estrogen. It is a very important herb for FEMALE COMPLAINTS. It helps the adrenal glands to function more smoothly in conditions of STRESS AND EXHAUSTION. Because of this quality naturopaths have used licorice in treating HYPOGLYCEMIA, DIABETES, and ADDISON'S DISEASE, which latter results from a deficiency in the secretion of adrenal hormones. It is a specific for FLU, COLDS, and LUNG CONGESTION and is added to cough syrups. Its ANTI-INFLAMMATORY ACTION is due to suppression of the enzyme which breaks down the hormone CORTISOL, the body's natural anti-inflammatory product. This results in a longer life of this hormone. Licorice also possesses ANTIBACTERIAL and ANTIVIRAL action due to it's active compound GLYCYRRHIZIN which induces INTERFERON and activates WHITE BLOOD CELLS to fight infection. Studies show that it is effective in treating chronic active VIRAL HEPATITIS.

✓ NETTLE—In Dr. Vogel's opinion, no other plant can equal the nettle in cases of ANEMIA, CHLOROSIS, RICKETS, SCROFULA, RESPIRATORY DISEASES, and LYMPHATIC TROUBLES. Dr. Fox explains that HIVES arises from an impure state of the blood, and is generally connected with a disordered condition of the stomach and bowels. This is taken care of if one takes a teaspoon full of the juice of nettles three times a day. It also has diuretic properties. It contains alkaloids that help in RHEUMATISM by neutralizing URIC ACID. The TANNIN in the root has been used as an astringent enema to shrink HEMORRHOIDS and reduce excess MENSTRUAL FLOW. Dr. Weiss of Germany says, "Nettle juice is definitely useful in diuretic therapy. It has the advantage of being well tolerated and safe, as distinct from the drug THIOZIDES now so widely used." It has been said that the "sting of the Nettle is but nothing compared to the PAINS that it heals." The tea has also been used for rheumatism, by using it as a FOOTBATH. A tea of the seeds has been used for coughs and shortness of breath, and were used for many years to treat CONSUMPTION. Nettle provides significant relief from the symptoms of hay fever, and another study suggests that nettle juice might relieve the symptoms of PROSTATE ENLARGEMENT or BENIGN PROSTATIC HYPERTROPHY. It also helps relieve the pain of GOUT.

A woman of more than 70 years was diagnosed as having a number of fatal cancerous growths in her abdomen. Because of her advanced years her physician felt that she could not withstand the necessary operation. A neighbor suggested that she take STINGING NETTLE TEA. She began sipping the infusion throughout the day. After a few months she went to the doctor for her regular check-up and he expressed amazement. The growths had disappeared, and she was more vigorous than she had been in years. Many respected European herbalists regard the stinging nettle as a possible CANCER-PREVENTIVE. It is said that long-term ingestion of stinging nettle tea prevents any malignancy from finding a favorable environment in the body.

✓ PARSLEY—Parsley has maintained it popularity as a garnish since earliest times. It was used medicinally for GRAVEL, BLADDER and KIDNEY STONES, and DISORDERS of the URINARY SYSTEM. It is very rich in vitamins A and C which are recognized as nutrients which help prevent CANCER, and the high chlorophyll content of the leaves makes it an excellent treatment for cancer itself. It contains 22,500 units of vitamin A per ounce, while carrots have 1275 units per ounce. It has 4 times as much vitamin C as an equal weight of oranges. Its iron content is 5 times as much as spinach. Parsley tea has been used with very good effect for URINARY and PROSTATE problems, as well as problems of the GALL BLADDER, LIVER, SPLEEN, and HIGH BLOOD PRESSURE.

Cases of DIABETES have responded well to the use of parsley tea. Some biological medicine exponents discovered that the deterioration of the pancreas in diabetes was due chiefly to a deficiency of SODIUM SULFATE in minute quantities. It is reputed to act as a SOLVENT for URIC ACID when used as a tea. It has been used as a medicine for MENSTRUAL IRREGULARITIES, CRAMPS, and in general for "WOMEN'S COMPLAINTS." It is excellent for the GENITO-URINARY TRACT and for the STONES of the KIDNEYS, BLADDER, and GALL BLADDER, and other kidney troubles. According to Dr. Kirschner it has "properties essential to OXYGEN METABOLISM, and for maintaining the normal action of the adrenal and thyroid glands." It is especially recommended as food for the elderly. Hippocrates said: "Let foods be your medicine, and medicine your foods." A poultice of chopped fresh Parsley is used to prevent painful swollen breasts in nursing mothers.

Parsley should be used as a preventative herb. It is so nutritious that it increases resistance to infections and diseases. It has a tonic effect on the entire URINARY SYSTEM. It has been used as a CANCER PREVENTATIVE. It is said to contain a substance in which cancerous cells cannot multiply.

Parsley contains one of the highest levels of chlorophyll of any herb, and chlorophyll is the active ingredient in breath fresheners, such as Chlorettes. Parsley inhibits the secretion of HISTAMINE, hence, its anti-histamine action may help those with HAY FEVER or HIVES. It also contains PSORALEN, a chemical which shows promise in the treatment of a form of cancer called CUTANEOUS T-CELL LYMPHOMA.

✓ PEPPERMINT—The MINTS such as PEPPERMINT, SPEARMINT, HORSE-MINT, CATNIP, ROSEMARY, etc. have been popular herbs from the earliest times. The people even paid "tithe of mint" as indicated in Matt. 23:23 and Luke 11:42. Peppermint has been used for ages as a remedy for INDIGESTION, NAUSEA, GAS PAINS, or to modify the bitter effects of other medicines. The Indians used peppermint tea as a VERMIFUGE. The early settlers employed it for DYSPEPSIA. In Jamaica it was used for COLIC. In early times the mints were placed in a bath for a calming and strengthening effect for the NERVES and MUSCLES. It is also used for DIARRHEA, HEADACHES, and SEASICKNESS. Due to the presence of several essential oils Peppermint prevents congestion of the BLOOD supply to the brain, stimulates circulation, and strengthens and calms NERVES. This calming effect allows the patient to apply himself to the task at hand.

It is the MENTHOL in peppermint that is responsible for the herb's beneficial effect. Menthol stimulates the flow of bile to the stomach which promotes digestion. Menthol has considerable anesthetic power. It is in many pain-relieving skin creams such as Solarcaine™, Unguentine™, Ben-gay™, and Noxzema™. Menthol vapors help relieve nasal, sinus, and chest congestion, hence, it is an ingredient in Mentholatum™ and Vicks Vaporub™. Peppermint oil in the test tube kills several BACTERIA and the HERPES SIMPLEX virus, which cause cold sores and genital herpes, as well as the TUBERCULOSIS BACILLUS. Several herbals recommend peppermint as a treatment for MORNING SICKNESS.

✓ RED CLOVER—RED CLOVER TOP was Mrs. White's herb drink. Jethro Kloss, who was a friend of Elder and Mrs. White, in his book *Back To Eden*, says that he was told that Mrs. White cured herself of cancer by using RED CLOVER blossoms, and that she used them all during her life as a beverage. Red clover is specified by herbalists as one of the four home remedies of CANCER. The other three being CARROT JUICE, CONCORD GRAPE JUICE, and RED OAK BARK. Red clover tea has been used as a SPRING TONIC for purifying the blood, and to treat chest complaints such as COLDS, ASTHMA, and BRONCHITIS. It is a SEDATIVE for those suffering from chest constriction

Red clover tea is recommended for ULCERS in general. Researchers from the National Cancer Institute have found anti-tumor properties in the herb. They found that red clover contains four anti-tumor compounds including GENISTEIN. In addition red clover contains some TOCOPHERAL, a form of vitamin E that has been shown to prevent chest tumors in animals. One study showed red clover effective against several BACTERIA in the test tube, including the TUBERCULOUS BACILLUS. One author says that it has a positive effect on CANCER PATIENTS when taken with CHAPARRAL.

✓ RED PEPPER/CAPSICUM/CAYENNE

◆ *A Good Heart Medicine*

Red pepper is said to be unequaled for warding off diseases and equalizing blood circulation. It is called a 'SUPREME AND HARMLESS INTERNAL DISINFECTANT'. It increases the heart action but not the blood pressure. It is said to PREVENT STROKES and HEART ATTACKS. Its official name, CAPSICUM, is derived from the Greek word meaning "to bite." While it is biting to the tongue, it is nonetheless benign and gentle within the body, it is considered to be a reliable restorative and internal stimulant.

The red peppers are given three categories of strength: a. those with 1 BTU of heat rating are labeled PAPRIKA; b. those with a heat rating of under 25 BTU are labeled RED PEPPER; c. those with a rating above 25 BTU are labeled CAYENNE. It is one of the greatest of all herbs and can be used with any other herb, in fact, it increases the power of all other herbs. These peppers are full of vitamins and minerals. It will increase the healing properties of other herbs. It heals STOMACH ULCER and stops the HEMORRHAGING. It is fine food for the HEART. It will stop and prevent HEART SEIZURE, SHOCK, increase the CIRCULATION, and CAUTERIZE an open wound. For a HEART ATTACK give cayenne tea, hot if possible, and the attack will stop in about 2 minutes. Adventist herbalist Al. Wolfsen keeps a vial of cayenne with him at all times. He has seen people lying on the sidewalk with a heart attack, has asked for a glass of water, has mixed his cayenne into it, and has given it to the afflicted, and they have recovered rather quickly.

◆ *It Has Analgesic Properties*

Herbalists prescribe red pepper for COLDS, GASTRO-INTESTINAL and BOWEL problems, as a DIGESTIVE AID, for ARTHRITIS, and SORE MUSCLES. It STIMULATES the flow of SALIVA as well as STOMACH SECRETIONS. It helps to reduce blood CHOLESTEROL levels, and the tendency for BLOOD TO CLOT internally, and it thereby ALLEVIATES A HEART ATTACK. It has anti-bacterial properties that help relieve infectious diarrhea. Recently, RED PEPPER has been shown to possess real PAIN RELIEVING or ANALGESIC properties for certain types of chronic pain, especially in arthritis cases. It renders the skin insensitive to pain by depleting SUBSTANCE P, a neurotransmitter, the chemical in the peripheral nerves that send the pain message to the brain. The effective chemical in red pepper is called CAPSAICIN, which acts as a powerful stimulant. It is the "hot stuff" part in hot peppers, and it has lowered CHOLESTEROL in lab animals.

In another experiment, after rats were fed capsaicin, it doubled the rate at which cholesterol was removed from the body. Jethro Kloss called cayenne "One of the most wonderful herb medicine that we have." Another author calls cayenne "a supreme and harmless internal disinfectant." Herbalist R.C. Wren calls it "the purest and most certain stimulant in herbal materia medica." He says that a COLD may usually be removed by one or two doses of the powder taken in warm water. It is found to interfere with the action of what is called "substance P," the chemical in the peripheral nerves that sends pain messages to the brain. It is so effective for reasons not well understood that two over-the-counter capsaicin creams called ZOSTRIK and AXSAIN have won FDA approval.

◆ *It Reduces Cholesterol—*

ZOSTRIK is the most effective pain treatment for SHINGLES, or HERPES ZOSTER. Shingles in adults is caused by the same virus that causes chicken pox in children. The virus remains dormant in the body until later in life, when, for unknown reasons, it appears in some people as a shingles rash. In basically healthy adults shingles clears up by itself within three weeks. Two recent studies indicate that RED PEPPER may help reduce cholesterol and PREVENT HEART DISEASE. Some herbalists have advised adding red pepper to socks or shoes to TREAT COLD FEET. It will keep them warm. It can be applied externally in poultices as a stimulant for chilled skin, and as a remedy for painful joints. It stimulates the blood flow which reduces the inflammation. It helps to drop the BODY TEMPERATURE so that the natives in hot climates can tolerate the heat much better.

PREVENTS CANCER—The Spirit of Prophecy has spoken against the use of condiments which are injurious in their nature, which irritate the stomach, and which make the blood feverish and impure.(CD339). Cayenne certainly irritates the stomach. That is why some people have spoken out against it. It should therefore be used mixed with food, and the stomach will gradually adjust itself to its "hot" nature. For FLU PREVENTION there is nothing like CAYENNE PEPPER, or CINNAMON BARK, or CINNAMON OIL TEA. Because of its great many benefits health-wise, we must consider it as one condiment that is generally beneficial.

The Eppley Cancer Institute presented the idea that CAYENNE PEPPERS may help reduce the risk of CANCER. They found out that HOT RED PEPPER contains a substance called CAPSAICIN which changes into a chemical that absorbs FREE RADICALS in the liver, and thereby prevents them from turning into cancerous substances.

✓ SAGE—In former times sage was used medicinally for so many ailments that a 14th century writer asked, "How can a man die who has sage in his garden?" John Wesley claimed that the use of sage tea had fully satisfied his expectations of it as a remedy for PALSY. He said, "My hand is as steady now as it was at fifteen." In herbal lore, the plant was associated with the health of the SPLEEN, and was venerated as a sacred herb capable of increasing the LIFE SPAN. It has a rejuvenating effect on the EYES, BRAIN, GLANDS, and NERVOUS SYSTEM. Suppurating wounds washed with a decoction of sage will heal quickly. Sage tea purifies the LIVER and KIDNEYS according to Father Kneipp. The tincture and volatile oil have been used for BRONCHITIS, inflammation of the THROAT, and makes an excellent GARGLE for it. It is a BACTERICIDE and FUNGICIDE of penetrating power. It contains a volatile oil, TANNIN, RESIN, and a bitter principle. The oil is composed of PINENE, CAMPHOR, SALVENE, and CINEOL.

Many people use SAGE as a HAIR CONDITIONER, and to darken GRAY HAIR. Also SAGE TEA with equal parts of rosemary is said to stimulate the growth of hair. It contains powerful antioxidants which slow spoilage. One study shows that SAGE reduces blood sugar glucose levels in DIABETICS who drink the infusion on an empty stomach.

A lady tells of how sage acted on the TONSILLITIS afflicting her son. When her son, Tom, awakened one morning with inflamed and infected tonsils, she prepared a tea of sage and had Tom use the infusion as a gargle every other hour all day long. By the following morning, Tom's tonsils were back to normal. She was surprised at his speedy recovery, and resolved never to be without sage in her household again.

✓ SARSAPARILLA—Sarsaparilla is the dried root of a genus of climbing vines native to tropical America. The name is derived from two Spanish words, SARZA and PARILLA, meaning a small, thorny vine. The plant grows only in moist places and develops long, slender roots. Sarsaparilla was the wonder remedy of bygone days, and was considered a necessity by many people for good health. Old time drug stores carried a wide variety of sarsaparilla preparations. Sarsaparilla is a BLOOD PURIFIER and an ALTERATIVE. It acts kindly and freely on the kidneys, stimulating the sudoriferous glands as well as the sebaceous glands of the skin. It is a strong DIURETIC and stimulates the excretion of wastes such as URIC ACID and excess CHLORIDE. It promotes SWEATING, and with it even more toxins are removed from the lymph and circulatory systems. It contains an important male hormone TESTOSTERONE and the female hormone PROGESTERONE.

It increases the appetite and gently counteracts a constipated condition of the bowels. When taken freely for a considerable length of time it will overcome the majority of our troublesome SKIN diseases in general. When a person takes it freely he will find that it will act on the KIDNEYS similar to watermelon, and the sweat of the skin will be of a greasy, waxy nature. In a case of SCROFULA, caused by a bad vaccine virus, where the flesh seemed as though it would fall off the bones, the doctors had given her up and said that she would probably die. The mother of the girl made a strong tea of sarsaparilla root and made her drink it instead of water. It worked, and the girl completely recovered.

Sarsaparilla is also used for IMPOTENCE, LIVER PROBLEMS, RHEUMATISM, GOUT, and SYPHILIS, It reduces FEVER, CLEARS SKIN DISORDERS such as ECZEMA and PSORIASIS, and CONTROLS DIABETES,

STOMACH and KIDNEY DISORDERS. Sarsaparilla contains the hormones TESTOSTERONE, PROGESTERONE, and CORTIN. TESTOSTERONE prolongs youth and prevents premature aging. PROGESTERONE is necessary for the development of the mammary and genital organs, and is essential for reproduction. CORTIN is one of the hormones of the adrenal glands, and if the adrenal glands secrete only a small or insufficient amount of cortin, the individual becomes easy prey to infectious disease and also develops nervous depression and general weakness.

✓ SASSAFRAS—Sassafras is a remedy for BLADDER, KIDNEY, and THROAT AILMENTS. It is a TONIC for STOMACH and BOWELS. The bark of the root is used for medicine. It is a BLOOD THINNER and PURIFIER, and acts gently on the KIDNEYS. It stimulates the action of the liver to clear TOXINS from the system. It has been used as a PAIN reliever, especially the afterpains from childbirth, and to bring down a FEVER. People who drink its tea are more resistant to COLDS and THROAT infections. It was a popular drink among the early colonists who used it as a "spring tonic." The bark of the root contains a volatile oil, resin, wax, camphor, tannic acid, starch, gum, lignin, and salts. It has been found to possess general ANTISEPTIC powers.

✓ SLIPPERY ELM—Slippery elm has been regarded by herbalists as an excellent food for convalescents. It is nutritious, easy to digest, and helpful to the stomach and intestines. Today it is most often used in lozenges for alleviating SORE THROATS and COUGHS due to colds.

Slippery elm was well known by the Indians for its DIURETIC, EMOLLIENT and DEMULCENT qualities. It has MUCILAGINOUS as well as NUTRITIVE value. In the treatment of inflammation of the stomach, it acts as medicine and food, given as a gruel flavored with honey. One writer says that it contains as much nutritive value as oatmeal. It is regarded today as one of nature's most excellent DEMULCENTS, and is employed for its ability to NEUTRALIZE STOMACH ACIDITY. The poultice is recommended for BURNS, ULCERS, CHILBAINS, and SKIN DISEASES. Because of its strengthening effect on the body, and its soothing action on the lungs, it is considered valuable for the debilitating conditions of BRONCHITIS, COUGHS, and other PULMONARY COMPLAINTS.

One man reported that he had had a WART on his hand for 30 years, which one day grew larger and became inflamed. A friend recommended having it surgically removed, but his wife suggested that he try slippery elm instead. He made a "blob" with the powder, placed it on the wart, and kept it covered with cotton and secured with a bandage. He changed the bandage every other day for about four weeks. The inflammation was gone and the wart had shrunk to the size of a pin head. He then put a slice of lemon peel on it in the same manner, and in another week the rest of the wart could be detached and there was a perfect healing.

✓ VALERIAN—The plant contains VALERIC, FORMIC, AND ACETIC ACIDS, in addition to STARCH, RESIN, a GLUCOSIDE, and two ALKALOIDS. It is reputed to act as a SEDATIVE to the entire nervous system, and has been so used for hundreds of years. It is said to allay PAIN and promote SLEEP. It is known as a CALMATIVE for nervousness and hysteria. The scent of some Asian species is strong and pleasant. It is said that SPIKENARD was the Biblical name of valerian, and was called a perfume from the east.

The drug VALIUM is derived from the valerian root. Valium has many side effects which are much greater than its benefits. When the VALERIAN ROOT as a whole is used there are no side effects. The body can use only what is NATURAL. Scientific studies show that the active ingredients of valerian, the VALEPOTRIATES, do act as tranquilizers in small animals and in humans. It is called "one of the most relaxing herbs." It is also used for anxiety, insomnia, headaches, and intestinal cramps. Animal studies show that it reduces BLOOD PRESSURE. Valerian also has anti-convulsant effects, which lends credence to its traditional use in treating epilepsy. In some cases 400 IU of VITAMIN E stopped epilepsy seizures from 70 to 100%. Studies also show that it has some anti-tumor effect.

✓ WILLOW BARK—In 1763 the bark was recommended specifically for FEVERS. The fresh bark contains SALICIN, which is converted into SALICILIC ACID in the body. It is called "natural aspirin." It interferes with the production of PROSTAGLANDINS which trigger inflammation. In the 1700's it was used to treat MALARIA. In 1838, salicilic acid was produced through the oxidation and hydrolysis of salicin. In 1893 chemists produced ACETYLSALICILIC ACID from salicilic acid. This new product became known as ASPIRIN. ASPIRIN is derived from salicylic acid by a slight change in its formula. Down through the ages before the discovery of salicin, Willow Bark was used to combat PAIN of various types, including of RHEUMATISM, ARTHRITIS, GOUT, and ANGINA. Indian tribes boiled the inner root bark and drank strong doses of the resulting tea to promote sweating in cases of chills and fever. Willow bark is used by herbalists as an ANODYNE, ANTIPYRETIC, ASTRINGENT, and ANTISEPTIC. It is useful for HEADACHES, NEURALGIA, HAY FEVER, FEVER, and INFLAMMATION of the JOINTS, just like aspirin. In animal studies aspirin is associated with an increased risk of birth defects. The bark is not as powerful as aspirin itself, but it is safer. Sip the tea regularly to strengthen your immune system and to resist painful reactions.

A young woman had been diagnosed as having CANCER of the BLADDER. The disease had progressed to the point where she was hospitalized and was suffering great pain. Her doctor allowed the use of the WILLOW-HERB INFUSION, but said that he was doubtful anything could help. She drank one cup in the morning and one in the evening for two weeks, and found that she was actually feeling better at the end of that period. Even the doctor had to admit that the herb helped.

A man was in the hospital with a HEART INFARCTION, but he also suffered from PROSTATE DISORDER. Because of the heart condition the doctor did not believe that he could withstand an operation. He began to drink three cups of the WILLOW-HERB TEA daily. After several days he had no more complaints. He said that it is unbelievable that medicinal plants give such results.

Flower Remedies—Aroma Therapy

Dr. Edward Bach of England gave up his medical practice in order to research plant remedies for the emotions through flowers. He discovered a new system of herbal medicine based upon the principle "treat the patient and not the disease." Remedies are prescribed, not for the physical disorders but for the patient's state of mind—his fear, anxiety, sense of failure, regret, or whatever might be the underlying cause of the patient's illness. He gave patients a specific herbal remedy for a specific emotional state of mind. As the negative emotion disappeared, the physical complaint cleared up, and the patient was restored to health. We are told that "There are life-giving properties in the balsam of the PINE, in the fragrance of the CEDAR and the FIR, and other trees also have properties that are health-restoring" (MH264).

The scents of flowers influence the physiological, emotional, and mental moods of people. "The delicately tinted flowers in their perfection perfuming the air" (SC10). The use of perfumes is one branch of aroma therapy. Flowers embody influences of joy, peace, inspiration, strength, purity, and harmony. Emotional patterns change in the ill person when beholding flowers. "Fruit and flowers are nothing in comparison with what they will be in the earth made new, yet even today the sick may find health and gladness and joy in the field and orchard. What a restorative this is'. What a preventive of sickness.'

"The leaves of the tree of life are for the healing of the believing, repenting children of God who avail themselves of the blessing to be found in tree and shrub and flower, even marred as nature is by the curse" (MM234). "In flower garden and orchard, the sick will find health, cheerfulness, and happy thoughts" (MM232). "Seeing the flowers, plucking the ripe fruit from the trees, hearing the happy songs of the birds, have a peculiarly exhilarating effect on the nervous system" (MM231). Of her own attitude Mrs White says, "I love the beautiful flowers. They are memories of Eden, pointing to the blessed country into which, if faithful, we shall soon enter. The Lord is leading my mind to the health-giving properties of the flowers and trees" (AH147).

Mrs. White's Use Of Herbs

◆ *Her Use Of Red Clover Tea*

Mrs. White had always used RED CLOVER tea as a good and wholesome drink. At one time she took a little Java tea as a medicine in a case of severe vomiting. During another illness, she drank a cup of very strong coffee with a raw egg broken into it as a medicine (2SM302–3). She has all along placed the emphasis upon the eight natural remedies and herbs. Throughout her writings she states that we should use these natural remedies now, which are simple and easy to use by everyone, and which are nonpoisonous. They were of prime importance in her health program. She does not state anywhere that we should in the future use other remedies which are less simple and more poisonous. We cannot say that in the future there would be found substances that God hadn't thought of, that would be better than the herbs which he has created. In the modern methods of healing men have created many inventions, but we must believe by faith that none of them are as good as the herbs which God has created for us.

Mrs. White says: "If you come to my house I will show you the bag that contains my herb drink. I send to Michigan, across the mountains, and get RED-CLOVER TOP.... I have always used red-clover top, as I stated to you. I offered you this and told you it was a good, simple, and wholesome drink." (2SM302).

◆ *Catnip and Hop Tea*

"A cup of tea made from CATNIP herbs will quiet the nerves. HOP tea will induce sleep. Hop poultice over the stomach will relieve PAIN.... When the head is congested, if the feet and limbs are put in a bath with a little MUSTARD, relief will be obtained. There are many more simple remedies which will do much to restore healthful action of the body. All these simple preparations the Lord expects us to USE FOR OURSELVES, but man's extremities are God's opportunities. If we neglect to do that which is within the reach of nearly every family, and ask the Lord to relieve PAIN when we are too indolent to make use of these simple remedies within our power, it is simply presumption." (2SM297).

In connection with these modern inventions Mrs. White says: "After seeing so much harm done by the administering of drugs, I cannot use them, and cannot testify in their favor. I must be true to the light given me by God" (2SM293). So the reason she did not speak of any other medications that might be found in the future, is because there would not be any more effective one produced by man. Anything that man would produce would combine benefit and harm at the same time, and people would be taking risks on their life which they otherwise would not have to take. Science has since her time developed stronger, and more powerful so-called "medicines" which help while harming presently or in the future.

◆ *God's Medicines Cover All Diseases*

If God had not given us a complete range herbal medicines for our health and for every disease that might come along, then His help in our behalf would have been incomplete. Such incompleteness would have allowed some persons to die which would have lived if God's help and assistance in our behalf would have been complete. It would have been unfair for God not to give us relief from every possible disease. But contrary to this He has given us substances which will bring us complete relief if we have faith in them and make use of them. Let us not be so bold as to believe that God did not know what poisonous drugs would be developed in our day or in Mrs. White's day. He knew them all even before they were developed. For this reason Mrs. White said: "I do not think that I can give you any definite line of medicines compounded and dealt out by doctors, that are perfectly harmless. And yet it would not be wisdom to engage in controversy over this subject. The practitioners are very much in earnest in using their DANGEROUS CONCOCTIONS and I am decidedly opposed to resorting to such things. They NEVER CURE; they may CHANGE the DIFFICULTY to create a WORSE ONE. Many of those who practice the prescribing of drugs, would not take the same or give them to their children. If they have an intelligent knowledge of the human body, if they understand the delicate wonderful human machinery, they must know that we are fearfully and wonderfully made, and that NOT A PARTICLE of these strong drugs should be introduced into this human living organism" (2SM289–90).

Today we cannot give as an excuse the fact that our drugs are different from what they were in Mrs. White's day. But when God talks about drugs and says that "THEY NEVER CURE," he makes a statement for all time, present, past, and future, for He knows the end from the beginning. Today's drugs are faster acting, purer, more powerful, and therefore more damaging to the constitution than before. They have not been getting better, just more harmful.

◆ *A Pledge In Regard To What We Can Do For Ourselves*

"In regard to that which we can do for ourselves, there is a point that requires careful, thoughtful consideration. I must become ACQUAINTED WITH MYSELF, I must be a LEARNER always as to how to take care of this BUILDING, the body God has given me, that I may PRESERVE IT in the very best CONDITION OF HEALTH. I must EAT those things which will be for my very BEST GOOD PHYSICALLY, and I must take SPECIAL CARE of my CLOTHING such as will conduce to a healthful CIRCULATION of the BLOOD. I must not deprive myself of EXERCISE and AIR. I must get all the SUNLIGHT that it is possible for me to obtain.

"I must have WISDOM to be a faithful GUARDIAN of my BODY. I should do a very unwise thing to enter a COOL ROOM when in a PERSPIRATION; I should show myself an UNWISE STEWARD to allow myself to sit in a DRAFT, and thus expose myself so as to take a COLD. I should be unwise to sit with COLD FEET and LIMBS, and thus drive back the blood from the extremities to the BRAIN or the INTERNAL ORGANS. I should always protect my feet in DAMP WEATHER.

"I should EAT REGULARLY of the most HEALTHFUL FOOD which will make the best quality of blood, and I should NOT WORK INTEMPERATELY if it is in my power to avoid doing so.

"And when I VIOLATE the LAWS God has established in my being, I am to REPENT and REFORM, and place myself in the most favorable condition under the doctors God has provided—PURE AIR, PURE WATER, and the healing precious SUNLIGHT" (2SM296–7).

◆ *Other Remedies (2SM295–300).*

✓ CHARCOAL—Mrs. White says, "Teach nurses and patients the value of those health-restoring agencies that are freely provided by God, and the usefulness of simple things that are easily obtained."

"I will tell you a little about my experience with CHARCOAL as a remedy. For some forms of indigestion, it is more efficacious than drugs. A little OLIVE OIL into which some of this powder has been stirred tends to cleanse and heal. I find it is excellent. PULVERIZED CHARCOAL from EUCALYPTUS WOOD we have used freely in cases of inflammation" (2SM298). A man suffering from inflammation of the bowels was given pulverized charcoal in water to drink, with bandages of charcoal over the bowels and stomach. In half an hour there was a change for the better. An eighteen months old child had a painful swelling on the knee from the bite of some poisonous insect. Pulverized charcoal, mixed with FLAXSEED was placed upon the swelling, and this poultice gave relief at once. (2SM299–300). It possesses the wonderful power of withdrawing POISON from the system (Letter 326, 1906).

Charcoal poultices are used for FEVER, SNAKE BITES, STING OF REPTILES, INFLAMMATION OF THE BOWELS, BLOODY DYSENTERY, POISONOUS INSECTS, to FILTER WATER, to ELIMINATE FOOT ODORS, and to RELIEVE GAS PAINS. The charcoal is to be made from the wood of the eucalyptus tree, and we are told that God's blessing may be expected to follow the use of these means, but other types of charcoal were also used.

In 1831 a French pharmacist swallowed CHARCOAL at the same time that he took STRYCHNINE to show that charcoal was an effective remedy for all kinds of POISONS.

Today, specially processed or ACTIVATED CHARCOAL is used to treat POISONING and OVERDOSES. Unlike regular charcoal, activated charcoal has extremely large surface areas, as much as a 1000 square meters per gram, that readily absorbs or binds toxins from the stomach and intestines and takes them out of the body.

- ✓ EUCALYPTUS OIL—Mrs. White cannot advise any remedy for cough which is better than EUCALYPTUS OIL and HONEY. Into a tumbler of honey put a few drops of the eucalyptus. Stir it well and take whenever the cough come on. Take a teaspoon of this mixture, and relief comes almost immediately. Also good for pains in the chest and lungs.
- ✓ GRAPE JUICE AND EGGS—For a poverty-stricken diet get eggs from healthy fowls and drop a raw egg into a glass of grape juice. This will supply the system with what it needs. Eggs contain properties which are remedial agencies in counteracting poisons. (2SM303).
- ✓ CATNIP HERB—will quiet the NERVES
- ✓ HOP TEA—will induce SLEEP. Hop poultices over the stomach will relieve PAIN.
- ✓ WEAK EYES—If the eyes are weak, if there is pain in the eyes, or inflammation, soft flannel cloths wet in HOT WATER and SALT, will bring relief quickly.
- ✓ HEAD CONGESTED—When the head is congested, if the feet and limbs are put in a bath with a little MUSTARD, relief will be obtained. These simple preparations the Lord expects us to USE FOR OURSELVES. They are within the reach of every family.
- ✓ FIGS—When Hezekiah was sick, God sent him a message that he should die. When the king cried to the Lord, the Lord promised him that He would extend his life by fifteen years. He was given direction to make a poultice of FIGS, and lay it upon the part affected. This was done and Hezekiah was restored to health. We are told that it would be well for us to treasure this prescription which the Lord ordered to be used, more than we do (2SM300).

Back To Eden—Jethro Kloss

Jethro Kloss was a man who in 1939 wrote a book entitled *Back To Eden*. He wrote this book as a result of having become acquainted with Mrs. White's books on health. After having read them he decided to become an herbalist. He left home at an early age, lived in boarding houses, eating little except devitalized foods, until his health began too fail. He suffered a complete breakdown and became so weak, that at one time he was in bed for three months with pain he says "no tongue can describe." "Death would have been a welcomed release." He tried every remedy known to the medical profession, and none of his doctors gave him one ray of hope. He had no thought of ever getting well again, and had made his will. It was then that he came across the books written by Mr. and Mrs. James White, he says, who although they were not physicians, were great medical missionaries, as he put it. In those books he says he found statements like these, "Nine out of ten would get well if they used simple God-given means." And "Do not eat food robbed of its life-giving elements." "Do not eat food that makes you sick." This was an entirely new line of thought to me, he said.

He recalled when in his youth his parents were called to a neighbors house after someone had been given up to die, and his parents, with their herbs, fruit juices, and vegetable broths, helped the sick one back to health again. He began to accept many of the suggestions in Mrs White's books until he was a well man again.

One time there was an epidemic of typhoid fever in the locality where he was living, and many died. Someone told him of a family who had no one to wait on them. He went to the house, and when he approached he met the doctor outside. He asked the doctor if he had any objections if he tried to help these folks. He said that he didn't and then added that the women would recover but that the man would die. The man had pain and hemorrhage in the bowels, and ulcers from his mouth through the entire digestive tract. He treated the man with simple remedies, gave him plenty of water, fruit juices, and fomentations. In six weeks the man was up and around.

He was so pleased and happy that he had been successful that he continued nursing with good results. He also nursed for several doctors who were surprised that one having had no medical training of any kind could get such results. He found that the healing art as God gave it was to be practiced by ministers and gospel workers, and that God had never changed that plan. He said that when we heed God's principles and methods, God will do for us what we cannot. He said that God has provided a remedy for every disease that might afflict us.

That Satan cannot afflict anyone with any disease for which God has provided a remedy. Our creator foresaw the wretched condition of mankind in these days, and made provision in Nature for all the ills of man. He said, "No matter how many germs get into the body, if the blood stream is clean and the blood corpuscles are in a healthy condition, you will be safe. Everyone comes in contact with many kinds of germs, but these organism's will not harm you or cause you sickness and death unless they have a place in which to propagate themselves" (p. II). He finally said that "The fundamental principle of true healing consists of a return to natural habits of living" (p. IV).

THE HEALING FOODS

What Is A Healing Substance

One cannot really talk about a healing substance because the process of healing is exclusively the province of God, of Christ, of Nature, of the internal laws of body wisdom and power. Substances can aid the healing process, and those substances are those that help to cleanse the system. They are the ones that will help speed the healing process along. These are God's 8 DOCTORS, the many NATURAL HERBS, RAW FOODS, FRUITS, VEGETABLES, and their JUICES. Any practice which would add POISONS to the system in order to heal it must be classified more under the category of MALPRACTICE. This may be a TRUTH which will be very difficult to swallow. Dr. Trall has said: "The presentation of new truths so as not to offend old errors are often regarded as arguments directed as attacks upon people's reason, because they mistake their own ingrained prejudices as being established principles."

When poisons are called medicines we believe that they are healing substances, when actually they are not. What the most virulent poisons, taken in the name of medicines, often accomplish is to reduce the red and white blood cells to a fatal minimum. But these blood cells represent our IMMUNE SYSTEM, which is the system that fights our diseases. And here we are fighting the system that is fighting our enemy, and is endeavoring to keep us in health.

Apple—The King Of Fruits

◆ *The King And Queen Of Fruits*

The apple is called the "KING OF FRUITS," and the statement that "AN APPLE A DAY WILL KEEP THE DOCTOR AWAY" represents a reputation on the part of the apple that seems to be well deserved. It comes from an old English verse which says: "An apple before bed makes the doctor beg his bread." It is an all-around health food. It is ANTI-CARCINOGENIC and ANTI-VIRAL. Dr. Ronowalchuk says that apple juice from the grocery shelf is strong enough to eradicate the POLIO VIRUS with 100% effectiveness. It is a food, beverage, tonic, medicine, cosmetic, and bowel regulator all in one. It acts as a natural stimulator for all body secretions. It is a health-builder and a disease-killer. If the apple is the king of fruits, then the title of queen of fruits would have to go to the GRAPE. The Spirit of Prophecy tells us that "Apples are superior to any fruit for a standby that grows" (CD312). And it also says that "apples and grapes are God's gift; they may be put to excellent use as healthful articles of food" (5T361). So to call them the king and queen of fruits is not entirely out of line. Tradition holds that the apple was the forbidden fruit in the Garden of Eden. Apocryphal literature says that it was the grape.

◆ *Pectin And Vitamin C*

Apples are one of the most readily available sources of vitamin C. Most of the vitamin C in apples is right under the skin, which has five times as much as the rest of the apple, so that peeling them may not be such a good idea. Small apples are generally richer in vitamin C than larger apples, but only because they have more area of skin per unit weight. Human beings, monkeys, and guinea pigs, and one or two other animals are the only ones which cannot manufacture their own vitamin C, and must therefore get it from outside sources in the food they eat. We get a large part of our vitamin C from the citrus fruits, and fresh vegetables. In Europe where there is only a limited supply of citrus fruits, except for the country of Spain, the people drink a lot of vitamin C content teas such as rose hips tea. The SUNNY SIDE or red side of an apple contains more sugar and more vitamin C than the green side. Apples lose some of their vitamin C food value when in storage.

The negative side about eating apples are the insecticide residues they may carry. Cooking does not destroy them. Hence, if possible eat only organically grown apples. A worm in an apple is a lot less of a menace to health than a few grains of LEAD or ARSENIC. Natural food supplements such as vitamins and minerals will protect you against these poisons. Apples are an alkaline food, and also an eliminative food. They contains PECTIN which has the ability to take up excess water in the intestines and make a soft bulk. Pectin is an important factor in jelly making. Pectin also stimulates the growth of tissue. It also has been successfully used on VERICOSE VEINS.

◆ *An Anti-Cancer Fruit*

The pectin in apples relieves diarrhea because intestinal bacteria transform it into a protective coating for the irritated intestinal lining. It adds bulk to the stool which helps both the DIARRHEA and CONSTIPATION, because of the kind of fiber that slows digestion and fills you up quickly, so it becomes an ally in weight control. Pectin is the "pectate" in the diarrhea preparation KAOPECTATE. It helps control blood sugar levels in DIABETES. European studies suggest that pectin helps eliminate LEAD, MERCURY, and other toxic heavy metals from the body. It helps remove poisonous substances from the system by supplying GALACTURONIC acid. It also helps protein matter in the intestines from spoiling. Pectin binds cancer-causing compounds in the colon, thereby speeding their elimination from the body. Apples contain an acid which blocks CANCER formation in lab animals who are dosed with cancer-causing agents, and may therefore have an anti-cancer action on humans. These anti-cancer agents are also located just under the skin.

◆ *They Reduce Cholesterol Levels*

Apples reduce CHOLESTEROL in hamsters and other animals with genetically high cholesterol levels, and it can do the same for man. It has reduced the cholesterol levels in persons from 10 to 30%, when the patient switched to a high fiber diet. It contains a soluble fiber which prevents sharp swings in the blood sugar level. Because of this, eating apples is found to be better than drinking apple juice. The good high density LIPIDS, HDL, increased, and the destructive artery clogging low density lipids, LDL, decreased. The researchers believe that it is the PECTIN in apples that brings this about, since pectin is a well-known anti-cholesterol agent. Apples can prevent cholesterol-induced GALLSTONES from forming. It seems that women get a greater lowering of blood cholesterol from eating apples than men. It has even been reported that the act of SMELLING apples has a calming effect on many people which tends to lower blood pressure. Fresh apple juice can knock out stomach FLU and POLIO viruses. It ranks tops with GRAPE JUICE in destroying these viruses.

◆ *Apples Fight Disease*

The apple is a neutralizer of all of the body's excess acids. It is therapeutically effective in all conditions of ACIDOSIS, GOUT, RHEUMATISM, JAUNDICE, LIVER AND GALL BLADDER TROUBLES, NERVOUS and SKIN DISEASES, and STATES OF AUTOINTOXICATION, CONSTIPATION, DYSPEPSIA, SKIN ERUPTIONS, and ARTHRITIS. It counteracts THROAT INFECTIONS, RELIEVES TENSION, FORTIFIES THE IMMUNE SYSTEM, and PREVENTS HEART DISEASE. It lowers CHOLESTEROL 10% on 2 apples a day. It has been said that an APPLE eaten after dinner will clean your teeth better than anything else. A Japanese study reports that people who eat three or more apples a day will not develop HIGH BLOOD PRESSURE as they get older. Apples contain minerals and vitamins which strengthen the blood. They also contain MALIC and TARTARIC acids which help disturbances of the LIVER and digestion in general. Apple juice prevents the formation of KIDNEY STONES and GALL STONES. The low acidity of apples stimulates salivary flow and thus helps remove debris from the teeth and stimulates the gum tissues. Apples are also recommended for OBESITY, SKIN ERUPTION, POOR COMPLEXION, INFLAMMATION OF THE BLADDER, GONORRHEA, ANEMIA, TUBERCULOSIS, NEURITIS, INSOMNIA, CATARRH, WORMS, HALITOSIS, and PYORRHEA.

◆ *Apple Juice And Cider*

Like apples, apple juice is an excellent food as long as it is fresh. As a drink it may have lost some of its PECTIN fiber. As it gets older it ferments, which means that it gradually develops more and more alcohol. until it turns into what is called "hard cider" which contains a certain percentage of alcohol, and is therefore no longer a healthful drink. Apple juice or sweet cider may be harmless, so that people have no scruples in buying it. "But it remains sweet for a short time only; then fermentation begins. The sharp taste which it then acquires makes it all the more acceptable to many palates, and the user is loath to admit that it has become hard or fermented." (CD436).

When this occurs, one can become just as intoxicated on the cider as on stronger drinks. We are told that "A few quarts of CIDER OR WINE may awaken a taste for stronger drinks." "Moderate drinking is the school in which men are receiving an education for the drunkard's career" (CD433).

"Licentiousness, adultery, and vices of almost every type, are committed as the result of indulging the appetite for WINE AND CIDER" (CD433). It is therefore not safe for some people to have cider around the house. It becomes a stimulant which Satan is encouraging them to indulge.

There is also another danger in the use of sweet cider. "Often those who manufacture cider for the market are not careful as to the condition of the fruit used, and the juice of wormy and decayed apples is expressed. Those who would not think of using the poisonous rotten apples in any other way, will drink the cider made from them and call it a luxury; but the microscope shows that even when fresh from the press, this pleasant beverage is wholly unfit for use" (CD436).

Apricots

In folk medicine, the apricot's primary medicinal part is the kernel, which is a source of the ANTI-CANCER agent LAETRILE. The apricot is cherished by the HUNZAS as a source of exceptional longevity. It is said to be equal to liver in hemoglobin regeneration. Apricots have little or no fat, sodium, or cholesterol. They have plenty of POTASSIUM, VITAMINS A and B_2. They rate high in ALKALINITY. They contain COBALT which is necessary for treating anemic conditions. They are high in iron and richer in minerals than most fruits. They are good body cleansers. They are said to help prevent cancer because of their content of BETA CAROTENE or pre-vitamin A, which has been very successful in thwarting cancer in laboratory animals. People who eat lots of fruits and vegetables, high in beta carotene, have lower rates of CANCER of the LUNG, SKIN, LARYNX, PANCREAS, STOMACH, BLADDER, and ESOPHAGUS. They are also indicated in cases of ANEMIA, TUBERCULOSIS, ASTHMA, BRONCHITIS, GALL STONES, DIARRHEA, and TOXEMIA.

Bananas

◆ *Work Against Ulcers*

Plantains, a larger type of banana, which are often eaten unripe and cooked, contain powerful medicinal properties against stomach and duodenal ULCERS, ulcerative COLITIS, and HEMORRHOIDS. It works the same way as the anti-ulcer drug CARBENOXOLANE, but without that drug's serious side effects. Plantains strengthen the surface cells of the stomach lining, and form a sturdy barrier against noxious juices.

◆ *Lower Blood Pressure And Cholesterol*

Ordinary bananas LOWER BLOOD CHOLESTEROL because of their high PECTIN content, which on a weight basis is even higher than that of apples. One medium sized banana contains about as much pectin as a medium sized apple. Two small bananas provide about as much fiber as a slice of whole wheat bread, but unlike bread, bananas contain a significant amount of soluble fiber. They contain almost NO SODIUM and a very modest amount of vitamin C, and about one fifth of a man's daily requirement of vitamin A. A banana has about 100 calories, is almost fat free, and is high in POTASSIUM which is important in converting sugar into GLYCOGEN, which is then held in storage for future energy needs. Potassium also helps in LOWERING BLOOD PRESSURE. Bananas are as good source of VITAMIN B_6, which helps fight a form of KIDNEY STONE disease, as well as CARPAL TUNNEL SYNDROME.

◆ *Feeding Young Children*

Baby specialists make considerable use of well-ripened bananas in the feeding of young children, It is the cornerstone in the treatment of DIARRHEA, SPRUE, or CELIAC disease. They are a regulator in diarrhea as well as in constipation. Bananas feed the natural ACIDOPHILUS bacteria of the bowel, and their high potassium content benefits the muscular system. It has been said that the inner surface of the BANANA SKIN may be applied directly to burns or boils for a good healing effect.

Barley

When Christ fed the five thousand, He used five barley loaves and two fishes, and multiplied them many times to feed the multitude. On the 2nd day of the feast of unleavened bread the first fruits of the year's harvest, a sheaf of barley was presented before the Lord.(DA77). Barley was the earliest grain in Palestine, and it began to ripen at the opening of the Passover feast. It is probably the oldest grain used for food. It was used as flour for bread-making extensively in Egypt and Palestine (Deut. 8:8). In the Middle East, barley is a staple as a cereal and flour grain. As a result of eating it, heart disease rates are low. In Pakistan barley is referred to as the "MEDICINE FOR THE HEART."

Barley can drive down blood CHOLESTEROL. There are compounds in barley which reduce the liver's ability to manufacture the bad LDL-type cholesterol that damages blood vessels, and leads to heart attacks and strokes. Barley is a cereal grass that is an excellent source of fiber and protein. It therefore raises the levels of high density lipoproteins, HDL, that keep CHOLESTEROL under control and guards against ARTERIOSCLEROSIS. Some researchers believe that barley contains PROTEASE INHIBITORS which SUPPRESS CANCER-causing agents in the intestinal tract and thereby act as antidotes to cancer formation.

It is helpful for underweight people to increase their body weight. It may be useful in cases of ASTHMA because of a substance called HORDENINE, which relieves bronchial spasms. It is a body builder, and is valuable in cases of STOMACH ULCERS, DIARRHEA, and is good for TEETH, HAIR, and NAILS. A poultice of it is good for SKIN DISEASES.

Beans And Peas

◆ *Eating Beans Is Good For Your Heart*

Legumes, beans, peas, and lentils, are good medicines for the CARDIO-VASCULAR SYSTEM. When you eat dried beans they are not entirely digested. The undigested substance is attacked by bacteria in the colon, and in this process a lot of chemicals are liberated. These chemicals act like medicines such as telling the liver to cut down its production of CHOLESTEROL, and the blood to speed up clearing out dangerous LDL cholesterol. That is one reason why experts think that eating beans is good for your HEART. This process can also produce cancer-blocking chemicals. In several studies Dr. Anderson has seen cholesterol levels drop 60 points in 3 weeks when beans were added to the diets of men with high cholesterol. A major therapeutic substance in dried beans is thought to be SOLUBLE FIBER. In a case where GREEN PEAS were a major gas producer, adding a little GINGER or GARLIC to the peas showed them to be potent GAS BLOCKERS.

◆ *Beans Help Diabetics*

Type I DIABETICS, those who need daily insulin shots, have cut their insulin needs by 38% by eating a cup of COOKED BEANS a day. Those with type II diabetes, (adult onset diabetes), who do not produce enough insulin, virtually eliminated the need for any injections. The reason is that BEANS produce such a slow rise in blood sugar, that the body needs to release much less insulin to keep the glucose level under control. It appears that less insulin stifles hunger, and through a complicated mechanism may facilitate the excretion of sodium, thereby lowering blood pressure. Eating high fiber foods like beans does lower blood pressure substantially according to numerous studies. Vegetarians, for example, had a diastolic blood pressure that was 18% lower than that of meat eaters. Even people with normal blood pressure have brought it down another five or six percent by increasing their intake of high fiber foods like beans.

◆ *Beans Are Anti-Cancer Agents*

Beans are said to be good cancer preventers. The reason for this is that beans are concentrated carriers of PROTEASE INHIBITORS, enzymes that can counteract the activation of cancer-causing compounds in the intestines. Feeding animals protease inhibitors also blocked the development of colon and breast cancer. Beans are more nutritious when sprouted. SOY BEANS and MUNG BEANS are the most popular beans for SPROUTING. Soybeans especially help prevent deficiency diseases because they contain iron, calcium, and B-vitamins. When sprouted most of the B vitamins are increased, and vitamin C is produced within the bean. After 7 days of storage in the refrigerator the vitamin C content of soybeans doubles. After this it deteriorates. With sprouted soy and mung beans the riboflavin content increased 4 times, and the niacin content doubled. With reference to Daniel and his companions, beans produce a vibrant look of radiant health.

Folk medicine as well as numerous scientific studies have shown that PEAS are anti-fertility agents. Fresh garden peas are slightly diuretic in action. They also give relief to ulcer pains in the stomach because they help use up the stomach acids. They are an outstanding source of vitamins A, B, and C. The pea pods are very high in chlorophyll, iron, and calcium.

◆ *Beans And Flatulence*

The most notorious universal gas producers are sugars, notably RAFFINOSE, which is highly concentrated in beans. They reach the large intestines in great amounts because we lack the enzyme to digest them properly. Eating baked beans, one study found, increased the amount of gas produced by 12 times. One remedy is to use plenty of GARLIC. SORBITOL, a low-calorie sweetener, is also a great gas producer.

◆ *De-Gassing Your Beans*

To degas your beans, rinse the beans, add them to boiling water and boil them for 3 minutes. Let stand for 2 hours. Pour off the water and add new water at room temperature to cover the beans. After 2 hours pour off the water and add new water at room temperature to just cover the beans. after 2 hours pour the water off, add more water and let soak overnight. Rinse again with room-temperature water, then add water and cook till done in 75 to 90 minutes. Also a supermarket product, called BEANO, added to gaseous foods, is effective in reducing gas.

Broccoli—The King Of The Cabbage Clan

◆ *Cruciferous Vegetables—The Anti-Cancer Family*

Broccoli is the king of the cabbage family consisting of BROCCOLI, BRUSSELS SPROUTS, CABBAGE, CAULIFLOWER, COLLARD, KALE, KOHLRABI, and MUSTARD. They are called CRUCIFEROUS VEGETABLES because the reproductive apparatus of the flowers of these plants contain two components that are arranged like a cross, which is the reason for the name. Scientists place these vegetables at the top of the list when it comes to PREVENTING CANCER. The cabbage family can inhibit the growth of TUMORS, prevent cancer of the COLON and RECTUM, DETOXIFY HARMFUL CHEMICALS, LOWER "BAD" CHOLESTEROL (LDL), HEAL GASTROINTESTINAL TUMORS, and they give RADIATION PROTECTION. They are rich in known CANCER ANTIDOTES. The whole family is high in ANTI-CANCER ACTIVITY, but broccoli tops them all. Broccoli contains 33 compounds that help prevent cancer. It counteracts the carcinogen NITROSAMINE, as well as the steroids which cause BREAST CANCER. Like spinach and kale it is endowed with CAROTENOIDS, which may give it added powers against lung cancer. It is very potent in blocking cell mutations which foreshadow cancer. Those people eating broccoli up to ten times a month were nearly twice as likely to have colon cancer than those who ate broccoli more than twenty times a month. It was shown that broccoli kept guinea pigs from succumbing to otherwise lethal doses of radiation.

◆ *America's Favorite Vegetable*

According to a poll BROCCOLI is America's favorite vegetable. CAULIFLOWER was second. A cup of fresh cooked broccoli contains two and one half times the recommended daily allowance for vitamin C. It is one of the best vegetable sources of calcium. All of the foods in the cabbage family are best eaten with proteins, because the combination is said to drive amino acids to the brain. It is said that there are 900 compounds in whole foods with the ability to prevent cancer. But only 9% of Americans eat enough vegetables to qualify as having a balanced diet.

Brussels Sprouts—The Queen Of The Cabbage Family

Brussels Sprouts is extremely high in vitamin C. It is richer in protein than most vegetables. It is low in sodium and fat. It is moderate in vitamin A, riboflavin (B_2), and iron. It is moderately high in potassium and fiber. It is a good general tonic food, and is recommended for CATARRH, OBESITY, ACIDOSIS, HARDENING OF THE ARTERIES, AND BLEEDING GUMS. It seems to detoxify AFLATOXIN, a fungus linked to high rates of liver cancer. It frequently contaminates peanuts, corn, and rice, and is a special threat in third world countries. VITAMINS A and B_2 work against aflatoxin.

Cabbage

◆ *The Anti-Ulcer Vegetable*

Cabbage is hailed as an anti-ulcer remedy. In a study a quart of raw cabbage juice was given to fifty-five patients with gastric, duodenal, and jejunal ulcers. It healed all of them, and reduced the otherwise normal healing time 72%. It also prevents cancer of the colon. Cabbage's known anti-cancer compounds include CHLOROPHYLL, FLAVONOIDS, CAFFEIC AND FERULIC ACIDS, as well as VITAMINS C AND E. Cabbage is said to contain an ANTIBIOTIC capable of destroying bacteria and viruses. It boosts the immune functioning of animal cells growing in test tubes. A study in Japan showed in a year-long survey that those people who ate the most cabbage had the lowest death rates from all causes. This lifts cabbage to a status along with yogurt and olive oil, as a potential LIFE EXTENDER.

◆ *A Blood Purifier*

Cabbage is therapeutically effective in conditions of SCURVY, GOUT, RHEUMATISM, PYORRHEA, ASTHMA, TUBERCULOSIS, CANCER, GANGRENE, KIDNEY AND BLADDER DISORDERS, OBESITY, DIABETES, TOXEMIA, LUMBAGO, SKIN ERUPTIONS, AND POOR COMPLEXION. It is a BLOOD PURIFIER and an anti-scorbutic agent because of its vitamin C content. People who don't eat cabbage are 3 times more likely to develop colon cancer. It is best eaten raw in order to preserve all of the enzymes. Because cabbage is a sulfur food, it can cause intestinal distress. It also contains a great deal of roughage, and some people find that they cannot eat raw cabbage. Raw cabbage juice may be drunk when for some reason citrus fruits are not available for their vitamin C content. The darker outside leaves of the cabbage have as much as 40% more calcium than the inside leaves.

Fresh raw cabbage juice is very helpful for STOMACH and DUODENAL ULCERS and inflammations, because of its content of vitamin U. It contains adequate amounts of calcium, phosphorus, iron, cobalt, vitamin A, inositol, choline, pyridoxine, and vitamin K. It contains many minerals. The sulfur in cabbage destroys the ferments in the blood, and is especially good for any skin trouble when used both internally and externally. SAUERKRAUT JUICE stimulates the body in general because it is high in LACTIC ACID. It is one of the best foods for keeping a clear COMPLEXION.

Carrot

◆ *A High Source Of Vitamin A*

The name "Carrot" comes from the Celtic and means "red of color." Carrots are an important source of vitamin A. They contain almost all of the vitamins which the body needs. Carrots contain CAROTENE, which is the precursor of vitamin A, also called provitamin A. It is the plant form of vitamin A. There is no direct vitamin A in plants, and there is no carotene in animal livers. Carotene is changed to vitamin A by the liver. Tests have shown that more of the carotene is converted into vitamin A when the carrot is shredded or juiced, than when it is eaten whole, or cooked. Experiments have shown that only 2 to 5% of carotene is absorbed by the body when raw or cooked carrots are eaten, no matter how well they are chewed, but that from 4 to 36% of the carotene is absorbed when the carrots are well shredded before eating. This suggests that it is a good idea to juice carrots, for in juicing them the cell walls are broken down so that a lot of carotene can be absorbed. Carrot juice has also been recommended for nursing mothers, in order to enhance the quality of their breast milk. Older people have a harder time converting carotene into vitamin A. Hence, they should take additional COD LIVER OIL in order to get a sufficient amount of vitamin A.

◆ *It Has Potential Against Cancer*

✓ IT DISSOLVES TUMORS—Carrots are the champion disease fighter on every level. A high intake of carotene has shown a potential for preventing cancer of the lung, esophagus, stomach, intestines, mouth, throat, bladder, pancreas, and prostate. Dr. Kirschner tells the story of a woman with stomach cancer whose weight went down to 67 pounds. At that point she heard about carrot juice, and started to drink it a little at a time, and at first diluted with water. She gradually raised the amount to a gallon or more a day and ate or drank nothing else. She kept this up for 18 months until she was healed of the cancer. It is said that carrot juice contains almost every vitamin and mineral which the body needs. Carrots are particularly good as a supportive treatment for DIABETICS, and when used regularly in the diet it helps to ease the pain of GOUT, RHEUMATISM, and ARTHRITIS.

✓ COOKED CARROTS ABSORBED AS WELL AS RAW CARROTS—A cup of raw shredded carrots provides 31,000 international units of vitamin A when the carotene is converted. Because carrots become denser with cooking, a cup of cooked carrots provides 38,000 international units of vitamin A. Furthermore, it has been found that the carotene in cooked carrots is actually better absorbed than that in raw carrots. 5,000 IU of carotene is the recommended daily dietary allowance. One researcher says that 12,500 IU would be desirable for preventing cancer. A woman with SPLENIC LEUKEMIA recovered completely on RAW CARROT JUICE.

✓ PROTECT FROM CHEMICAL POLLUTANTS—Carrots can protect the skin from ULTRAVIOLET RAYS, OXYGEN, and CHEMICAL POLLUTANTS. Chemical pollution accelerates the decomposition of the OZONE LAYER by allowing more ultraviolet light through. Then molecules in the atmosphere combine with ultraviolet rays and oxygen to form SINGLET OXYGEN which can attack the cells of the skin leading to CANCER. It also works to activate CARCINOGENS. Carotene helps to break down the singlet oxygen when it touches the skin.

✓ VITAMIN A AND NIGHT-BLINDNESS—Carrots act to improve resistance to infections of all types, especially the EYES, THROAT, TONSILS, as well as the SINUSES and the entire RESPIRATORY SYSTEM.

The story is told of a young mother of two who had night-blindness because of a deficiency of VITAMIN A. She arranged her life so that she would never have to drive a car at night for fear of having an accident. One time one of the children went into convulsions. She was terrified but bundled both children into the car and drove to the hospital at 15 miles per hour. This happened during the day. After this trip she realized that she would have to do something about her night-blindness in case she might be forced to drive at night in an emergency. The following day she bought a juicer and started drinking a fresh full quart of carrot juice per day. Her husband joked that she was "turning yellow," but she persisted. After only a few weeks, she found that her night-blindness was clearing, and finally she developed complete confidence in night driving.

Cherries

Cherries cleanse the system. The darker cherries are more valuable than the lighter ones as they contain a greater quantity of MAGNESIUM, IRON, AND SILICON. Cherries are high in iron, and are a wonderful blood builder. Their high alkaline content gets rid of toxic waste. They have a wonderful effect on the glandular system. They stimulate the secretion of digestive juices, and are effective CLEANSERS of the liver, kidneys, and gall bladder because of their HIGH IRON CONTENT. Cherries were found to be potent bacterial agents against TOOTH DECAY. ELLAGIC ACID which is found largely in cherries and strawberries, is a cancer preventative in that it counters many man-made carcinogens.

In one study cherry juice blocked 89% of the enzyme activity leading to plaque formation, which is a prelude to decay. They are valuable in cases of anemia, bad blood, poor complexion, high blood pressure, rheumatism, asthma, and especially GOUT and ARTHRITIC gout. Gout is a disease that is characterized by excessive uric acid in the blood, and by attacks of arthritis. A half pound and more of cherries a day has been found to bring relief to sufferers of gout. Twelve gout patients who ate one-half pound of cherries per day reduced their URIC ACID level to normal. Uric acid is largely an end-product of meat digestion. It was found that canned cherries work as well as fresh cherries.

Corn

Corn is one of the easiest foods to digest. It is high in roughage, and high in MAGNESIUM which is a bowel regulator. Yellow corn is higher in PHOSPHOROUS than white corn, which makes it an excellent food for the brain and nervous system. It is rated with brown rice and barley as on of the best balanced starches. It is a respectable source of IRON and ZINC, a fine source of POTASSIUM, and it is very low in sodium. Corn has been recommended in cases of anemia, emaciation, and as a general body building food. The vitamins and minerals in corn are largely contained in the germ which is removed in milling. Chewing and eating a lot of corn has been shown to reduce dental cavities. Corn oil lowers blood CHOLESTEROL, and it is a rich source of LINOLEIC acid, which is essential to good health.

Celery

◆ *An Alkaline Protective Food*

Celery is popular among vegetable juice drinkers. Raw vegetables and their juices are most healthful foods, because they are raw and fresh, and maintain all of their vitamins and minerals. It is high in roughage and low in calories. Natural juice should be sipped and not drunk like water, for it is a food. It is an ALKALINE protective food with a high mineral content. It is rich in sodium, chlorine, potassium and magnesium. Celery is generally known as a SODIUM FOOD. Because of its high sodium content, it is the best food to counteract the effects of EXTREME HEAT. But we must remember that it contains sodium in organic form, and in ORGANIC FORM sodium is beneficial to the body, and is called the youth maintainer, for it helps keep us young and active. On the other hand, common table salt, which is inorganic sodium chloride, is generally detrimental to the system in the quantities in which it is commonly used.

◆ *It Keeps Calcium In Solution*

Celery NEUTRALIZES ACIDS, and thereby counteracts acidosis and aids digestion. It also purifies the blood stream. The overindulgence of concentrated sugars and starches has the tendency to leave deposits of inorganic calcium in the system. The organic sodium in celery aids in maintaining such inorganic calcium in solution until it can be eliminated from the body before it settles in the arteries and tissues and causes trouble.

Japanese physicians prescribe celery for rheumatism, caused largely by acid forming foods which in excess quantities dissolve calcium from the bones. Food chemists have demonstrated that because of its high alkalinity celery neutralizes the calcium in the blood, and thereby helps in the treatment and prevention of arthritis. Arthritis being a disease in which excess calcium produced by excess acidity, is not eliminated from the blood stream by the lack of neutralizing substances and therefore settles out of the bloodstream into tissues and joints.

Celery helps sleeplessness if one drinks one or two glasses of celery juice a day. For people who drink one or two glasses of celery juice a day are said not to suffer as much from heat as those who do not do so. Hippocrates said: "Nerves distraught? Let celery be your food and medicine."

Cranberry

Recent research finds that only one half cup of cranberry juice cocktail a day can ward off urinary tract and bladder infections in individuals at high risk of infections The reason is that cranberries increase the urine acidity with HIPPURIC acid which kills the bacteria. Cranberries deodorize urine by helping to rid it of E. Coli bacteria, and preventing them from releasing ammonia. In one study 16 ounces a day caused the odor to disappear. It prevents bacteria to stick to the surface of the urinary tract. One doctor suggests that cranberries help to retard the formation and even help dissolve calcium type KIDNEY STONES. Cranberries are helpful in cases of skin disorders such as pimples, high blood pressure, obesity, poor appetite, fevers, for kidney and liver disturbances, and for rectal disturbances such as piles and hemorrhoids.

Date

The date tree was cultivated long before Christ in Mesopotamia and in the Nile Valley of Egypt. These old date trees ranged in height from 40 to 80 feet. Dates were then known as "the candy that grows on trees." Spanish missionaries introduced the date to the Western World, and especially into Mexico and California

Dates are a highly concentrated food, nourishing, and easily digested. They are a source of quick energy. They contain from 35 to 75% sugar, Hence, they are a valuable substitute for candy, and are not acid-forming. They are beneficial for COUGHS, SORE THROAT, BRONCHITIS, ANEMIA, LOW VITALITY, and COLITIS. Dates can be eaten with whole RAW MILK for ULCERS of the STOMACH. For an upset stomach soak a few dates in a cup of hot water. The water dates are soaked in can be used with milk for children who have sensitive stomachs, as it helps them to digest the milk. They are especially recommended for NURSING MOTHERS. They are a good source of copper, which is a diet essential, even though it is needed only in small amounts.

Figs

◆ *God Recommends Their Use*

When God heard HEZEKIAH'S prayer to keep him alive, God called Isaiah to have him tell Hezekiah that he would extend his life by fifteen years. Isaiah then told Hezekiah that he should take a lump of figs, and put it on the boil. When this was done he recovered (2 Kings 20:7). One word from God or one touch of the divine finger, would have been enough to cure Hezekiah instantly. But in this connection we are told that it would be well for us to treasure the prescription which the Lord ordered to be used in this case (2SM300). God here ordered one of His natural medicines to be used for the purpose of healing, again to give us an example of what we should do under similar circumstances. Figs will be in the NEW EARTH. (EW19).
Among the Hebrews the fig tree was associated with the vine as a symbol of peace and plenty. In Bavaria figs are cooked in milk for use in treating ulcerated gums. Among the Hindus the milky juice of the tree is given to relieve a toothache, while in the U.S. the juice is used in the treatment of ringworm.

◆ *An Anti-Cancer Agent*

Figs are also today recognized as being good for BOILS and ABSCESSES. Some country folks use powdered figs in a paste and apply it to WOUNDS and SORES. Figs are a traditional ANTI-CANCER agent. In recent times Japanese scientists have isolated the active fig agent as BENZALDEHIDE. They injected a fig distillate into human advanced cancer patients with dramatic results. 55% improved, 7% went into complete remission, and 29% into partial remission. With the fig distillate patients generally lived longer. The fig juice also killed bacteria in test tubes. Radioactive bodies are reported to be present in figs which give them their special property.

Figs have a high calcium content, and are also richer in iron and copper than most foods. Their total mineral content is 2 to 4 times that of most foods. There have been reports that cancer is rare in regions where lots of figs are eaten. According to French scientists, it is thought that figs can prevent the formation of PRECANCEROUS CONDITIONS in the body. Figs should be bought unsulfured. Like dates they make an ideal healthful "candy" for both children and adults. In spite of their high sugar content they are not acid-forming. In fact they are one of the most alkaline forming foods there is. However, one must remember that sugar in the organic form does not act the same way in the body as refined table sugar. Table sugar splits up in the body and forms an acid, while organic sugar does not do so.

◆ *A Quick Energy Food*

When the fig is broken off the tree before it is ripe, a milk escapes which has wonderful healing properties. If the milk is put freely on WARTS, it removes them. A tea made of the leaves will take spots off the face or body. Figs are helpful in the treatment of joint inflammation and swelling such as in RHEUMATOID ARTHRITIS. The sulfur compound responsible for this is an enzyme called FICIN. It is also found in pineapple and papaya. Figs are of considerable value in the prevention and treatment of NUTRITIONAL ANEMIA and

CONSTIPATION. In general figs are beneficial for low blood pressure, anemia, emaciation, skin disease, Raynaud's disease where there is poor circulation, poor complexion, and skin eruptions. Fig juice is also beneficial for sore throats, coughs, and ulcers in the digestive system. They are LAXATIVE because of the MUCIN and PECTIN they contain, as well as being a good low fat source of FIBER. They are a high CALCIUM food, high in CARBOHYDRATES, and turn into ENERGY very quickly. The BLACK MISSION figs are high in POTASSIUM, and they are a remedy for ARTHRITIS.

Garlic

◆ *An Excellent Antibiotic*

In Numbers 11:5 we are told that the children of Israel, while in Egypt, ate freely of CUCUMBERS, MELONS, LEEKS, ONIONS, and GARLIC. So they must have been in good supply there. Miraculous healing power appears to exist in common garlic. Research shows that for 4000 years or more garlic has been used to cure many ailments that are being studied today in modern scientific laboratories. The Babylonians knew of its CURATIVE POWERS, and it was highly honored and esteemed in ancient Egypt, where thousands of slaves working on the great Cheops pyramid were fed garlic daily. They all claimed that garlic cured INTESTINAL DISORDERS, FLATULENCE, WORMS, INFECTIONS of the RESPIRATORY SYSTEM, SKIN DISEASE, WOUNDS, and the SYMPTOMS OF AGING.

Garlic is reportedly the oldest, safest, and surest remedy for ASTHMA, BRONCHITIS, and other RESPIRATORY AILMENTS. The Greek physician DIOSCORIDES specified garlic for all LUNG DISORDERS. PLINY, that first century Roman naturalist maintained that garlic cured CONSUMPTION (TB). Against garlic, COLD, FLU VIRUS, and ALLERGY GERMS don't stand a chance. The ETHERS of garlic are so potent that they DISSOLVE MUCUS in the sinuses, bronchial tubes, and lungs. Garlic is a widely used ANTIBIOTIC which has no harmful side effects, as might be evident with PENICILLIN. It is NATURE'S OWN ANTIBIOTIC. It contains a bacteriocide called CROTONALDEHYDE. There is no limit to the dosage, and no danger of disrupting the delicate relationships among the various bacteria that exist in our bodies. At the turn of the century, garlic ointments, compresses, and inhalents were the drug of choice against TUBERCULOSIS.

ALLIIN, which is the first substance isolated from garlic, is effective against the germs of SALMONELLA, DYSENTERY, STREPTOCOCCI, SCARLET FEVER, SEPSIS, DIPHTHERIA, ERYSIPELAS, and RHEUMATIC FEVER. ALICIN, another garlic ingredient, fights CONJUNCTIVITIS, PUTREFACTION, TYPHOID, CHOLERA, and TB. It destroys some germs even PENICILLIN won't touch, such as BACILLUS PARATYPHOID—A, which creates dysentery, rheumatism, and kidney complications. GARLIC VAPORS halt germs at a distance of 20 cm, and its germ killing power remains in the bloodstream for 10 hours.

◆ *It Heals Without Side Effects*

Garlic has the ability to kill dangerous organisms without attacking the organisms vital to the body's health. There are many compounds used as medications which kill germs, but they have side effects which harm the body. For example, FORMALDEHYDE inactivates all viruses, but it also reacts with the body's own protein, and is therefore a deadly poison to the body. Many drugs used today are antagonistic to body processes, but because the reaction is not immediate, they continue to be used.

A Japanese researcher discovered that garlic increases the capacity of the body to assimilate vitamin B_1 or thiamin. It becomes available quicker and in greater amounts. Blood concentrations of thiamin increase ten-fold to a level otherwise impossible to achieve except through injections.

Garlic contains VITAMIN C, and has the ability to increase its absorption from other foods. Vitamin C is said to act like INSULIN according to Dr. Bamerjee of Calcutta, India. Vitamin C, like insulin, helps to metabolize the carbohydrates in foods.

Garlic is rich in MUSTARD OILS which have a cleansing effect upon the entire system from stimulating the APPETITE and the secretion of gastric juices to the promotion of PERISTALSIS and DIURETIC action. The ETHERS in garlic are so potent and penetrating that they help to dissolve the accumulations of MUCUS in the sinus cavities, and thereby clear a STUFFED NOSE. Their MITOGENETIC RADIATION or "GURWITCH RAYS" which they give off are able to dislodge toxic wastes and then prepare them for elimination. It also helps to eliminate intestinal parasites as well as the poisons from the body through the pores of the skin. The oil of garlic is composed in part of SULFIDES and DISULFIDES and these unite with virus matter in a certain way which inactivates the virus organism. This is accomplished so perfectly that absolutely no harm is done to any beneficial organism in the body.

◆ *It Heals Many Diseases*

✓ A UNIVERSAL REMEDY—One doctor said that garlic is the best treatment found to get rid of GERMS, and that it is a specific for the TUBERCULOSIS BACILLUS. Dr. McDuffie used garlic to cure hopeless TB cases, and called it "A UNIVERSAL REMEDY." Thus nature by diet, rest, exercise, baths, climate, and garlic furnishes sufficient and specific treatment for the medical aspects of tuberculosis. In World War I garlic was used to fight TYPHUS, DYSENTERY, and ENTERITIS, to PREVENT INFECTION and GANGRENE in battle wounds. IN WORLD WAR II British physicians treated battle wounds with garlic with total success in warding off SEPTIC POISONING and GANGRENE.

✓ SEPTIC POISONING AND GANGRENE—It was reported that not one case of SEPTIC POISONING or GANGRENE occurred among those treated. Even Dr. Albert Schweitzer used garlic against TYPHUS, CHOLERA, and LEPROSY. It has helped cure 82% of special MENINGITIS cases as compared with only 15% for the drug AMPHETERICIN.

✓ POLIOMYELITIS—It has also reduced the incidence of POLIOMYELITIS by more than 30% compared with an untreated control group. During a POLIO EPIDEMIC in Sweden, out of 1204 children who took garlic, not a single case of polio occurred. We are told that during the great plagues that swept Europe during the Middle Ages, those who ate garlic were immune.

✓ EARACHE—Garlic oil helps make EARACHES disappear within 10 to 15 minutes, by pouring a garlic oil into the ear, and then stopping it with cotton.

✓ ANEMIA—One woman claimed that garlic cured her ANEMIA. She says that it completely relieved her symptoms of WEAK DIGESTION, NUMBNESS, TINGLING, FATIGUE, SHORTNESS of BREATH, LACK of APPETITE, DIARRHEA, WEIGHT LOSS, and FEVER. Anemia can result from inadequate PROTEIN, IODINE, COBALT, COPPER, VITAMIN C, or any of the B-VITAMINS—all of which are contained in garlic.

✓ ARTHRITIS—One wheelchair patient consumed 5 to 6 cloves of garlic daily along with a raw vegetable salad. Within 2 weeks the inflammation "just went away." In 4 weeks the joints healed and she had a remarkable restoration of flexibility. During the 5th week she left her wheelchair, needing neither cane nor walker. At the end of the 6th week she joined a jogging club and started jogging. She said that it was GARLIC that saved her from ARTHRITIS.

✓ CONTROLS MEASLES AND HBP—In 450 B.C. Hippocrates ranked garlic as one of the most important of his 400 therapeutic remedies. CRUSHED GARLIC on the soles of your feet can alleviate MEASLES. Over 80% of HIGH BLOOD PRESSURE (HBP) cases can be controlled by diet alone. Garlic can make such a diet very effective.

✓ HEART ATTACK AND STROKE—Stroke or heart attack risk increases with reduced blood clotting time. It increases in proportion with higher blood pressure, because HBP forces platelets to clump more easily. Garlic contains substances that reduce both PLATELET CLUMPING and FIBRIN ACTIVITY which develops clots. High volume garlic consumers have the lowest platelet aggregation and clot formation.

✓ CANCER—the active materials in garlic also have anti-cancer properties. The active ingredient ALLICIN has reduced cancer according to its dose. At high doses garlic is 100% effective as shown in experiments with animals.

◆ *It Is An Infection Fighter*

Garlic destroys insects, eliminates bacteria, fungus, tumors, lowers blood sugar levels as well as fat levels, it eliminates plaque buildup in the arteries, and lowers cholesterol and triglyceride levels, and lowers blood pressure.

Garlic contains an amino acid called ALLIIN. When garlic is crushed an enzyme ALLIINASE is released which converts the alliin to ALLICIN, an antibiotic with an antibacterial action equivalent to 1% penicillin. Garlic destroys bacteria because of its compound allicin. It does this without upsetting the organism, that is, without any side effects. Tests have shown that raw garlic destroys bacteria better than PENICILLIN and TETRACYCLINE. It is a broad-spectrum antibiotic against a long list of microbes that spread diseases including BOTULISM, TUBERCULOSIS, DIARRHEA, STAPH, DYSENTERY, and TYPHOID. It is effective against 72 separate infective agents. One researcher said that garlic has the broadest spectrum of any antimicrobial substance we know. It is ANTISEPTIC, ANTI-INFLAMMATORY, ANTIBACTERIAL, ANTIFUNGAL, ANTI-PARASITIC, ANTIPROTOZOAN, and ANTIVIRAL. It is better than the drug CLOFIBRATE in lowering cholesterol.

It is also an EXPECTORANT, DIURETIC, DIAPHORETIC, and VERMIFUGE. It is one of the richest sources of GERMANIUM, an anti-cancer agent, and a mineral which strengthens the IMMUNE SYSTEM. It is also a potent stimulus to INTERFERON production. It contains SELENIUM, an excellent ANTIOXIDANT and overall IMMUNE ENHANCER. Garlic can lower serum CHOLESTEROL levels, and can have dramatic effects on ATHEROSCLEROTIC heart disease. Garlic controls INTESTINAL PUTREFACTION, and the consequent prevention and absorption of toxic substances from the digestive tract. If garlic is cooked, it is no longer a microbe killer, for then all of the allicin is destroyed.

Garlic also contains MANGANESE (Mn). There is evidence that a lack of manganese can actually affect GLUCOSE TOLERANCE, the ability to remove excess sugar from the blood. Its deficiency may therefore contribute to DIABETES. Plant extracts which are good sources of Mn have been used as home remedies in diabetes. They are BLUEBERRY, ONION, BREWER'S YEAST, and GARLIC. The mineral which gives garlic its odor, namely SULFUR, is found in the pancreatic insulin.

◆ *Russian Penicillin*

In Russia garlic is used so much as an infection fighter that it has come to be known as "Russian Penicillin," where 500 tons of garlic were used to combat an outbreak of INFLUENZA. Garlic is also a Russian remedy for COLDS, WHOOPING COUGH. and INTESTINAL DISORDERS. Certain Slavic people still eat a clove of garlic with each meal during the winter months to prevent COLDS and FLU. In 1973 Japanese researchers showed that garlic is in fact able to prevent infection by the INFLUENZA virus. Chinese physicians recently used it in high doses to cure CRYPTOCOCCAL MENINGITIS, a fungal infection that is frequently fatal. The Chinese physicians concluded that part of the cure was due to garlic's stimulation of the patients' IMMUNE SYSTEM. In an experiment 9 people ate 12 to 15 cloves of garlic a day, while 9 other people took no garlic. The immune system's natural killer cells of the garlic eaters destroyed from 140% to 160% more CANCER CELLS than did the killer cells of the non-garlic eaters. The experimenter says that he eats a couple of garlic cloves a day, and he reports that he hasn't had a COLD since he started the regimen. It is said that in case of the onset of a cold, put a clove of garlic in the mouth on both sides of the cheek. The cold will disappear in a matter of hours, or at most within a day.

◆ *It Does Wonders To The Cardiovascular System*

Garlic lowers blood cholesterol in humans and creates other blood changes protective against heart disease. It proved far more protective than the standard drug CLOFIBRATE. In a Loma Linda study of Japan's cold-pressed, odorless, raw garlic substance, KYOLIC, 1 gm a day lowered the unfavorable LDL blood cholesterol and triglycerides in about 60 to 70% of the volunteers. Onion and garlic fight HEART ATTACKS by inhibiting the formation of blood clots, by making the platelets less sticky. Garlic consistently LOWERS BLOOD PRESSURE in laboratory animals. It was also shown to work on humans in the same manner. The Bulgarian Academy of Science reported that garlic in humans produces a systolic blood pressure drop of 20 to 30 points, and a diastolic drop of 10 to 20 points. Dr. Pouillard of France says that garlic juice taken over a period of 10 days produced improvement both in HEART RHYTHM and HEART ACTION. It relieved DIZZINESS, ANGINA PAINS, and BACKACHES in 3 to 5 days.

Garlic and onions are full of potent CLOT-FIGHTING COMPOUNDS. They block the detrimental blood-clotting proclivities of FATS. So when you eat fatty foods, add some garlic or onions as a safeguard against blood-clotting. AJOENE is the anticoagulant compound in garlic. Garlic releases a strange type of ultraviolet MITOGENETIC emission referred to as GURWITCH RAYS. They stimulate cell growth and strengthen the immune system.

Garlic dissolves the crystals whose accumulation causes HARDENING of the ARTERIES. It accelerates and regulates blood circulation by stimulating the heart muscles, and it purifies the blood at the same time. It therefore gives excellent results in troubles due to INSUFFICIENT CIRCULATION such as in VARICOSE VEINS, PILES, RHEUMATISM, etc.

◆ *Garlic Works Against Tumors And Cancers*

Russian scientists successfully used garlic extracts against human tumors. Dr. Gurwitch discovered that garlic and onions emit a peculiar type of ultraviolet radiation that have the property of stimulating cell growth, and have a rejuvenating effect on all body functions. Numerous animal studies show that fresh garlic can immunize animals against tumor development or reverse it, once under way. In a Japanese study fresh garlic completely wiped out BREAST CANCERS in mice. In U.S. experiments in 1987, garlic in animals was found to be more effective in warding off BLADDER CANCERS than a well-known cancer vaccine called BCG. A Chinese study suggests that ALLIUM vegetables such as onions and garlic may reduce the risk of stomach cancers. Garlic fulfills all of the requirements of a perfect therapeutic agent:
- It is absolutely safe.
- It has no bad aftereffects
- It has no dosage limits.
- Blood pressure is reduced gradually without any sudden shock.
- It does not interfere with any other medication.
- It also relieves weakness, dizziness, headaches, ringing ears, chest pains, and gas pains.
- Good results are obtained regardless of age.
- It is now easy to take in odorless tablet form.

Grapes

◆ *Grapes Are God's Gift*

We are told that "Apples and grapes are God's gifts. They may be put to excellent use as healthful articles of food" (5T361). We are to eat freely of grapes as well of many other fruits (7T134). Even the redeemed will eat grapes, for the tree of life will have grapes on it (EW19). They are the "Queen of Fruits." At the marriage feast at Cana, "the wine which Christ provided for the feast, and that which He gave to the disciples as a symbol of His own blood, was the PURE JUICE of the grape. To this the prophet Isaiah refers when he speaks of the new wine 'in the cluster', and says, 'Destroy it not; for a blessing is in it'" (DA149; Isa. 65:8). Christ did not contradict Proverbs 20:1, where it says "Wine is a mocker, strong drink is raging: and whoever is deceived thereby is not wise," for that text speaks of fermented wine. Christ Himself gave this warning to Israel (MH333), "The unfermented wine which He provided for the wedding guests was a wholesome and refreshing drink. Its effect was to bring the taste into harmony with a healthful appetite" (DA149). "The Bible nowhere sanctions the use of intoxicating wine" (Te97). Fermentation is a symbol of SIN and DEATH (DA653), but Christ Himself is the embodiment of righteousness and life (Jo. 14:6). He is the true vine from whom all of the blessings of the fruit of the vine flow (Jo. 15:1).

◆ *Grapes Destroy Disease-causing Viruses*

Grapes are used throughout the world for curative purposes. Grapes are ANTIVIRAL and ANTI-TUMOR AGENTS because of their concentrations of certain phenols and tannins. They are powerful killers of disease-causing viruses in test tubes. Grape juice has the power to fight viruses. It does so by changing the surface of a virus so it can't hook onto a cell and begin to multiply. They have been shown to be potent against the POLIO virus and against the HERPES SIMPLEX virus.

According to Dr. Cleve, Dean of the University of Wisconsin, grapes possess high levels of CAFFEIC acid, a polyphenol compound with strong powers to prevent CANCER in animals. During the grape season in France, people use grapes as their sole diet for many days. The low incidence of cancer in these areas has been attributed to the high percentage of grapes in the daily diet.

◆ *Grapes Have Great Cleansing Properties*

Grapes have great internal body cleansing properties. The therapeutic value of grapes is also due to their high MAGNESIUM content; which is very beneficial in cleansing the intestinal tract. They are a good BLOOD and BODY builder. Grape juice is easily assimilated, and is called the "Nectar of the Gods." It is indicated in cases of CONSTIPATION, GOUT, RHEUMATISM, SKIN and LIVER disorders. It aids in the elimination of URIC ACID from the system. Crushed grapes can be used as a pack on a tumor or growth with good effect.

GRAPE SKINS and SEEDS are good for bulk. When chewed well grape skins make a good laxative. There is also a laxative element found in the seeds. Grapes are good at cleansing the liver and at aiding kidney function. They are ALKALINIZING to the blood. They are very SOOTHING to the nervous system. Their high content of grape sugar gives QUICK ENERGY. Dark grapes are high in iron which makes them good blood builders. They are wonderful for KIDNEY and BLADDER. As grapes do not mix well with other foods, it is best to eat them alone. The dark Concord grapes are thought to be the best. When purchasing bottled grape juice, be sure that it is unsweetened.

Dr. L.L. Schneider, N.D., recovered from PLEURISY and a COLLAPSED LUNG by using a GRAPE JUICE DIET. It cleansed the blood of poisonous substances as well as MUCUS and PHLEGM. He claimed no cure but amazing relief.

Grapefruit

◆ *The Citrus Family*

The members of the family are citron, grapefruit, kumquat, lemon, lime, orange, and tangerine. They all have definite anti-cancer capabilities. The National Cancer Institute officials say that the year-around availability of citrus fruits is probably a major reason for the drop in STOMACH CANCER in this country. This is exactly what was found in a Dutch study. The vitamin C in them is known to counteract powerful CARCINOGENS called NITROSAMINES. In a Swedish study, citrus fruits ranked tops along with carrots as food most favored by people with the lowest rates of PANCREATIC cancer. Florida researchers found that citrus fruits have the power to lower BLOOD CHOLESTEROL. A body ACID CONDITION resulting from a high protein diet can best be neutralized and eliminated by the ALKALINE MINERAL ELEMENTS in citrus fruits for they are all alkaline reacting. All acid fruits can be eaten with vegetables. That includes pineapples too. Those who are ill with a cold will find that a citrus diet is the next best thing to a complete fast and rest in bed.

◆ *Grapefruit Reduces Cholesterol*

Grapefruit is an acid fruit, which is highly alkaline in reaction. It is a natural antiseptic for wounds, when used externally. Grapefruit is an amazing medicine for the heart. It contains compounds that lower cholesterol, and help to reverse atherosclerosis. Grapefruit pectin is fully as powerful as the drug CHOLESTYRAMINE in reducing BLOOD CHOLESTEROL. The therapeutic PECTIN resides in the cell walls, so to get the cholesterol-lowering effect, one must eat the chewy part. Grapefruit juice as such is not high in pectin and does not depress blood cholesterol. Grapefruit rind contains the valuable VITAMIN P, an important vitamin for healthy gums and teeth. To extract this vitamin, simmer the rind in water for about 20 minutes, then strain and drink the water. Grapefruit is rich in CITRIC ACIDS and their salts, such as POTASSIUM and CALCIUM salts. It is excellent as an acid in the digestion of protein. It is also an excellent aid in reducing FEVERS from COLDS and FLU.

Grapefruit helps dissolve inorganic calcium in the cartilage of joints, as in arthritis, as a result of an excessive consumption of devitalized white flour and white sugar products, which are acid-reacting products. Fresh grapefruit contains ORGANIC SALICYLIC ACID, which aids in DISSOLVING INORGANIC CALCIUM in the body. It works against any hardening of body tissue, such as hardening of the liver and the arteries. It also helps in preventing STONE FORMATIONS. In Japanese studies, when grapefruit extract was injected under the skin of mice, it stopped their tumor growth and caused a partial or complete remission of the malignancy, thereby counteracting the cellular changes that can lead to CANCER. Grapefruit is indicated in cases of OBESITY, SLUGGISH LIVER, GALLSTONES, FEVERS, PNEUMONIA, POOR DIGESTION, POOR COMPLEXION, and is valuable as a DRUG POISON ELIMINATOR.

◆ *Orange*

University of Florida scientists found that drinking a liter of orange juice did combat the RUBELLA, OR GERMAN MEASLES, by accelerating the appearance of rubella-fighting antibodies in the blood. Other scientists have found that the components of ORANGE PEELS help kill bacteria and fungi, and tend to lower blood cholesterol. It is the pulp of the orange which contains the pectin. The U.S. Dept. of Agriculture has shown that frozen orange juice concentrate has almost the same VITAMIN C content of the orange it came from. Due to their HIGH FIBER content, whole oranges have proved more filling than orange juice. In Canadian tests some orange juice bought at supermarkets did not display antiviral activity in test tubes.

Oranges are excellent for treating OVERACID BODY CONDITIONS, CONSTIPATION or a SLUGGISH INTESTINAL TRACT. In case of ACIDOSIS drink orange juice or eat oranges after meals. In case of insufficient stomach acid, start the meal with a peeled orange or a glass of orange juice. Those who suffer from TOOTH DECAY or poor gums are probably lacking in vitamin C, as may be people with GASTRIC or DUODENAL ULCERS, and their diet should be supplemented with high potency vitamin C. In cases of FEVERS or ARTHRITIS, drink orange juice freely.

◆ *Lemons, Limes, And Scurvy*

Lemons and limes gained fame for their ability to prevent SCURVY. At the time of the great ocean voyages by slow sailing ships during the 15th, 16th, and 17th centuries, the disease of scurvy ravaged the early explorers who had no fresh food on board. During Vasco da Gama's famous voyage of 1497–98, 100 of a total crew of 160 perished of scurvy. In 1577 a Spanish galleon was found adrift with all aboard dead of this malady. On one of Columbus voyages a group of Portuguese sailors, sick with scurvy, asked to be put ashore to die on land. They were left on an island where hunger drove them to eat wild plants and fruits. Later this vessel returned by the same route and their shipmates were astonished to find them all recovered and in good health. The island later came to be called Curacao, which means "cure" in Portuguese. In 1753 the Scotch physician James Lind in his book on scurvy showed how it could be overcome with CITRUS FRUITS. It took the British Navy over 40 years until 1795 before they ordered daily rations of citrus fruits for its seamen. As a result they came to be nicknamed "Limeys." During this time of neglect 200,000 seamen still died of this disease. It has been said that more sailors have died of scurvy than have been killed in all the naval battles ever fought.

Both lemons and limes contain 5 to 6% CITRIC ACID as compared with oranges and grapefruit which contain from 1 to 2%. Lemons are ideal for getting rid of toxic materials in the body, because their mineral content is highly alkaline-forming. Lemons can be used effectively in cases of INFLUENZA. They seem to have the property of increasing elimination through the skin, and therefore help reduce fever. LEMON JUICE is also a wonderful GERMICIDE, which has destroyed at least 20 different types of germs. A SORE THROAT clears up by gargling it with lemon juice. Lemons are wonderful for FEVERS, because a feverish body responds to citric acid fruits better than to any other food. LIMES are a cross between lemons and oranges and partake of the qualities of both.

URATE STONES have been dissolved through the ingestion of LEMON JUICE. Drinking the juice of one or two lemons a day has been effective in 50% of the cases.

Jacques Cartier, the French explorer, explored the St. Lawrence river and found that the needles of the WHITE CEDAR are high in vitamin C content. In the early days a ship stopped at a port in the St. Lawrence river. On board half of the crew was sick with scurvy. An Indian chief looked at them and then made a brew out of pine needles and gave it to the sick sailors. With this brew they all recovered.

Nuts

◆ Can Replace Meat

One of the foods in the diet given us by our Creator was nuts. They were given us as a food which satisfied our protein and fat requirements. Today in our encouraged return to God's original diet, they are to represent a displacement of meat in the diet of those who have been partaking of meat. We are told that "Nuts and nut food are coming largely into use to take the place of flesh meats. With nuts may be combined grains, fruits and some roots, to make foods that are healthful and nourishing. Care must be taken, however, not to use too large a proportion of nuts. Those who realize ill effects from the use of nut foods may find the difficulty removed by attending to this precaution" (CD 364).

◆ They Have Complete Proteins

Nuts are a rich concentrated food that has its place when used judiciously.

Possibly no more than 10 to 16% of the meal should be composed of nuts (CD365). Nuts also vary in their nutritional value. Some are more wholesome than others. We are told that "ALMONDS are preferable to PEANUTS; but peanuts in limited quantities, may be used in connection with grains to make nourishing and digestible food" (CD364). It has been determined by a famous research organization that from the standpoint of complete proteins, peanuts and other nuts, have COMPLETE PROTEINS, which means that they contain all of the essential amino acids which must be obtained from food, because the body itself cannot manufacture them.

◆ They Block Cancer In Test Animals

All nuts contain high amounts of PROTEASE INHIBITORS which are known to block cancer in test animals. They are therefore possible antidotes to cancer in humans. The anti-cancer agent BENZALDEHYDE, which is found in figs is also in almonds. Bitter almonds also contain a substance called AMYGDALIN or LAETRILE, and the oil contains mostly benzaldehyde. That may be the reason why some people have said that eating 8 almonds a day will prevent cancer. It may therefore be a possible antidote to cancer in humans. Nuts are also rich in POLYPHENOLS, which are other substances which are known to have thwarted cancer in animals. The oil from WALNUTS, like that from vegetables, is considered healthful because it is polyunsaturated, and therefore tends to lower blood cholesterol. Peanuts ranked highest on the "glycemic list," meaning that they are least likely of fifty foods tested to cause sharp rises in BLOOD SUGAR. They promote a steady slow rise in blood sugar and insulin, making them good food for those who may be worried about blood sugar levels and DIABETES.

◆ Peanuts And Aflatoxin

Peanut oil has caused ATHEROSCLEROSIS or clogged arteries in monkeys and other laboratory animals. It is therefore not recommended by heart-disease authorities even though it does lower blood cholesterol levels. Peanuts, as well as peanut butter, may, when not fresh, become contaminated with a mold called AFLATOXIN, which is a carcinogen, or cancer producing substance. It has been shown to produce LIVER CANCER. The high fat, carbohydrate, and protein content of all nuts make them an ideal food for strengthening the body. The CALCIUM content, especially of ALMONDS makes them valuable for the teeth and bones. They are also an all-around body builder, in cases of EMACIATION, and for NURSING MOTHERS.

◆ They Reduce Stress

Nuts act as a natural antidote to STRESS. When a handful of nuts is chewed thoroughly, the rich source of MAGNESIUM will soothe the hyperirritability of the nerves and muscles, as well as stabilize the HEARTBEAT, and make you feel more relaxed. Magnesium is the natural tranquilizer that acts as a speedy antidote to stress.

Oats

◆ An Old-fashioned Remedy

Oats have been "old-fashioned" for a long time. But suddenly someone shows us that this food has health benefits that are well suited to modern times. It has become a food that has health benefits that overcome the health hazards of so-called "junk foods" which moderns eat. Dr. Anderson of the University of Kentucky gave an OAT BRAN test to a group of people. The test indicated that those who participated in it also lost an average of 3 pounds of weight. Oat bran is also a rich source of DIETARY FIBER, especially CELLULOSE, HEMICELLULOSE, and PECTIN. It acts like a sponge in absorbing excess cholesterol and preparing it for elimination. The mechanism is due to oat bran's knack for binding BILE ACIDS in the intestines and breaking them down.

◆ *It Lowers Cholesterol*

Oats are a potent tonic for heart and blood. They suppress blood cholesterol significantly. One half cup of oats—a large bowlful when cooked—lowers the detrimental LDL CHOLESTEROL an average of 20%. Beneficial HDL cholesterol usually rises about 15% over a period of time, thereby preventing HEART ATTACKS and HYPERTENSION. Plain oatmeal is about as potent as pure oat bran. In one experiment healthy young men who added four oat bran muffins daily to their regular diet lowered their blood cholesterol an average of 20%. Oats work best with those whose blood cholesterol count is between 240 and 300. They usually see a 23% reduction in about 3 weeks. Oat bran does not seem to work with about 15% of the population, especially with those with abnormally high cholesterol in the 300 to 400 range who may have a genetic defect. Oat bran also works as a LAXATIVE even though it is not as rich in insoluble fiber as wheat bran. Both oat bran and oatmeal increase FECAL BULK.

◆ *It Solves Internal Infection Problems*

Oats have an anti-inflammatory effect on certain skin problems like contact ECZEMA, which gives credence to the long-time recommended use of OAT FACIAL PACKS as beneficial to the skin. Some physicians recommend oatmeal PACKS for treating PSORIASIS. Oats are high in PROTEASE INHIBITORS, those chemicals that dampen the activation of certain viruses and cancer-causing chemicals in the intestinal tract. It is therefore likely that oats have ANTI-INFECTIOUS and ANTI-CANCER capability, as well as against a variety of internal problems such as DIVERTICULITIS and HEMORRHOIDS. Oats and cereal grains reduce the amount of insulin required each day by DIABETICS. When oats are milled, the germ and the bran remain in the portion used for food. So oatmeal is a WHOLE-GRAIN CEREAL, like brown rice.

Olives

◆ *God's Anointing Oil*

It is said that 8 of the original olive trees in the Garden of Gethsemane are still in existence. This may be true since the olive tree can attain to an age of over 2000 years. Since time immemorial the olive tree has been regarded as a symbol of peace, an emblem of the benignity of the Divine nature, in almost every land in the world. The olive leaf was chosen by DIVINE PROVIDENCE as a sign to Noah of the abatement of the deluge (Gen. 8:11). Also olive branches were ordered as one of the materials for constructing the booths at the Feast of Tabernacles (Neh. 8:15). According to Zech. 4:14 "the two anointed ones that stand by the Lord of the whole earth" are represented by the olive trees, and two candlesticks which also represent the Old and the New Testaments. Usually olive oil was placed upon a person who was anointed at God's direction, and such oil was symbolic of an endowment of the Holy Spirit.

◆ *Better Than Any Animal Fat*

We are told that "Olives may be so prepared as to be eaten with good results at every meal. The advantages sought by the use of butter may be obtained by the eating of properly prepared olives. The OIL in the olives relieves CONSTIPATION, and for CONSUMPTIVES, and for those who have inflamed and irritated stomachs, it is BETTER THAN ANY DRUG. As food it is better than any oil coming secondhand from animals." (CH477). "When properly prepared, olives like nuts, supply the PLACE of BUTTER and FLESH MEATS. The oil, as eaten in the olive is far preferable to animal oil or fat. It serves as a LAXATIVE" (MH298). It is one of the mildest laxatives there is, and should always be used with little children where castor oil is now used. One or two tablespoons before bedtime should be sufficient for most people. The oil is also a remedy for KIDNEY diseases (CD360). Olive oil mixed with charcoal tends to cleanse and heal (2SM298).

◆ The Best Heart Disease Fat

The residents of the Island of Crete get 45% of their calories from fat and 33% of their calories from olive oil. In spite of such high fat consumption, the population of Crete has one of the world's LOWEST RATES of HEART DISEASE and CANCER. Crete consumes more olive oil per person than any other nation. Not far behind are the Italians, Greeks, and Spaniards. In general people living around the Mediterranean die of heart disease only half as much as American do. Ancel Keys of the University of Minnesota found that death rates from heart disease and from all causes, were exceptionally low in men who consumed olive oil as their major source of fat.

Olive oil contains 60% fat and is considered a good cleansing and healing agent due to its high content of POTASSIUM. It is also rich in SODIUM and CALCIUM. It is easily digested and imparts a soothing and healing influence to the digestive tract. It also retards the stickiness of blood platelets in its artery protecting tendency, due to its high content of OLEIC ACID.

Olive oil contains chemical components that work wonders on the blood, such as blocking the tendency of the blood to clot, improving good HDL cholesterol ratios, and combating dangerous arterial buildups of cholesterol. Olive oil is a MONOUNSATURATED FAT which COMBATS high CHOLESTEROL just as effectively as a low fat diet. Dr. Grundy advises Americans to substitute olive oil for other oils and fats to prevent cardiovascular disease. It has an even better effect than the polyunsaturated oils such as CORN OIL, SAFFLOWER OIL, and SUNFLOWER OIL.

A study of 5000 Italian men and women, ages 29 to 59 showed that those who used olive oil extensively had significantly lower cholesterol, and their BLOOD SUGAR levels were 6.6% lower in men. Those who used polyunsaturated fat showed no reduction in cholesterol. Those who used BUTTER, which is high in saturated fats, had higher levels on all counts—CHOLESTEROL, BLOOD PRESSURE, and BLOOD SUGAR.

◆ Slows The Aging Process

Dr. Berg of the University of Milan found that one chemical in olive oil, called CYCLOARTHANAL neutralizes CHOLESTEROL during the absorption cycle, by keeping it out of the bloodstream. He also found out that one tablespoon of olive oil wiped out the cholesterol raising effect of two eggs. University of Kentucky researchers found that olive oil LOWERS BLOOD PRESSURE. A mere of a tablespoon a day reduced blood pressure by 5 systolic points, and 4 diastolic points. In a study in France which lasted 4 months, hospital patients suffering from high blood cholesterol were given as much olive oil to drink as they wanted, but no other oil or fat was allowed. After the 4 months the cholesterol level of 7 patients dropped 26%. In ten others it dropped 14%.

◆ It Serves Many Purposes

Olive oil is used for culinary purposes, salad dressings, the manufacture of cosmetics, soaps, and cleaning solutions. It is used in SUNBURN lotions, plasters, and ointments. The antioxidants in OLIVE OIL, by destroying free radicals, seem to help the AGING PROCESS by keeping cells alive longer, and by fighting off attacks of these harmful substances so as to produce an anti-cancer effect. J. Rodale said, "One of my hunches is 'Go all out on olive oil. Italians consume a lot of olive oil, and look at the wonderful HAIR of Italian women. I have been to Italy many times and I would say that one could see with the naked eye fewer naked heads than in the U.S.'"

Olive oil has been found to stimulate the GALLBLADDER by stimulating bile secretions and thereby eliminating GALLSTONES. It should be pointed out that in an experiment reported by Dr. E.M. Brockbank, a gallstone lost 68% of its weight in two days when immersed in pure olive oil. Olive oil also takes away STOMACH ULCERS. Dr. Dewitt Fox suggests that olive oil be used for stomach ulcers instead of cream which is generally advised as a part of an ulcer diet. Some doctors say that OLIVE OIL contains vitamin U, which is believed to have healing power against stomach ulcers. It was found to be helpful in disorders of the LIVER, in DIABETES, for it reduces blood sugar levels, and with INDIGESTION problems.

It is reported that a woman soaked her feet for 10 minutes every day in a hot footbath with shavings of CASTILE SOAP which is made of pure olive oil. It reduced her blood cholesterol which fact was confirmed by a doctor. Pure olive oil has been shown to reduce CHOLESTEROL by 26%.

◆ *Grades Of Olive Oil*

Olive Oil is not generally treated to remove its taste and odor. For this reason some people feel that olive oil is far superior to other oils. Peanut oil, sunflower seed oil, soybean oil, and sesame oil are refined—which means deodorizing them so that they have practically no odor or taste. There are several grades of olive oil:

- ✓ VIRGIN—designates the top grade of olive oil. By international agreement, it may not be mixed with refined oils and still be considered virgin.
- ✓ EXTRA VIRGIN–is olive oil that has "absolutely perfect flavor." It must have no more than 1% free oleic acid.
- ✓ FINE VIRGIN—meets the same standards, except that it may have up to 1.5% free oleic acid.
- ✓ SEMI-FINE—or ordinary virgin oil, labeled simply "virgin," must have good flavor and no more than 3% free oleic acid.
- ✓ REFINED—olive oil comes from processing oil that is too high in acidity or has an "off" flavor. Refining the oil removes extra acid along with color, odor, and much of the flavor.
- ✓ PURE—olive oil is a mixture of refined and virgin oils. Manufacturers add enough virgin oil to give the mixture the desired flavor.

Potatoes

◆ *Folklore*

For a long time most people had the idea that potatoes were an unhealthful and fattening food loaded only with calories and starch. But they were far from the truth. Not only were potatoes falsely accused, but their good points went virtually unnoticed. At one time women had special pockets in their dresses where they carried raw potatoes to ward off rheumatism. Raw potato juice and hot potato water are supposed to relieve gout, rheumatism, lumbago, sprains, and bruises. Eating potatoes was once recommended by American physicians to purify the blood, cure dyspepsia, and aid digestion.

◆ *One Of The Most Alkaline Foods*

Potatoes along with other vegetables, are an alkaline reacting food, in fact they are one of the most alkaline reacting foods. That is why they have been used frequently against diseases caused by a too highly acid diet. Potatoes are about 20% CARBOHYDRATES, and 2% PROTEIN. If a person ate 3 pounds of potatoes a day, he would obtain all of the necessary 30 grams of protein. In addition they contain so many vitamins and minerals, that they are quite capable of alone sustaining life over a period of time. The story is told of a lady who was allergic to all foods except potatoes. She lived for many years on only potatoes, without exhibiting any noticeable harm from them.

◆ *A Good Source Of Potassium*

The POTASSIUM in the potatoes is strongly alkaline, which makes for good liver activation, elastic tissues, and supple muscles. Potassium is the healer of the body and is very necessary in rejuvenation. The potassium makes the potato a good food for the HEART. Recent research has linked potassium intake directly to protection from stroke. Researchers of the University of California found that an extra 400 milligram of potassium per day caused a 40% reduction in the risk of having a stroke. Half a baked potato is all you need to pick up that additional amount. It was found that boiled potatoes may lose from 10 to 50% of potassium, while baked potatoes lose only from 3 to 6%. A baked potato is a good body-building food and is easily digested.

◆ *They Exhibit Anti-Viral Activity*

WHITE POTATOES, especially when raw, have high concentrations of PROTEASE INHIBITORS which neutralize viruses and carcinogens. Of all the foods examined by investigators, the inhibitors extracted from potatoes have the strongest anti-viral powers. Especially the SKINS of potatoes are rich in CHLOROGENIC acid, a polyphenol, that prevents cell mutations leading to cancer. Investigators at Florida State University found that potato skins had ANTIOXIDANT activity, which neutralizes the damage done by so-called free radicals. When potatoes are peeled, the alkaline part is cut away, and there is practically nothing left but the starch which is acid-forming. The eyes and the skin of the potato contain its life-giving properties.

When the skin is not eaten, the best part is lost. Also when the skin is baked too brown, the life-giving properties are destroyed.

◆ *Medicinal Value*

The application of a raw crushed potato for the relief of BURNS, as well as a poultice of raw potatoes for the relief of sore eyes, boils, and inflammation of the skin is very beneficial. Eating raw potatoes has cleared up a case of ECZEMA in one individual. This is no doubt due to the fact that potatoes alkalinize the blood. Scientists have found some substance in potatoes that may help the body in the assimilation of protein. Potato soup can be used to great advantage in cases of URIC ACID, STOMACH DISORDERS, and for replacing MINERALS in the system. To control DIARRHEA cook soup with milk. The milk controls diarrhea by having a constipating effect, if boiled, and the potato adds bulk which is also necessary to control it. Potatoes FRIED in fat are not only quite indigestible, but also have a tendency to create a disturbance of the liver and gall bladder. SWEET POTATOES contain PEPTIDE substances that bind heavy metals such as cadmium, copper, mercury, and lead, thereby detoxifying them.

Rice

◆ *The Kempner "Rice Diet"*

Rice has a long history as a treatment for HIGH BLOOD PRESSURE, KIDNEY PROBLEMS, and DIABETES. Dr. Kempner of Duke University in the 1940's pioneered the "rice diet" for the treatment of high blood pressure, and kidney problems, and there is ample evidence that it works. Those on the rice diet also found that PSORIASIS cleared up dramatically, even where years of systemic and local medications had failed. Psoriasis is skin growth gone awry. Normally skin cells mature in 28 to 30 days. In psoriasis new skin cells develop 7 times faster than normal. As the dead cells are pushed farther from the skin surface, they form silvery white scales over the plaques.

He prescribed the rice diet to a 33 year old woman who had high blood pressure, failing eyesight, kidney disease and an enlarged heart. After a few days on the diet she was sent home to continue it there. She returned in 2 months and her blood pressure checked normal, her eyesight had significantly improved. After two years she reported that she was feeling "young and strong." Dr. Rosati of Duke University says: "I have seen people who were TOO SICK for the bypass surgery get well on the diet. People who were BLIND from diabetes go away able to see. Others have avoided KIDNEY DIALYSIS. THE RICE DIET is made from 2 CUPS of RICE, 1 CLOVE of CHOPPED GARLIC, CUP OF APPLE JUICE, and 1 or 2 teaspoons of LEMON JUICE.

◆ *Anti-Tumor Substances In Rice*

Japanese scientists in 1981 discovered three anti-tumor substances, isolated from rice bran, which were found to suppress tumors in mice. A missionary who had toured most of the Orient reported that he never saw a case of CANCER among people who lived mostly on rice. In animal experiments rice bran reduced the risk of bowel cancer, but not nearly as much as wheat bran did.

◆ *Rice—A Kidney Stone Fighter*

Japanese investigators found that eating rice bran reduced the calcium in the urine, and also lowered calcium-type KIDNEY STONES in seventy patients. They believe that the PHYTIC ACID in the rice blocks the absorption of unwanted calcium so that it doesn't get into the urine to form stones. They believe it to be as effective as certain pharmaceuticals, but without adverse effects.

◆ *The Nutrients In Rice*

About of the world's population considers rice their basic food. Rice, being a cereal, has an ACID reaction in the body's metabolism. Brown rice contains FAT, MINERALS, and VITAMINS. When it is POLISHED, these nutrients are greatly reduced. Polishing the rice eliminates most of the B_1 vitamin, and hence causes BERI BERI in Oriental countries. In 1884, when people reverted to brown rice, it completely cured the disease. The THIAMIN (B_1) in rice is needed by the body to digest the starch. By polishing the rice, it becomes a peril to health because the thiamin has been removed. When rice is polished into white rice, 10% of the protein, 85% of the fat, and 70% of the minerals are removed, as well as large amounts of the B-vitamins contained in the bran and germ. So most of the real food value of the rice is taken out in the polishing. It has been said that brown rice has 8 times more nutrition than white rice.

◆ *Rice Against Disease*

Rice is reported as beneficial for STOMACH ULCERS and for the relief of DIARRHEA. Because of its mineral content, it is said to supply important nutrients for the HAIR, TEETH, NAILS, MUSCLES and BONES. It also works against HEART DISEASE. Rice is gluten-free and non-allergic. Always use brown rice with all of its FIBER and B-vitamins.

Soybeans

◆ *An All-Purpose Food*

Rodale asks us to imagine a food grown easily on most soils and in most climates, which contains more first class PROTEIN than meat, will keep for years without spoiling, is easily prepared, and can be made into almost any kind of dish for any course of a meal. Imagine such a food endowed with large amounts of CALCIUM, IRON, and other important minerals, as well as the B-vitamins and vitamin E. Finally, imagine a food rich in UNSATURATED FATTY ACIDS which keep CHOLESTEROL in its place so that it will not be found in harmful deposits in the gall bladder, kidneys, and blood vessels. Such a food is the soybean. It is now believed that vitamin B_{12} may also be present in fermented soy foods such as MISO and TEMPEH, instead of being found only in animal foods. Some of one of the fatty acids in soy bean oil, namely LINOLENIC ACID, is converted in the body into the same OMEGA-3 fatty acid as those in fish oil. The three established fatty acids are ARACHIDONIC, LINOLEIC, and LINOLENIC acids. They are found in PEANUT, SAFFLOWER, and SOY oils, the three richest sources.

◆ *Rich In Protein*

Soybean flour is between 40 and 50% protein. In comparison meat is about 20% protein. Soybeans yield more protein per acre than any other crop. The crop closest to this in protein yield is peanuts. Soybeans are one of the few non-animal proteins which are complete— that is, they contain all of the essential amino acids. For this reason they can take the place of meat, eggs, fish, or milk in the diet. Soybeans are richer in POTASSIUM than any other food except brewer's yeast. They contain more PANTOTHENIC ACID than any other food except egg yolk, brewer's yeast, liver, rice bran, and wheat bran. The IRON in soybeans is 96% "available" — that is, digestible and used by the body. The OIL in soybeans is 51.5% LINOLEIC acid — the fatty acid which is believed to be the most effective of all in emulsifying cholesterol in the blood so that it does not form unhealthful deposits. The calcium of soybeans is about as well digested as that of milk.

◆ *They Lower The Risk Of Cancer*

Women eating soybeans regularly tend to have lower rates of BREAST CANCER than those who don't. When a group of Japanese men and women ate a bowl of MISO or soybean paste soup a day, they had a lower risk of STOMACH CANCER than those who never ate it. Soy beans have a high amount of anti-cancer PROTEASE INHIBITORS. They can prevent the development of CANCER due to X-RAYS.

◆ *Soybean Lecithin*

The lecithin contained in soybeans is an unsaturated fatty acid. It has the ability to clean out VEINS and ARTERIES, soothe the LIVER and GALLBLADDER, dissolve CHOLESTEROL, increase the CIRCULATION, heal KIDNEY DISORDERS, and some forms of ARTHRITIS. it has cured many DIABETICS, as well as BRAIN CLOTS, STROKES, and PARALYZED LIMBS. It was reported in the Journal of the Mt. Sinai Hospital that one woman, age 38, had a cholesterol reading of 1370. This was reduced to 445 when she took 2 teaspoonfuls of lecithin daily for 3 months. Other readings of from 300 to 600 were cut in half.

One man's eyesight was so bad, he could not read the printed page. Even large letters were blurry. His doctor said that it was OLD AGE and POOR CIRCULATION. Then he heard how LECITHIN cleans out the bloodstream. He thereupon took 3 tablespoons a day. In 2 weeks his vision had cleared up.

A man complained of DEAFNESS and RINGING in the EAR for many years. When he began to use soybean lecithin every day, the ringing stopped and his hearing cleared.

A nurse reports using ordinary LECITHIN, purchased at a health food store, to heal BEDSORES of a man patient at the hospital where she worked. Three times a day the sores were cleaned with (H_2O_2), then coated with liquid lecithin, and bandaged. The patient did not lean on the sore area. In two days everyone was surprised to find that the sores were healing nicely.

Spinach

◆ *The King Of Vegetables*

Spinach has been called the "King of Vegetables," and is beneficial in KIDNEY problems, and in all conditions of LOW VITALITY. It tops the list of foods eaten more often along with carrots, by people worldwide with lower rates of all types of CANCER. Spinach is hailed by scientists as a promising LUNG CANCER ANTIDOTE because of its extremely high concentration of CAROTENOIDS, including BETA CAROTENE. It also contains CHOLINE and INOSITOL, the substances that help prevent ARTERIOSCLEROSIS, or hardening of the arteries. Spinach juice was found by Italian scientists to block the powerful carcinogens known as NITROSAMINES. It was shown to be more potent in this regard than carrots, cauliflower, lettuce, and strawberry. It is an excellent source of vitamins A and C and IRON, and contains about 40% POTASSIUM. It is a good source of vitamin K, which aids in the formation of the blood substance required for the clotting of blood. It leaves an alkaline ash in the body. It is good for LYMPHATIC, URINARY, and DIGESTIVE problems. It has a LAXATIVE effect, and is wonderful in weight-loss diets. It has also been found valuable for ANEMIA, NERVE EXHAUSTION, ARTHRITIS, HIGH BLOOD PRESSURE, DYSPEPSIA, and BRONCHITIS.

◆ *Spinach Contains Oxalic Acid*

The body cannot metabolize OXALIC ACID. In order for the body to get rid of oxalic acid, it calls for a reserve of calcium. If there is no reserve, the body will take it from the bones and teeth. This forms CALCIUM OXALATE. Normal kidneys will extract these crystals from the bloodstream and develop them into KIDNEY STONES. If an individual is eating too much cholesterol-containing foods, in addition to acid foods, he may develop GALL STONES, which are largely composed of calcium oxalate and cholesterol.

Spinach is BEST EATEN RAW in salads, as cooking frees the oxalic acid in it, which has the effect of limiting the availability of CALCIUM. When spinach is cooked, the ORGANIC form of oxalic acid is changed to an INORGANIC form which then may form oxalic acid crystals in the kidneys. The organic form of oxalic acid is helpful in stimulating the peristaltic action of the intestines. It is not only beneficial but essential for the physiological functions of the body. The inorganic oxalic acid readily forms an interlocking compound with calcium, even combining with the calcium in other foods eaten during the same meal, destroying the nourishing value of both. This can result in such a serious deficiency of calcium, that it has been known to cause decomposition of the bones. It should be noticed that the minerals in our foods, such as iron, frequently cannot be assimilated and used completely if they have become inorganic through cooking, and they often prevent the utilization of other elements through chemical action. Thus, the iron in fresh spinach juice may be utilized 100%, but only 20% or less of it would be utilized in cooked spinach. Cooking makes the beneficial substances in RAW VEGETABLES break down into less beneficial chemicals.

The most abundant supply of organic oxalic acid is found in fresh raw SPINACH, SWISS CHARD, TURNIP and MUSTARD GREENS, KALE and COLLARDS, and the broad-leafed FRENCH SORREL, and RHUBARB. Because of its high concentration of oxalic acid, cooked rhubarb is probably responsible for more kidney trouble among children than any other single factor.

Tomatoes

Dr. Coldity of Harvard Medical School interviewed more than a thousand people about their diets, and then tracked their health for five years. What he found was that the chances of dying from CANCER was lowest among those who ate TOMATOES or STRAWBERRIES every week. Tomatoes are rich in vitamins A and C, and contains some fiber which fits right in with the cancer prevention recommendations of the national cancer prevention groups.

Tomatoes are eaten most by Hawaiians with a lower risk of stomach cancer, by Norwegians with a lower risk of lung cancer, by Americans with less prostate cancer, and by elderly Americans with lower death rates from all cancers. Tomatoes increase the alkalinity of the blood and help remove TOXINS, especially URIC ACID, from the system. Their detoxifying substances are the trace elements CHLORINE and SULFUR, which stimulate the liver to eliminate toxic wastes from the system. They are wonderful as a LIVER and BLOOD cleanser, in elimination diets, and are very high in VITAMIN value.

Fresh raw tomato juice is most beneficial and has an ALKALINE reaction if digested when no starches or sugars are present in concentrated form; but if they are present, and eaten during the same meal, then the reaction is definitely ACID. Tomatoes have a fairly high CITRIC and MALIC acid content, and some oxalic acid. When tomatoes are cooked or canned, these acids become inorganic, and, as such they are detrimental to the system, although their injurious effect is insidious, and may not manifest itself immediately. Some instances of kidney and bladder STONES are the result of taking cooked or canned tomatoes or its juice and eating it particularly with starches and sugars. Fresh, raw, tomato juice is rich in SODIUM, CALCIUM, POTASSIUM and MAGNESIUM.

SPECIAL FOODS

Carob and Chocolate

◆ *The Diet Of John The Baptist*

According to Mark 1:6 we are told, "And John was clothed with camel's hair, and with a girdle of a skin about his loins; and he did eat LOCUSTS and WILD HONEY." The word "locust" can denote either a short-horned grasshopper or the locust tree, and the edible pods of that tree. It has been a puzzle to some scholars as to which of the two types of food he ate. We are told the following in CH72, "His diet. PURELY VEGETABLE, of locusts and wild honey, was a rebuke to the indulgence of appetite, and the gluttony that everywhere prevailed." Since he was a vegetarian, this fact leads us to the conclusion that the "locusts" which he ate were the pods of the locust tree, which are also known as CAROB pods. In German the carob pods are called "St. John's Bread."

In Luke 15:16 we read with reference to the experience of the PRODIGAL SON, "And he would fain have filled his belly with the husks that the swine did eat: and no man gave unto him." The Greek word for husks is "keratia," which means "little horns." The shape and appearance of the locust pods are as little horns. Hence, scholars agree that these husks were the pods of the carob or locust tree.

◆ *The Nutritional Value Of Carob*

Carob is a well-balanced food full of vitamins and minerals. The sugar in carob is a natural sugar, such as occurs in honey, fruits, and vegetables. Natural sugars carry their own B vitamins with them for purposes of digestion, so that other parts of the body are not robbed of these vitamins. Carob has an alkaline reaction within the body. Its pH value is 10.6, which is extremely ALKALINE. Carob powder looks and tastes a lot like chocolate, and is generally used, by health-minded people, as a substitute for chocolate.

◆ *Health Benefits Of Carob*

From the health maintenance point of view, carob is good for BONES, TEETH, and GUMS. It is useful for stopping vomiting in infants by adding carob power to their milk. From the disease standpoint it is indicated in case of LOW VITALITY, LOW BLOOD PRESSURE, POOR CIRCULATION, GOITER, ULCERATION, DYSENTERY, and DIARRHEA. Carob syrup is also valuable in cases of SORE THROAT, COUGHS, STOMACH and BOWEL INFLAMMATIONS, and DIARRHEA.

◆ *The Composition Of Chocolate*

Chocolate is made from the cocoa bean which is largely grown in Central Africa in the Gold Coast. It is very high in calories, about 2500 calories in one pound of processed chocolate. Cocoa as used in a breakfast drink, contains 1 to 2% THEOBROMINE which is an alkaloid drug and a stimulant like caffeine. The fat is pressed out of cocoa and is sold as cocoa butter. Cocoa butter's main type of fat is STEARIC ACID, which tests show does not elevate CHOLESTEROL. It seems to be neutral. The cakes that are left still contain 20 to 30% cocoa fat. This is bitter chocolate. which when ground produces cocoa powder. For sweet chocolate, sugar is added. An average size chocolate bar contains 78 mg of CAFFEINE — about half as much as a cup of coffee. It also contains OXALIC ACID which has the property of combining with CALCIUM in the human digestive tract, rendering the calcium useless for human nutrition, and also robbing the body of stored calcium, and allowing it to be excreted in the urine rather than being absorbed by the body.

◆ *Health Hazards Of Chocolate And Cocoa*

The caffeine in cocoa stimulates the HEART, raises the BLOOD PRESSURE, lowers the BLOOD SUGAR, and creates a FALSE SENSE of SECURITY in that it appears to relax tired nerves.

It can cause damage to genetic material, and can therefore genetically lead to the development of CANCER by altering the DNA. The THEOBROMINE in chocolate produces these same undesirable effects. In ACNE cases, it is usually one of the first foods forbidden by the doctor. Chocolate has been established as one of the positive causes of ACNE because of its high fat content. It is also said to be the cause of the itching of PURITUS AND CHOCOLATE MILK also is not recommended, because it robs the milk of some of its calcium.

Many people do not realize that most of the popular drinks such as TEA, COFFEE, CHOCOLATE, and COCOA, as well as the popular soft drinks contain CAFFEINE. Adventists seem to like to drink cocoa at Ingathering time to warm people up who come in from the cold. Cocoa is one of the sources of ALLERGIES in children. They eat it as chocolate candy, or as chocolate syrup in milk. Cocoa in any form is habit forming in the same way that tea and coffee are habit forming. Children love it in spite of the fact that it causes ASTHMA ATTACKS, VOMITING, ITCHING MOUTH, ABDOMINAL PAIN, COUGH, CLOGGED NOSE, ITCHING HIVES, SORES AROUND THE MOUTH, and NAUSEA. One doctor found that of 100 children chosen at random, 76 were found to be allergic to chocolate. Chocolate contains THEOBROMINE, a drug which is used as a heart stimulant. It is a frequent cause of gastrointestinal distress.

◆ *Giving Up Chocolate*

Chocolate is not especially good for you. Besides being fattening, it also contains a chemical—TYRAMINE—which can trigger headaches. And since it is nearly all fat, and contains caffeine, it should be avoided at all costs, especially if a person is suffering from HEARTBURN.

It must be explained, especially to the young, that the use of chocolate may produce poor teeth, soft bones, bad hearts, nervousness, and bad complexion. In place of chocolate substitute DATES, FIGS, CAROB CANDY, ALMONDS, SUNFLOWER SEEDS, and RAISINS. Use CAROB POWDER in place of where cocoa was formerly used. If there is a calcium deficiency, supplement the diet with BONE MEAL, the richest and best natural source of calcium.

Honey

◆ *Honey And Inspiration*

The goodness of honey was recognized by King Solomon when he said, "My Son, eat thou honey; because it is good; and the honeycomb, which is sweet to thy taste" (Prov. 24:13). At the same time he mentioned that the eating of honey can be overdone when he said, "It is not good to eat much honey" (Prov. 25:27). Too much of a good thing is not good. One can overeat on good food. The excess then becomes poison to the body. The promised land of Canaan was called a LAND FLOWING with MILK and HONEY (Ex. 3:17). So milk along with honey was considered to be a good food. John the Baptist even ate honey along with his carob pods (Matt. 3:4). The MANNA which God gave to the children of Israel in the wilderness tasted like wafers made with honey (Ex. 16:31). God promised the Israelites that if they would keep His commandments, He would give them the finest of the wheat, and bring them honey out of the rock (COL289).

◆ *The Nutritional Qualities Of Honey*

Besides the Bible, the most interesting medical notes on ancient medicine come from the records of the Egyptians who were really honey addicts. One finds that no fewer than 500 out of 900 known Egyptian medical formulas are based on honey.

The Greeks called honey the "nectar of the gods." The NECTAR which the bees gather from the flowers is composed of SUCROSE, a double sugar, the same as table sugar or a DISACCHARIDE. The double sugar is changed to single sugars or MONOSACCHARIDES, in the bees' honey sack, consisting for the most part of dextrose and levulose, 34 to 42%. DEXTROSE is GLUCOSE, also called GRAPE sugar, and LEVULOSE is FRUCTOSE. They are as different from each other as the right hand is from the left hand, which isn't very different in structural arrangement. Honey has a high content of fructose, which does not need INSULIN for its assimilation, because it is absorbed slowly. That is why DIABETICS can eat it without any problems. Honey consists of 9 ACIDS, PROTEINS, MINERALS, VITAMINS, ENZYMES, and POLLEN, which is largely protein. 15 different sugars have been identified in honey, the result of enzymatic and acid action. Honey increases the

HEMOGLOBIN COUNT, and the FATTY ACID content of honey stimulates PERISTALSIS.
- ✓ GLUCOSE—or DEXTROSE, is found in RIPE FRUITS, FLOWERS, LEAVES, ROOTS, and SAP, and it is prepared by the HYDROLYSIS OF STARCH.

  FRUCTOSE—or LEVULOSE, is found in RIPE FRUIT, HONEY, MOLASSES and SYRUPS. In most fruits glucose exceeds fructose; in apples and pears fructose is higher; in oranges, grapes, and strawberries, they are in about equal amounts. Fructose is 50 times sweeter than sucrose. Fructose is a MONOSACCHARIDE, or simple sugar.
- ✓ GLYCOGEN—consists of repeating glucose units. It is hydrolyzed to GLUCOSE, MALTOSE, and DEXTRINS.
- ✓ SUCROSE—TABLE SUGAR, a double sugar or DISACCHARIDE, is what NECTAR is largely composed of. Through enzymatic action it changes to a mixture of glucose and fructose, which mixture is called INVERT SUGAR. This represents a partial digestion of the nectar. Sucrose is DEXTROROTARY, meaning that it rotates the plane of polarized light to the right. Invert sugar, on the other hand, is LEVOROTARY, for it rotates the plane of polarized light to the left. Invert sugar is the principal component of honey.

◆ *Honey Produces Quick Energy*

Honey is a rapidly acting source of MUSCULAR ENERGY, and has great value as a RESTORATIVE. There is no better food to meet MUSCULAR FATIGUE and EXHAUSTION. Honey itself contains some VENOM, because the bees use their stings also for the preservation of honey.

Honey should be natural, raw, unheated, unfiltered and unprocessed. Carbohydrates such as sugars need the B-vitamins in order to be assimilated properly. Honey contains sufficient of the B-vitamins to digest them properly. CLARIFYING honey reduces the vitamin content from 35 to 50%. Honey contains all of the VITAMINS which nutritionists consider necessary to health. The DARK HONEYS, such as BUCKWHEAT and HEATHER, are richer in minerals than the lighter ones, and are also more alkaline. Dark honey added to a milk diet will increase the HEMOGLOBIN or RED BLOOD CELL count. Amino acids are present in honey as minor components. Honey is rapidly assimilated, and is an excellent source of QUICK ENERGY. It produces energy faster than either starch or sugar, without taxing the digestive system. For nutritional value on a scale from 1 to 10, honey is 9, glucose 7, corn syrup 7, brown sugar 6, white sugar 4. COMB HONEY WAX is essential for the development and maintenance of the breathing tract. Individuals who ate honey comb honey in their diet until they were 16, seldom had a cold, hay fever, or other nose disorders. The chewing of honey comb produces an immunity to breathing tract troubles that lasts for four years.

It has been determined by research that DARK honey added to a milk diet will increase the hemoglobin count in rats, whereas LIGHT honey lowers the count. When the honey was replaced by SUGAR, the rats became anemic. Honey was also found to contain an ANTI-HEMORRHAGING FACTOR, which suggests the presence of vitamin K. In a test of CALCIUM RETENTION for infants, it was found that such retention was always higher if honey had been included in the formula rather than corn syrup. Honey is SLIGHTLY ACID to the taste, but it is an ALKALINE food.

◆ *Honey Is Rich In Enzymes And Minerals*

Honey and minerals are essential for normal digestion and assimilation. Honey contains the following enzymes: DIASTASE, which is in the digestive juice that converts starch into sugar. INVERTASE, which changes sucrose into a mixture of the simple sugars of dextrose and levulose, called INVERT SUGAR; CATALASE, speeds up the decomposition of hydrogen peroxide to water and oxygen; PEROXIDASE, which hastens the transfer of oxygen from peroxide to a tissue that requires oxygen; and LIPASE, which changes the fats of cream and egg yolk in the stomach to fatty acids and glycerol. Not only do we find the usual food minerals in ionized form such as CALCIUM, POTASSIUM, MAGNESIUM, IRON, PHOSPHORUS, SULFUR, and IODINE, but also the highly important TRACE MINERALS such as BORON, CHROMIUM, COPPER, LITHIUM, NICKEL, TITANIUM and many more. These trace minerals are needed in only very small amounts, but honey contains them in the right quantity. All are derived from the soil in which the plants grow from which the honey is taken. Heat or pasteurization is equally destructive of both enzymes as well as minerals in their ionized state.

◆ *The Hygroscopicity Of Honey*

The word "hygroscopicity" means "an attraction for moisture" This quality gives honey a great natural healing power, for disease germs cannot thrive nor live in it. The reason for this is that honey is an excellent source of potassium, and the potassium withdraws from the bacteria moisture which is essential to their existence. They will shrivel up and die in it. Through experiments it was found that typhoid fever germs died within 48 hours in honey, pneumonia germs in 4 days, dysentery germs within 10 hours. This potentially keeps a lot of diseases from getting a foothold. For this reason it has also been found that CAKES made with honey rather than with sugar KEEP LONGER.

◆ *The Anti-Bacterial Qualities Of Honey*

In ancient times it was well known that honey possesses anti-spoiling properties. Even meat used to be preserved in honey, because it had ANTI-BACTERIA and ANTI-MOLD properties. That is why long before PENICILLIN, doctors used honey to heal seriously infected wounds. Such ANTI-SPOILING factor, however, is immediately destroyed by heat or pasteurization. In modern Russian clinics, honey is used for hard to heal sores of nose, mouth, and throat ailments, EYE diseases, HEART, LIVER and KIDNEY diseases, STOMACH and INTESTINAL ULCERS, as well as certain NERVOUS diseases. Father Kneipp claimed that small ulcers in the stomach are quickly contracted, broken, and healed by honey. Honey is often mixed with lemon juice as a soothing COUGH SYRUP. Folk medicine is entirely correct in declaring honey to be a potent DESTROYER of BACTERIA, an ANTISEPTIC, and a DISINFECTANT. The ACIDS in honey also renders it an unfavorable medium for bacterial growth. The acids are: ACETIC, CITRIC, FORMIC, SUCCINIC, and AMINO acids.

◆ *Honey Hastens Healing*

Honey possesses miraculous NUTRITIONAL and MEDICINAL PROPERTIES, and has been used for healing purposes since early history. Honey increases CALCIUM RETENTION in the system, prevents NUTRITIONAL ANEMIA, is beneficial in KIDNEY and LIVER DISORDERS, COLDS, POOR CIRCULATION, and COMPLEXION PROBLEMS. It has been found that most CENTENARIANS in Bulgaria and Russia have used honey liberally in their diet. Honey is said to HASTEN HEALING and at the same time keeps the wounds sterile. On such wounds it is found to work BETTER THAN ANTIBIOTICS.

Honey is used in modern Russian clinics to treat patients with hard to heal SORES, NOSE, MOUTH, and THROAT AILMENTS, EYE DISEASES, LIVER AND KIDNEY DISEASE, STOMACH and INTESTINAL ULCERS, and certain NERVOUS INVOLVEMENTS. The usual daily dose is 3 ounces. Honey destroys all kinds of bacteria, such as SALMONELLA, SHIGELLA, E. COLI, and V. CHOLERAE which cause DIARRHEA. When eaten, honey retains its bactericidal power in the intestinal tract. The antibiotic properties of honey are active in dilutions as low as 13%.

The bees secrete an enzyme in which one of the active principles is INHIBINE. This substance breaks down chemically to produce HYDROGEN PEROXIDE or H_2O_2, which is a common household disinfectant, which is almost identical to a mild antibiotic. Inhibine is destroyed by light and heat. For this reason it is worthwhile to obtain honey extracted only by centrifugal force without any processing or heating. When the sugar in honey was removed, the remaining distillate of honey still killed a broad range of bacteria as effectively as STREPTOMYCIN, and the germs also did not develop a resistance to honey as they did to streptomycin. Ingesting the POLLEN found in honey desensitizes children to ASTHMA and HAY FEVER. The pollen in honey has a higher vitamin C content than almost any fruit or vegetable. Better than any other food, honey fulfills Hippocrates' requirement for an ideal food: "OUR FOOD SHOULD BE OUR MEDICINE, AND OUR MEDICINE SHOULD BE OUR FOOD."

◆ *Honey For Long Life*

The sweetening substances in honey are about a dozen or so simple sugars, of which the most plentiful are glucose and fructose. These sugars do not require to be digested but are immediately absorbed by the bloodstream as "energy fuel." The father of medicine, HIPPOCRATES, lived to a ripe old age and ate honey all his life. The famous medical scientist AVICENNA said: "If you want to remain young, eat honey." A lecturer on beekeeping once said, "Bee keepers live longer than anybody else." There are more than 25,000 men and women in Russia that have passed their 100-year birthday. They have singled out honey for their food and medicine more than any other substance for long life.

A lady reported that as a young girl she was given up by her physicians as a hopeless CONSUMPTIVE with TB. A friend of hers then prescribed a diet of HONEY and GOAT'S MILK with the result that she became free of her illness for the rest of her life, and she was still well in her 90th year. The benefits derived from the daily use of honey cannot be explained by the known elements of honey. They always exceed what the chemical facts would suggest. Here, the whole is greater than the sum of its parts.

◆ *Honey And Disease*

Up to the end of the 19th century, honey enjoyed a great reputation as a THERAPEUTIC SUBSTANCE. Then the modern sulfur drugs and antibiotics came in, and the natural healing agents lost their respect. These drugs have given patients serious kidney disorders, and have given many people violent reactions and even death. No one has ever mentioned having suffered serious consequences as a result of having used honey internally and externally. In some parts of the world, honey in the form of eye drops is used for treating TRACHOMA. Two teaspoons of honey at each meal will make twitching eyelids disappear. Dr. Bodag Beck said that he had cured a STONE-BLIND horse with HONEY AND SALT.

A young man suffering from POISON OAK had a doctor tell him to let a nanny goat eat the poison oak which they love, and then have him drink the milk. In doing so the young man immunized himself against the poison oak. A HONEY-COD LIVER OIL salve for healing has been used in Germany with excellent results. It has healed WOUNDS, ULCERATIONS, BURNS, FISTULES, BOILS, CARBUNCLES, and FELON in the shortest possible time. Honey as a SURGICAL DRESSING was used by the Egyptians and others. It is NON-IRRITATING, NON-TOXIC, SELF-STERILE, BACTERICIDAL, NUTRITIVE, CHEAP, and EFFECTIVE. Honey has been hailed as a cure for HAY-FEVER and ALLERGIES. Honey, besides its value as a food, also has MEDICINAL values. Dr. Jarvis, in his book *Folk Medicine*, points out that honey is a wonderful medicine for producing SLEEP; that a teaspoon of honey before going to bed prevents BED-WETTING; that it is one of the best COUGH remedies; that it is a cure for BURNS, and an ALLEVIAND for HAY FEVER sufferers. Mrs. White says that honey and EUCALYPTUS OIL are good for throat troubles (2SM301). Honey is also a fine HEART STIMULANT. It has a long-lasting effect because of its slow-absorbing sugar LEVULOSE.

Some medical researchers in New Zealand claim that they have found the cause of ULCERS. They feel that the bacterium HELICOBACTER PYLORI is to blame. Instead of using antibiotics they have found an alternative to them called HONEY. With the use of biopsies of gastric ulcers, They discovered that this bacterium could be easily destroyed with a 20% solution of MANUKA HONEY. Practically all bee products such as HONEY, POLLEN, PROPOLIS, and ROYAL JELLY, have at one time or another been reported to be effective at preventing and curing ulcers. Honey's strong antibacterial properties have been made use of for ages as a folk medicine.

◆ *Honey For Diabetics*

Mr. L.M.D. Edmeston of New York writes that he not only cured many cases of RHEUMATISM with BEE STINGS, but he also has a list of people who were cured of DIABETES. In one home both the man and his wife suffered from diabetes. They went to various doctors for a long time without improving. Finally they went on a diet consisting of large amounts of honey and plenty of fruit, and today both are recovered. In the medical profession Dr. F.C. Ameiss advocated TUPELO honey for diabetics, as having a minimum percentage of dextrose and a MAXIMUM of LEVULOSE.

Dr. Beszedits of Mexico says that giving honey to diabetics may seem anti-scientific and anti-medical or rather silly to a superficial observer. But we must remember that bees gather honey from medicinal plants also, RED CLOVER, for example, being a medicinal plant. It has always been believed that the curative properties of certain plants are transmitted by the bees from the blooms into the honey they produce. The natives of India drop LOTUS honey into the eyes to cure CATARACTS, and the belief in the ANTI-TUBERCULOTIC effect of EUCALYPTUS HONEY is world-wide.

Dr. Davidov of Russia has found honey to be a good substitute for sugar in DIABETES. He believes that honey prevents ACETONEMIA and that it diminishes the amount of sugar in the urine in spite of the fact that honey contains 75% sugar. One of his patients used one pound of honey in ten days without an increase of the sugar rate in the urine. When the use of honey was stopped for a while, the sugar percentage in the urine rose, but after again taking 4 teaspoonfuls of honey daily, the rate dropped again. One man cured himself of DIABETES with a special diet that he asked for, but which the doctors refused to give him. It consisted of mostly raw SPINACH, LETTUCE sweetened with honey and lime juice, RAW CARROTS sweetened with honey to taste, RAW CABBAGE salad with lime juice and honey, RIPE TOMATOES, raw or canned, sweetened with honey, and WHOLE WHEAT BREAD. After over a year on this diet, the doctors could find not a trace of sugar.

Sugar

◆ *The Composition Of Sugar*

There are some Adventists who say that honey is the same as sugar. Such a statement is quite far from the truth.

Sugar is a pure carbohydrate,(99.5%), called SUCROSE, consisting of carbon, hydrogen, and oxygen in a chemical union. It is produced from sugar cane and sugar beets. It is a pure chemical, because during the refining process all vitamins and minerals are taken out. That is why some hygienists don't call it a food but a DRUG to which Americans have become addicted. It OVERSTIMULATES the ISLANDS OF LANGERHANS in the pancreas, causing a condition called HYPER-INSULINISM, which means that they are secreting too much insulin, and are burning up too much of our blood sugar, thereby causing HYPOGLYCEMIA. This means that the brain, which lives solely on blood sugar or glucose, is not getting enough. The average American takes in directly or indirectly as hidden sugar about 120 pounds a year. This is almost the highest intake in the world except for the country of Colombia, where they imbibe a national drink which is made mostly of sugar. As a chemical all it can give us is CALORIES for energy of 5 calories per gram, and not nourishment. The nectar which the bees gather represents largely sucrose, the double sugar. This double sugar is changed in digestion to single or simple sugars. In the case of honey, the bees in their nectar sacs, will change the nectar to the simple sugars of glucose and fructose, which means that before we get the honey, it has already been partially digested. This process is called INVERSION.

◆ *Sugar's effect Upon The System*

Since sugar must be changed from a double sugar to simple sugars, when used in excess it places a heavy burden upon the pancreas. In many people therefore, sugar ADDICTION leads to the exhaustion of the PANCREAS, and hence to DIABETES. Sugar addiction represents a craving for the stimulation of artificial sweets. Any type of artificial sugar product should not be taken upon an empty stomach, because such sugar is a powerful stimulant which oxidizes in the stomach upon the slightest contact with oxygen, producing an explosive shock effect upon the digestive system without providing the body with nutriments. It gives a short-lived LIFT to the system, followed by a slump which then craves for another lift. The desire for "just one more piece" finally becomes a compulsion, and the individual is on his way to becoming a sugar addict. That is why some people can eat one piece of candy after another until the whole box is consumed. Poorly nourished children and adults are very susceptible to sugar addiction, and people who suffer from nerve fatigue are the most susceptible of all. Since sugar doesn't provide nourishment, a dependence upon it leads to MALNUTRITION.

◆ *White Sugar—A Drug*

White sugar is often called a DRUG because in the refining process everything of food value has been removed except the carbohydrates, which are pure calories without VITAMINS, MINERALS, PROTEINS, FATS, ENZYMES or any other elements that make up food. Pure carbohydrates do not exist in nature. So white sugar is extremely harmful, as harmful as a drug, especially in the quantities in which present-day Americans consume it, which is around 120 pounds per year. Natural foods come equipped with all of the things necessary for their metabolism. Did you ever hear of a cattle grower feeding this cattle on white sugar? He knows what the consequences will be. Yet he will feed his children and himself on a food so deadly, he knows that his stock could not survive on it.

◆ *Natural Sugars Come With Vitamins*

Naturals sugars such as in fruits and vegetables, have with them a full assortment of B-vitamins that are necessary for the assimilation of the sugars. None of these B-vitamins is present in WHITE SUGAR. But if the sugar is to be used by the body, they must be present. So they are drafted from NERVES, MUSCLES, LIVER, KIDNEYS, STOMACH, HEART, SKIN, EYES, and BLOOD. This leaves these organs of the body deficient in B-vitamins. The vitamin B deficiency produced by eating refined sweets can contribute to many other disorders such as BERIBERI and PELLAGRA, which are two extreme examples, but also to HEART TROUBLE, CONSTIPATION, COLITIS, many SKIN DISEASES, and MOUTH DISORDERS like VINCENT'S DISEASE.

◆ *Honey's Advantages Over Sugar*

☞ Honey is a natural unrefined food, containing vitamins, minerals, enzymes, and acids.

☞ It is a food and not a non-food.

☞ It is non-irritating to the delicate membranes of the digestive tract.

☞ It is assimilated rapidly and easily.

☞ It spares the kidneys, thereby lessening tissue destruction.

☞ It provides a maximum of energy units with a minimum of shock.

☞ It enables the athlete to recuperate rapidly from severe exertion, and show less evidence of fatigue.

☞ It has a natural, gentle laxative effect.

☞ It is highly alkaline rather than acid-forming.

☞ It has its own vitamins and minerals, while sugar robs the body of B-vitamins necessary to digest sugar, as well as calcium.

☞ It increases the hemoglobin count.

☞ Useful in arthritic conditions—sugar causes arthritis.

☞ Useful for kidney and liver disorders.

☞ Asthma and hay fever are improved by eating honey containing pollen to which patients are allergic.

◆ *Sugar And Inspiration*

We are told that "Far too much sugar is ordinarily used in food. Cakes, sweet puddings, pastries, jellies, jams, are active causes of INDIGESTION. Especially harmful are the custards and puddings in which milk, eggs, and sugar are the chief ingredients. The free use of milk and sugar taken together should be avoided" (CD113) "They impart IMPURITIES to the system" (2T369). The reason given for this is that such a combination causes FERMENTATION in the stomach, and they are therefore harmful, and the less of them are put on the table, the better it will be for all. The fermentation clouds the BRAIN and brings peevishness into the disposition (CD327). And when largely used, sugar is more injurious than MEAT (CD328). We are also told that sweet foods produce IMPATIENCE and IRRITABILITY in those who accustom themselves to their use. (CD321).

Another thing that sugar itself, as well as in combination with milk, does is to CLOG THE SYSTEM, thereby causing constipation and all kinds of diseases (CD197). "It hinders the working of the living machine" (CD331). One basic reason we might mention as the cause is that sugar doesn't have any fiber to allow it to be pushed through the system readily. The story is told of a man who left off meat, and was in its place substituting large quantities of sugar, because he didn't know what else to substitute. Science also tells us that milk and sugar together produces OXALIC ACID, which then converts the soluble lime salts into an insoluble oxalate of lime, and thereby produces a condition known as DECALCIFICATION or LIME STARVATION. In this manner it robs the body of calcium from bones, causes teeth to DECAY, causes RICKETS among the young, as well as ADENOID NASAL GROWTHS, and INFLAMED TONSILS. Natural sugars are surrounded by many vitamins and minerals, and therefore do not react like pure sugar. For example, FIGS contain 60% sugar, but they are among the most alkaline of all foods.

◆ *The Assimilation Of Sugar*

In order to assimilate the sugar in the body, certain B-vitamins must be present. If they are not taken in with the sugar, your body must steal them from other parts of the body. To this extent sugar will create a VITAMIN B DEFICIENCY, unless extra B-vitamins are supplied through foods rich in these vitamins. Even though the FRUCTOSE in fruit is metabolized to GLUCOSE just like all other sugars, the sugar in fruit does come in a "package" with vitamins, minerals, and food fiber. It is said that pure sugar gives us "naked" or EMPTY CALORIES, and therefore leaves less room for "well-clothed" calories. Sucrose must first be broken down into monosaccharides by enzymes, to glucose by INVERTASE, to maltose by MALTASE, to lactose by LACTASE. Then they can be absorbed through the intestinal wall. This absorption happens very fast, and if too much sugar has been eaten it may upset the glucose balance of the blood

POLYSACCHARIDES or multiple sugars, have to pass many digestive processes to be turned into glucose. For this reason they will be absorbed more slowly than the mono- or disaccharides. Hence, the glucose produced from polysaccharides, such as in GRAINS, will not upset the glucose balance of the blood.

The LIVER can accommodate only a small amount of refined sugar, up to an ounce a day and turn it into glycogen. Any additional amount is immediately absorbed by osmosis into the blood, and is converted to CARBONIC ACID (H_2CO_3). In order for the body to neutralize the corrosive action of this acid, calcium is withdrawn from the bones, and in the form of calcium hydroxide, it combines with this acid to give us CALCIUM CARBONATE and water. The calcium carbonate thus formed then settles in muscles, tissues, and blood vessels to cause HARDENING OF THE ARTERIES, (ARTERIOSCLEROSIS), DIABETES, and ARTHRITIS. If as a result blood vessels burst in the brain we have a STROKE. If damage occurs in the heart we have a CORONARY OCCLUSION.

◆ *Sugar Causes Caries And Other Diseases*

Starch is a carbohydrate with a formula very close to that of sugar. In the mouth starch is changed to sugar almost as soon as you eat it with the help of the enzyme PTYALIN, so that eating refined and bleached white flour is almost the same as eating white sugar. Excessive sugar consumption causes the teeth to decay, because they are weakened by the withdrawal of calcium from them. But even more teeth are lost from periodontal or gum disease. Dr. Weston A. Price studied the teeth of many people in many places, and came to the conclusion that eating a diet of natural fresh foods provides nearly complete protection against tooth decay, while eating a diet of sweet, refined, processed, and canned foods creates nearly complete vulnerability to tooth decay. He found that the diets of cavity-free people were rich in vitamins A and D, and in the minerals calcium and phosphorous.

There also appears to be a relationship between high sugar consumption and MIGRAINE HEADACHES, POLIO, RHEUMATIC FEVER, ARTHRITIS, DIABETES, CANCER, GALL BLADDER DISEASE, AND OTHER DEGENERATIVE DISEASES. It is estimated that 80% of tooth decay could be prevented by not eating refined sugar. It was found that persons who take in lots of VITAMIN B_1, and leave off all sugars, are not bothered much by stinging insects such as MOSQUITOES and BLACK FLIES. Insects simply do not bite people who eat no sugar. Indians in Canada leave all sugars from their diet before the black fly season to keep from being bitten. It is said that individuals with diabetes do not get bitten either.

Sugar is suspected of contributing to the cause of CANCER. TUMORS are known to have a great appetite for sugar. A study showed that a carbohydrate meal with sugary food has a bad effect on LEARNING ability and BEHAVIOR. Extra sugar will quickly create a nutritional deficiency, unless protein foods are also taken. CRIME can be traced to the malnourished and demineralized condition of individuals who live largely on sugary foods, such as doughnuts and candy bars. We must remember that the same amount of sugar is a higher percentage for a lower weight child than for an adult. If at a dinner we say that each individual can have one piece of pie, that one piece represents a higher percentage of sugar for the child than for an adult, unless the child gets a proportionately smaller piece. The average adult takes in about 150 gm of sugar per day.

◆ *Sugar Needs Vitamin B_1 for Assimilation*

All NATURAL FOODS contain nutritive elements — VITAMINS, ENZYMES, MINERALS, TRACE ELEMENTS, FATTY ACIDS, ETC. — which are necessary for effective digestion and assimilation of the nutrients. Vitamins E, A, and D cannot be assimilated unless they are accompanied by fatty acids. Conversely, OIL cannot be properly utilized without a certain amount of vitamin E. CARBOHYDRATES are not digested properly without vitamin B. When WHITE SUGAR is consumed the body will use its own storage of vitamin B, particularly B_1, in order to digest it, because sugar is totally void of all vitamins necessary to digest it. This leads to a VITAMIN B_1 DEFICIENCY. It also depletes several trace minerals necessary for healthy JOINT CARTILAGE and SYNOVIAL FLUID.

◆ *The Relation Between Sugar And Thirst*

Nutritionist A. Colbin in her book *Food and Healing* uses mother's milk as a standard to determine the relationship between the amount of carbohydrates in the diet and the amount of water necessary to balance it. In mother's milk the ratio between protein, carbohydrates and water is 1:9.5:90, or roughly 1x9x90. This means that for 1gm of protein there are 9.5gm of carbohydrates, and 90 gm of water. This may be the reason that those people who eat meat eat a lot of sweets also. This also means that for 1gm of carbohydrate you need 9gm of water. For every gram of sugar, a carbohydrate, you need 9gm of water. For this reason sweets MAKE YOU THIRSTY. Here you find the cause for the popularity of SOFT DRINKS. When they are ice-cold, they numb the taste buds, while the liquid fools us into thinking that thirst is being quenched. However, the 7 teaspoons of sugar in each bottle create a need for more water, and thereby keep us reaching for more of these drinks. This would not quite be so true if the drinks were at room temperature.

As a food honey is vastly superior to white sugar which is devoid of any nutritional value. Honey is a perfect food. It contains large amounts of vitamins and minerals, rich particularly in vitamins B and C. It contains practically all of the B-complex vitamins which are necessary for digesting sugar. These natural sugars are easily digested, converted by the enzymatic action of the bee's salivary glands.

It is best not to sweeten BERRIES with sugar, because they will then cause fermentation in the system, resulting in an ACID REACTION. When sweetening is required, only HONEY should be used, for honey does not have the strong acid reaction of sugar. Honey contains certain ORGANIC ACIDS which react in the body to produce ALKALINITY.

◆ *Sugar Creates An Acid Condition In The Body*

Pure sugar creates an acid condition in the body, and acidity DEMINERALIZES the system. This is due to the fact that when sugar is metabolized, it creates various acids within the body. The acids formed when sugar decomposes in the presence of protein create a form of ACID INTOXICATION or SELF-POISONING, which manifests itself in various types of CATARRH or RHEUMATISM. The body works to neutralize these acids, and it does so by withdrawing calcium from the bones in the form of CALCIUM OXIDE which combines with water to form calcium hydroxide. It also throws the CALCIUM-PHOSPHORUS BALANCE (2 Ca: 1P) out of kilter in the blood by causing the phosphorus level to drop. When not enough phosphorus is present, calcium cannot be absorbed by the body. The result is nervousness, skin troubles, digestive troubles, and a host of other troubles. It also uses up B-vitamins, iron, and other nutrients directly from our own reserves. Then our teeth are weakened as calcium is withdrawn from them and thereby become more susceptible to bacterial attack. This "Syphoning Effect" of sugar is also what lies behind the gnawing hunger it can produce in some people, since the hunger then is for missing elements such as fiber, vitamins, minerals, protein and water. Quitting sugar suddenly can bring on WITHDRAWAL SYMPTOMS in the form of STRONG CRAVINGS. Such cravings can bring on CRIMINAL BEHAVIOR which has been described by several researchers.

◆ *Sugar Makes Bones Softer And Longer*

It has been estimated that a Japanese child, that is brought to the U.S. in infancy, would grow 2 to 3 inches taller than it would have grown in Japan. The bones have become longer but also softer. Such extra growth can be attributed to the extra growth stimulation of the greater amount of REFINED SUGAR such a child would be absorbing. Someone has also suggested that the extra growth hormones it would obtain from the extra MILK it would drink would add to this effect. The amount of refined sugar which could be tolerated by the human organism is less than 20 gm/day; for a child it is 6 gm/day; for an infant 1 gm/day. The average American gets about 150 gm/day or 7 times more than he can properly assimilate. Any amount above 20 gm/day is absorbed by osmosis into the circulation to be converted to free CARBONIC ACID. To neutralize this acid, calcium is taken from the bones and in the form of CALCIUM CARBONATE is precipitated into the soft meshes of muscles, tissues, and vessels. Blood and lymph vessels become coated with calcium carbonate. ARTERIOSCLEROSIS, hardening, and brittleness of vessels is underway. Arteries may easily burst. If damage occurs in the brain we have a STROKE; if in the heart we have a CORONARY OCCLUSION.

◆ *Low Blood Sugar Caused By High Sugar Intake*

✓ POLIO—AN EFFECT OF LOW BLOOD SUGAR

Some years ago Dr. Sandler of North Carolina brought to a standstill a POLIO EPIDEMIC that had frightened the residents so badly, that they were willing to try out the diet he recommended. In his diet Dr. Sandler forbad all forms of REFINED SUGARS, such as DESSERTS, SOFT DRINKS, CANDIES, and so forth. His theory was that LOW BLOOD SUGAR (Hypoglycemia) makes people susceptible to POLIO. Low blood sugar is brought about by eating lots of sugar, paradoxical as this may sound. Eating sugar brings up the blood sugar level for a short time, but then it plunges down far below the normal level. This makes one feel uncomfortable and one craves something sweet again. So you have a soda, a piece of candy, or a doughnut, and the blood sugar shoots up again and makes you feel better. A vicious cycle has now been created. Polio is related to low blood sugar, which is far more prevalent in this country than high blood sugar, which is DIABETES. With a diet similar to Dr. Sandler's, Dr. Abrahamson in his book *Mind, Body, and Sugar*, relates spectacular cures for ASTHMA, ALCOHOLISM, NEUROSES, RHEUMATIC FEVER, ULCERS, EPILEPSY, and DEPRESSION. Dr. Fred Klenner cured polio patients by giving them 28 to 42 gm of VITAMIN C for a 150 lbs. person, and he repeated this process every 8 to 12 hours.

✓ HEADACHES—CAUSED BY LOW BLOOD SUGAR.

The brain cannot function without GLUCOSE. When there is insufficient sugar in the blood, the resulting condition is similar to that of OXYGEN STARVATION. To meet the demands of the brain, more blood is needed; hence, the blood goes pounding through your head at a faster clip, and the result is a throbbing headache. Also, if you are EXCITED, NERVOUS, or UNDER PRESSURE, your ADRENAL glands go into high gear and consume sugar at a faster rate, thus further depriving your blood of the sugar it needs, thereby causing headache discomfort. People who get hungry between meals may develop a headache because of low blood sugar. While eating between meals is not recommended, the headache may go away if a snack of FRESH FRUIT, NUTS, or SUNFLOWER SEEDS is taken to boost the energy stores. Persons who are constantly eating CANDY for "energy" will feel more tired and headachy at the end of the day than those who eat nothing at all between meals.

◆ *Artificial Sugar Substitutes*

✓ SACCHARIN—Dr. Uglow found that saccharin is 12 times as deadly to bacteria as carbolic acid. It is a COAL TAR derivative and a deadly poison. Saccharin is a protoplasmic poison, that is, regardless of how long the process may take, saccharin eventually poisons protoplasm. It was found that dry seed peas did not sprout in a saccharin solution, while they sprouted in sugar and salt solutions. Dr. Uglow found that when placing some cyclops, one-celled animals, in a solution of one part of saccharin to 8000 parts of water, that it took only 24 hours to kill all of the cyclops. Saccharin has the tendency to build up concentrations in the bladder, and thereby has induced BLADDER CANCER in mice and rats, and has produced deformities in developing chicks. Incidentally, a relation of saccharin to water of 1:10,000 is approximately the solution one gets when one slips a saccharin tablet into a cup of tea or coffee.

Certain coal tar products are known to produce CANCER through their effect on the cells of the body. We should not need further proof of the harmfulness of saccharin and all other synthetic sweeteners. Although saccharin is illegal in food and drink as far as interstate commerce is concerned, there is nothing to prevent local food processors from using it in all their sweet products, unless the state has a law which forbids it.

✓ ASPARTAME—NUTRISWEET

This artificial sweetener is not suitable for foods that are heated for any length of time, as it breaks down into chemicals that are no longer sweet. One out of 20,000 babies is born without the ability to metabolize PHENYLALANINE, one of two amino acids that make up aspartame. This can result in MENTAL RETARDATION. It may cause BRAIN TUMORS, HEADACHES, DIZZINESS, and MENSTRUAL PROBLEMS. Aspartame can actually lead to OBESITY, because it triggers the body's conversion of blood glucose into saturated fats. This causes LOW BLOOD SUGAR, which in turn causes the signal to eat, and such a response will ultimately lead to weight gain.

◆ Brain Food

ALPHA LINOLENIC ACID or ALENA is an essential fatty acid. It is present at a level of about 1% in GREEN LEAFY VEGETABLES, WALNUTS, and COLD WATER FISH. Fish is often referred to as "brain food." It is also present in CANOLA OIL. A particularly rich source of this brain food is ground fortified FLAXSEED which contains from 16% to 22% Alena. The type of omega-3 oil found in flax seed can prevent TUMOR growth. It counteracts the effects of other dietary fats that promote the growth of cancer. Flax seed oil can be used in baked goods. Alena and its derivatives comprise 65% of some parts of the brain.

Milk

◆ *The Milk Of The Word*

All animals as they are born will take in milk from the mother that gave them birth. So milk from the mother is the proper food substance for the growing infant. Similarly, new children of God must assimilate the basic principles of the Bible as the "milk of the Word" (1 Pet. 2:2), for beginning Christians are not able as yet to assimilate the meat or solid food of doctrine of the Word, which nourishes the experienced Christian. "As newborn babes, desire the sincere milk of the word that ye may grow thereby" (1 Pet. 2:2). Paul further says, "I have fed you with milk, and not with meat: for hitherto ye were not able to bear it, neither yet now are ye able" (1 Cor. 3:2). "For everyone that useth milk is unskillful in the word of righteousness: for he is a babe"(Hebr. 5:13).

◆ *The Land Of Milk And Honey*

When God led Israel out of Egypt into the promised land, he led them into a land "flowing with milk and honey" (Ex. 3:8). By relating the promised land to milk and honey, God emphasized milk and honey as excellent foods. He did not then mean for the Israelites to sterilize their milk, for the proliferation of bacteria was not then as great as it is today. Also, we should not assume that the "milk" referred to means necessarily cow's milk, for GOAT'S milk was most frequently used, as well as the milk from COWS, CAMELS, and SHEEP (Gen. 32:15; Deut. 32:14; Prov. 27:27). Since fresh milk did not keep very well in Palestine's hot climate, it was processed into BUTTERMILK, CURDS, and CHEESE. Milk was poured into goat skins where it soured and thickened.

◆ *Cow's Milk As Food*

Man appears to be the only organism which habitually consumes milk after the period of lactation has ended. Most authorities on nutrition also consider milk a food for which there is no adequate substitute. Milk is no doubt one of the most COMPLETE single foods. It contains COMPLETE PROTEINS, CARBOHYDRATES in the form of milk sugars, the MINERALS, and many VITAMINS. The sugar is predigested, the fat is already emulsified. It also gives the ordinary diet a better-balanced mineral content. Without milk, few dietaries would contain enough calcium for the adult, and still less for the child. Of the vitamins in milk, IRRADIATION damages vitamin A, PASTEURIZATION destroys the vitamin C, and vitamin D is extremely variable. Authorities have pointed out some disadvantages in the use of milk, but to discourage its consumption on that basis might be dangerous to the general public health, since few have enough knowledge of nutrition to supply their requirements without milk.

IRON is in very low supply in milk, so that a diet which consists entirely of milk will produce ANEMIA. Cow's milk has to be supplemented with iron foods as the child grows. Enough iron is held in the liver to meet the needs of the child during the first year. After that the milk can be supplemented by adding BLACKSTRAP MOLASSES to it. Also it is not recommended to feed children SKIM milk during the first year, for MOTHER'S milk has even more fat in it than cow's milk. Removing the fat from milk also removes the VITAMIN D, although this is usually added to milk. Mother's milk contains VITAMIN C while cow's milk that has been pasteurized contains practically none. Also Vitamin E is more abundant in mother's milk than in cow's milk, hence, most infants who are deprived of breast feeding do not get enough vitamin E, since their formula is usually not supplemented with vitamin E. Studies of BOTTLE-FED infants indicate that they require 2.5 to 5.0 mg of vitamin E daily. However, they get only 0.3 to 0.7 mg daily in a 24 oz. feeding. Cow's milk has 4 times as much PROTEIN and only one half as much CARBOHYDRATES as human milk. This may explain the custom of sweetening cow's milk. It means that consuming cow's milk provokes a CRAVING for SWEETS. Milk will neutralize stomach acid. It also contains TRYPTOPHAN, an amino acid that induces SLEEP.

All protein foods must be chewed. Milk should be taken in little sips and chewed in the mouth before it is sent to the stomach. Heating milk not only kills the pathogenic bacteria, it kills the living vitality of the milk also. The calcium becomes less assimilable. It is the cream factor that is most harmful in milk. It is mucus forming in the human system. Nearly all children who have tendencies to COLD, BRONCHIAL COUGHS, NASAL and NOSE PHLEGM FORMATIONS do better when milk is abandoned altogether. This is why SKIM MILK is better than WHOLE MILK.

ALLERGIES are caused largely by milk. HEART DISEASE and ATTACKS have also been traced to the use of milk. STOMACH IRRITATIONS may be due to the fact that the protein in cow's milk differs from the protein in human milk. Many cases of ECZEMA, BLOATED STOMACH, ARTHRITIC JOINT PAINS, ASTHMA, NASAL CONGESTION, EAR INFECTIONS, and even PERSISTENT VOMITING, are to some extent milk derived. It is suggested that we do not use milk as a thirst quencher.

◆ *Mother's Milk*

✓ BREAST-FEEDING IS BEST—For an infant there is no better milk than mother's milk. Besides this the next best milk is said to be RAW GOAT'S MILK. Most animals are BREAST-FED until they have tripled their birth-weight. Right after a baby is born, the mother's milk contains COLOSTRUM which contains ACIDOPHILUS bacteria needed for normal bowel function. It also contains substances known as IMMUNOLOGICAL FACTORS that help an infant fight infections, and may also stimulate the baby's own immune system, encouraging various types of white blood cells to produce protective ANTIBODIES. Also breast-fed babies use their mouth muscles more effectively and are therefore less likely than bottle-fed babies to end up with crooked TEETH. At this point cow's milk is five times harder for the baby's liver to handle, as the fat globules are five times larger. In a Harvard study it has been suggested that breast-feeding may protect against pre-menopausal BREAST CANCER, perhaps by interrupting ovulation, by changing the hormonal balance, or by affecting the physical structure of the ducts in the breast where cancers are most likely to develop. These ideas remain yet to be proven.

✓ COW'S MILK INCREASES CHOLESTEROL — A University of Illinois study indicated that infants fed by FORMULA similar to cow's milk had higher levels of CHOLESTEROL and TRIGLYCERIDES in their blood than breast-fed babies. Both human and cow's milk are rich in cholesterol. It is believed that the reason for this is that the cow's milk has almost 4 times as much protein as human milk. Mother's milk contains just 7% protein instead of 25% for cow's milk. The HIGH FAT CONTENT of mother's milk may help in the assimilation of calcium from the milk. It has also been found that the level of VITAMIN D in breast milk is directly related to the amount of vitamin D in the mother's diet.

✓ MOTHER'S MILK SPURS MENTAL DEVELOPMENT—There is very strong evidence that an unknown substance in MOTHER'S MILK spurs MENTAL DEVELOPMENT, thereby giving the breast-fed children an advantage here. It has been suspected that too much ANIMAL FAT may dim the mental faculties. Rats fed LARD did not find their way through mazes as readily as rats fed SOYBEAN OIL. Some experts believe that it is the OMEGA-3 fatty acid in mother's milk which brings this about, for omega-3 has been found critical in fetal and infant BRAIN DEVELOPMENT.

◆ *Raw Milk*

Raw milk is better than pasteurized milk for human consumption if the disease germ count can be kept low. CERTIFIED RAW MILK is available in health food stores. It is higher in enzymes, hormone growth factors, proteins, minerals, fats, and natural vitamins than pasteurized milk. Certified raw milk has an ANTI-STIFFNESS benefit, which is destroyed in pasteurization. It is important for easing ARTHRITIS distress, and also helps against RHEUMATOID ARTHRITIS.

◆ *The Chemicals In Milk*

There is developing a PENICILLIN sensitivity in people due to the large amount of penicillin we drink in our milk. When cows get sick with MASTITIS, a disease of the udder, they are treated with penicillin. Antibiotics are now incorporated into the food of cows. This increases the clotting of blood, which can cause HEART ATTACKS. Reactions to penicillin are represented by ACNE, HIVES, FEVER, JOINT PAINS, SHOCK and DEATH. Penicillin also counteracts the development of MILK CULTURES for making CHEESE. Some infants fed on cow's milk develop ANTIBODIES to the protein in the milk. This indicates that the protein is not compatible with the bloodstream, and that the body is defending itself against it. Breast-fed infants do not develop antibodies to mother's milk.

Dairy herds exposed to DDT pass it along in their milk. When part per million is included in their diet, the body fat may reach concentrations of 150 times as much, because DDT accumulates in the fatty tissues. DDT is toxic. There is no antidote. It is absorbed by plants and grass. The cows eat the grass, and that is how it gets into the milk. Low levels of antibiotics in milk is building up a sensitivity to the drug. Those people who do not have any adverse reaction from a dose of penicillin are likely to develop a sensitivity to it from milk-drinking. Allergic reaction to PENICILLIN is the most common cause of ANAPHYLACTIC SHOCK, which is considered to be a cause of CRIB DEATH. So here we have a reason for blaming penicillin for crib deaths.

RADIOACTIVE FALLOUT covers the whole earth. It gets into the grass which the cows eat. It then gets into the milk which we drink. In this manner STRONTIUM 90, a radiation product, gets into our system. It attaches itself readily to calcium. All types of these radiations can cause cancer. It has been estimated that RADIOLOGISTS have a life span which is 6 years less than that of the average of the population.

It is no doubt for many of these reasons that we have been told that the time will come and may now be already at our doorsteps, when there is no longer any safety in drinking the milk of cows, so that milk will have to be excluded from our diet (CD411). This is also due to the fact that "DISEASE in animals is INCREASING in proportion to the WICKEDNESS AMONG MEN" (CD356). Basically Mrs. White never denounced the use of milk for she used it herself. She realized that a moderate use of milk is not objectionable, but that the free use of it might be injurious to health (CD 357, 468). She mentioned that "If milk is used, it should be thoroughly sterilized; with this precaution, there is less danger of contracting disease from it use. But if the cows are healthy and the milk thoroughly cooked, there is no necessity of creating a time of trouble beforehand"(CD357). Thorough sterilization means destroying 100% of all bacteria that might be in the milk. She acknowledged that it was the responsibility of the health food business to supply the people with substitutes for milk (CD350). This it has done with the production of SOY MILK. She also mentions that people with weak blood-making organs may need to use milk and eggs to build themselves up (MH320). She recognized the fact that some people cannot use milk while others thrive on it (CH154).

◆ *Pasteurized Milk*

PASTEURIZATION is the process of heating milk at a temperature of 140 degrees Fahrenheit for 30 minutes, which process destroys about 95% of the bacteria. When we say that the process destroys bacteria, we must realize that it will destroy the BENEFICIAL BACTERIA that may be present as well as the HARMFUL ONES, but not quite all of the harmful ones. This may be the reason why the Spirit of Prophecy has told us that "if milk is used, it should be thoroughly STERILIZED; with this precaution, there is less danger of contracting disease from its use. The difference between pasteurization and sterilization is that sterilization refers to the destruction of all bacteria.

Pasteurization destroys vitamin C, makes calcium salts insoluble, interferes with the PHOSPHORUS element which is closely allied with the CALCIUM element to prevent RICKETS. As we have said before, heat never increases the nutritional value of any food. So what does pasteurization accomplish? It causes a loss in the soluble calcium and phosphorus content of milk. It destroys all of the enzymes including PROTEASE, LACTASE, DIASTASE, LIPASE, CATALASE, AMYLASE, and PHOSPHATASE, which are required for good assimilation, and results in ALLERGIES and DIGESTIVE PROBLEMS. It destroys 50% of the vitamin C. It drives out some of the iodine which helps prevent RICKETS. It causes DEFECTIVE TEETH, IRRITABILITY, CONVULSIONS, and CONSTIPATION. It destroys LECITHIN. It changes the chemical structure of the protein and renders it and some of the minerals less digestible and assimilable. A bottle of milk left standing on the porch in daylight loses from 50 to 70% of its RIBOFLAVIN within two hours, and 5 to 15% of the vitamin B_2 is lost in pasteurization.

◆ *Pasteurization And Disease*

Experiments with calves have demonstrated that they cannot live on their own mother's milk, if that milk has been subjected to the heat of pasteurization. The calves died within one to two months from diseases born of malnutrition and systemic poisoning. Dr. Pottenger of California fed cats and kittens pasteurized milk. Some of the conditions that developed were BRITTLE BONES, LUNG and BRONCHIAL DISORDERS, and STERILITY.

When he fed them raw natural milk as it comes from the cow or goat, every animal lived a normal life span. The same experiment with cats on a farm in New York developed in them in addition TUMORS, CANCER, NEPHRITIS, and DIABETES. Similar results were obtained when cats were fed COOKED MEAT instead of raw meat. They died in a short time of ATHEROSCLEROSIS. On a diet of raw meat they thrived.

◆ *Milk Tolerance*

Milk is an excellent food for those who are milk tolerant. 70% of the world's population just can't drink milk or eat dairy products except YOGURT, without getting an upset stomach. 75% of White Americans have no problem in digesting milk, but 75% of American Blacks have been found to be intolerant of milk, a condition called LACTOSE INTOLERANCE. Normal people absorb about 92% of milk lactose; those with lactose intolerance absorb only from 28% to 58%. Many people have acute reactions to milk, including CRAMPS, BLOATING, INTESTINAL GAS, and DIARRHEA Those who are tolerant have sufficient of the enzyme LACTASE in their intestines, which breaks down the milk sugar LACTOSE, into a form that the body can use. The others may be deficient in the LACTASE which is needed to digest the lactose, and therefore have difficulty in digesting milk. All normal mammals stop producing the enzymes needed to digest their baby food once they have been weaned. A few populations who had to rely on the milk of their herds for food seemed to keep the ability to continue producing the lactase enzymes, and thereby remain able to digest milk during their adult years. Almost everyone else, including 70 to 90% of blacks, Chinese, Japanese, some Jews, and most Mediterranean people, have lost that ability.

Dr. Robert D. McCracken believes that descendants of the ancestors who historically herded dairy animals and lived on lactose-rich milk and cheese are usually tolerant to milk. Their intestines seem to contain plenty of lactase, so that milk for them is an excellent health food. On the other hand, those whose ancestors seldom used milk, are usually intolerant to milk, because their intestines do not contain sufficient lactase.

For those who are lactose intolerant, YOGURT comes with its own digestive enzyme which allows yogurt's lactose to be digested in the small intestines. There are also milk products which contain added lactase, the enzyme which your body lacks, such as LACTAID, a lactase treated milk. Lactaid also comes in capsule form.

If one is lactose-intolerant, one can also drink lactose-reduced milk which is generally available. It has about 70% less lactose in it, but it tastes sweeter than regular milk. One can make it oneself by buying LIQUID LACTASE and add it to regular milk. Five drops per quart can break down over 70% of the milk sugar in 24 hours. If you want even greater reduction, then let the milk stand for 2 or 3 days. In this way one can eliminate nearly all of the lactose. One can also use lactase tablets or capsules, and take them just before one consumes the milk. But they are usually less effective than adding the drops to the milk.

Rats lack an enzyme to properly use GALACTOSE, a sugar in milk produced from LACTOSE. Without this enzyme they generally get CATARACTS when they are fed lots of milk or milk products. Dr. Williams of the University of Texas fed 18 groups of rats 18 different diets. All diets except one contained large amounts of galactose up to 20%. At the end of 9 weeks cataracts had formed in the eyes of the rats which got plain chow without vitamins. The rats which received the vitamin supplements in addition had no cataracts. The group without galactose also had no cataracts.

To overcome lactose intolerance, a person can buy lactase enzymes or raw unpasteurized milk in the health food store. The WULZEN FACTOR, an anti-stiffness element, is abundant in raw milk, but it is not in pasteurized milk.

◆ *Homogenized Milk*

HOMOGENIZATION deals only with the fat globules in milk. Normally their size allows 4000 of them to cover the length of an inch, which makes them large enough to rise to the surface as cream. By homogenization these fat globules are made so small that they no longer rise, but remain scattered through the milk. Homogenization is a purely mechanical process, and nothing is changed except for the distribution of the fat

Dr. Kurt Oster feels that the process of homogenization of milk breaks down the normal-sized fat particles and allows an enzyme called XANTHINE OXYDASE (XO), found in milk fat, to pass through the intestinal wall, without being changed by the digestive process. It enters the blood stream, which it normally would not, and in turn destroys vital body chemicals that would normally protect the arteries of the heart. It helps to break down proteins in the digestive tract. Upon entering the bloodstream it will attack the heart and the arteries. The body then collects FAT and CHOLESTEROL and builds them up at the damage sites, narrowing the vessels. This does not happen with RAW MILK.

It is the breakup of the fat in homogenized milk that allows XO to go through the walls of the intestines into the bloodstream. In non-homogenized milk the XO is excreted. To back up his idea Dr. Osler claims that the DEATH RATE from HEART DISEASE in different countries is proportionate to how much homogenized milk people drink, and is also far less in countries where people normally boil their milk, for boiling destroys the xanthine oxidase. Pasteurizing milk to 173 degrees destroys 30% of XO. At 183 degrees all of the XO is destroyed. At any higher degree such as boiling, which would represent sterilization, again all of the XO would be destroyed. Most of the vitamin A is destroyed when milk is homogenized.

◆ *Soured Milk—Buttermilk*

The best way to take milk is in its soured form as YOGURT, KEFIR, ACIDOPHILUS, or regular CLABBERED milk. Soured milks are superior to SWEET milk, as they are in pre-digested form, and are very easily assimilated. They also help to maintain a healthy INTESTINAL FLORA and prevent intestinal PUTREFACTION and CONSTIPATION.

◆ *The Function Of Enzymes*

ENZYMES are complex substances which enable us to digest food and help us absorb it into our bloodstream. They are sensitive to temperatures above 118°F, and are destroyed at 130°F, at which point most of the vital force needed for nourishment is dissipated.

There are 3 types of enzymes: FOOD ENZYMES from raw food, DIGESTIVE ENZYMES, and METABOLIC ENZYMES. Most metabolic enzymes are produced in the pancreas. When cooked food is eaten the body's enzyme supply is used for digestive enzymes rather than metabolic enzymes. This puts a strain upon the pancreas, and causes it to enlarge. As a result the pancreas of humans on a diet of cooked and raw food is 300% larger than of those who eat raw food only.

The breakdown of food into nutrients is done by enzymes which are chemical reactors in the food we eat, or which are made in our bodies from the food we eat. Different enzymes work on three different food groups—PROTEINS, CARBOHYDRATES, and FATS. Each group has its own set of enzymes. A protein enzyme can only work on proteins. A carbohydrate enzyme can only work on carbohydrates, and a fat enzyme can only work on fats. Enzymes are often antagonistic to one another.

The word ENZYME comes from the Greek meaning FERMENT. Man uses enzymes to make sour milk and cheese. He ferments bread and makes it rise with the help of enzymes. He preserves vegetables by the enzymatic process of PICKLING them, and makes SAUERKRAUT. All these foods are storehouses of enzymes. There are many enzymes which the body itself produces. The METABOLIC enzymes run our bodies; the DIGESTIVE enzymes digest our foods; and the FOOD enzymes start our digestion. More enzymes are needed on a cooked food diet than on a raw food diet. On a cooked food diet the PANCREAS become enlarged due to the body's increased need for digestive enzymes.

◆ *Cooking Destroys Enzymes And Vitamins*

COOKING not only destroys enzymes, but also vitamins, and changes proteins and fats to a form more difficult to digest. During this process, proteins, starches, and fats are broken up into simpler compounds.

◆ *The Medicinal Properties Of Lactic Acid Fermented Foods*

Fermentation is the DECOMPOSITION or ACIDIFICATION of organic substances produced by the action of living organisms and enzymes. LACTIC ACID FERMENTATION is the formation of LACTIC ACID from carbohydrates by the action of BACTERIA, which usually involves the STREPTOCOCCUS and LACTOBACILLUS BACTERIA. It must be distinguished from ALCOHOLIC FERMENTATION, which is the action of YEAST on carbohydrates which produces ALCOHOL. An excellent way of increasing the amount of raw food in the diet is to eat lots of fermented lactic acid foods. Fermenting foods is an excellent way of preserving foods for winter use, and not only preserve them, but also increase their nutritive value without cooking.

SAUERKRAUT, PICKLES, PICKLED VEGETABLES, MISO, and YOGURT are examples of predigested or fermented foods due to the development of lactic acid. Honey is a food predigested by nature. Such foods require less enzyme output and digestive work than more complex or cooked foods. It completely changes the character of a food. It improves their keeping qualities. It makes bland foods tastier, stronger, so that when no refrigeration is available it can still be wholesome. It increases nutritional richness. The bacteria synthesize additional enzymes and vitamins, and create a more digestible amino acid balance. They are especially helpful in the synthesis of vitamin B_{12}. Fermented foods improve the INTESTINAL FLORA, thereby aiding in the digestion of protein and carbohydrate foods.

Dr. JOHANNES KUHL, the foremost expert on the therapeutic value of lactic acid fermented foods, indicates that fermented foods and juices possess extraordinary medicinal properties, and should be used in the biological treatment of many diseases. CANCER, ARTHRITIS, DIGESTIVE DISORDERS and diseases of the KIDNEYS and LIVER, are especially suited for treatment with fermented juices.

Lactic acid destroys harmful bacteria in the intestines and contributes to the better digestion and assimilation of nutrients. It is best not to use commercially fermented foods, as they are always prepared with vinegar, toxic chemicals, and preservatives.

In the Pottenger cat experiments, a group of cats was divided into two parts. One group was fed only COOKED FOODS and PASTEURIZED MILK, while the other group was fed RAW MEAT and UNPASTEURIZED MILK. The cats fed the cooked diet developed all of the symptoms of the major degenerative diseases found in humans. The raw food group did not develop any diseases.

When bacilli have converted the MILK SUGAR into LACTIC ACID, the milk becomes sour. It can be made from pasteurized, skimmed, or partly skimmed milk to which a BACTERIAL CULTURE is added to SOUR the milk. After the milk has soured, the growth of disease producing bacteria ceases, and the MILK PROTEINS change into a more digestible form. FERMENTED MILK is one of the best neutralizers of putrefaction in the colon with the help of acidophilus bacilli WHEY is the liquid left after the milk curds have been used to make cheese. It consists of WATER, LACTOSE or MILK SUGAR, MILK PROTEIN, and most of the MINERALS in the original milk. It is effective in normalizing and changing the INTESTINAL FLORA so as to work against CONSTIPATION and DYSENTERY, to the extent that harmful bacteria are discouraged, and helpful ones are encouraged. Its action is similar to acidophilus milk and yogurt.

BUTTERMILK has less fat per serving than 1% low-fat milk. 2% low-fat milk is 2% fat by weight, but actually contains 35% of calories from fat. 1% milk has 23% fat calories. Less than 5% of the calories in skim milk are from fat. Buttermilk is a fine calcium food, good for teeth and bones, and easily digested. It is indicated in cases of CONSTIPATION, ACIDITY, PIMPLES, INSOMNIA, and helps destroy putrefactive BACTERIA in the bowels.

◆ *How To Get Enough Enzymes*

- Eat as much raw food as possible, up to of diet.
- Eat foods as soon as possible after they have been harvested
- In winter under scarce RAW FOOD conditions, use FROZEN FOODS. Freezing does not destroy enzymes, it only inactivates them.
- If you cook some vegetables, cook them as fast and as little as possible. CHINESE COOKING by steaming vegetables, which leaves them still crisp and half raw, preserves most of the enzymes.
- CHEW all foods, especially carbohydrates, well. Enzymatic action starts in the mouth.
- Use unpasteurized raw milk if possible. PASTEURIZATION destroys enzymes. Goat milk is particularly rich in enzymes, and raw milk is available at better health food stores.
- Use as many as possible of the fermented enzyme foods such as HOMEMADE SAUERKRAUT, HOMEMADE SOURED MILK, HOMEMADE YOGURT, HOMEMADE KEFIR, and HOMEMADE COTTAGE CHEESE. They are all extremely helpful for the healthy condition of the bacterial flora in the digestive tract.
- RAW GRAINS, especially WHEAT and SEEDS are rich sources of enzymes. Since baking requires high temperatures, bread is void of enzymes. Use grains raw by sprouting them.
- Buy a JUICE EXTRACTOR and make your own enzyme-loaded drink of fresh raw fruit and vegetable juices. Drink juices before meals and immediately after they have been prepared. Brewer's yeast, raw honey, papaya, rose hips, and kelp are, in addition to the enzymes, rich in vitamins and minerals.

◆ *Yogurt*

Years of medical research has determined that FERMENTED MILK PRODUCTS such as YOGURT can help keep people in good health. Yogurt is a good source of CALCIUM, especially for people who cannot drink milk because they have trouble digesting the milk sugar LACTOSE. Yogurt contain's less lactose than milk, which makes it easier to digest. Fermented milk products are beneficial in treating other conditions such as INDIGESTION, HIGH CHOLESTEROL LEVELS, BOWEL IRREGULARITY, HIGH BLOOD PRESSURE, and even FOOD POISONING. Fermented milk is identified by the bacteria it contains, and not all types are equally beneficial. THERMOPHILUS MILK, for example is effective in reducing lactose intolerance, but BUTTERMILK is not. ACIDOPHILUS milk has slowed the growth of TUMORS in mice. YOGURT BACTERIA, injected directly into MOUSE TUMORS made the growths shrink.

YOGURT is defatted milk soured with LACTOBACILLUS ACIDOPHILUS bacilli, and contains a high concentration of those bacteria which are vitally necessary for the health of the intestines. By reducing PUTREFACTION, it helps to protect us against the bacteria causing DYSENTERY, TYPHOID, PNEUMONIA, and numerous other diseases. Very close to yogurt is another soured milk preparation known as ACIDOPHILUS MILK. It looks and acts as yogurt does, but the taste is not nearly so pleasant. Both yogurt and acidophilus milk contain live cultures of BENEFICIAL BACTERIA. They initiate the fermentation process that transforms plain milk into tart-tasting yogurt. Some experts believe that these bacteria solve GASTROINTESTINAL PROBLEMS, lower blood CHOLESTEROL, and even help prevent CANCER.

Yogurt has all of the advantages that milk has and is without several of milk's disadvantages. People who show an allergy to milk can usually tolerate yogurt. The CURDS formed by yogurt are much finer than those of ordinary milk. The difference in digestibility is shown by the fact that milk is only 32% digested after an hour in the digestive tract, while 91% of the yogurt has been digested in the same amount of time. A large percentage of people who show an ALLERGY TO MILK are able to tolerate yogurt with no ill effect whatsoever. The yogurt organism converts the protein molecules in milk which are blamed for the allergic reactions, thus eliminating the source of the problem.

Yogurt bacteria convert the LACTOSE in milk into LACTIC ACID. This acid supplements the action of the hydrochloric acid in the stomach, causing digestion in a natural fashion. The stomach's production of hydrochloric acid decreases with age, but the acidophilus bacillus stays in the stomach long after the cultured milk itself has been eaten and digested. BABIES also respond to the use of yogurt when treating INFANTILE DYSPEPSIA, DIARRHEA, and CONSTIPATION. This seems to indicate that there is a problem created for them by the use of uncultured cow's milk. BELCHING, STOMACH RUMBLING, and FLATULENCE are also said to be remedied with yogurt.

Yogurt is safe because it is predigested. The bacteria in yogurt take over for the missing lactase enzyme, and help to digest much of the lactose. Commercially frozen yogurt is sometimes re-pasteurized or reheated, and this extra heat may kill the helpful bacteria. It must contain the live, active culture in order to be effective.

◆ *Yogurt Is A Natural Antibiotic*

Normally GOOD BACTERIA in the system outnumber the BAD BACTERIA by about 99 to 1. An ounce of yogurt or acidophilus has several hundred million active helpful microorganisms. But when you take ANTIBIOTICS, this ratio shifts in favor of the bad bacteria. Antibiotics kill bacteria, but they kill the good bacteria more readily than the bad ones, because the good ones are more susceptible to them. Killing the good bacteria in the intestines immediately causes diarrhea. But the good bacteria destroy the bad ones if enough of them are present. It is also believed that the bad bacteria make enzymes which produce cancer-causing compounds such as NITROSAMINES. Since the yogurt culture destroys these bad bacteria, they are therefore also believed to PREVENT CANCER. Yogurt cultures are called PROBIOTICS which means "for life," as compared to ANTIBIOTICS which means "against life." Women who take antibiotics, for example, are at risk of VAGINAL YEAST INFECTIONS, because antibiotics destroy the beneficial lactobacilli which keep yeasts and other pathogenic organisms in check. When the lactobacilli are destroyed, the yeasts proliferate. The result:—VAGINITIS.

Dr. Metchnikoff of Russia in the early 1900's advocated the theory that much disease is caused by microbial putrefaction in the intestines, which poisons the body by releasing toxins that destroy artery walls and cause senility and early death. He believed that these microbes could be counteracted by yogurt, which contains ANTIBIOTIC FACTORS. When mice were injected with SALMONELLA and INFLUENZA bugs, they all remained alive on a diet of yogurt, while the mice without such a diet all died. The fermentation process seems to spawn unique antibiotics, just as moldy bread yields penicillin.

Investigators have found at least SEVEN NATURAL ANTIBIOTICS in yogurt. These are as potent as STREPTOMYCIN, PENICILLIN, and others. They have destroyed AMOEBAE, TYPHUS, S. DYSENTERIAE, E. COLI, STREPTOCOCCUS, and STAPHYLOCOCCUS bacteria. It is very important to note that while yogurt destroys the harmful bacteria, it does NOT HARM any of the BENEFICIAL BACTERIA, but rather assists in their growth. Yogurt increases the immune system's production of antibodies and other infection fighting agents. It triples the amount of INTERFERON manufactured by the cells. It has potent ANTI-TUMOR activity, and it reduces the growth of CANCER CELLS in mice by 30%.

It is also believed that yogurt cultures can reduce CHOLESTEROL in the bloodstream. This idea is based on tests of the Finns and the Masai tribe of Africa, both of which eat a huge fat diet of cultured milk products. The Finns eat more yogurt per person than does any other people in the world.

◆ *Goat's Milk—Best Animal Milk For Man*

Besides mother's milk raw goat's milk is the most beneficial milk for humans of all ages to drink. It is one kind of milk that is COMPATIBLE with HUMAN NUTRITION. Proverbs 27:27 says, "And thou shalt have goat's milk enough for thy food, for the food of thy household, and for the maintenance for thy maidens." The Bible "land of milk and honey" statement (Ex. 3:8), may refer as much to goat's milk and sheep milk than to cow's milk. (Deut. 32:14). The quality of goat's milk is far SUPERIOR to that of cow's milk. It is NATURALLY HOMOGENIZED, for the FAT GLOBULES are SMALLER than those in cow's milk and is therefore more easily assimilated. It is NOT MUCUS FORMING like cow's milk.

Goat's milk must be USED RAW, and must not be heated above 118 degrees Fahrenheit, and should not be pasteurized. Like in the case of calves, if pasteurized goat's milk is fed to the kids of the goat, they will likely be dead within six months. Goat's milk was designed for a baby goat which weighs about 8 pounds at birth, the same as a human infant. It has a better quality of PROTEIN, with a much higher amount of NIACIN and THIAMIN than almost any other food product. It is beneficial in cases of DIARRHEA in small children due to its high niacin content. It is also better than cow's milk as an infant food because its protein and mineral ratio is closer to that of mother's milk. It is a highly concentrated source of ENZYMES. It contains both ANTI-ARTHRITIC and ANTI-CANCER factors, and is therefore recommended for these conditions. An Englishman who died at age 152 ate a diet entirely of goat's milk, goat's milk cheese, whey, and raw vegetables.

A man with ulcers was pronounced "incurable" by 15 doctors. After this an old-timer suggested that he live largely on GOAT'S MILK. He tried this suggestion and, as proven by x-rays, his ulcers disappeared completely.

◆ *Soy Milk*

Soy bean milk has been successfully used as a substitute for cow's milk in the feeding of children who are allergic to cow's milk, that is, they cannot tolerate either the protein or lactose, or both. It is far richer in IRON, THIAMIN, and NIACIN, but less so in CALCIUM and PHOSPHORUS content. Human milk contains 1% protein, 6% carbohydrate, and 3% fat. Cow's milk contains 3% protein, 5% carbohydrates, and 3% fat. Soy milk contains 33% protein, 33% carbohydrates, and 17% fat. Soy milk is very much higher in the basic substances, which means that it can be diluted more to make it compatible with cow's milk. In one study of 102 infants, soy milk took away the symptoms of ECZEMA, STOMACH DISORDERS, IRRITABILITY, ASTHMA, and CHRONIC NASAL DISCHARGE. Acidophilus milk can also be made with soy milk with the same good results. Dr. Tiling of Hamburg Germany, has treated hundreds of children who were suffering from ECZEMA, ASTHMA, DIARRHEA, and SPRUE. They were all allergic to COW'S MILK. He found that when he substituted soy milk for cow's milk that it promoted GROWTH, IMPROVED APPETITE, REVIVED DIGESTIVE FUNCTION, and restored the general DISPOSITION of the children, NORMAL BEHAVIOR, and MENTAL ALERTNESS.

◆ *Cottage Cheese*

Cottage cheese is made from soured milk which is heated to 140 degrees Fahrenheit until it curdles. Then it is strained and what is left is wholesome cottage cheese. It is recommended that the milk be unpasteurized raw milk. Cottage cheese has all the benefits of soured milk. It is a good protein dish for Adventists who are advised through the inspired counsels of the Testimonies not to consume any other kind of processed cheese. The important thing about cottage cheese is that it be fresh, and the best kind of cottage cheese is the one that is freshly home-made.

One day an FDA research chemist lady came to Adventist Al. Wolfsen's sanitarium in Hawaii and asked him if he was using any cheese. He said that they were using cottage cheese. She said that cottage cheese is one of the worst foods in the grocery store. When it has been on the shelf for quite a while, under the microscope one can see a lot of things wiggling around in it. This may be the reason why every few weeks the super markets have a sale on cottage cheese, because it doesn't stay fresh very long.

◆ *Milk And Disease—Crib Deaths—SIDS*

In spite of strong efforts and precautions, the best milk delivered from the dairies continues to show the presence of some pathogenic bacteria. Milk is such a good culture medium, that it is easily contaminated. It was largely implicated in the great epidemics of TYPHOID and CHOLERA that occurred in the days before pasteurization was employed. Because of these precautions these epidemics are no longer in evidence. However, there may be other problems that are now in evidence.

✓ CRIB DEATHS—Milk may explain the problem of crib deaths. Up to about 25,000 babies die sudden unexplained infant deaths each year. They fall asleep and never wake up. Such a sudden death syndrome occurs in ANIMALS as well as in humans. Evidence from a study in New Zealand gives an indication that crib death may be a DEFICIENCY SYNDROME. It has been found that vitamin E deficiencies in young pigs will cause sudden death. This may also be true of infants. Very few babies even partially breast-fed during the first 5 months are known to die in this manner. Breast-fed babies get plenty of vitamin E, while infants fed on cow's milk may get very little. In a study of 2500 crib deaths only three were reared on mother's milk.

✓ ALLERGIC REACTION TO COW'S MILK—According to Dr. Stowens of Louisville Medical School, a deputy coroner, the critical point relates to the difference in vitamin E levels between human and cow's milk. He came to the conclusion that crib deaths are due to an ALLERGIC REACTION to cow's milk, due to ANAPHYLACTIC SHOCK. The body produces antibodies to fight against the type of protein which it cannot absorb. It is these antibodies that produce a sudden shock reaction which results in death. Crib deaths never occur in infants which are totally breast-fed, and even seldom when they are only partially breast-fed. It is because some infants do not digest the protein in cow's milk, but absorb it whole from the intestinal tract. This sensitizes them, causing kidney damage without any outward signs. In a Chicago study of the 1930's, of the infants who were breast-fed, 1.5 per 1000 died, while of those fed cow's milk 85 per 1000 died during the first 9 months of life.

PENICILLIN has been shown to cause anaphylactic shock in some people. This may be the reason as to why SIDS occurs in some babies. The cow's milk may still have some penicillin in it from penicillin shots given to the cows.

✓ DEFICIENCY IN VITAMIN E—Human milk contains an average of 1.14mg of vitamin E per quart, while cow's milk averages from .21mg in the early spring to a maximum of 1.06 mg per quart in mid fall. It is in the winter months, when the vitamin E level in cow's milk is at its lowest that most crib deaths occur. The function of vitamin E is to combine with polyunsaturated fatty acids to prevent the formation of toxic peroxides within the metabolism. Vegetable oils in synthetic formulas for baby milk have had their fats refined and stripped of their vitamin E content. After vitamin E was given to young pigs, the fatalities ceased. Vitamin E keeps a greater oxygen supply in the system, by keeping other substances from combining with oxygen.

✓ COW'S MILK DEFICIENT IN IRON—Milk causes IRON DEFICIENCY ANEMIA in children sensitive to the protein in milk. Iron loss is produced by inducing gastrointestinal bleeding. Milk fat, a saturated fat, may produce HARDENING OF THE ARTERIES. An oversupply of cow's milk gives us an oversupply of CALCIUM which causes blockage in the kidneys so as to form KIDNEY STONES. Cow's milk has 4 times as much calcium as mother's milk. Pasteurized, homogenized milk, is one of the major causes of HEART DISEASE. 55% of people in the U.S. die of heart disease in some form. Pasteurization kills the vital parts of milk. Cow's milk is the most MUCUS-FORMING food used by human beings. The CASEIN content of cow's milk is exceedingly high, being about 300% more than is contained in mother's milk. It can result in COLDS, RUNNING NOSES,

TONSILLITIS, ADENOIDS, and BRONCHIAL TROUBLES. As a result most experts and the American Academy of Pediatrics recommends that babies up to the one year old should be BREAST-FED or given an IRON-ENRICHED FORMULA.

✓ MILK AND GROWTH—About 150 years ago doctors realized that they could not increase the period of lactation between mother and child for much more than a year. By selective breeding it was realized that cows can be induced to give far more milk than is needed for their calves, so that the surplus could be fed to our babies, in order that the lactation period for them could be extended almost indefinitely, to the benefit of the children and the race. This idea worked somewhat against nature which allows the mother's milk to dry up after weaning. From the standpoint of the infants and children the doctors appeared to be correct. Babies fed on cow's milk appeared to grow better, bigger, and healthier than breast-fed babies, and this seemed to be true also as the period of lactation was extended into childhood.

So the present results of the period of lactation with cow's milk appeared to be beneficial. The question to be asked is why cow's milk is apparently so successful in rearing human babies and children. The answer to this question turns out to be quite obvious if we remember that God designed that the milk of every species was designed for that specie especially, and that the rate of growth of the specie is largely determined by the nature of the PROTEIN MOLECULE of that specie. Approximately therefore, the percentage of protein in any milk is an index of the rate of growth. A rabbit, for example doubles its birth weight in 6 days, a kitten in 9 days, a calf in 47 days, and a human baby in about 180 days or 6 months. From these figures we see that a calf grows at 4 times the rate of a baby. It also receives about 4 times the amount of protein which the baby receives. For this reason, if we use cow's milk for the baby's food, we would increase its weight and rate of growth beyond what would naturally take place with mother's milk.

✓ MILK AND CANCER—The Roswell Park Cancer Institute made a study of 3,334 cancer patients and 1300 subjects without cancer. They found that the people who drank 2% MILK had a significantly lower risk of cancer than those who drank WHOLE MILK. The effect of SKIM MILK was lower yet. Whole milk has 2 times as much fat as 2% milk, and 2% milk has 2 times as much fat as skim milk. Whole milk is the third largest source of FAT in the American diet, after ground beef foods, such as hamburgers, meat loaf, and hot dogs lunch meat.

Bread

◆ *The Preparation Of Bread*

We are told that classes should be formed to teach people how to make good bread, and to put the ingredients together to make healthful food combinations from grains and vegetables (MM267). "Religion will lead mothers to make bread of the very best quality.... Bread should be thoroughly baked, inside and out. (so as to destroy the yeast germs) The health of the stomach demands that it be light and dry. Bread is the staff of life, and therefore every cook should excel in making it" (CD315). The health of the family requires it. Also in the making of bread MILK should not be used in the place of water. It makes the bread much less wholesome. Milk bread does not keep sweet as long after baking as does bread made with water, and it ferments more readily in the stomach (CD316). We are told that "all wheat flour is not best for a continuous diet. A mixture of WHEAT, OATMEAL, and RYE would be more nutritious than the wheat with the nutritive properties separated from it" (CD321). Our present day MULTIGRAIN breads should be highly recommended if all of the grains are whole grains which have all of the nutriments retained. While two meals a day is preferable to three meals a day, if a third meal is taken it should be light so that it will be digested by bedtime. It is suggested that it consist of FRUIT and BREAD (CD178). Fruit juices mingled with bread is also recommended.

ZWIEBACK is a German name meaning twice-baked. BISCUIT is a French name meaning twice-cooked. However, the way the latter is made, it isn't always cooked twice. Nevertheless, twice-baked means being first baked, and then being baked again by being thoroughly dried out. Such bread is the most EASILY DIGESTED and the most palatable of foods. If this bread is kept in a dry place it keeps much longer than ordinary bread, and if reheated before using it will be as fresh as when newly made.

◆ *The Flour Used In Bread*

About 50% of the American diet today consists of products made of white sugar and refined chemicalized white flour. This fact may be an important reason for the great increase in degenerative diseases. In nature every substance used for food contains vitamins and minerals. Our bodies must have these elements if we are to properly assimilate STARCH, PROTEIN, and FAT. In the milling of flour, the GERM is removed because it has a low keeping quality, and because its fat content easily gets rancid. This eliminates the vitamin E it contains, which deficiency can cause heart trouble. What is left is almost pure starch. This is treated with one bleaching chemical after another, all of which render the flour more and more unfit for human consumption. Then the flour is "enriched" with a few of synthetically produced B-vitamins and iron, after all of the natural vitamins have been taken out, and also preservatives are added to it.

In the baker's WHOLE WHEAT FLOUR, in most cases a preservative has been added to keep insects from consuming the flour before it reaches the baker, and to keep the bread from molding before it reaches the consumer. These preservatives are strong chemicals and so toxic that insects know better than to eat them. This is the reason why baker's whole wheat bread may be worse for you to eat than baker's white bread.

In 1901 we were classified as the healthiest nation in the world among a statistical study of 100 nations by the United Nations. In 1920 we dropped to 2nd place. In 1950 we were in 3rd place. From 1940–45 was the healthiest time in the U.S. Sugar, meat, white flour, gasoline, alcohol, and cigarettes were rationed. So from 1945–50 we were in 1st place again. In 1970 we were in 41st. place. In 1978 we were in 83rd place. In 1981 we were 95th.

◆ *Milling Removes Vitamins And Minerals*

Today the wheat is ground in the STEEL ROLLER process which heats up the flour and removes a large amount of the valuable nutrients it contains. The first known cases of POLIO emerged after the steel roller mill process began a little over 100 years ago. In the old days the grain was ground in STONE MILLS, which revolved slowly and kept the flour at a low temperature. It maintained 75% of the vitamin B_1, while the modern process maintains no more than 10% of the vitamin B_1.

In the milling process the BRAN or outer coat is removed. It contains large amounts of vitamins and minerals and especially iron. Then the GERM is removed from the wheat. It is the very heart and life of the seed. It is one of the richest sources of vitamins B and E and contain valuable proteins and fat. Then the flour is bleached with CHLORINE DIOXIDE or NITROGEN TRICHLORIDE in order to age it. That is why this latter chemical is also called AGENE. This chemical ages the flour at once instead of waiting two or three weeks in order to age it naturally. By it a part of the protein of the flour is converted to a substance that is poisonous to all species of animals. BLEACHING increases the acidity of the flour, and it enables the miller to use inferior flours. It makes the flour pure white. Unbleached flour has a gray appearance. Bleached flour changes a good protein into a bad one which causes nervous instability, and it gives dogs FITS. In the past a little jingle was heard which said, "The whiter the bread, the sooner you're dead." Psychiatrists claim that bleached flour contributes to MENTAL DISEASES.

◆ *Commercial Bread Is Almost Unfit For Food*

When the bran and the germ is removed from the grain, this process removes some 20 natural vitamins and mineral elements. In the enrichment process 4 or 5 vitamins and minerals are replaced. But the vitamins that are replaced are synthetic vitamins which often do not have the same beneficial effect as natural vitamins. Experiments seemed to show that synthetic vitamin C does not cure SCURVY while natural vitamin C does. It has been found that commercial whole wheat bread that contains the wheat germ is a worse product than commercial white bread for the simple reason that the whole wheat flour must be treated with up to 400% more of the poisonous preservative chemicals than the white flour.

◆ How Not To Make Bread

When God gave us the grains to eat, He did not want us to take them apart, throw some of it away, and eat the rest. All foods should be eaten whole according to the way God made them with the proper preparation. We should not use fine flour. We are told that "FINE-FLOUR BREAD cannot impart to the system the nourishment that you will find in the unbolted wheat bread.... For use in bread-making, the super-fine white flour is not the best. Its use is neither healthful nor economical. Fine-flour bread is lacking in NUTRITIVE ELEMENTS to be found in bread made from whole wheat. It is a frequent cause of constipation and other unhealthful conditions" (CD320).

We should also not use SODIUM BICARBONATE, or the mixture called BAKING SODA in BREAD-MAKING. Mrs. White gives us the reason for this when she says, "The use of soda or baking powder in bread making is harmful and unnecessary. Soda causes inflammation of the stomach, and often poisons the entire system" (MH300). "HOT BISCUITS raised with soda or baking powder should never appear upon our tables. Such compounds are unfit to enter the stomach. Hot raised bread of any kind is DIFFICULT OF DIGESTION" (CD343). She says that they are breaking down the digestive system of tens of thousands. "Bread should never have the slightest taint of SOURNESS. It should be cooked until it is most thoroughly done. Thus all SOFTNESS and STICKINESS will be avoided.... bread two or three days old will be more healthful than fresh bread" (CD108). It can also be bought more cheaply.

◆ Baking An Essential Practical Art

We are told that "there is more religion in a good loaf of bread than many think."(CD316). She also says that "It is a religious duty for every Christian girl and woman to learn at once to make good, sweet, light bread from unbolted wheat flour. Mothers should take their daughters into the kitchen with them when very young, and teach them the art of cooking" (CD262). "Cooking is no mean science, and it is one of the most essential in practical life.... Scanty, ill-cooked food depraves the blood by weakening the blood-making organs. It deranges the system and brings on disease, with it accompaniment of irritable nerves and bad tempers. The victims of poor cookery are numbered by thousands. Over many graves might be written: 'Died because of poor cooking;' 'Died of an abused stomach'" (CD257)

◆ Bread And Disease

Many persons suffer from gastric irritation due to the large amounts of bran in whole wheat bread. Wheat is probably one of the greatest substances for causing allergic effects. Dr. R.H. Rowe checked on 500 persons with allergies. He found that at least of these allergies were caused by WHEAT. Bread is a common cause of HIVES, ECZEMA, and MIGRAINES. Dr. Alvarez of the Mayo Clinic said that according to allergists the commonest cause of migraines is wheat. Bread that has not been thoroughly baked, that is clammy and soured should not be placed in the human stomach. We are told that "Many have been brought to their death by eating heavy, sour bread" (CD318). The story is told of a girl who made a batch of sour, heavy bread. In order to get rid of them she threw them out to a couple of very large hogs. The next morning the hogs were found dead. Bread is an acid food, and one must be careful as to how much of it one is eating, and whether or not one is eating enough alkaline foods to balance the acid foods. Outside of meats and cheese, acid foods are FILBERTS, WALNUTS, CRANBERRIES, GRAINS, PLUMS, and PRUNES.

◆ Unleavened Bread

When Christ sat down at the Passover table, unleavened cakes were before him. When the Israelites celebrated the Passover in Egypt with the institution of the Feast of Unleavened Bread on the eve of their departure from Egypt, they also partook of unleavened bread. Such bread had a great significance. The use of such bread "was expressly enjoined in the law of the Passover, and as strictly observed by the Jews in their practice, that no leaven should be found in their houses during the feast" (PP278). Leaven was a symbol of sin, which was to be put away from all who would receive life and nourishment from Christ. Hence, the feast was to be kept with the unleavened bread of sincerity and truth. (1 Cor. 5:8). Today we are continuing the use of unleavened bread as the only correct representation of the Lord's Supper. (6BC1090).

◆ *The Bread Of Life*

"When we pray, 'Give us this day our daily bread', we ask for others as well as ourselves. And we acknowledge that what God gives us is not for ourselves alone. God gives us in trust, that we may feed the hungry. Such prayer includes not only food to sustain the body, but also that spiritual bread which will nourish the soul unto life everlasting. Christ says, 'I am the LIVING BREAD which came down from heaven: if any man eat of this bread, he shall live forever' " (MB111–2). Christ will see to it that none of his children go hungry. A comforting statement is the one that David made in Psalms 37:3, 25, "Trust in the Lord and do good; so shalt thou dwell in the land, and verily thou shalt be fed"...."I have been young, and now am old; yet I have not seen the righteous forsaken, nor his seed begging bread."

CHOLESTEROL, FATS, AND OILS

Cholesterol—An Important Body Substance

◆ *The Body Produces Its Own Cholesterol*

Cholesterol is a substance closely related to fats. and is widely distributed in animal tissues and occurs in various fats and oils, the yolk of eggs, nerve tissue, the liver, kidneys, and the adrenal glands. Various organs of the body can manufacture cholesterol as needed, such as MUSCLES, SKIN, and LIVER. The body can synthesize its own cholesterol from non-cholesterol containing foods. The less cholesterol a person eats, the more the body itself produces. The body's production of cholesterol is slowed down if the blood cholesterol level is increased by the cholesterol in the foods we eat. The KEY to keeping cholesterol from depositing where it is not wanted is to have UNSATURATED FATTY ACIDS from UNSATURATED FATS in your diet. Cholesterol is necessary for many body functions among them the formation of VITAMIN D, the SEX HORMONES, ADRENOCORTICAL HORMONES, and the BILE SALTS.

EXCESS FAT in the DIET increases blood cholesterol and causes the red blood cells to CLUMP. It thereby lowers the oxygen carrying capacity of the red blood cells which is a cause of ANGINA, RESPIRATORY INSUFFICIENCY, HEART DISEASE, PLAQUES, STROKE, CLAUDICATION, and GALLSTONES,

◆ *The Body Manufactures All HDL Lipoprotein Cholesterol*

There exists high density lipoprotein cholesterol (HDL), as well low density lipoprotein cholesterol (LDL). The HDL is the GOOD kind of cholesterol, and the LDL is the BAD kind of cholesterol. The body manufactures only the good kind of cholesterol. Oils, fats, and grease of animal origin contribute to the LDL cholesterol. According to the National Heart, Lung, and Blood Institute, your LDL level should be below 130mg%, your HDL level should be above 35mg%, and your total cholesterol level should be below 200mg%. It has been estimated that 1 gm of vitamin C per day could increase HDL levels by 8%.

The majority of cholesterol in the body is manufactured by the liver, and smaller amounts by the small intestines and the individual cells. The body produces between 1500 mg and 1800 mg every day. The average diet gives the individual between 200 mg and 800 mg daily. It has been shown many times that the cholesterol obtained from the diet has only a very low influence on the cholesterol in the blood. If you were to avoid any cholesterol in your diet, the body would still manufacture cholesterol at the rate of about 1 grams per day. Only or 20% of the cholesterol found in the body is derived from diet, the rest is made by the body.

◆ *Cholesterol Is Only Found In Products Of Animal Origin*

Animal fats — all of them, including MILK, BUTTER, the FAT in MEAT and so forth — contain cholesterol which appears to be responsible for HARDENING of the ARTERIES, HEART DISEASE, GALLSTONES, and so forth. Vegetable fats contain no cholesterol, but they contain unsaturated fatty acids, as opposed to the saturated fatty acids which are in foods of animal origin. Vegetable fats are also more easily digested than animal fats.

Cholesterol is absolutely essential to life. It is in every cell, and is vital for normal cellular metabolism. It is also necessary as a conductor for the nerves to transmit their impulses throughout the body, from and to the brain. It is also necessary for the production of a number of substances such as sex hormones and other steroids. Outside the body cholesterol is found only in products of ANIMAL ORIGIN, and is usually associated with ANIMAL FATS which are SATURATED fats, and which usually contain the LDL cholesterol. Foods high in animal-saturated fats are BUTTER, WHOLE MILK, CREAM, ICE CREAM, and CHEESE. So a VEGETARIAN could not get any cholesterol into his system, even though he may get the saturated fats of palm oil and coconut oil into his system.

◆ *Triglycerides*

TRIGLYCERIDES represent a combination of GLYCEROL and three FATTY ACIDS. They are produced in the liver from carbohydrates. They provide the body's major source of energy from fat. Most of the fat and oil we eat is composed of triglyceride molecules. Much of the fat, sugar or carbohydrates that we don't quickly burn as energy is converted to triglycerides and moved through the bloodstream to be stored. They become an independent risk factor for heart disease. In women over the age of 50, triglycerides are a better predictor of heart disease than LDL cholesterol according to Dr. Castelli, the medical director of the Framingham Heart Study. Experiments with pure air have shown that when animals are given a concentration of oxygen, they showed a decrease of triglycerides and cholesterol in their blood. On the other hand, when FAT was increased in the blood, the triglycerides were increased.

Low levels of triglycerides are a sign of good health, because they almost always occur with low levels of other fatty particles like CHOLESTEROL. The normal range is from 85 to 250mg%. Triglycerides increase after a meal. Eating sugary foods will raise the triglyceride levels significantly in some people, says Dr. Sheldon Reiser of the U.S. Department of Agriculture. There is good evidence that FISH OIL lowers triglyceride levels.

◆ *The Lecithin In Eggs Controls The Cholesterol*

Eggs, besides containing cholesterol, also contain LECITHIN, which is a cousin of the fat family. It is contained in all natural oils and in the FAT of egg yolk. Lecithin is a HOMOGENIZING AGENT capable of breaking fat and cholesterol into tiny particles which pass readily into the tissues, so that larger particles do not get stuck in the walls of the arteries. It is when cholesterol is not EMULSIFIED that it deposits on the artery walls. In egg yolk lecithin emulsifies the cholesterol to reduce its particle size, so that egg yolk alone should not be given as a cause of the hardening of the arteries. The word "lecithin" itself means "the yolk of an egg."

◆ *Cholesterol And Heart Attacks*

High concentrations of cholesterol in the blood is associated with HEART ATTACKS. In the Framingham study it was shown that men with an average of 260 milligrams (mg) of cholesterol per 100 milliliters (ml) of blood, indicated as 260mg%, were three times as likely to have heart attacks as men with a reading below 195mg. The average adult male cholesterol level in the U.S. is 210–220 mg, which is considered too high by the experts. There is a tendency on the part of the body to keep the relation between cholesterol and lecithin on a 1:1 constant relationship. If something occurs to cause a rise in cholesterol, the level of lecithin rises accordingly. If there is an UNBALANCED FOOD INTAKE for a long time, then the body is short on lecithin, and cholesterol, deprived of its biological mate, may be deposited where it is not wanted and may cause harmful disturbances.

◆ *Cholesterol And Drugs*

Many drugs cause false results when blood cholesterol is measured. CORTISONE and INSULIN will cause the blood cholesterol to go way up. Animals exposed to severe protracted cold have high cholesterol levels. When drugs are used to lower cholesterol levels, it is at times possible to measure an increased amount of cholesterol coming out of the body. In other instances one can show that an increased amount of cholesterol is being deposited in the heart and other organs as the blood cholesterol is reduced. The most recent long term studies reveal that even if the cholesterol is lowered through the use of drugs, there is no indication that there is a lessening of heart attack deaths. No one knows for sure if the use of these drugs might have a detrimental effect on the patient. The serenity of daily life in ROSETO, Pennsylvania, was the real reason for the virtual absence of heart attacks there, in spite of the fact that the people ate an excessive amount of saturated fats, were overweight, and smoked. The men of Roseto were the unchallenged heads of their households, and everyone had great civic pride. Most of all there was mutual support and understanding throughout the entire community.

◆ *How To Lower The Cholesterol In The Blood*

☛ NIACIN—NICOTINIC ACID—VITAMIN B_3—Various VITAMINS have been shown to lower blood cholesterol, but these vitamins must be taken in large amounts as compared to what is usually prescribed. Vitamins C and E are two such vitamins, but the one used the longest is NIACIN, which is NICOTINIC ACID or vitamin B_3. One study showed that niacin lowered the cholesterol level from 72% to 52%.

- VITAMIN C—ASCORBIC ACID—Vitamin C or ascorbic acid, definitely normalizes the cholesterol count of the blood stream. According to Dr. F.R. Klenner, results from the first intravenous injection of 500mg vitamin C show that the cholesterol count goes down towards normal. The hospital regime includes 500 mg in the morning and another 500 mg in the evening. Emil Ginter showed that vitamin C controls cholesterol, by converting it to BILE ACIDS, while Dr. Ralph Mussma of the University of Pennsylvania showed that vitamin C can increase cholesterol excretion. Take 1 to 3 gm per day.

- VITAMIN E—VITAMIN E performs an important service of retention of oxygen in the blood. A shortage of oxygen in the blood leads to an improper synthesis of PHOSPHOLIPIDS. With sufficient oxygen the proper distribution of cholesterol in the bloodstream is accomplished. The more polyunsaturated vegetables oils one eats, the more vitamin E is required in the diet. Processed polyunsaturated oils tend to lose much and sometimes all of their vitamin E, which also causes abnormal blood conditions. The excessive use of polyunsaturated oil, without sufficient vitamin E, destroys the red blood cells. Ancel Keys found that giving PECTIN to patients resulted in a decrease in the amount of cholesterol in the blood. It prevents SCAR TISSUE formation in burns, sores, and post-operative healing. It reduces the absorption of cholesterol from the intestines, thereby allowing the cholesterol to pass through the body to be excreted. Soluble fiber, especially of OAT BRAN and BEANS, flush cholesterol from the body. Dr. Paul D. White states that EXERCISE reduces the cholesterol level of the blood, and takes the fat out of the walls of the important arteries. Garlic, onions, avocados, and fish oils all decrease cholesterol levels. 400 to 800 IU per day are usually prescribed.

- EATING BREAKFAST—A government study of 12,000 people compared those who ate a ready-to-eat CEREAL and those who SKIPPED BREAKFAST. It was found that the cereal eaters had the lowest cholesterol by an average of 6.6 points.

◆ *Other Natural Ways For Lowering Cholesterol—*

- APPLES—eating apples daily has reduced cholesterol by 10%.
- BARLEY—lowers the liver's ability to produce cholesterol.
- BEANS—a cup of cooked beans per day has lowered cholesterol by 19%.
- CARROTS—eating 3 carrots per day has lowered cholesterol by 11%.
- CHILI PEPPER—is said to lower cholesterol.
- EGGPLANT—seems to block cholesterol from being used when fatty foods have been eaten.
- GARLIC—5 fresh cloves of garlic mixed with other food has lowered cholesterol by 10% in 25 days. Scientists at Loma Linda University fed 4 capsules of liquid garlic to patients with high cholesterol readings. 6 months later their cholesterol had dropped 44 points.
- GRAPEFRUIT PECTIN—Capsules of grapefruit pectin have reduced cholesterol by 8% in 4 months without adverse side effects. This pectin is just as effective as the anti-cholesterol drug CHOLESTYRAMINE which can cause a long list of problems.
- HERBS—The cholesterol reducing herbs are FENUGREEK, GINGER, and RED PEPPER.
- LECITHIN—1 ounce of lecithin daily has reduced cholesterol by 18%. The lecithin in egg yolk is largely saturated and therefore does not have the benefits of vegetable-source lecithin, such as from soybeans.
- YOGURT—3 cups of yogurt a day has reduced cholesterol levels by as much as 5% to 10% in a week.
- VITAMIN C—1000 mg daily has decreased cholesterol in one case from a reading of 230 to 140.
- OTHER FOODS—that have played a part in lowering cholesterol are SKIM MILK, OAT BRAN, OLIVE OIL, PLANTAINS (large green bananas), SEAWEED, KELP, and SOYBEANS.

☞ VEGETABLE DIET—A vegetable diet will reduce the cholesterol level 25% or more in 4 to 6 weeks.

Vegetable Oils Verses Animal Fats

✓ FAT—Fat is the carrier for the fat-soluble vitamins A, D, E, and K, as well as a source of essential fatty acids which are necessary for proper cell function. Fat has twice as many calories as protein and carbohydrates, which means that it develops twice as much heat in the body, and helps to maintain body temperature in cold weather better than proteins and carbohydrates. Eskimos consume a high proportion of animal fat in the form of seal oil, in their cold climate, but their largely one-sided nutrition gives them an average life span of hardly more than 30 years.

Lev. 7:23 says: "Ye shall eat no manner of fat, of OX, or of SHEEP, or of GOAT." This means no animal fat.

✓ POLYUNSATURATED OILS—Polyunsaturated vegetable fats include CORN OIL, COTTONSEED OIL, SAFFLOWER OIL, SESAME SEED OIL, SOYBEAN OIL, and SUNFLOWER OIL. Vegetable oils are rich in UNSATURATED FATTY ACIDS, vitamins F and E, and LECITHIN. The harmfulness of animal fat was recognized in the statement "It shall be the perpetual statute for your generations throughout all your dwellings, that ye eat neither fat nor blood." "BUTTER is less harmful when eaten on cold bread than when used in cooking; but, as a rule, it is better to dispense with it altogether" (CD349). However, we are also made aware that "the time will come when we may have to DISCARD some of the articles of diet we now use, such as MILK and CREAM and EGGS, but it is not necessary to bring upon ourselves perplexity by premature and extreme restrictions. Wait until the circumstances demand it, and the Lord prepares the way for it" (CD355–6). Disease among animals is increasing in proportion to the increase of wickedness among men (CD356). When oil is refined, it becomes virtually a pure chemical which is robbed of its associated nutrients. In this state it is likely to be eaten in excess. There is then in the diet too much fat and too little of vitamins, minerals, bulk, and fiber.

✓ MONOUNSATURATED FATS—OLIVE OIL and CANOLA OIL are considered to be the main monounsaturated fats. They are considered to be even better than polyunsaturated fats. We are told that "the oil, as eaten in the OLIVE is far preferable to animal oil or fat"(MH298). This statement recognizes the advantage of vegetable oil over animal fat.

✓ SATURATED FATS—These fats are mostly animal fats, except for COCONUT OIL and PALM OIL, which as vegetable oils are classified as saturated fats. Animal fats tend to develop heart disease, whereas unsaturated fats can reverse it. However, research has shown that HEATED UNSATURATED FATS can cause CANCER. COLON CANCER is due largely to high fat consumption. A high fat diet is proportional to the incidence of cancer in many countries. The average American gets 40% of his calories from fat, and if he eats out, the total can go as high as 70%. The suggestion has been made by various agencies that we reduce our fat intake to 30% or less. The IDEAL DIET is 10% fat, 10% protein, and 80% carbohydrates. The process of HYDROGENATION turns an unsaturated liquid oil into a saturated solid fat by adding hydrogen atoms to its chemical formula. This destroys most of the ESSENTIAL FATTY ACIDS. It has been found that hydrogenation can alter the cell membrane function so as to make them more permeable to carcinogenic substances.

All fat contains chains of carbon atoms. If the fat is saturated, the chain is straight. An unsaturated fat has at least one bend in it. But when manufacturers hydrogenate, or add hydrogen to it, some of the unsaturated fats become saturated. Others lose their bend and become what are called TRANS FATS with straight chains, like all saturated fats. These straight chain fats can fit closer together, which is what makes them MORE SOLID. Hydrogenated fat is less likely to become rancid. It can be reused many times for deep fat frying; it makes margarine spread more easily; and it makes baked goods tender and flaky. That is why companies like them. These straight chain fats have been found to raise your cholesterol quite a bit.

When animals eat a low fat diet of 5% of calories, they experience to the BREAST TUMORS of animals on higher fat diets. It has also been determined that women whose diets are lowest in fat have the lowest BREAST CANCER rates. The Japanese have half the breast cancer incidents in women than the Americans. They also consume only 20% or half of their calories in fat as compared to American women.

✓ RANCIDITY—The oxidation of fats turns them rancid. This forms free radicals which have been implicated in the development of CANCER, ARTHRITIS, CARDIOVASCULAR DISEASE, STROKE, and the AGING PROCESS. Rancid fat is also responsible for the destruction of the fat-soluble vitamins.

◆ *The Processing Of Fats—Heating*

The processing which various oils and fats go through before they appear on grocery shelves destroys the LECITHIN content, but leaves the CHOLESTEROL. In general we may say that all polyunsaturated vegetable oils are good foods for us to partake of. Through heat the polyunsaturated fats become more saturated, and their goodness vanishes to a large degree. THE LONGER A POLYUNSATURATED OIL IS HEATED, THE MORE DANGEROUS IT BECOMES. When heated UNSATURATED corn oil was fed to animals, the female animals had a 127% increase in BREAST CANCER. This also could explain a cause of breast cancer in women. In the same experiment, when heated SATURATED fat was fed to a similar group of animals, there was NO INCREASE in breast cancer, and these animals lived much longer. The reason is that saturated fats are not appreciably changed by heat, but unsaturated fats are. Dietary animal fat promotes and initiates CANCER. It increases BILE ACIDS and BILE STEROIDS, as well as ANAEROBIC BACTERIA in the colon which then form bile acid CARCINOGENS.

◆ *Use Cold-pressed Vegetable Oil*

A study of 6500 Chinese by Dr. T.C. Campbell of Cornell University, showed that while the Chinese averaged 2636 calories daily, and Americans averaged 2360 calories daily, the American diet was 3 times higher in calories from FAT. As a result, Americans have 5 times the incidence of BREAST CANCER.

High quality fresh, crude, and unrefined COLD-PRESSED VEGETABLE OILS are recommended as an addition to a wholesome diet. The average daily amount should not exceed 2 tablespoons. Vegetable oils are rich in UNSATURATED FATTY ACIDS. One must make sure that the oils are NOT RANCID. One can taste rancidity in oils, and one must also make sure that they are actually cold-pressed. Most oils so marked are not cold-pressed, but CHEMICALLY EXTRACTED or HEAT EXTRACTED. The safe cold-pressed oil is actually OLIVE OIL, SESAME OIL, or SUNFLOWER SEED OIL.

◆ *Heated Fats Neutralize Vitamin A*

Fats used in deep-fat-frying develop an anti-vitamin A factor when heated which destroys part of the vitamin A activity of foods eaten at the same time. Such people may suffer from a vitamin A deficiency, and a vitamin A deficiency is definitely known to be a factor in the cause of cancer. Reheating fats and oils also increases their rancidity, and increases free-radical activity as well as their carcinogenic potential. Hence it has been clearly established that all processed or commercial oils are carcinogenic, and MARGARINE is an ultra processed oil. It actually raises LDL cholesterol levels the same way that saturated fat does because of the HYDROGENATION PROCESS which converts liquid fats into solid fats. It does this by converting naturally occurring CIS-FATTY-ACIDS into TRANS-FATTY-ACIDS.

◆ *Hydrogenated Vegetable Oils Behave Like Animal Fats*

Dr. Kritchevsky has demonstrated that when CORN OIL is heated for no more than 15 minutes, and then fed to animals, it actually enhances rather than reduces ATHEROSCLEROSIS. Furthermore, when a polyunsaturated oil is heated, the oil forms a POLYMER, which is the same chemical formula connected into a long chain, which turns the oil into VARNISH. Animals that were fed such heated fats were found stuck to their cage floor by their varnish feces. Some suffered total intestinal obstruction. Now we can more clearly understand what the Spirit of Prophecy means by GREASE when it says, "You should keep grease out of your food" (CD200). It would mean largely heated vegetable oils.

According to Dr. Rosenvoldt of Hope, Idaho, HYDROGENATED vegetable oil behaves like animal fats. The fats were originally unsaturated essential fats, but when hydrogenated they lost their unsaturated essential qualities. Accordingly, the common solid cooking fats of vegetable origin may be almost as detrimental to the welfare of our arteries as the animal fats. Even the jar of peanut butter is now filled with hydrogenated peanut butter.

◆ *Vitamin E And Lecithin Removed From Processed Oils*

When oils are processed as cooking oils, VITAMIN E as well as LECITHIN is removed. Such removal will increase the oil's clarity as well as its keeping qualities or shelf life. What is then done with these nutrients is that doctors use them for treating HEART DISEASE which is caused to a large extent from eating the oils from which the vitamin E and lecithin have been taken away. Such oil can now be sold cheaper for it lasts almost indefinitely, and it is now affordable to almost everybody. As everybody now switches from the natural food to the "improved and fortified" version, nutritional deficiencies and illnesses will now begin to appear. Now there are two moneymaking products instead of just one, one of which even makes those modern day illnesses, which are caused by their deficiencies, to disappear. And the doctors in hospitals are kept busier curing those illnesses. The general public is getting sicker, but the hospitals are enlarging their facilities to take care of the greater onslaught of patients. This is the price we pay for "progress."

◆ *Monounsaturated Fats—Olive Oil*

MONOUNSATURATED fats are abundant in OLIVE OIL, CANOLA or RAPESEED OIL, SAFFLOWER OIL, SUNFLOWER OIL, AVOCADOS, and NUTS. Scientists are finding out that they are doing our arteries a lot of good. Canola oil contains a kind of fatty acid that is converted in the body to a type of fat abundant in fish oils. It has the second highest percentage of monounsaturated fat of any oil. Olive oil is the highest. In the U.S. heart disease is our greatest disease calamity. People living around the Mediterranean sea die from heart disease only half as often, even though they get about 40% of their calories from fat, the same as Americans. Scientists found that "monos" lowered cholesterol. The "monos" were found to lower the bad cholesterol while leaving the good kind in tact. The difference therefore between us and the Mediterranean people is the mainstay of their diet which is olive oil. Olive oil is about 75% monounsaturated fat. This confirms what the Spirit of Prophecy has told us about the benefits of olive oil (CD359–60). In a study of 8000 Italian men and women, those who used olive oil had lower BLOOD PRESSURES, as well as lower BLOOD SUGAR levels than those who used BUTTER or POLYUNSATURATED OIL. Monounsaturated oil is less likely than polyunsaturated oil to turn rancid.

A high fat consumption, when accompanied by plenty of essential nutrients does not cause arteriosclerosis or heart disease. The Masai men of Tanganyika live almost exclusively on milk and meat. They have low cholesterol levels, and give no evidence of arteriosclerotic heart disease. According to Dr. Rosenvoldt it has been shown in animal experiments that a deficiency in LINOLEIC ACID results in visible bleeding from the KIDNEYS and early death. Olive oil is rich in linoleic acid, and Mrs. White has said that it is a remedy for kidney disease (CD360).

Fish Oils

✓ THEY CONTAIN ESSENTIAL FATTY ACIDS—About 15 years ago two Danish medical doctors discovered, that Greenland Eskimos had very few heart attacks and deaths due to heart disease despite eating an extraordinarily high-fat diet. Their diet contains a large amount of the polyunsaturated OMEGA-3 essential fatty acid, especially two acids which are abbreviated as EPA and DHA. As essential fatty acids (EFA's), they cannot be made in the body and must be obtained from food. A high concentration of EFA's are found in the ocean plants called PLANKTON. Deep-sea fish such as SALMON, HERRING, and MACKEREL are especially rich in omega-3 EFA's. One study showed that a daily intake of fish oil reduced blood triglycerides by 64%, cholesterol by 8%, and diastolic blood pressure by 9%.

- ✓ OMEGA-3 HELPS THE HEALING PROCESS—OMEGA-3 fish oil helps the healing process by making the blood cells less sticky, and keeping them from piling up and blocking the artery. Increasing fish oil in the diet leads to a slight lowering of the LDL cholesterol, and it sometimes reduces high blood pressure as well. It also helps to cut down on arthritis discomfort, and even reduces the PAIN of MIGRAINE HEADACHES and even prevents them. Mice on omega-3 lived twice as long as normal mice, had half the normal inflammatory diseases, showed a complete absence of kidney disease, and had blood cholesterol levels half that of normal mice. Appreciable levels of omega-3, are contained in CANOLA OIL, RAPESEED OIL, and LINSEED OIL. Since fish were not in God's original diet, we can get omega-3 oil from WALNUTS, SOYBEANS, and COMMON BEANS.

  Fish oils, which are rich concentrates of polyunsaturated fatty acids and vitamin D, stimulate the lymphatic system. They energize the lymphocytes to release substances such as MACROPHAGES which devour the wastes and speed their elimination. The vitamin D from the fish oils increases the number of lymphocytes, accelerates the creation of antibodies, and manufactures a powerful cleanser known as INTERFERON.

- ✓ IT REDUCES DEATH FROM HEART DISEASE—The DEATH RATE of 2000 previous heart attack patients was reduced by 30% when they ate the essential fatty acid fish oil. The essential fatty acids also inhibit TUMOR GROWTH by increasing the oxidation of fatty acids in tumor tissue. Investigators feel that omega-3 fish oils exert their therapeutic effect in RHEUMATOID ARTHRITIS and PSORIASIS by suppressing the body's formation of interleukin-1 and the tumor necrosis factor, which are both mediators of inflammation. The director of the Framingham study, Dr. Castelli, stated that "The overall benefit of seafood is far better than chicken or turkey. EPA and DHA are not in chicken, and seafood doesn't have the saturated fatty acids of poultry.

- ✓ 4. IT SUPPRESSES PRE-CANCER GROWTHS—Studies have shown that fish oil consistently decreases the size of animal tumors, their number, as well as their tendency to spread. It also suppresses pre-cancer growths, as well as thwarting the spread of BREAST cancer after surgery and defeats the attempts of cells to metastasize.

PROTEIN AND MEAT

INSPIRATION AND A MEAT DIET

God's Original Diet Did Not Include Meat

God's original diet was a pure vegetarian diet. All of the food elements which were necessary for man's health and well-being were in this diet. God would not give man a diet which is somewhat devoid of vital elements. "God gave man no permission to eat animal food until after the flood" (CD373). Even so, those people who did not listen to God did eat animal food before the flood "until their cup of iniquity was full, and God cleansed the earth of its moral pollution by a flood" (CD373).

After the flood most of the people who did not acknowledge God continued to eat flesh food, and so God decided to allow them to continue to eat flesh food "to shorten their sinful lives" (CD373). As a result the race began to decrease in size, and length of years. Even then God allowed his people to eat only certain types of meat which he called clean meat, and of these meats, the eating of the fat and the blood was strictly forbidden (CD374). So today God wants His people to return to His original diet and "among those who are waiting for the coming of the Lord, MEAT EATING will eventually be done away with; flesh will cease to form a part of their diet" (CD380). Animal food is not the most healthful food for man (CD374), and it was never the best food (MH313). God wants us to take a firm stand against meat eating. We have been told for many years that if we desire to have PURE BLOOD and CLEAR MINDS, we must give up the use of flesh meat (CD383).

Meat is Secondhand Vegetables

We are told that "The diet of the animals is vegetables and grains. Must the vegetables be animalized, must they be incorporated into the system of animals, before we get them? Must we obtain our vegetable diet by eating the flesh of dead creatures?.... Those who eat flesh are but eating grains and vegetables second hand; for the animal receives from these things the nutrition that produces growth. The life that was in the grains and vegetables passes into the eater. We receive it by eating the flesh of the animal. How much better to get it direct by eating the food that God provided for our use" (CD396). "It is a mistake to suppose that muscular strength depends on the use of animal food. The needs of the system can be better supplied, and more vigorous health can be enjoyed without its use" (MH316).

The Composition Of Meat

"We are composed of what we eat. God's people are to take a firm stand against meat eating" (MM277–8). Meat contains many products of EXCRETION which are harmful. The chemical composition of BEEF BROTH is like that of human URINE. It has been known for a long time that a high protein diet is harmful to health. "Animal food shortens life" (4SpG121). One reason is that the breakdown of protein develops a lot of acids such as URIC, HIPPURIC, SULFURIC, and PHOSPHORIC acids. These acids are one of the basic causes of disease.

Pesticides are sprayed on plants, and on some of the plant that we eat. Animals eat the plants including the pesticides. The pesticides become part of the constitution of the animal. In the animal they are concentrated often more than 10 fold. Meat therefore becomes a concentrated source of pesticides, even though the pesticides are originally applied only to the food plants and grains that the animals eat.

What Meat Eating Does To Our Nature

We are told that "Not an ounce of flesh meat should enter our stomachs. The eating of flesh is UNNATURAL" (CD380). When the children of

Israel murmured in the wilderness because they were hungering for the fleshpots of Egypt, they said, "We shall DIE WITHOUT MEAT" (CD379). When God gave them the meat, they died WITH THE MEAT, because God's curse was with the gift of meat simply because His blessing was not on it. Since the directions given to Israel also apply to us today, and the warning is for us not to do as they did, we would have to say that God's curse is still on the eating of meat. To follow God's direction is for our own good. Mrs. White was shown that "the follies of Israel in the days of Samuel will be repeated among the people of God today, unless there is greater humility, less confidence in self, and more trust in the Lord God of Israel, the ruler of the people" (HL283).

We are told that meat is an unhealthful food. It "strengthens the appetites that war against the soul, developing the lower propensities. A diet of flesh meat tends to develop ANIMALISM. A development of animalism LESSENS SPIRITUALITY, rendering the mind incapable of understanding TRUTH" (CD382). Pythagoras said 2500 years ago, "Only living fresh foods can enable man to apprehend the truth." The ANIMAL NATURE is strengthened and the SPIRITUAL NATURE is weakened (CD383). The Bible admonishes us to "abstain from fleshly lusts that war against the soul" (1 Pet. 2:11). "Its use is contrary to the best development of the physical, mental, and moral powers" (CH477). It should also not be placed before our children, for "its influence is to excite and strengthen the lower passions, and has a tendency to deaden the MORAL POWERS" (CD389).

Meat Eating And Disease

We are told that "meat is the greatest disease breeder that can be introduced into the human system"(MM266). When the Israelites received their meat and ate it, a large number became sick and died. Eating meat today will make our BLOOD IMPURE, and many diseases follow from such impure blood. "God's curse is resting upon the animal creation. Many times when meat is eaten, it decays in the stomach, and CREATES DISEASE. CANCERS, TUMORS, and PULMONARY DISEASES are largely caused by meat eating" (CD383), and many die of disease caused wholly by meat eating.... Some of the processes of fattening animals for the market produce disease (CD385). Many HORMONES and DRUGS are used to fatten cattle for the market by putting them in their feed, and the people who eat the meat get them into their system. People who have ingested a lot of hormones from meat eating often have a PUFFY APPEARANCE. One of those drugs used for fattening cattle and chickens today is DIETHYL STILBESTROL, which has been shown to be a CARCINOGEN. It has produced cancer in humans who ate such meat. Hence we are told that "many die of disease caused wholly by meat eating" (2SM218). Flesh was NEVER THE BEST FOOD, but its use is now doubly objectionable, since disease in animals is so rapidly increasing (CD384).

Why Meat Is Not A Good Food

"Meat is not essential for health or strength, else the Lord made a mistake when He provided food for Adam and Eve before their fall" (CD395). The blood and flesh of the animals contain POISONS of the worst kind, and yet this fact is not realized (CD385). "Some are not immediately affected, while others are attacked with severe pain, and die from FEVER, CHOLERA or some unknown disease. In others it produces CRAMPS, CONVULSIONS, APOPLEXY, and SUDDEN DEATH" (CD386). But people do not realize that it is the meat that is doing this. One of the attractions of meat is that it is a NERVE STIMULANT, and can give a person a "HIGH" like TEA and COFFEE.

Dr. Visek of Cornell University implicated a high protein diet in the development of CANCER. He found that AMMONIA, which is a by-product of meat metabolism, is highly CARCINOGENIC, and can cause cancer development. A high protein diet also breaks down the pancreas and lowers our resistance to cancer, as well as contributing to the development of DIABETES.

The FLAVOR in meat is due to the presence of URIC ACID, which is the major cause of GOUT. Uric acid is one of the by-products of protein metabolism. It is poisonous to living tissues. When it is not properly removed from the body by the kidneys, it is often deposited in the kidneys and causes KIDNEY DISEASE. An excess also causes BLADDER STONES. A high protein diet is a high acid diet.

This thickens the blood and puts a strain on the arteries and the heart. The kidney of a dog, which we could say was created as a meat eater, has 10 times the capacity to eliminate uric acid from the system than has the human kidney. This fact suggests that the human body was not basically made for meat consumption.

Meat is also loaded with putrefactive bacteria. They often multiply readily so as to overpower the ACIDOPHILUS BACILLI which one is born with, and as a result the colon becomes constipated.

A Tenfold Liability To Take Disease

We are told that "The LIABILITY to take disease is increased TENFOLD by meat eating" (CD386). "Meat eating creates disease" (CD383). It develops a poor quality of blood and flesh, and produces a condition of INFLAMMATION in which the body is prepared to take on disease. (CD386–7). If life is in the blood, good blood, then death is in bad blood, and bad blood is what meat will give us. This is not the only problem according to Dr. Lloyd ROSENVOLDT, for in *Science and Modern Manna* he says, "Other problems arise because new diseases arise. Some diseases just appear. Often we do not know where they come from. They strike suddenly without warning." Mrs. White also speaks about unknown diseases being caused by meat eating (CD386). "People are continually eating flesh that is filled with TUBERCULOSIS and CANCEROUS GERMS. Tuberculosis, cancer, and other fatal diseases are thus communicated" (CD388). It has been estimated that there are 1 million decay producing bacteria in one gram of beefsteak, 31 million in beef liver, 75 million in ground beef, and 125 million in one gram of fish. This probably explains the strong odor of fish. With the reference to cancerous germs we would today probably speak of VIRUSES, for research has shown that viruses are one of the causes of cancer. Meat eating is not to be made a test in our church, but ministers are strongly requested to follow the principles of HEALTH REFORM in this regard as an example to others (CD401). "Many who are now only half converted on the question of meat eating will go from God's people to walk no more with them" (CH575).

KIDNEY DEGENERATION and BRIGHT'S DISEASE can be induced in rabbits and humans by the use of meat. Meat eating is especially harmful upon the kidneys. In Bright's disease the blood stream carries to the kidneys toxins that give rise to degenerative changes. Carnivorous animals avoid the flesh of other carnivorous animals, and prefer the purer meat of vegetarian animals. Meat eating can cause HYPERTROPHY, or enlargement of the LIVER, KIDNEYS, and the ADRENAL glands, and it gives rise to an increased incidence of NEOPLASMS or TUMORS, and a decreased life span.

The Use Of Eggs

We are told that eggs are less objectionable than meat and that they contain "properties which are remedial agencies in counteracting poisons" (CD204). If a person is physically weak, it is of benefit to him if he drops an EGG INTO GRAPE JUICE, and this combination will strengthen the body and supply the substances that are needed to build up the body. Because of the fact that disease is increasing among all animals according to the wickedness among men (CD366), in time eggs will need to be given up as part of our diet. We are told that "When the time comes that it is no longer safe to use MILK, CREAM, BUTTER, and EGGS, God will reveal this" (CD353). But while we are eating them they should not be classed with flesh meat (CD351). Eggs represent high quality protein. The white of the egg is almost 100% protein. That is no doubt the reason why the German word for protein is "eggwhite." It contains all of the ESSENTIAL AMINO ACIDS. The egg is the seed for a new life, and all of the nutrients necessary for such a new life are included in it. Aside from the protein, eggs are rich in all essential vitamins and minerals in the yolk, with the exception of vitamin C. Adelle Davis mentions a study at the Alameda County Hospital in which the fat from egg yolks equivalent to 36 eggs was given to patients daily, and their blood cholesterol never rose above normal. The reason is that the fat contains lecithin and the B vitamins CHOLINE and INOSITOL necessary for the proper use of cholesterol by the body.

Egg Yolk Contains Lecithin

It has been discovered that large amounts of

egg-white eaten every day produces illness. A substance in raw eggs called AVIDIN, destroys the B-vitamins in the intestinal tract, but cooking destroys the avidin. Egg yoke contains cholesterol which sometimes collects on the walls of the arteries and interferes with blood flow. This does not necessarily mean that too much cholesterol has been eaten, but it may indicate a disorder caused by an unbalanced diet. The egg YOLK also contains LECITHIN, a fatty substance upon which cholesterol depends to keep it in a state of emulsion so that it does not collect on the walls of the blood vessels, or form stones in the gall bladder. Lecithin is largely found in SEEDS. If you don't eat seeds, or if you eat foods from which the lecithin has been removed by processing, then cholesterol may collect in the arteries. Dr. Chen suggests that it may be possible to correct the condition of too much cholesterol in the blood with SOYBEAN LECITHIN. This should also improve HEART DISEASE and HARDENING of the ARTERIES. Apparently God intended for us to obtain a large part of our cholesterol from the body itself.

Cholesterol Without Lecithin Can Be Harmful

It can be harmful to eat cholesterol without the presence of lecithin. We are generally not getting enough lecithin from our food because the processing which fats and oils go through destroys the lecithin content, but leaves the cholesterol. Without the lecithin to emulsify it, cholesterol gathers in lumps. One researcher reported that giving lecithin and vitamin E to patients with DIABETES reduced their insulin requirement considerably, and their diabetes improved.

Almost everything you eat in a restaurant gives you cholesterol without lecithin. Hence, it is no wonder that hardening of the arteries, directly or indirectly, kills more Americans than any other disease. MARGARINE also goes through a dozen or so processes at high heat, which guarantees that no vitamins or lecithin remains in it. Margarine is made of polyunsaturated oils, and some of them are converted into saturated fats during the manufacture of the margarine, thereby negating some of advantages in terms of cancer risk.

MEAT EATING AND THE WORLD'S MORAL DILEMMA

Man Is Not Made For Meat Eating

The physiological makeup of man does not lend itself to the digestion of meat. Among the animal world MEAT EATING or CARNIVOROUS ANIMALS are constituted differently from herbivorous animals. Carnivorous animals possess a short digestive system which is 3 times the length of their bodies. This is so because flesh decays very rapidly, and the products of decay quickly poison the bloodstream if they remain too long in the body. Their stomachs have 10 times the amount of hydrochloric acid than herbivorous animals for the efficient digestion of meat. They do not have molars for grinding food. Unlike grains, flesh does not need to be chewed in the mouth to predigest it, for it is digested in the stomach and in the intestines. Meat eating animals also have an almost unlimited capacity for handling saturated fats and cholesterol.

Vegetarian animals have 24 molars for grinding food. They have much larger digestive systems which are 10 times the length of their bodies. The human digestive system is 12 times the length of the body.

The kidneys of meat eaters have to do 3 times the amount of work to eliminate poisonous nitrogen compounds such as UREA and URIC ACID. When the kidneys cannot handle all of the uric acid, it is deposited throughout the body. When it is in saturated form it crystallizes and settles in the joints to form ARTHRITIS. When it collects in the nerves it develops NEURITIS and SCIATICA.

Meat Is Low In Fiber

Meat is low in fiber, hence, it moves very slowly through the system, about 4 times slower than grains and vegetable foods. This fact makes chronic constipation a common ailment in our society. The natural fiber of vegetarian food is a significant deterrent of APPENDICITIS, CANCER OF THE COLON, HEART DISEASE, and OBESITY. The SCOTS who eat 20% more beef than the BRITISH also have 20% more cancer of the bowels. This is one of the world's highest rates of bowel cancer. The meat eating ESKIMOS have one of the shortest lifespan in the world.

Vegetarians Live Longer

In the U.S. 50% of the people are overweight, but on the average vegetarians weigh about 20 pounds less than meat eaters. They live longer, have lower incidence of heart disease, and a much lower rate of cancer. They are stronger, more agile, and have more endurance than meat eaters. Also the world's longest lived animals, the horse, the oxen, the buffalo, and the elephant are all vegetarians. The HUNZAS have one of the highest lifespan in the world. Besides them, those people who live on low protein or meat diets are the BULGARIANS, the RUSSIAN CAUCASIANS, the YUCATAN INDIANS, and the EAST INDIAN TODAS, also have the highest life expectancy in the world, from 90 to 100 years. Their diet consists mainly of whole grains, fresh fruit, vegetables, and goat's milk. Those people who live on high animal protein diets such as the ESKIMOS, the GREENLANDERS, the LAPPLANDERS, and the Russian KURGIS TRIBES have the lowest life expectancy in the world, from 30 to 40 years. Dr. McGarrison, a British general, who lived among the Hunzas for over 10 years, stated that he never saw a case of APPENDICITIS, COLITIS, or CANCER among them. He said "they know no sickness." They live up to 90, 100 and over a 100 years of age; are virile, strong, and active long after they have reached the usual three score and ten. Dr. A. Leaf related that the factors most responsible for the Hunzas long life expectancy are: 1. Their total low calorie diet of 1900 cal./day, and 2. their predominantly vegetarian diet. Their average daily intake of protein is about 30gm.

Vegetarianism Can Save The World

It has been estimated that if we conserved our grain supply and gave it to the poor and malnourished instead of to cattle, we could easily feed all of the chronically underfed people in the world. Today more than half of the world's population is hungry all the time, and nearly half of them are starving. The poor man's grain is being syphoned off to feed the rich man's cow. One author said that if we were all vegetarians, we could banish hunger from the earth. The grain that we feed to animals should be fed to hungry people. MAHATMA GHANDI said that the earth has enough for everyone's need, but not enough for everyone's greed.

One acre of land used to raise a steer will provide only about one pound of protein, This same acre of land planted in soybeans will produce 17 pounds of protein. Hence, raising animals for food is a tremendous waste of the world's resources. 80 to 90% of all the grain grown in the U.S. is used to feed meat animals. Eating meat therefore is one of the main problems of the world's food shortage. Because of eating meat, most people eat two to four times the recommended protein requirement, from 60 to 120 gm. The cost of one pound of meat is about 20 times higher than the cost of one pound of equally nutritious plant protein. Only 10% of the protein of the grain fed our livestock is recovered in the meat we eat. 90% goes down the drain. Raising food for a meat diet also uses 8 times as much water as growing vegetables and grains. Americans consume a ton or 2000 pounds of grain per person per year through the feed for meat-producing livestock, while the rest of the world averages about 400 pounds of grain or 20% of that amount

It appears that the world is destroying itself by means of the raising of cattle for meat, instead of using available land for the raising of vegetable food. The production of beef requires that a cow be fed 10 calories of grain and hay for every calorie of meat that is produced. A cow must be fed 21 pounds of plant protein in order to produce 1 pound of meat protein for human consumption. of our harvest acreage is fed to livestock so that in a single year 18 million tons of protein suitable for human consumption becomes inaccessible to man. Cows are the most inefficient producers of food nutrients. Frances Lapp has computed that an acre of cereals can produce 5 times more protein than an acre devoted to meat production. Legumes can produce 10 times more, leafy vegetables 15 times more, spinach 26 times more. Much land is wasted on producing non-nutritional MONEYMAKING crops such as COFFEE, TEA, RUBBER, COCOA, and FIBERS.

The American Attitude Toward Health is CURE-MINDED

Dr. Paava Airola in his book *Health Secrets From Europe,* says that Americans are basically CURE-MINDED, while Europeans are basically PREVENTION-MINDED. He had studied the health methods in both Europe and the U.S., by spending half of his life in each. A cure-minded person does not worry about his health until he gets sick. A prevention-minded person is concerned about preserving his health and preventing disease while he is well by his own effort. He says that we are always looking for some CHEMICAL AGENT which will cure or control the disease. European research is directed largely toward the discovery of the CAUSATIVE FACTORS of disease and in finding the means of preventing the causes. In the past we have largely ignored NUTRITION as the possible CAUSATIVE as well as PREVENTIVE and CURATIVE FACTOR in disease. When during Ingathering time I knocked on a door and handed the person one of our magazines dealing with nutrition and cancer, the person responded by saying, "I don't believe that diet has anything to do with cancer," when as a matter of fact it has a great deal to do with cancer. ARTHRITIS, PROSTATE PROBLEMS, COLDS, HIGH BLOOD PRESSURE, MULTIPLE SCLEROSIS, ULCERS, PSORIASIS, MISCARRIAGES, and HEART DISEASE are a few of the diseases European doctors treat with dietetic restrictions and vitamin-mineral therapies.

Our View Of Health Is ADOLESCENT

We believe that the reason for our view of health can be found in the fact that as a nation, and as far as the life of a nation goes, we are a relatively young nation with young ideas. This is indicated by the fact that when a group of men get together, they call each other "boys," and when a group of women get together they call each other "girls" regardless of age. If we take as a rule of thumb the idea that 10 years in the life of a nation is equivalent to 1 year in the life of a person, then as a nation we are about 20 or 21 years of age, just growing out of adolescence. In Europe many nations have existed from 700 to a 1000 years. Now a young person doesn't think about PREVENTION. He takes things as they come and reacts to them on the spot. In medicine this means that we don't do much about maintaining our physical well-being until we get sick, and then we want something that will quickly relieve us of our discomfort. Drugs are the substances that can quickly relieve us of such discomfort, but cannot cure us of what ails us.

Knowledge Is The Basis Of Prevention

To practice prevention takes KNOWLEDGE, a lot of knowledge. In prevention we must perceive the cause and effect relations between what we do and the future effect of our actions, and this causal relation a young person does not as yet perceive. It is wisdom for us to perceive the future effect of our present action. One basic way in which such wisdom is obtained is to have had many experiences in the past from which to learn such relationships. But many experiences of living take time to happen and to be experienced. That is why we say that wisdom comes with age, and the young do not have as yet the experiences in their background from which to draw such wisdom. Such wisdom is the result of many repetitive experiences from which we learn the fundamental facts of life. An American author by the name of Van Wyke Brooks once said, "Of all the good qualities which Americans possess, WISDOM is not one of them."

Medical Facilities Created By Wealth Do Not Create Health

In spite of spending billions of dollars on health care, having more hospitals, being served by more physicians per capita, using more synthetic drugs, having the finest medical scientists working in the most elaborately equipped laboratories, endowed by great wealth, in the most magnificent educational and research centers found anywhere, yet more than 40% of the nation's potential military manpower had to be rejected for physical unfitness. 9 million men of military age were unfit to serve in World War I

It is estimated that there are still over 80 million chronically ill people in the U.S. This situation seems to be getting worse with every passing year. There seems to be an epidemic increase in such diseases as HEART DISEASE, CANCER, ARTHRITIS, ALLERGIES, MULTIPLE SCLEROSIS, and BIRTH DEFECTS. Our mortality rate is higher than that of most civilized countries, and in life expectancy the U.S. ranks 22nd for men and 10th for women. Some scientists call the health conditions in the U.S. catastrophic. Only half of American households are found to have an adequate diet, and the other half are perhaps overfed but undernourished.

Pure Chemicals Do Not Develop And Maintain Health

Why should this be in a country which has the best medical system in the world and the most abundant food supply? The causes can be found in the form of devitalized, factory produced, and chemicalized food, loaded with poisonous residues from additives and pesticides. To this can be added the physical surroundings in the cities which are often a peril to health. There is the prevalence of the air poisoned with deadly chemicals, polluted water, unhealthful dwellings, and the great consumption of toxic drugs. All of these give us most of the reasons for the nutritional state of affairs. Chemical fertilizers have depleted our soil, and although the quantity of crops still remains high, the nutritional quality of foods produced on depleted soil is lowered.

The end result of CHEMICAL FARMING METHODS is always disease; first in the LAND itself, then in the PLANTS, then in the ANIMALS, and then in MAN. SYNTHETIC FERTILIZERS stimulate plant growth and force-feed the plants, creating an imbalance and producing a bloated product. Vegetables grow fast and large, but they lack many of the essential elements. Their quality is low. Plants treated with chemical fertilizers are more susceptible to PESTS and DISEASE.

In addition to pesticides, our foods are loaded with toxic chemicals which are added during processing. They are PRESERVATIVES, DYES, BLEACHES, MOISTENERS, ACIDIFIERS, ALKALIZERS, EMULSIFIERS, and others too numerous to mention. Many of these are harmful and unfit for human consumption. The air in our larger cities is polluted by the poisonous gases from automobiles and industries, and has become a major health hazard. Our water is as unfit for drinking as our air is for breathing. Almost half of the American public is drinking fluoridated water in spite of the mounting evidence of the toxic effect of the sodium fluoride added to it. Aerosol cans of various cleaning and utility products, give off a fine mist of toxic chemicals. Use instead the pump versions of the same products.

HOUSE PLANTS help clean the indoor air. 15 to 20 plants would do the work of a high efficiency air cleaner. They can clear FORMALDEHYDE fumes from new carpeting, BENZINE and CARBON MONOXIDE from the air. PHILODENDRONS are very good at this, also ALOE VERA, PEACE LILIES, SNAKE PLANT, POTTED IVY, and CORN PLANT (dracaena).

THE BODY'S NEED FOR PROTEIN

The American Protein Craze

When Dr. Aly of Sweden returned from one of his American lecture tours he was asked about his most memorable experience on his trip. He said that it was the AMERICAN HIGH PROTEIN CRAZE. After his lectures people would look closely at his face to see if he had rouge on it. They couldn't believe that a man could look so healthy without eating meat. They kept asking, "But where do you get your protein?"

All Foods Contain Some Protein

All disease is due in some measure to ENERVATION and LOWERED RESISTANCE caused by wrong food consumption—excess food, deficient food, incompatible food, and acid-forming food. Restoration is produced by right food—vital food, balanced food, building food, and healing food. Any form of illness indicates a disturbed state of body chemistry, generally an acid state. Correcting this state should be done with food, not drugs.

It is a scientific fact that our bodies are made up largely of protein. Does this mean that we need to eat a lot of protein in order to supply the needs of the body? Hardly. Nevertheless, protein is necessary for good nutrition. Every plant, every vegetable, every fruit, every seed, every nut contains some protein. On the average fruits contain about 1% protein, and vegetables average somewhat over 3% protein. Meats have about 17% protein, while soybeans have up to 40% protein, lentils 25%, lettuce 1.2%, orange .9%, peach .5%, potatoes 2% etc. Researchers from all over the world have studied the need for protein in our diet and have come to the conclusion that on the average 30gm of protein or 1 ounce a day is sufficient for the average person's needs. In the U.S. the average person gets 71% of his protein from meat, in Russia the people get only 25% of their protein from meat.

It is difficult to eat any natural food, no matter what it is, that does not have protein in it. If it is deficient in amino acids, it does not matter. The body only requires about one ounce per day, and if its requirement for essential amino acids is not in the food supply, it makes them up by scrapping its own metabolic wastes. The body is not only very provident, but it is also very conservative of its resources. The AMINO ACIDS produced from the breakdown of body proteins are re-utilized by the body and are combined again to form new PROTEINS. The nonessential amino acids can be synthesized within the body. One can fast many weeks in accord with our capacities, and the body suffers no protein deficiencies, no vitamin C deficiency, or any other deficiency. Rather it is more likely to restore balance and to correct deficient conditions under a fast than when eating. The witness to this is the nearly 100% restoration of SCHIZOPHRENICS to mental wholesomeness through fasting. Researchers say that schizophrenia is a disease of protein imbalance in the brain.

Raw Protein Is Better Than Cooked Protein

If a person ate 3 pounds of potatoes during one day, he would supply the body's need for protein for that day. Potatoes have complete proteins. Many other vegetables, grains, and nuts have complete proteins such as SOYBEANS, SESAME, PUMPKIN, SUNFLOWER SEEDS, ALMONDS, MILLET, AND GREEN VEGETABLES. You need less protein if you obtain it from RAW VEGETABLE sources than if you obtain it from meat sources. RAW PROTEINS have a higher biological value than COOKED PROTEINS. You need only the amount of protein if you eat raw vegetable proteins as compared with cooking them. Furthermore, raw protein is utilized twice as well as cooked protein. Several foods with incomplete proteins will COMPLEMENT one another if eaten at the same time to produce a result that represents complete protein. Also some seeds and grains which do not contain complete proteins, become complete proteins after they are SPROUTED. Vegetable proteins were formerly believed to be incomplete and inferior to animal proteins, but are actually biologically as good or better than animal proteins. For example, the protein in POTATOES is biologically SUPERIOR to that of meat, eggs, and milk. Studies in Germany showed that the performance of athletes improved after they switched from a daily 100gm animal protein diet to a 50gm vegetable protein diet. Proteins in excess of body needs are burned as fuel for energy, and as an energy food proteins are inferior to carbohydrates and fats.

Balancing The Amino Acids

AMINO ACIDS are the building blocks of which PROTEINS are constructed, and they are the end-products of protein digestion. When it comes to getting a sufficient amount of especially the essential amino acids, it is not necessary to get a balance of them at the same meal. It is necessary only to get a balance of all of the amino acids for all of the meals on the same day, because the body has internal reserves of amino acids. Most vegetarians who eat a wide range of food have no real problems in meeting their protein requirements. A rule of thumb is to get about 50–60% of calories from complex carbohydrates, no more than 30% from fat, and about 15% from proteins.

How To Obtain Complete Proteins

The foods of animal origin are considered "complete" with regard to proteins because they contain all of the ESSENTIAL AMINO ACIDS, which are the amino acids which we must obtain from food because the body does not manufacture them. Many plant foods also have complete proteins such as ALMONDS, SESAME SEEDS, SOYBEANS, BUCKWHEAT, PEANUTS, SUNFLOWER SEEDS, PUMPKIN SEEDS, POTATOES, and all LEAFY GREEN VEGETABLES. Those which are considered "incomplete" have some but not all of the essential amino acids. By combining plant foods in the same dish, it is possible to make the dish have complete proteins. An example is beans-and-grains, or specifically beans-and-rice, which is a dish that is popular in various parts of the world where animal foods are in short supply. The proteins in grains such as rice are deficient in the essential amino acids LYSINE and ISOLEUCINE but contain sufficient amounts of the essential amino acids TRYPTOPHAN, METHIONINE, and CYSTEINE; the proteins in beans are exactly the opposite. When we put them together in the same dish they represent complete proteins. Other "complete" combinations are lentils-and-barley, couscous-and-chick-peas.

The Benefits Of a Low Protein Diet

The digestion of protein in excess of metabolic need leaves toxic waste products which contribute to self-intoxication and disease. One of the by-products of protein metabolism is AMMONIA, which is considered to be a strong CARCINOGEN. Too much protein also causes mental disorders such as SCHIZOPHRENIA, as well as severe deficiencies of vitamins B_3, B_6, and MAGNESIUM. Protein metabolism results in higher blood content of URIC ACID, UREA, and PURINES which have a toxic, paralyzing effect on muscles and nerves. Protein insufficiency is almost unheard of in developed societies. Even in undeveloped societies, the major dietary problem is usually not related to getting enough protein, but rather in getting enough calories. Protein insufficiency in the absence of calorie insufficiency is very rare.

Excess Animal Protein Acidifies The Blood

Vegetable protein yields a greater percentage of ALKALIES and is low in bacterial content. Animal protein yields a greater percentage of ACIDS with a high bacterial count, and has a greater tendency to putrefaction. A diet high in animal protein content acidifies the blood much as sugar does, and an acidified blood will dissolve CALCIUM from the bones. The more protein is eaten the more calcium is excreted. The urine of a potato eater is almost ALKALINE; that of a meat eater is highly ACID, as a result it has been determined that POTATO URINE will dissolve URIC acid. Vegetable proteins have only one half the putrefactive effect of animal protein. The proteins of CEREALS and LEGUMES were found to be the least putrefactive of all proteins.

Animal protein introduces URIC ACID into the blood due to the preformed uric acid they contain, and due to the uric acid they form in the system in the course of their metabolism. This explains the observation made by westerners in Hong Kong harbor where the little Chinese coolies carry 200-pound rice bags all day long, eating nothing but rice and vegetables. Asked why they don't eat meat, one of them said, "If I ate meat I would not be able to carry these bags all day long." Meat eating leads to the desire for TOBACCO, the effect of which is to cause a temporary precipitation of the excessive uric acid formed in the blood, thus relieving distress and creating a false sense of ease and well-being. It is the URIC ACID that gives the flavor to meat.

Adventists Live Longer Than The General Population

In the study conducted by Dr.'s Lemon and Walden of those Adventists in the State of California who had died, it was determined that Adventists as a group have better health and live longer than people in the the general population by 5 to 6 years. 70% fewer Adventists die from all types of CANCER, 68% fewer from RESPIRATORY DISEASES, 88% fewer from TB, and 85% fewer from PULMONARY EMPHYSEMA. Our rate of LUNG CANCER is practically zero. Research revealed that there had been only 9 cases of CANCER OF THE LUNG, and each of these had at some time been a smoker. Adventists have 46% less STROKES, and 60% less HEART DISEASE. Our rate of CORONARY disease is 40% less than the general population. The SDA mortality rate from all causes is two times lower than that among the general population. In a study in Colorado SDA children were shown to have 50% fewer cavities than other children in the area. A by-product of Adventist abstinence from ALCOHOL is the fact that they have only about 35% as many accidents. All of these advantages in health may be due to the fact that 50% of Adventists are VEGETARIANS.

Vegetarians Have More Endurance than Meat Eaters

Studies have shown that ENDURANCE increases with a lower protein intake, and that the endurance of vegetarians surpasses that of meat-eaters. A high natural carbohydrate/low animal protein diet holds the greatest potential for optimum health. Tests show that a low protein vegetarian diet can prevent 97% of CORONARY OCCLUSIONS. Studies in the tropics have shown that the majority of digestive disorders such as DYSPEPSIA, DIAR-

RHEA, and DYSENTERY, are caused by overeating, and that APPENDICITIS is caused largely by fermentation after excessive eating of meat. CENTENARIANS are low protein eating people. The Bulgarians have 1600 centenarians to every million population as compared to 9 in the U.S. and 50 in Russia. Their diet consists largely of BLACK BREAD, RYE, BARLEY, VEGETABLES, and SOURED MILK in the form of YOGURT and KEFIR. They eat little meat.

Results Of A High Protein Diet

The metabolism of proteins consumed in excess of the actual need leaves TOXIC RESIDUES of METABOLIC WASTES in the tissues, causing AUTOTOXEMIA, OVERACIDITY, NUTRITIONAL DEFICIENCIES, accumulation of URIC ACID and PURINES in the tissues, INTESTINAL PUTREFACTION, and contributes to the development of many of our most common and serious diseases, such as ARTHRITIS, KIDNEY DAMAGE, PYORRHEA, SCHIZOPHRENIA, OSTEOPOROSIS, ATHEROSCLEROSIS, HEART DISEASE, and CANCER. It also causes PREMATURE AGING and a lower LIFE EXPECTANCY.

Research by Dr. Lennart Krook shows that overindulgence in meat leads to a mineral imbalance in the system — too much PHOSPHORUS and too little CALCIUM, for meat has 20 times more phosphorus than calcium, which leads to severe CALCIUM DEFICIENCY, and a resultant loss of teeth or PYORRHEA. Another study showed that the more meat you eat the more deficient you become in VITAMIN B_6, as well as in MAGNESIUM, CALCIUM, and NIACIN or Vitamin B_3. MENTAL ILLNESS and SCHIZOPHRENIA are often caused by a niacin deficiency, and have been successfully treated with high doses of niacin.

Protein From Soybeans

Soybean Proteins contain all of the essential AMINO ACIDS in good proportion. That is why they can take the place of meat, eggs, fish, and milk. They are richer in POTASSIUM than any other food except brewer's yeast. They contain more PANTOTHENIC ACID than any other food except egg yolk, brewers yeast, rice bran, wheat bran, and liver. The IRON in soybeans is 96% available, that is, digestible and used by the body. The OIL in soybeans is 51.5% LINOLEIC ACID, the fatty acid which is believed to be most effective in emulsifying CHOLESTEROL in the blood so that it does not form unhealthful deposits. The CALCIUM in soybeans is as well digested as is that of milk.

Soybeans yield more protein per acre than any other crop. One acre of soybeans will provide the requirement of protein for one person for 2224 days according to Rodale, while peanuts will provide 1785 days of protein requirement. Crude soybean oil is our best source of LECITHIN at present. Lecithin is the substance which emulsifies fats. Soybean lecithin has been shown to reduce blood cholesterol, and is believed to help ameliorate CORONARY disease and ARTERIOSCLEROSIS. Soybeans contain twice as much FIRST CLASS PROTEIN as meat, four times that of EGGS and WHEAT, five or six times that of BREAD, twice that of lima and navy beans, and most nuts, and twelve times that of milk. They will keep for years without spoiling. They are easily prepared into almost any kind of dish for any course of a meal. They have large amounts of iron and other minerals, as well as B-vitamins and vitamin E. They are rich in unsaturated fatty acids which keep CHOLESTEROL in its place so that it will not settle as harmful deposits in the GALL BLADDER, KIDNEYS, or BLOOD VESSELS.

The Relation Between Protein, Carbohydrates, And Fluid Intake

One author has used MOTHER'S MILK as a standard of relationships between food substances. If we use it as a standard for the sake of illustration, then the ratio between its protein and carbohydrate content by weight is 1:8, one part of protein to eight parts of carbohydrate. The amount of WATER in meat is only TWICE the amount of PROTEIN (2:1). The amount of water in mother's milk is 80 times the amount of protein (80:1). We can now see why diets high in protein, especially animal protein, recommend the drinking of 8 glasses or more of water a day. It is to flush out the kidneys. VEGETARIANS do not need that much additional water in their diets because plant foods already contain a very high proportion of water. COOKED BEANS, for example, have 13 times as much water as protein.

Now we can also see why a high protein diet creates a craving for carbohydrates, especially sweets or sugar products. Proteins need 8 times their weight in carbohydrates, in order to create a balance, and the amount of carbohydrates in meat is practically ZERO. We can also see the reason why some people seem to be able to live on a diet of hamburgers and candy bars, for the carbohydrates in the candy bars will balance the protein in the hamburgers, even though such a combination represents otherwise very poor nutrition due to the absence of many vitamins and minerals. Speaking of minerals, a high protein diet will also deplete the body of minerals and especially of CALCIUM.

Why Adventists Substitute Sweets For Meat

Now we can also see that when ADVENTISTS give up meat, they may overemphasize desserts. A craving for SWEETS, accompanied by a craving for FATS signals a protein deficiency. People who switch to a vegetarian diet crave SWEETS, BREAD, BUTTER, PEANUT BUTTER, and NUTS. Such a craving disappears when more protein foods, such as BEANS, are added to the diet. An excess of ALKALIZING FOODS such as fruits, vegetables, salads, and potatoes, will create a demand for ACID-FORMING FOODS. Since the acid-forming food of meats has been discarded, often sweet products will replace them, since they are acid-forming. A meal with 30gm of proteins demands about 240gm of carbohydrates. If the carbohydrates are not supplied by bread, beans, grains, or starchy vegetables, a craving for sugared desserts is almost inevitable. This is exactly what the Spirit of Prophecy tells us in the following statement, "When flesh food is discarded, its place should be supplied with a variety of grains, nuts, vegetables, and fruits, that will be both nourishing and appetizing" (CD315).

If enough complex carbohydrates are supplied by the main meal, a dessert often becomes less attractive. A similar logic presents itself in the combining of MILK and SUGAR products such as ice-cream. The protein-carbohydrate ratio in cow's milk is 2:3, when it should be 2:16 or 1:8. This means that a lot of sugar with milk will bring it closer to the balance of the ideal ratio. But the high amount of refined sugar will create a deficiency in vitamins and minerals. So again the counsel is correct that the free use of milk and sugar should be avoided.

Protein Consumption And Aging

Two doctors, Schwartz and Bircher, of Germany and Switzerland, have reported that the aging process is triggered by AMYLOID, a by-product of protein metabolism. This explains why people who traditionally eat low protein diets such as the HUNZAKUTS, BULGARIANS, RUSSIAN CAUCASIANS, YUCATAN INDIANS, and EAST INDIAN TODAS, also have the highest average LIFE EXPECTANCY in the world, from 90 to 100 years. Also too much animal protein leads to PREMATURE AGING by causing a BIOCHEMICAL IMBALANCE, OVERACIDITY in the tissues, INTESTINAL PUTREFACTION, CONSTIPATION, and DEGENERATION of the vital organs. This also explains why the people who live on high animal protein diets, such as the ESKIMOS, GREENLANDERS, LAPPLANDERS, and RUSSIAN KURGIS TRIBES, have the lowest life expectancy in the world, from 30 to 40 years. Americans lead the industrialized world in per capita meat consumption, and they are also in 21st place in life expectancy among industrialized nations.

VITAMINS

Vitamins Are Organic Food Substances

◆ *Vitamins are Catalysts For All Living Cells*

As catalysts vitamins speed up the processes in all living cells, plant and animal. They are food substances contained in all living organisms and as such are absolutely necessary for proper growth and maintenance of health. PLANTS manufacture their own vitamins. ANIMALS obtain theirs from eating plants or other animals that eat plants. Like hormones they regulate body processes. Their presence or absence even in very small amounts may mean the difference between good and bad health. They combine chemically with OXYGEN, ENZYMES, MINERALS, and HORMONES to form other chemical compounds. If vitamins are not present then certain chemical reactions will not take place. All vitamins are SYNERGISTIC in their action: that is, they are more effective when taken simultaneously.

From the standpoint of SOLUBILITY, there are two different types of vitamins—those that can be dissolved in FATS, and those that can be dissolved in WATER. All vitamins found in liver and eggs are FAT-SOLUBLE, and those that are in fruits and vegetables are WATER-SOLUBLE. One reason why fat-soluble vitamins are expressed in INTERNATIONAL UNITS (IU) is that each of them consists of several compounds. Thus one IU of vitamin A includes RETINOL, some RETINYL ACETATE, and some CAROTENE. The IU is a measured amount of each of these three substances.

There are two forms of vitamin E, the NATURAL and the SYNTHETIC form. The natural form is D-ALPHA TOCOPHEROL, and the synthetic is called DL-ALPHA TOCOPHEROL. One IU of the synthetic form equals 1 mg, but 1 IU of the natural form equals 1 mg. In tests the natural vitamin E was found to be 3 times as potent as the synthetic vitamin E.

The only potentially natural toxic vitamins quantitatively speaking are the fat soluble vitamins A, D, and K. The safe upper limit of vitamin A is 300,000 U.S. Pharmacopeia or USP units. The limit of vitamin D is 80,000 U.S.P. units, and of vitamin K is 12 mg.

◆ *The Need For Vitamins In Health*

When man began to mill flour to make white bread, a lot of diseases cropped up which could only be explained by something that was missing from the food people were eating. When scientists began to search for this important missing link, they discovered vitamins. The name comes from VITA, meaning life, and AMINES—which are chemical compounds that were originally thought to be vitamins. When it comes to eating, especially vegetable foods, it is best to eat them whole as they come from the garden without much cooking or processing. However, in this day of the world's history there seems to have developed in the modern diet a need for vitamins above the amount that is eaten in the food. There seems to exist a need for taking vitamin supplements because the vitamin content of our food has been reduced for the following reasons: 1. SOIL DEPLETION due to modern methods of farming; 2. The increasing use of TOXIC PESTICIDES on crops; 3. The PROCESSING and CHEMICALIZING of our food; 4. the overuse of PURE SUGAR up to of all of our calories; 5. the CHEMICAL ADDITIVES put in our food.

◆ *Kitchen Handling Can Destroy Vitamins*

We need more vitamins because of the way we destroy them in the kitchen. When we pick up a CARROT we throw away the GREEN TOP which has greater nutritional value than the root, for it contains additional vitamin K. STORING the carrot for some time causes it to lose vitamins. SCRAPING the skin loses a large part of the minerals. SOAKING it causes a loss of natural sugar, all of the B-vitamins, vitamins C and P, and many of the minerals except calcium. If the carrot is

SHREDDED there is a loss of 20% vitamin C, and another 20% if allowed to stand for an hour before eating, which loss is due to oxidation. Cooking destroys vitamin C, and if salt is placed in the water, the greatest loss of vitamin C occurs. If the carrot is frozen and thawed, more vitamin C is lost. So not many vitamins are left which you can pick up with a knife and fork. Furthermore, the decline of almost 20% in our consumption of green and yellow vegetables can have a drastic effect on the amount of vitamin A we get.

◆ *Drugs And Chemicals Destroy Vitamins*

We know that the drugs of PENICILLIN and CHLOROMYCETIN destroy NIACIN. ARSENIC and SULFA COMPOUNDS destroy PARA-AMINOBENZOIC ACID a B-vitamin. MINERAL OIL destroys vitamins A, D, and K. FLUORIDES destroy the enzyme PHOSPHATASE upon which many vital body processes depend. Americans by the millions are using these drugs regularly, and so for them there is a great need to restore the vitamins which they have removed from their bodies, and we hope that none of our Adventists are using these drugs.

Many chemicals in our environment destroy or inactivate vitamins, such as CARBON DIOXIDE and CARBON MONOXIDE from car exhausts, SULFUR COMPOUNDS from chimney smoke, TOBACCO SMOKE, a miscellaneous poison in the air. In SELF-DEFENSE we must take extra B and C vitamins, as these are known to aid in excreting poisons from the body. In factories food is BLEACHED, COLORED, DEHYDRATED, HYDROLIZED, HOMOGENIZED, GASSED, EMULSIFIED, PASTEURIZED, HEATED, AND CHEMICALIZED. Some of the toxic qualities of these processes are known to destroy vitamins. We also absorb many elements harmful to vitamins in our drinking water, such as CHLORINE, FLUORINE, ALUMINUM, SULFATES, CARBON, LIME, and others. COFFEE drains some of the B-vitamins out of our body. Also artificial sweets cut down on B-vitamins.

The Sources Of Vitamins

Vitamins occur naturally in all foods. A food rich in carbohydrates contains plenty of vitamins and minerals necessary for processing that carbohydrate. The same is true of protein foods and fatty foods. All vitamins are needed in only extremely small amounts. It is for the most part impossible to relate any one vitamin to any one disease, except for those disorders which we know are directly caused by a shortage of some vitamin. SCURVY results from a lack of vitamin C; RICKETS from a lack of vitamin D; PELLAGRA from a deficiency of niacin(B_3), BERIBERI from a lack of thiamin(B_1) NIGHT BLINDNESS results from lack of vitamin A. The GREEN LEAVES of plants are the laboratories in which plant vitamins are manufactured. They are therefore full of vitamins. SEEDS contain the vitamins which the plant has stored there to nourish the next generation of plants. The organs of animals contain vitamins which the animal's digestive system has stored there. The YOLK of eggs contain vitamins which the mother animal provides for the use of her young. Fish store vitamins in their LIVERS.

The Daily Requirements Of Vitamins

The amount of vitamins necessary for the body are given in terms of milligrams (mg). A gram is of an ounce. They are also expressed in terms of INTERNATIONAL UNITS. For vitamin A one international unit (IU) equals mg. The MINIMUM DAILY RECOMMENDATION (MDR) is really a minimum. It represents the least amount that will keep the average person from developing a deficiency disease due to the lack of that vitamin. Actually from 2 to 4 times that amount of any vitamin will produce the most abundant growth and health. 30mg of vitamin C daily will keep the average person from getting SCURVY; one mg of thiamin (B_1) will keep one from getting BERIBER However, Everyone admits that what will protect you from a deficiency disease is not the amount that will keep you at your best. So there is a second set of official figures, the RECOMMENDED DAILY ALLOWANCE (RDA). Getting this amount is supposed to keep one in a good nutritional state. The RDA of vitamin A is 5000 IU. Some nutritionists say that for perfect health and protection from disease, you may need as much as 20,000 units.

Our richest source of vitamin A is FISH LIVER OIL, and people can get too much of it. Polar bear liver is richer in vitamin A than any other substance. A pound of polar bear liver may contain as much as

8 million units of vitamin A. Some explorers have become poisoned from eating it. The symptoms of such poisoning are NAUSEA, VOMITING, DIARRHEA, and DROWSINESS. A researcher reported that it takes at least 50,000 IU of vitamin A a day for 18 months to produce symptoms of hypervitaminosis for vitamin A. Another reported that 2 million IU in a single dose is the only way to create hypervitaminosis symptoms for vitamin A.

Natural Versus Synthetic Vitamins

◆ *Synthetic Vitamins Do Not React Like Natural Vitamins.*

Artificially prepared synthetic vitamins do not react in the body the same as natural vitamins. It is not sufficient to say that their chemical formulas are exactly alike. For even this isn't quite true. There are still two important differences between them. First, natural vitamins come with supplementary substances such as other vitamins, minerals, and micro-elements whose total synergistic effect within the body is different from that of the single vitamin. After all, God wouldn't say that only the vitamin C in rose hips is important, but rather would he say that all of the elements as well as the supernatural way in which he put them together is important.

◆ *Left-handed And Right-Handed Forms Of Vitamins*

Man, in his analytical way of looking at things wants to say that the element which is most active or reactive in substances is the element that is most important. But modern nutritional research has determined that some elements contained in a natural food product, almost too small to be measured, are important in the total beneficial effect of that food upon the body. Secondly, a synthetically produced compound is not necessarily chemically equivalent to the natural one. The reason for this is the fact that there are left-handed and right handed forms of molecules, which have the same formula, but react differently. Is a left-handed glove exactly like the right-handed one? Not quite, because they cannot be properly interchanged.

◆ *Some Synthetic Vitamins Are Toxic*

In the book "Vitamin And Mineral Therapy," by Dubin and Funk, the latter being the discoverer of vitamin B_1, it states that the synthetic product is far more toxic than the natural one. It has been determined that if only the right-handed form of a vitamin exists naturally, such as vitamin D, then producing vitamin D artificially will give us only the left-handed form, and that the left-handed form is then toxic, while the natural form is not. If both the right-handed and the left-handed forms exist naturally, as in the case of the sugars DEXTROSE and LEVULOSE, then neither of them is toxic. For example, SYNTHETIC VITAMIN D sold as 'Viosterol' and 'Vigantol' causes blood in the urine by its distinctive action on the kidneys. Deaths have been reported from ordinary dosages used to 'protect' children from rickets. When in one case the synthetic form of LACTIC ACID was given to some babies to modify their milk, a few of them died. Dr. W. Held found that the dextrolactic acid, the right rotary sugar of milk, is a food, while the levolactic acid is a poison. He says that the moral for mothers is to use only the natural dextrolactic acid for milk modification. It is said that where a food product is composed of right-handed molecules, the left-handed ones may be as useless as in the case of left-handed and right-handed nuts and bolts in machinery. The artificial is never the same as the natural, for in the natural there are always necessary and possibly unknown elements which are lacking in the artificial form.

The Need For Vitamins In Disease

◆ *Disease Increases The Body's Need For Vitamins*

With our present knowledge of vitamins it can be stated that there is evidence that many diseases not primarily due to nutritional vitamin deficiency can be related to a defective supply of vitamins, and that some of those conditions respond to massive doses of vitamins, especially the B-complex and vitamin C. FEVERS increase the body's need for vitamins. Vitamin A is very low in fever diseases, and also in TUBERCULOSIS patients. Low vitamin C levels have been found in tuberculosis as well as in ARTHRITIC and RHEUMATIC DISORDERS. There is also an increased need for the B-vitamins during INFECTIONS of any kind. The requirements of rats for Vitamin B_1 and two other B vitamins is twice as high at a temperature of 91 degrees as at a temperature of 65 degrees. This may indicate that we need more vitamins during SUMMER HEAT. It is customary in some hospitals to give as much as 1000 to 2000 mg of vitamin C before and after surgery to prevent or treat SHOCK.

◆ *Massive Doses Of Some Vitamins Are Helpful*

HERPES ZOSTER or SHINGLES, the stubborn and painful clustering of small blisters near the ear was effectively treated with thiamin in 25 cases. The patients were given intramuscular injections of 200 mg of thiamin (B_1) daily, but the doctors thought that even a lesser dosage would have been equally effective. Dr. Bock says that dental postoperative PAIN is promptly and completely relieved in most patients by the administration of vitamin B_1, and that much pain can be prevented by using the B_1 before the operation. The low pain threshold of many dental patients may be indicative of a thiamin deficiency. There is evidence that replacement of free thiamin to injured and diseased NERVES not only restores proper functioning, but also relieves pain.

The Need For Vitamins In Counteracting Poisons

◆ *Man-made Vitamins Have Side-effects*

Many people today do not EXERCISE sufficiently. As a result their ADRENALS do not produce sufficient CORTISONE, and for the lack of it many come down with ARTHRITIS. Then they are given artificially made cortisone in which there are many gaps. No pharmaceutical chemist can make cortisone the way the adrenals can. As a consequence deadly side-effects result from this man-made cortisone—such as WEAKENING of the SPINE and BRAIN.

A doctor warned that some infants recently had been born with DEFORMED HEARTS, MENTAL RETARDATION, and accompanying IN-BORN DEFECTS that she believed were caused by doctors administering EXCESSIVE DOSES of VITAMIN D during pregnancy. Pure vitamin D can be obtained only synthetically. In nature vitamin D is always accompanied by vitamin A as in the case of COD LIVER OIL. It has been known for a long time that large amounts of vitamin D in the system, if not balanced by proportional amounts of vitamin A will lead to HYPERCALCEMIA, or an excess of calcium in the blood serum, caused by its being drained from the bones. This does not occur with vitamin D from fish liver oils.

◆ *Artificial Vitamins Are Deficient Vitamins*

The Journal of Immunology told the story of a group of guinea pigs who were given a diet deficient in vitamin C. Guinea pigs cannot produce their own vitamin C. As a result they developed SCURVY. They could not be entirely cured of it by synthetic vitamin C. When they were fed fresh cabbage which is rich in vitamin C and the things which accompany it in nature, they were quickly brought back to normal.

Three groups of CHICKS were fed the same diet. The first group received no vitamin D; the second group received synthetic vitamin D; and the third group received natural vitamin D from Cod liver oil. The first group gained 259 gm of weight; the second group gained 346 gm; and the third group gained 399 gm. Of the no-vitamin chicks 60% died; of the synthetic group 50% died; and of the natural vitamin D group there was not a single death.

Vitamin Interrelationships

Eddy and Dahldorf show that the inter relationships among B-vitamins are complicated and numerous. For example, RIBOFLAVIN (B_2) is poorly absorbed unless THIAMIN (B_1) is present. Giving large amounts of NIACIN (B_3) by itself produces sudden and unexpected symptoms in laboratory animals. This indicates that the so-called "enrichment" of cereals is bound to have a devastating effect eventually, for all of the B-vitamins are removed when flour is refined, and only two or three are replaced synthetically.

No nutrient by itself should be expected to prevent or cure any disease. Nutrients as such always WORK COOPERATIVELY in metabolism as a team. When a specific vitamin appears to cure a specific disease, it is because other vitamins in the system help to round out the incomplete team into a complete one.

Vitamins and minerals do not cancel each other out. Instead they work so closely together that some of them can actually substitute for others in emergencies. In the case of SCURVY, for example, laboratory animals which are getting enough of the B-vitamins can somehow substitute them for vitamin C, so that they do not get scurvy as soon as those animals which are not getting so much vitamin B. The causes of vitamin B_1 deficiency are INSUFFICIENT DIETARY INTAKE, DEFECTIVE UTILIZATION, INADEQUATE ABSORPTION, interference from ANTIBIOTICS, and increased demand in ILLNESS, FEVER, and PREGNANCY.

ALCOHOLISM and B-VITAMIN DEFICIENCY are often mentioned together, and rightly so. Alcohol does not inhibit the action of B_1, but the high caloric value of alcohol increases a person's requirement for all the B-vitamins. At the same time the alcoholic, from lack of appetite, reduces his dietary intake, and develops alcoholic psychosis which is probably due to a lack of B_1 and B_3, both of which are needed to process carbohydrates such as alcohol.

Vitamin A

◆ *Vitamin A And Beta-Carotene*

Vitamin A exists only in foods of animal origin, such as liver and dairy products. As such it does not exist in vegetables and fruits. Vegetables and fruits contain BETA-CAROTENE, which must be changed in the liver to vitamin A. Beta-carotene represents two molecules of vitamin A locked together. When the body needs vitamin A, it sends a special enzyme to unlock the amount it needs. Vitamin A in animal sources comes from the fact that animals have eaten plants and have converted the beta-carotene into vitamin A for their own use. CAROTENOIDS are naturally occurring pigments found in fruits and vegetables, notably alpha and beta-carotene which have "vitamin A activity," which means that they can be converted to vitamin A. True vitamin A is known as PRE-FORMED VITAMIN A. Beta-carotene is also known as PRO-VITAMIN A.

◆ *The Sources Of Vitamin A*

The foods containing the most beta-carotene are SWEET POTATOES, CARROTS. SPINACH, SQUASH, CANTALOUPES, APRICOTS, and PUMPKINS. The foods containing preformed vitamin A or RETINOL are FISH LIVER OILS, EGG YOLK, MILK FAT, and ORGAN MEATS. PINK or RUBY-RED GRAPEFRUIT contains up to 26 times more CAROTENOIDS, including BETA CAROTENE, than the white variety. The plant foods eaten today contain far less vitamin A due to the artificial fertilizers and nitrates which have a tendency to destroy vitamin A in foods, in the field, and in our bodies. Growing foods with natural fertilizers will maintain their vitamin A content. Vitamin A is also called "The Growth Factor," so-called by Dr. McCollum who noticed that it promoted growth in laboratory test animals. Many green vegetables contain the beta-carotene even though they do not have the yellow color of the carotenoids. Here that color is masked by the CHLOROPHYLL, which is nature's protection against harmful oxidation.

After the liver has changed beta-carotene to vitamin A, an excess of vitamin A can be stored in the liver for long periods of time and released whenever needed. People who drink a lot of carrot juice, and get more than they need of beta-carotene, find that their skin will turn yellow. They do not get HYPERVITAMINOSIS from vitamin A, because the excess is stored. This means that the body has no present need for the production of more vitamin A, and therefore stores the beta-carotene in the tissues. When the need again arises, the beta-carotene is turned into vitamin A, and the skin color turns back to normal. One person with yellow skin, who had taken too much carrot juice, found himself in the hospital because of an accident, and before the attendants found out what he had drunk they interpreted his condition as yellow jaundice.

◆ *The Need For Vitamin A In Health*

Since vitamin A is stored in the body, it is not absolutely necessary to eat some every day. The daily recommended allowance (RDA) is as follows: 5000 IU for moderately active adults; 1500 to 3500 IU for children up to 12 years of age; 6000 IU for pregnant women; 8000 IU for nursing mothers. Vitamin A has a vital effect on the COMPLEXION. When it is in short supply the cells on the surface shrivel up and die. The result is a wrinkly, dry, coarse appearance.

Dr. Roels of Columbia University proved that vitamin A in the diet is necessary for the proper absorption of PROTEIN. In a study of 500 Indonesian children suffering from KWASHIORKOR, A protein deficiency disease, he found that the same amount of protein in the diet produced a much greater increase in height and weight, when the diet also included vitamin A rich PALM OIL. A deficiency of protein also cuts down the absorption and utilization of vitamin A.

Vitamin A keeps the skin healthy and also helps to maintain the protective mucus that lines the mouth, alimentary canal, stomach, and intestines. It also activates disease-fighting T-cells. Beta-carotene may be even better than vitamin A. It stimulates the MACROPHAGES, the large cells that search out cancerous tumors and destroy them.

A compound which can take the sun's power and convert it into usable energy is in the retina of the human eye, and is called VISUAL PURPLE. Visual purple is essential for sight and can be made in the eye only if sufficient vitamin A is present. It is used up helping you see in bright light. It renews itself after dark while you are sleeping. A day in bright sunlight at the beach may use up so much visual purple, that you may have trouble with GLARE driving home after dark. In a test many drivers who failed their night vision tests had liver troubles, for the liver stores vitamin A. A lack of vitamin A may also cause difficulty in reading in dim light, and an inability to store fat. Research has discovered that rats given no vitamin A could manufacture enough visual purple to see well if they were kept in darkness all the time. Could it be that a deficiency in vitamin A and too few hours of darkness are sufficient reasons for some of our eye problems?

You require less vitamin A when you also take supplements of ANTIOXIDANTS such as vitamins E. C, and SELENIUM. Vitamin A will prevent SUNBURN with vitamins C, E, B_5, and PABA (para-amino-benzoic acid), a B-vitamin.

◆ *The Benefits Of Vitamin A*

Vitamin A builds resistance to all kinds of INFECTIONS. It is a MEMBRANE CONDITIONER. It keeps the mucous linings and membranes of the body in a healthy condition. It prevents EYE DISEASES by helping the development of visual purple in the eye. It plays a vital role in the nourishment of SKIN and HAIR. It promotes GROWTH and vitality. It aids in the secretion of GASTRIC JUICES and in the digestion of PROTEINS. It helps prevent PREMATURE AGING and SENILITY. It increases LIFE EXPECTANCY and extends YOUTHFULNESS. It protects against the damaging effects of POLLUTED AIR. It increases the permeability of blood capillaries by contributing to better TISSUE OXYGENATION.

A Minnesota study showed that those people who ate more beta-carotene rich foods were less likely to die of CANCER. Studies with rats indicate that doubling the normal amount of vitamin A increased the LIFE SPAN by 10%. Quadrupling the vitamin A increased the life span by 20%.

SYNTHETIC vitamin A does not have the same beneficial effect as natural vitamin A. When rabbits were treated with synthetic vitamin A, there developed indentations in the surfaces of the cells, and the cells became spherical and lost hemoglobin. When vitamin E was added to the synthetic vitamin A, this harm to the cells was prevented.

◆ *Vitamin A And Disease*

✓ INFECTION—Any infection alters the metabolism and increases our need for more nutrients. Physicians have observed that malnourished children suffer more infections than those who are adequately nourished. Vitamin A fights INFECTION not by killing the disease germs, but by providing for the health of the mucous membrane which the germs attack. Because of this it is a powerful agent against COLDS, SINUS TROUBLE, and PNEUMONIA. It contributes enormously to growth and DENTAL HEALTH in children. Our grandmothers knew how beneficial a daily dose of cod liver oil was, containing both vitamins A and D, even though they may not have known why.

✓ DIABETES—Two New York physicians discovered with rats that DIABETICS are unable to transform carotene into vitamin A. The diabetic rats had only as much vitamin A in their bodies as the non-diabetic ones.

✓ LEUKOPLAKIA—The white skin changes that occur on the mucous membrane inside the mouth are known as LEUKOPLAKIA, and indicate a vitamin A deficiency. It is cause for concern as leukoplakia is a frequent forerunner of skin cancer. In monkeys with leukoplakia 10,000 units of vitamin A a day for 30 days returned their affected gums back to normal.

- ✓ AIR POLLUTION—Dr. Saffioti in an experiment blew into the lungs of hamsters chemical particles that are found in urban AIR POLLUTION and in cigarette smoke. He found that the changes that occurred in the cells of the hamsters lungs were changes that precede CANCER. Eventually up to 100% of the animals got lung cancer. Giving hamsters Vitamin A prevented these changes in lung cells, and hence prevented lung cancer. There is every indication that human beings who are getting enough vitamin A would have the same experience.

- ✓ ACNE—ACNE is treated with a vitamin A preparation called RETINOIC ACID, as well as with another form of vitamin A called VITAMIN A ACID. It has been found that most acne can be treated by eliminating sugar or any food containing it. Acne is unknown to primitive people who have no access to sugary foods. It appears in their young people as soon as they move to civilization and begin to use soft drinks, candy, cakes, desserts, and sugary snacks. Taking YOGURT daily or the lactobacillus tablet preparation is a great help along with a no-sugar diet.

- ✓ BLADDER STONES—STONES in the BLADDER are common consequences of vitamin A shortage. Also GOITER has been linked to vitamin A deficiency.

- ✓ NEARSIGHTEDNESS—MYOPIA

Myopia may be due to a lack of VITAMIN A and CALCIUM in the diet. 5000 units of vitamin A daily is recommended, and 10 to 15 times that much in cases of deficiency. Foods rich in vitamin A are CHARD, BEET GREENS, and DANDELION LEAVES. A 4 oz. serving of these contain 15,000 to 20,000 units of vitamin A. These foods are also rich in calcium. Other good sources are WATERCRESS, KALE, MUSTARD GREENS, TURNIP GREENS, and PARSLEY.

◆ *The Interrelationships Of Vitamin A*

Vitamin A has a definite interaction with vitamin D. Neither is as effective without the other. Either can be toxic without the other. That is why fish liver oil contains both vitamin A and D. Hence, it is not recommended that anyone take a supplement that is exclusively vitamin A or D. Doctors have reported an association between those who take the PILL and LIVER CANCER. The pill is made of STEROID HORMONES which have been linked to cancer. It is known that contraceptives decrease the amount of vitamin A in the liver, and the hormones of which the pill is made influence the way the body uses vitamin A. It is also known that vitamin A participates in cell division in certain tissues of the body. Since cancer is a disorder of cell division, it is possible that a lack of vitamin A may be the cause of such tumors.

◆ *Substances That Destroy Vitamin A's Effectiveness*

An active THYROID is absolutely essential to the process by which our bodies convert carotene into vitamin A. But high NITRITE levels in the system depress thyroid activity and make carotene conversion impossible. The NITRATE from fertilizers is converted to nitrite in the stomach, and the nitrite in turn slows down thyroid activity. The nitrites also destroy the body's own storage of vitamin A

Gastrointestinal or LIVER DISEASES or infections limit our capacity to use vitamin A. For example, the continual taking of MINERAL OIL dissolves the store of vitamin A in the body and carries it away before it can be absorbed. The food value of vitamin A is lost if the fat in which it is contained becomes RANCID. Always keep your fish liver oil in the refrigerator. Vegetables containing vitamin A do not lose it when they are cooked, for vitamin A is not water soluble.

◆ *Deficiencies of Vitamin A*

In a Norwegian study it was found that smoking men having a low vitamin A intake were 4 times more prone to develop lung cancer than equally heavy smokers who take in a normal amount of vitamin A. Without sufficient vitamin A a person will get FREQUENT COLDS, his HAIR will turn GRAY sooner, his SKIN will WRINKLE SOONER, and his MUCOUS MEMBRANE will become HARD. Women with a low vitamin A intake have a threefold greater risk of developing CERVICAL CANCER. Reports from the University of Washington of the dietary habits of 416 women found that those women who consumed the most DARK GREEN AND YELLOW VEGETABLES had a 60% lower risk of cervical cancer, while an abundant intake of FRUIT JUICES was associated with a 70% lesser risk of cervical cancer.

Prolonged deficiency of vitamin A may result in increased susceptibility to INFECTION especially in the respiratory tract; RETARDED GROWTH in children; LOSS of APPETITE and vigor; DEFECTIVE GUMS and TEETH; PSORIASIS; DANDRUFF; dry dull HAIR and excessive hair loss; a poor sense of TASTE and SMELL; and NAILS which peel or are ridged. A study in India showed that MORTALITY of children with MEASLES was reduced by more than half when they were given extra VITAMIN A.

Vitamin B

◆ *What Are The B-Vitamins?*

Vitamin B is a complex of water-soluble vitamins and vitamin-like substances including THIAMIN (B_1), RIBOFLAVIN (B_2). NIACIN (B_3) PYRIDOXINE, PANTOTHENIC ACID, BIOTIN, FOLIC ACID, CHOLINE, INOSITOL, PARA-AMINO-BENZOIC ACID, and VITAMIN B_{12}. They are responsible chiefly for the health and maintenance of NERVES, EYES, DIGESTION, SKIN, as well as the processing of CARBOHYDRATES, FATS, and PROTEIN, APPETITE, GROWTH, the production of HORMONES and DIGESTIVE JUICES, the prevention of ANEMIA, the maintenance of the SEX GLANDS, SEBACEOUS GLANDS, BONE MARROW, and many other complex body functions.

B-vitamins are safe in very large amounts because they are water-soluble. They are NOT STORED to any extent in the body, so that whatever is not needed is rapidly excreted. However, a certain balance among them is advisable. It is best to use them together in food and supplements, for they complement one another. ORTHOMOLECULAR THERAPY, meaning restoring those chemical to the body which normally belong there, is helpful for ALCOHOLICS and DRUG ADDICTS. Large doses of NIACIN are used to offset the violent reactions to LSD. Diet and vitamins are now being used also to treat AUTISTIC CHILDREN, HYPERACTIVE CHILDREN, MINIMAL BRAIN DAMAGE, and LEARNING DISABILITY. A SWOLLEN TONGUE can result from lack of one or several of the B-vitamins pyridoxine, thiamin, and riboflavin.

B-vitamins are destroyed in food preparations by light, steam, long cooking, high temperatures, and long storage, as well as by antagonists in the form of drugs, chemicals, and also by alkalinity in the stomach caused by antacids.

◆ *Sources Of The B-Complex*

Biochemists call the B-vitamins the B-COMPLEX, because you do not find one of them in food or in living tissue without the others being close at hand. They go together, they help one another out. If one of them is a little short for some reason, another can often take its place and function. BREWER'S YEAST, which consists of tiny plants, contains all of the elements of the vitamin B-complex. It is also a rich source of PROTEINS, which proteins contain all of the ESSENTIAL AMINO ACIDS or building blocks of protein, In the present day U.S. there is a widespread deficiency in the B-vitamins, due partly to our overrefined food, and also due to the fact that refined sugar steals B-vitamins very rapidly from the system. In nature things are used as WHOLES. Removing all of the B-vitamins from our whole grain cereals and flour and only returning three synthetic ones is probably one of the worst things that could be done. The imbalances thus created are very complex, for all of the B-vitamins work together.

The B-vitamins are most abundant in WHOLE GRAINS, ALL SEEDS, NUTS, EGG YOLK, BRAN, WHEAT GERM, BREWER YEAST, LENTILS, BEANS, PEAS, SOYBEANS, and LEAFY GREEN VEGETABLES. In nature the B-vitamins are responsible for processing carbohydrates. By removing them from carbohydrate-rich foods like cereals and sugar, we invite nutritional difficulties. One half of all the food eaten in this country consists of depleted substances. For example, lesions in the mouth may be signs of advanced vitamin B deficiency.

◆ *Vitamin B_1—Thiamin*

✓ LOST IN MILLING—The main reason why a B_1 deficiency is quite general in the U.S. is that one of the richest sources of this vitamin is wheat germ which is in milling removed from the flour we use. At present most bread and flour is "enriched," meaning that thiamin and other B-vitamins have been added synthetically to the flour. However many researchers have shown that once a natural substance is removed from a food, it cannot be replaced by chemists in exactly the right proportions and combinations to produce the same nutritional effect as natural foods. It has furthermore been shown that synthetic vitamin preparations are quite ineffective in correcting vitamin deficiencies as compared to natural preparations.

✓ IMPROVES LEARNING—Vitamin B_1 is known as the ANTI-BERIBERI, ANTI-NEUROTIC, and ANTI-AGING vitamin. It is essential for effective protein metabolism. helps the body utilize CARBOHYDRATES by interaction with enzymes, promotes GROWTH, protects the HEART MUSCLE, stimulates BRAIN action, and helps maintain normal BLOOD COUNT. Added B_1 has been found to improve LEARNING and INTELLIGENCE in several experiments. Beriberi was formerly a common ailment of Oriental people who lived chiefly on polished rice. Any amount more than the body needs is excreted in the urine each day. The eating of SUGAR depletes the body's store of B_1.

✓ ADMINISTER ALL B-VITAMINS FOR BEST RESULTS—The best sources are BREWER'S YEAST, WHEAT GERM, WHEAT BRAN, RICE POLISHINGS, WHOLE GRAIN CEREALS, all SEEDS and NUTS. For best results with therapeutic doses of B_1, all other B-complex vitamins should be administered simultaneously. Prolonged ingestion of any one of the B-vitamins may result in high urinary losses of the others and thereby lead to deficiencies of these vitamins.

✓ B_1 CONTAINED IN COOKING WATER—When foods are heated with dry heat they lose less B_1 than if they are cooked in water. Adding SODA to beans that are cooking doubles the destruction of B_1. Toasting bread at high temperature destroys some B_1. When you cook vegetables, the cooking water should be saved. It contains valuable amounts of B_1 as well as other vitamins. Use it in soups or broths.

✓ B_1 STRENGTHENS HEART MUSCLE—Dr. Weiss of Harvard Medical School, proved that MYOCARDIAL HEART FAILURE or weakness of the heart muscle stems from a lack of vitamin B_1, by showing that even if the heart is greatly enlarged, it can be reduced in size in 48 hours with large doses of vitamin B_1. Dr. E. Brauer tells of relieving SCIATICA with injections of B_1. It was found that eating GARLIC along with B_1 gave the same effect as injections, according to a Japanese study.

✓ IT RELIEVES SHINGLES—SHINGLES or HERPES ZOSTER can be relieved by taking B_1. One man cured himself of shingles by taking lots of B-VITAMINS as well as VITAMIN E in liquid form. He applied them all over the red spots on back and chest. Two weeks later the spots were gone.

✓ DEFICIENCY—A deficiency of B_1 causes a loss of APPETITE, MENTAL DEPRESSION, "PINS and NEEDLES" sensation in feet and hands, and DNA changes which have been correlated with CANCER. This seems to indicate that hereditary factors can change with a change in mutation. The most severe deficiency of B_1 is BERIBERI, whose symptoms are WEAKNESS, PARALYSIS of leg muscles, HEART PAINS, CARDIAC FAILURE, NUMBNESS and STIFFNESS in the ankles. Lesser deficiencies lead to loss of APPETITE, loss of WEIGHT, MENTAL DEPRESSION, and NERVOUS EXHAUSTION. Deficiencies can be induced by excess of dietary sugar and by processed and refined foods.

◆ *Vitamin B_2—Riboflavin*

✓ PREVENTS LIVER CANCER—It is essential for GROWTH, GENERAL HEALTH, HEALTHY EYES, SKIN, NAILS, and HAIR. B_2 is found in NUTS, MILK, MILK PRODUCTS, ALMONDS, SUNFLOWER SEEDS, BREWERS YEAST, WHEAT GERM, WHOLE GRAIN BREADS and CEREALS. It helps to transform proteins, fats, and carbohydrates into ENERGY. It can be destroyed by light. Some relief of SKIN DISORDERS and CATARACTS has been attributed to B_2 therapy.

✓ In a study at the Sloan-Kettering Institute a group of rats was given a diet of rice plus a chemical known to cause cancer. In addition one group of rats was given a considerable amount of BREWERS YEAST. The unprotected rats had cancerous livers in 150 days, while the B_2 rats developed no cancer at all. It was later determined that the vitamin in Brewers yeast which was especially responsible for this result was RIBOFLAVIN. Although large amounts of brewers yeast cannot cure cancer, it was found that it can PREVENT LIVER CANCER from starting.

✓ DEFICIENCY DEVELOPS ANEMIA—Two Baylor University researchers put 8 volunteers on a diet without B_2. Then they were given vitamin supplements to make sure that they had enough of all other vitamins and minerals. They rapidly developed ANEMIA resulting in disorders of the blood cells and of the bone marrow where certain blood cells are manufactured. When B_2 was given them again the anemia was cured. There are cases of individuals who are unable to assimilate B_2 because of a faulty secretion of HYDROCHLORIC ACID in their stomachs or a lack of PHOSPHOROUS in their diets.

Its lack causes ANEMIA, BURNING SENSATIONS in HANDS, FEET, and EYES, loss of HAIR and WEIGHT, and difficulty in producing INSULIN. It aids in the absorption of IRON, has special CANCER-INHIBITING properties, and helps heal CRACKS on the LIPS. A deficiency of B_2 also results in a decrease in LYMPHOCYTES, and an increased susceptibility to INFECTION, as well as causing LIP, TONGUE, and MOUTH SORENESS and BURNING. The use of BORIC ACID in MOUTH WASHES can cause partial B_2 deficiency.

◆ *Vitamin B_3—Niacin, Nicotinic Acid, Niacinamide*

✓ THE ANTI-PELLAGRA VITAMIN — B_3 is the ANTI-PELLAGRA vitamin. It is important for proper CIRCULATION and healthy functioning of the NERVOUS SYSTEM. It is essential for proper PROTEIN, FATS, and CARBOHYDRATE METABOLISM. It helps maintain healthy SKIN. It is often prescribed in cases of COLD HANDS and FEET. In megadoses (massive doses), niacin has been successfully used in the treatment of SCHIZOPHRENIA. An extreme deficiency causes PELLAGRA, with the mental symptoms of HALLUCINATIONS and DEMENTIA, as well as SKIN RASHES, and NEURASTHENIA. Lesser deficiencies give rise to irritability, insomnia, backaches, headaches and so on. It is presently used to treat AUTISTIC children.

Not so long ago pellagra appeared mostly among the poor families in the South who lived largely on CORN and corn products. It has CHOLESTEROL as well as TRIGLYCERIDE-lowering potential. It also provides protection against POLLUTANTS and TOXINS. The three D's of pellagra in doctors terminology are DEPRESSION, DERMATITIS, and DIARRHEA.

Cow's milk contains little niacin. Good sources are RICE BRAN, NUTS and SEEDS, WHOLE WHEAT PRODUCTS, and GREEN VEGETABLES. Niacin, like other B-vitamins, is removed from our grains and cereals when they are refined. Some of it is then replaced in synthetic form. BREWERS YEAST, the richest source of all, was used by Dr. Tom Spies to cure cases of pellagra in the South. He found it much more effective than giving the isolated vitamin. He used to give his pellagra patients as much as cup of brewer's yeast a day with nothing but excellent results.

✓ A VASODILATOR—It dilates the blood vessels. It also has an essential role in TISSUE OXIDATION. When the body's need for niacin is not satisfied, a person may become TIRED, APPREHENSIVE, and PESSIMISTIC. He will constantly expect accidents, and disasters. His whole PERSONALITY may change. Nutritionists agree that foods containing all of the B-complex are superior in every way to any one of the B-vitamins taken separately. It also has been found that emphasizing one of the B-vitamins can cause a deficiency in some of the others. A deficiency of all of the B-vitamins causes CANKER sores in the mouth. A form of niacin was effective in treating 1000 patients at the New Jersey Neuropsychiatric Institute with

SCHIZOPHRENIA. 75% of the patients were cured. One patient who had been ill for 29 years was free of symptoms after only 5 days of treatment. Diets lacking in niacin can be tolerated if they contain enough of a protein called TRYPTOPHAN.

✓ IT CURES SCHIZOPHRENIA—One man had a sudden attack of acute SCHIZOPHRENIA, and was hospitalized for 3 months. He decided to do his own research and learned of the VITAMIN B_3 treatment for schizophrenia. Within hours after taking massive doses of NIACINAMIDE, a niacin derivative, his depression vanished, not to return. Self-confidence returned and fear left. He became vibrant, alert, and energetic. His friends were amazed.

◆ *Pantothenic Acid*

It is distributed in almost all plant and animal tissues. It is required in all energy producing reactions. It is essential for the proper functioning of the nervous system. It is needed for the formation of the red blood cells, and for healthy gums and teeth. It helps in the formation of protein and in the use of fats. A deficiency inhibits the formation of antibodies, decreases the T-CELLS, and decreases the destruction of CANCER CELLS. Women taking ESTROGEN need above normal amounts.

◆ *Vitamin B_6—Pyridoxine*

✓ IT ACTIVATES ENZYMES—Vitamin B_6 does not exist in natural form apart from other B-vitamins, so that any preparation which is sold just as pyridoxine would be synthetic. The need for pyridoxine is about the same as that for thiamin, about 1.5–1.8 mg per day. We can get our daily quota from 3 tablespoons of BREWER'S YEAST. It is essential for the metabolism of every amino acid PROTEIN. The more protein is consumed the more B_6 is required. It activates many ENZYMES and enzyme systems. It prevents NERVOUS and SKIN disorders such as ACNE, protects against degenerative diseases, and is also effective in OVERWEIGHT PROBLEMS caused by water retention. It regulates the balance between SODIUM and POTASSIUM in the body.

✓ IT PREVENTS TOOTH CAVITIES—Research determined that Cuban children who chewed sugar cane had fewer TOOTH CAVITIES and higher blood concentrations of B_6 than did a peer group in New York city. It was also demonstrated that young monkeys on a B_6 deficient diet had devastating tooth decay whereas a control group of monkeys had not. Some of the symptoms associated with DEPRESSION induced by oral contraceptives, were abolished by B_6. Women on BIRTH CONTROL PILLS need up to 30 mg of B_6 daily to neutralize the effects of the pill.

✓ IT TREATS PHOTOSENSITIVITY AND NAUSEA—A diet low in magnesium (Mg) but high in phosphorus (P) and moderate in calcium (Ca) tends to form STONES in the kidneys. B_6 has successfully treated a type of PHOTOSENSITIVITY characterized by intolerance to sunlight, and severe sunburn with little exposure. Cases of PARKINSON'S disease have responded to B_6 injections (in combination with magnesium). B_6 is required for the absorption of B_{12}, and for the production of HYDROCHLORIC ACID. It helps to overcome the NAUSEA and TOXEMIA of PREGNANCY, and some adverse effects of BIRTH CONTROL PILLS.

✓ BANANAS ARE A GOOD SOURCE OF B_6— BANANAS are a good source of pyridoxine, for they are about 5 times richer than any other fruit. Also AVOCADOS, EGG YOLK, SOYBEANS, WALNUTS, MOLASSES, GREEN VEGETABLES, CARROTS, and PEANUTS. The heat of cooking is especially destructive of this vitamin.

✓ DEFICIENCY OF B_6 CAUSES NERVE AND MUSCLE PROBLEMS—A deficiency causes many types of MUSCLE and NERVE PAINS, and swellings. It helps in reducing the level of CHOLESTEROL in the bloodstream. A deficiency of B_6 can also cause ANEMIA, EDEMA, ECZEMA, KIDNEY STONES, MIGRAINE HEADACHES, DISEASES of OLD AGE, and PREMATURE SENILITY. Some studies show that it can prevent or lessen EPILEPTIC SEIZURES. A lack of B_6 is suspected of being a probable cause of ARTERIOSCLEROSIS It is thought that a high fat and protein diet which is low in B_6 will cause DIABETES. An adequate amount of B_6 will help in keeping weight under control, because it is necessary for the functioning of the THYROID gland. A high percentage of B_6 is lost in cooking and refining. Any excess is excreted within 8 hours after ingestion. This makes B_6 a safe substance for which no harmful side effects have ever been reported.

✓ IT CURES CARPAL TUNNEL SYNDROME—A man consulted 6 doctors, and they all concluded that his problem was CARPAL TUNNEL SYNDROME. He found himself unable to stand the pain, and therefore found it impossible for him to work. The night before the operation he sneaked out of the hospital and consulted a nutritionist who prescribed for him 200 mg B_6 3 times a day. It took 6 weeks for the symptoms to vanish, but his hands became pain free and stronger than ever.

◆ *Vitamin B_{12}—Cobalamin, Cyanocobalamin*

It is also known as the "red vitamin." B_{12} is made in the digestive system of animals with the aid of intestinal bacteria. The mineral cobalt and the bacteria are necessary for its production. Some nutritionists say that man cannot produce it. Others say that if a person eats a pure vegetarian diet, man's intestines which produce many of the B-vitamins will also produce vitamin B_{12}. Since God instituted for man a vegetarian diet, would he leave such a diet incomplete by omitting from it a necessary factor? Some people say that a vegetarian has to eat brewers yeast or animal liver in order to get the necessary vitamin B_{12}. To those individuals one may say "Where do the animals, such as the cow, the ox, or the elephant get their vitamin B_{12} when they eat only grass"? It has been determined that all vegetarian animals can produce their own B-vitamins, including vitamin B_{12}, in their intestines, and this includes man also if he is a vegetarian. B_{12} IS THOUGHT TO ORIGINATE FROM BACTERIAL FERMENTATION OF VEGETABLE MATTER IN THE INTESTINES. There is also evidence that whole grains, such as WHEAT and OATS, supply the full complex of B-vitamins including B_{12}. Three ounces of OATMEAL for breakfast and three ounces of WHOLE WHEAT BREAD will supply enough B_{12} for the average adult for the day. While B_{12} is most abundant in foods of animal origin, it is believed that fermented foods such as SAUERKRAUT, MISO, SOURDOUGH BREAD, in fact any FERMENTABLE CARBOHYDRATE will help the intestinal bacteria synthesize B_{12}. Other foods that contain vitamin B_{12} also are GREEN BEANS, KELP, other SEAWEEDS, SOYBEAN MEAL, BANANAS, TEMPEH, EGGS, SUNFLOWER SEEDS, POLLEN, and MILK.

Those vegetarians who eat a lot of cooked vegetables may have a deficiency of B_{12}, but not those who eat raw fruits, vegetables, and grains. We are told that "in grains, fruits, vegetables and nuts are to be found all the food elements that we need" (CD313). B_{12} is essential for the production and regeneration of the RED BLOOD CELLS. It prevents ANEMIA, and PROMOTES GROWTH in children. A deficiency causes PERNICIOUS ANEMIA, CHRONIC FATIGUE, SORE MOUTH, NUMBNESS, and difficulty in CONCENTRATING. Other natural sources are BREWER'S YEAST, COMFREY LEAVES, KELP, PEANUTS, CONCORD GRAPES, WHEAT GERM, SOYBEANS, and OATS.

Pernicious anemia is a failure on the part of the body to manufacture enough RED BLOOD CELLS in the bone marrow. In some individuals this failure is believed to be caused by a lack of a certain secretion in the stomach, called "the intrinsic factor," whose job it is to extract B_{12} from food. It aids in blood cell formation, iron absorption, nucleic acid synthesis, and in the maintenance of nerve cells. It has a great effect on the growth of children. Since 1948 doctors have used B_{12} for MULTIPLE SCLEROSIS with great success. It is destroyed by drugs, heat, laxatives, alcohol, coffee, and tobacco.

◆ *Pantothenic Acid*

The name comes from the Greek word "panthos" meaning "universal." It occurs in all living cells of both plants and animals. Its exact function in human nutrition is still being debated. It occurs in YEAST, MOLDS, BACTERIA, EGG YOLK, PEANUTS, WHEAT GERM, LIVER, AND VARIOUS GRAINS. It is present in those foods which also contain other B-vitamins. It is present in lesser quantities in many other natural foods except for WHITE FLOUR and REFINED SUGAR from which it has been removed by processing. It dissolves in water. It is destroyed immediately when baking soda is added to food. For optimum health you should obtain between 5 to 10 mg of pantothenic acid daily.

The richest source of pantothenic acid in nature is ROYAL JELLY, which is the food fed to the bee larva to change it into a queen bee. Without royal jelly the larva would develop into a sterile worker bee.

A deficiency of pantothenic acid can produce DERMATITIS, ULCERS in the digestive tract, ANEMIA, WHITE HAIR, SPINAL CHORD DISORDERS, FATTY LIVER, HEART and KIDNEY damage, lack of WHITE BLOOD CORPUSCLES, SPINAL CURVATURE, and degeneration of the MYELIN SHEATH of the nerves.

It is involved in so many bodily processes that a deficiency also produces symptoms of "pins and needles" sensations in hands and legs, depression, apathy, abdominal pain, increased susceptibility to infection and muscle weakness.

Most children get a bad start in life by being fed a FORMULA rather than BREAST MILK. The pantothenic and thiamin contents of breast milk is about twice that of cow's milk, so most of our babies start out with less pantothenic acid than they would get from breast milk.

Dr. Williams gave two groups of mice the same chow except that in the water of one group he added some pantothenic acid. These mice lived about 20% longer than the other group. A number of black rats were fed a diet containing ample amounts of all vitamins except pantothenic acid. Within six weeks their black hair began to turn gray. With that effect they took on the appearance of OLD AGE. As soon as pantothenic acid was added to their diet, their hair turned black again. Two scientists who studied poorly nourished children in the tropics, reported that many of these children had gray hair. Their hair was restored to normal color when pantothenic acid was given them.

◆ *Biotin*

Biotin is involved in the metabolism of PROTEINS and FATS. It is Related to HAIR GROWTH and HEALTHY HAIR. It helps prevent hair loss. A deficiency may cause ECZEMA, DANDRUFF, SEBORRHEA, FATIGUE, MENTAL DEPRESSION, and HALLUCINATION. The best and richest natural source is BREWERS YEAST. Also UNPOLISHED RICE, and SOYBEANS. It is produced in the INTESTINES if there is a sufficient amount of healthy flora. SEBORRHEIC DERMATITIS and LEINER's disease, both skin diseases, which give the skin a red lobster appearance, were found to be due to a biotin deficiency. Cases of these diseases showed marked improvement when they were treated with biotin. Biotin is so potent that no human cell contains more than a trace of it. Still it is an essential constituent. The biotin molecule grabs a protein molecule which is then able with the help of other molecules to aid in the production of fat and other substances. But the protein that does this cannot function without biotin. So that without biotin the body's fat production is impaired.

◆ *Choline*

Its most important function is in its teamwork with INOSITOL as a part of LECITHIN. It is necessary for the synthesis of the NUCLEIC ACIDS, DNA and RNA. It is essential for proper FAT METABOLISM. It is useful in the treatment of NEPHRITIS. It can prevent the formation of GALLSTONES, as well as BEING USEFUL in the reduction of HIGH BLOOD PRESSURE. It has been used also in the treatment of ATHEROSCLEROSIS, KIDNEY DAMAGE, GLAUCOMA, and MYASTHENIA GRAVIS. Prolonged deficiency may cause CIRRHOSIS, the FATTY DEGENERATION of the LIVER, and HARDENING of the ARTERIES.

It is richly contained in COLOSTRUM, that extra-rich milk mothers give in their first days of nursing. It acts favorably in cases of HEART DISEASE. Only half as many choline treated heart patients died in a three year study as the non-choline treated patients. Foods rich in choline are SOYBEANS, PEAS, BREWER'S YEAST, WHEAT GERM, SPINACH, and EGG YOLK. Choline is also a successful agent in the treatment of HEPATITIS. A study of 37 patients found that treatment with choline reduced the duration of virus hepatitis to about half. In an experiment by Hamilton cirrhosis was produced in rabbits by diets deficient in choline. Only the B-complex in yeast but none of the pure vitamins inhibited the development of cirrhosis.

◆ *Inositol*

Inositol is vital for hair growth and can prevent thinning hair and baldness. As a part of lecithin, it participates in all of its functions. It is important for a healthy heart muscle. It helps in reducing cholesterol. It has been used in the treatment of OBESITY and SCHIZOPHRENIA. A deficiency may contribute to HAIR LOSS, CONSTIPATION, ECZEMA, EYE ABNORMALITIES, and HIGH BLOOD PRESSURE. It also seems to have a mild inhibitory action on certain types of cancer cells, and it retards the growth of tumors in mice to a degree directly proportional to the amount of inositol given. Natural sources are BREWER'S YEAST, WHEAT GERM, LECITHIN, GRAINS, NUTS, MOLASSES, and CITRUS FRUITS.

Vitamin C—Ascorbic Acid

◆ *Why Vitamin C Is Needed*

Vitamin C is essential for the healthy condition of COLLAGEN, the "intercellular cement" that holds our cells together. It is involved in the vital functions of all glands and organs. It is necessary for healthy teeth, gums, and bones. It strengthens all connective tissue, and is essential for the proper functioning of the ADRENALS and THYROID glands. It promotes healing in every condition of ill health. It helps prevent and cure the common COLD. It protects against all forms of STRESS, physical and mental. It protects against harmful effects of TOXIC CHEMICALS in the environment, in food, water, and air, for they make us use up vitamin C rapidly. It has been used successfully in RATTLE SNAKE bites which it has neutralized. It acts as a general natural ANTIBIOTIC. It is a specific against FEVER, and all sorts of INFECTIONS and GASTROINTESTINAL disorders. Signs which indicate a deficiency of vitamin C are EASY BRUISING, BLACK and BLUE SPOTS in the skin, BLEEDING GUMS, and LOOSE TEETH. Vitamin C stimulates the production of INTERFERON, a chemical that "interferes" with the production of viruses. It also triggers tumor destruction. It keeps the WHITE CELLS healthy, and these white cells produce antibodies which are needed to kill bacteria.

◆ *Massive Doses Are Now Recommended*

Physicians are now recommending MASSIVE DOSES of vitamin C to prevent COLDS, counteract CHOLESTEROL, and to perform many other beneficial acts. Dr. Fred Klenner has taken 10 to 20 grams of vitamin C daily for the past 10 years with nothing but beneficial results. He suggests that with these doses at least 3 glasses of milk, including buttermilk, should be taken. He has several hundred patients who have taken 10 gm or more of vitamin C daily for 13 to 15 years. 90% of these never have COLDS. Dr. Klenner sometimes gives as much as 150 gm of vitamin C intravenously in 24 hours to counteract such things as CARBON DIOXIDE (CO_2) and BARBITURATE poisoning, and VIRUS infections. Vitamin C in large doses can prevent many common disorders such as ALLERGIES, ASTHMA, CANCER, ARTHRITIS, ULCERS, and so on. Dr. Pauling estimates that large quantities of vitamin C can extend human life from 12 to 18 years.

It has been determined that all of the VITAMIN C necessary to prevent scurvy can be put on the head of a pin. So a little more than a tablespoon of lemon juice daily will prevent scurvy, which is a potentially fatal VITAMIN C DEFICIENCY DISEASE. With scurvy muscles waste away, wounds don't heal, black and blue bruises appear, and gums bleed and deteriorate. Lemon juice is an antioxidant, and lemon peel exhibits remarkable antioxidant activity. Antioxidants are believed to have a profound beneficial impact on human cells, including WARDING OFF CANCEROUS CHANGES and RETARDING AGING.

◆ *Most Animals Produce Their Own Vitamin C*

All animals except MAN, APES, GUINEA PIGS, some BATS and BIRDS produce vitamin C in their LIVER or ADRENAL glands from glucose.

Man and apes are also the main animals who catch cold. Compared with the amount of vitamin C produced by rats, it was found that a 150 pound person would have to produce a proportional amount of 4 gm of vitamin C each day under normal conditions. Under stressful conditions he would have to produce 15 gm. Those organisms who cannot produce their own vitamin C must get theirs from the foods they eat.

◆ *The Best Sources Of Vitamin C*

Vitamin C can be made synthetically, but the natural sources are to be preferred, for they come with extra food substances such as the BIOFLAVONOIDS RUTIN, CITRIN, and HESPERIDIN. Medically known as flavone glycosides, they are found mostly in GREEN PEPPERS, BUCKWHEAT, GRAPES, ROSE HIPS, APRICOTS, BLACK CURRENTS, ACEROLA BERRIES, and mostly in those fruits and vegetables containing vitamin C. These increase the therapeutic effect of vitamin C. The Russians have used bioflavonoids very successfully in the treatment of many diseases, particularly CAPILLARY FRAGILITY. They also protect against the harmful effects of X-RAYS. Synthetic vitamin C has also been used by some doctors with success in some specific cases.

The best natural sources of vitamin C are the CITRUS FRUITS, GREEN PEPPERS, CABBAGE, GREEN VEGETABLES, STRAWBERRIES, ROSE HIPS, and ACEROLA BERRIES. The last two are the greatest natural sources of vitamin C of any plant. RED PEPPERS have 1 times more vitamin C than GREEN PEPPERS and 11 times more CAROTENOIDS which the body converts into vitamin A. To get the most value from vitamin C foods, it is best to EAT THEM RAW. Steaming, stewing, baking and frying are all destructive of vitamin C. If you make stew or soup do not add the vegetables until a few minutes before serving. CAULIFLOWER has more vitamin C than oranges ounce for ounce. Fruits and vegetables left unrefrigerated for several days may lose most of their vitamin C. Open kettle HOME CANNING of tomatoes for example destroys practically all of the vitamin C. Commercially canned tomatoes are much richer in vitamin C, for they have been canned by vacuum pack so that no air enters to destroy vitamin C.

Vitamin C is the most highly perishable vitamin soluble in water. If a head of lettuce or cabbage is soaked in water in order to crisp it, most of the vitamin C content disappears into the water. SOAKING FOODS or discarding the cooking water destroys it. CUTTING, SLICING, GRATING, OR CHOPPING fruits and vegetables should be done just before they are eaten. FROZEN FOODS generally contain more vitamin C than canned ones. Baking soda or copper utensils destroy it. Someone has said that if you drop a pinch of soda into green beans or peas in order to give them a green color, you need not bother to eat them, for there will be little food value left.

◆ *The Need Of Vitamin C In Health*

For good health and normal function one should obtain from 75 to 150 mg of vitamin C per day. However, if one takes 3000 mg per day it will saturate the blood stream, and perform miraculous things such as neutralizing various TOXINS, KILLING PATHOGENIC BACTERIA, SPEEDING THE HEALING PROCESSES, and HELPING THE OXYGENATION OF TISSUES. Stress and exposure to poisonous substances use up vitamin C. It must be replaced every day, for the body does NOT STORE it to any degree. In severe stress most animals produce more vitamin C. Hence, it is suggested that man take more vitamin C, since he cannot produce his own.

The government's Recommended Daily Allowances or RDA's for vitamins are usually minimum standards and are set very low, and may therefore be inadequate for optimum health. They are, however, quite satisfactory for the food manufacturers who benefit from them. If, for example, a nutrition label reads that the product contains 100% of the RDA for vitamin C, the product "looks good" to a person. It looks good because of the RDA of only 60 mg per day. However, if we want to accept the optimal level of 3000 mg of vitamin C per day, then such a product has only 2% of the optimal intake of vitamin C.

Vitamin C is an outstanding aid to GOOD HEALTH and LONGEVITY. It is destroyed by LIGHT, AIR, and HEAT. It helps in the healing of WOUNDS, strengthens the IMMUNE SYSTEM, and helps protect the body against INFECTION. It is especially important in protecting NERVE CELLS from free radical damage. The phagocytic activity of the WHITE BLOOD CELLS depends upon the amount of vitamin C that is in the blood and tissues. In the battle to fight infections, vitamin C is destroyed. If the ascorbic acid levels are too low, the white blood cells will not attack the invading bacteria, nor ingest nor digest them. Ascorbic acid is one of the first substances that is synthesized in the growing seed to nourish the plant embryo. BEAN SPROUTS contain ascorbic acid while unsprouted beans do not.

Vitamin C is also necessary for the proper absorption of IRON in the body. Minerals such as CALCIUM and PHOSPHORUS are stored in our bones. If not enough vitamin C is present, the tissues of the bones will not retain the minerals and they are lost to us. Drinking ORANGE JUICE can boost the body's absorption of iron by as much as 400%, because vitamin C enhances iron's availability. The older we grow the more vitamin C we need. This is the very time when trouble with dentures or bad teeth causes many to stop eating fresh raw foods. Elderly institutionalized persons receive very little fresh fruit in their diet.

In the past and present surgeons have been using vitamin C after a serious operation to promote healing. More recent studies have shown that vitamin C is even more important before surgery than after. Vitamin C is an anti-stress vitamin, and since surgery is an extreme form of stress, vitamin C is the best kind of preoperative protection a person can get. Dr. Lewin of London proposes that vitamin C is more effective if it is taken in rather small doses during the day rather than in one or two larger doses, and if it is accompanied by a glass of grapefruit juice. Dr. Klenner's son received 10 gm of vitamin C per day ever since he was 10 years of age. By the age of 19, he had not developed a single TOOTH CAVITY.

◆ *Deficiencies Of Vitamin C*

For decades we have known that lack of Vitamin C causes impairment in many ways: Loss of WEIGHT, EXTREME WEAKNESS in MUSCLES, BONES BECOMING THIN and FRAGILE, LOOSE TEETH, the tendency to HEMORRHAGE etc. The effects of deficiency are so diverse, that practically every organ of the body is affected. Every BRUISING may indicate a lack of vitamin C. The discoloration that follows is the hemorrhaging of tiny capillaries. In experiments with guinea pigs it was found that the brain is that part of living creatures that suffers most from a lack of vitamin C. They found that the COPPER content of the brain is increased when vitamin C is lacking. It is well known that NEUROLOGIC and PSYCHIATRIC damage usually follows an increase in brain copper concentrations.

Dr. Frederick Reiss says that PRICKLY HEAT is associated with a vitamin C deficiency. He gave his patients 900 to 1000 mg of vitamin C which cured the condition. He says that small doses of 200 to 300 mg were effective only when hot weather subsided and perspiration decreased. He believes that HOT WEATHER depletes the body's store of vitamin C through perspiration. Dr. Pauling tells of a study in San Mateo County, California, which showed that people with a low intake of vitamin C had a DEATH RATE from all causes which was 2 times that of people who took some vitamin C. The study involved 577 people all over the age of 50. Two groups of people were given 50 mg and 1000 mg of vitamin C along with FERROUS SULFATE, a medicinal form of IRON. It was found that the 50 mg of vitamin C did not raise the level of iron in the blood, but the 1000 mg did.

Guinea pigs deprived of ascorbic acid were unable to convert GLUCOSE to GLYCOGEN for storage in their livers. But this condition was quickly remedied when vitamin C was added. When guinea pigs are progressively deprived of vitamin C, their tolerance to CARBOHYDRATES declines, and they are approaching a state of DIABETES in direct proportion. Lack of vitamin C affects the DENTINE of the teeth, causing it to wear away, thus increasing the likelihood of early decay.

A lack of vitamin C in cell walls seems to be the cause of RHEUMATOID ARTHRITIS. It seems possible that ASPIRIN may be one of the chief reasons why the patient is deficient in vitamin C. Hence, the continual taking of aspirin may guarantee that the arthritis victims would never recover.

◆ *The Need of Vitamin C in Disease.*

✓ SPEEDS WOUND HEALING — *JAMA, May 28, 1955, states that ascorbic acid is the only nutrient whose LACK has been proved to delay or prevent WOUND HEALING in man.* A study at Nebraska's Eppley Institute For Cancer Research showed that Vitamin C in large doses can effectively neutralize and destroy NITRITES in the stomach, and prevent their conversion into the cancer causing NITROSAMINES. It was also found that vitamins A, E, lecithin, and the B-complex had similar effects.

✓ KEEPS TERMINAL CANCER PATIENTS ALIVE—It was shown that 10 gm per day of vitamin C kept TERMINAL CANCER PA-

TIENTS alive 4 times longer. Vitamin C is toxic to a number of types of cancer cells, especially MELANOMA. gm of vitamin C three times a day was shown to reduce blood CHOLESTEROL levels by 35 to 40%.

✓ MASSIVE DOSES CURE DISEASES—There are physicians today who cure POLIO, PNEUMONIA, INFLUENZA, the COMMON COLD, and many other diseases with massive doses of vitamin C. One cannot really get too much of the natural vitamin C. People with the highest amounts of vitamin C in their diets had the lowest risk of cancer.

✓ DELAYS GROWTH OF TUMORS—Vitamin C delays the growth of tumors triggered by excess doses of hormones. It also blocks SKIN CANCER caused by ULTRAVIOLET LIGHT. BARLOW's DISEASE or INFANTILE SCURVY appeared in 1883. Breast-fed babies did not get the disease, but those fed with boiled or heated cow's milk did. It was cured by a speck of ascorbic acid. Scurvy in guinea pigs results in the rapid onset of ATHEROSCLEROSIS, because it was shown that vitamin C deprivation greatly increased CHOLESTEROL SYNTHESIS. Prolonged administration of ANTIBIOTICS results in vitamin C deficiency. Blood and urine levels of almost all vitamins fall during antibiotic therapy.

✓ REMOVES FATTY DEPOSITS—Dr. Carl F. Shaffer has shown in animal experiments that the FATTY DEPOSITS on the inside of the arteries can be removed by giving the animals vitamin C. A deficiency of vitamin C produces in guinea pigs a condition that is just like HARDENING OF THE ARTERIES in humans.

✓ HELPS CURE MUSCULAR DYSTROPHY (MD)—MD is caused by a lack of vitamin E in guinea pigs. When vitamin C was added to the diet 60% of the animals did not develop MD at all.

✓ PREVENTS GRAY HAIR—French scientists found that GRAY HAIR produced by a deficiency of PANTOTHENIC ACID, could be prevented for quite some time by giving vitamin C in large doses.

✓ REDUCES INTEROCULAR PRESSURE—The reduction of INTEROCULAR PRESSURE in GLAUCOMA, was accomplished by the injection of 20% SODIUM ASCORBATE solution with 70 mg per treatment. Dr. Dalton of Shelbyville, Indiana, gave patients with VIRAL PNEUMONIA, BRONCHITIS, SINUSITIS, FLU, and HEPATITIS massive doses of a preparation of vitamin C and B-vitamins which he injected daily. All responded almost miraculously.

✓ PREVENTS CATARACTS—CATARACT treatment with ascorbic acid gives dramatic results when the bloodstream is flooded with it. To prevent cataracts one doctor gives a formula of a special diet of vegetable greens, a pint of milk, 2 eggs, a chlorophyll tablet and vitamins A and C. A deficiency of vitamin C, B_2, and D, as well as calcium, can contribute to the development of cataracts, especially vitamin C. Vitamin C is concentrated 30 times more in the eyes than in the blood. In an experiment ultraviolet light was directed upon cultured eye tissue in order to cause oxidation. The more vitamin C was delivered to the tissue, the longer it took to form cataracts.

✓ PREVENTS BLADDER CANCER—It was demonstrated that the oral administration of large quantities of vitamin C will prevent the development of BLADDER CANCER. Dr. Schlegel of Tulane University believes that he can prevent bladder cancer with as much as 1500 mg of vitamin C. A Harvard researcher found that there is a greater incidence of bladder cancer among those men and women who drink COFFEE.

✓ RELIEVES POOR CIRCULATION—One physician gave 3 gm of vitamin C along with large doses of B-vitamins to patients suffering from POOR CIRCULATION so that their feet were constantly cold. In every case relief was obtained.

✓ PREVENTS AND CURES TETANUS—For TETANUS ascorbic acid dosages of 1gm/kg of weight for animals before or after the symptoms of tetanus had appeared saved all animals injected with tetanus toxins. Without the vitamin C all animals died. This dosage is equivalent to 140 gm of vitamin C for a 150 lb. man.

- ✓ VIRUS PNEUMONIA—Dr. Klenner gave a patient with VIRUS PNEUMONIA, a fever of 106 degrees, and unconscious, 140 gm of vitamin C within 72 hours. At the end of three days she was almost well.
- ✓ CARBON MONOXIDE POISONING—For CARBON MONOXIDE POISONING Dr. Klenner gives massive doses of vitamin C which is able to separate the carbon monoxide from the red blood cells which it is in the process of destroying.
- ✓ UNCONSCIOUSNESS — An UNCONSCIOUS man of 21 was taken to the hospital and was given 50 gm of vitamin C intravenously the first day, and 80 gm per day subsequently. Within a few hours life signs became normal, and his unconscious state changed into sleep. In another 8 hours he woke up. After 4 days he was taken out of intensive care, and on the 8th day he was released from the hospital.
- ✓ CURED CHICKEN POX—According to Dr. Klenner a man with CHICKEN POX was cured by taking 30 gm of vitamin C by mouth each day for 4 days.
- ✓ HEADACHES—A man decided to treat himself for a SINUS HEADACHE with VITAMIN C. He took 2 gm every hour for about 16 hours. The headache disappeared overnight and at the same time he realized that the spot in his eyes had disappeared as well. At other times SPOTS before the EYES have been cleared up with GARLIC and foods rich in B-vitamins.

◆ *The Benefits Of Vitamin C*

GUINEA PIGS, on whom weights were dropped which ordinarily would kill 100% of them, would always survive if given an ascorbic acid injection in doses above 100 mg/kg of weight shortly after. This was equivalent to 7 gm for a 150 lb. man. This could help wounded soldiers or accident victims. Exposure to X-RAYS lowers the level of ascorbic acid in the body. This fact could help RADIOLOGISTS, since it has been shown that they have an average life span which is 6 years less than the average of the population.

A 21 year study of 11,348 adults for their VITAMIN C intake was conducted at the University of California at Los Angeles (UCLA), beginning in 1971. It was to determine the effects of vitamin C supplementation on human LONGEVITY. It proved that men can expect a 6 year increase in LIFE EXPECTANCY by taking 500 mg of vitamin C daily. Using the same dose women can expect a life expectancy increase of 1 year. If the dose is increased to 900 mg per day, then the life expectancy increase for men is 10 years. Dr. Linus Pauling found that the risk from CANCER can be reduced 80% with an adequate intake of vitamin C. Other studies have found that vitamin C PREVENTS numerous types of cancer. Dr. Melvyn Werbach reported that CHOLESTEROL LEVELS dropped 41 points in only 6 weeks after beginning daily doses of 1000 mg of vitamin C. This health tip alone could save the lives of many people every year.

◆ *Vitamin C Counteracts Poisons*

Vitamin C is a potent detoxicant. It counteracts and neutralizes the harmful effects of many poisons in the body such as MERCURY, ARSENIC, DRUGS, BACTERIA, CARBON MONOXIDE (CO), SULFUR DIOXIDE (SO_2), and CARCINOGENS. Adelle Davis said that in a single year no less than 45 research projects reported that vitamin C rendered harmless a wide variety of BACTERIAL TOXINS, and that its action was nonspecific in that it was deadly to all types of viruses and bacteria, especially when given in large amounts. When mice were injected with 2 mg of STRYCHNINE, they all died. When injected with vitamin C before strychnine injection they did not all die. With 100 mg/kg of body weight 60% survived. With 1000 mg/kg of body weight, none of them died. This would be equivalent to 7 gm and 70 gm of vitamin C for a 70 kg or a 150 lb. man. A study of 63 women has shown that those who have been on the PILL for a year or more have less concentrations of vitamin C in their WHITE BLOOD CORPUSCLES than women not taking any contraceptives.

Laboratory animals were given DRUGS which caused CATARACTS. When they were given vitamin C at the same time no cataracts were formed. Rats are highly susceptible to cataracts when they are given large amounts of a sugar called GALACTOSE, which is produced from the milk sugar LACTOSE. If vitamin C is given along with the sugar, no cataracts appear. In 1938 Nitzesco showed that ascorbic acid when mixed with COBRA VENOM rendered it harmless. Guinea pigs injected with this venom died in 2 to 3 hours. With an injection of 25 mg of vitamin C they all survived. Researcher Dey needed 1 to 2 gm/kg of body weight to counteract the lethal effects of TETANUS TOXIN in guinea pigs. This is equivalent to more than 70 gm of vitamin C for a 150 lb. man. Smoking 1 CIGARETTE neutralizes approximately 25 mg of vitamin C, or the amount in a medium size orange.

A group of laborers exposed to FLUORIDE showed that the more vitamin C there is in the diet, the more is excreted in the urine every day. This indicates that vitamin C detoxifies fluoride by carrying it right out of the system. It means that fluorides use up the body's supply of vitamin C. Many researchers have found that SMOKING does indeed put certain cancer-causing substances into the bladder. They also showed that the formation of these substances could be entirely prevented by giving enough vitamin C. 1 gm per day completely prevented the formation of these cancer-causing substances.

◆ *Vitamin C Interrelationships*

Dr. King found that ample amounts of vitamin C in the intestines appear to encourage the intestinal bacteria to manufacture enough B-VITAMINS to make up for any not present in the diet. Indian scientists found that the right amounts of minerals ZINC, CHROMIUM, COPPER, and TUNGSTEN helped laboratory animals to use vitamin C to best advantage. With more or less of the right amount of minerals, the vitamin C activity was slowed down. The lesson is clear that the amounts of MINERALS found in natural foods seem to be the right amount for man as well as animals. As soon as we begin to subtract minerals by refining and processing foods we get imbalances. Nature balances things; man unbalances them.

◆ *Vitamin C For The Aging*

As we grow older, the process of aging causes us to develop nutritional needs which we did not have when we were younger.

Dr. McCormick developed the theory that DEGENERATIVE CHANGES in the body are caused by continued low levels of vitamin C in the body. Studies have shown that the majority of older people have notoriously low levels of vitamin C in their system, and it is believed that CANCER rarely grows in organs which have an adequate amount of vitamin C. Dr. Wilson of England surveyed the vitamin C status of elderly patients in his hospital. He noticed that men and women with higher levels of vitamin C lived longer than those with lower levels. The low vitamin C levels did not seem to produce any specific disease or condition of ill health, but those persons died sooner from all diseases.

◆ *Vitamin C And The Mind*

Dr. Milner found that all 40 of his PSYCHIATRIC patients had a severe vitamin C shortage. A 1000 mg of vitamin C every day for 3 weeks improved their overall personality functioning. It took that amount and time to saturate their tissues. It normally takes only from 24 to 48 hours. When a normal person is given 5 gm of vitamin C, his tissues are saturated—he can't absorb any more. But studies show that it takes from 20 to 40 grams of vitamin C to saturate the tissues of SCHIZOPHRENICS. However, they can get better on less. One doctor gave 40 schizophrenics, who had had the disease for years, 1 gm of vitamin C a day. Even at this rate many showed significant improvement.

Vitamin D—The Sunshine Vitamin

◆ *Vitamin D Is Formed In The Skin*

Vitamin D is formed when the ultraviolet rays of the sun, hitting the skin change ERGOSTEROL into vitamin D. It is needed for the absorption of CALCIUM and PHOSPHORUS. There are two forms of vitamin D. One is ERGOCALCIFEROL (D_2), and the other is CHOLECALCIFEROL (D_3), The latter is the one used to enrich milk. It appears that God intended man to obtain his vitamin D mainly from sunshine, from being out in the open air and exercising.

◆ *Sources Of Vitamin D*

Foods generally recognized as rich in vitamin D are MILK, BUTTER, FISH, and EGG YOLK. Fish liver oil is the richest source of vitamin D. Many people don't eat any of these foods for months at a time. In large cities the effective rays for creating vitamin D from the skin are absorbed by buildings and glass, so that people who don't go outside can fall short of vitamin D requirements.

There appears to be a substance in FUR and FEATHERS which is converted to vitamin D in sunlight. It is believed that animals with thick fur get their vitamin D by licking their coats. Rats which have rickets from lack of vitamin D can be cured by exposure to sunlight, but they must be allowed to lick their fur, else the sunshine does no good. If animals, who normally hibernate in winter when there is little benefit derived from sunlight, are given daily doses of vitamin D, they will not hibernate. Dark-skinned people absorb less ultraviolet light than fair-skinned people, so that they need a longer exposure to sunlight to produce the same amount of vitamin D.

◆ *Requirements of Vitamin D*

An average dose of vitamin D is from 400 to 1000 IU. When the National Institute of Health made a study of people hypersensitive to Vitamin D, it found that 10,000 IU per day would induce a toxic reaction. The Merck Index says that the danger level of a toxic reaction comes at prolonged daily use of 50,000 IU or more. Another estimate is that amounts on the order of 1000 to 3000 units per kilogram (2.2 lbs.) of body weight are toxic. So for a 150 lb. person, the toxic amount of vitamin D is somewhere between 100,000 and 300,000 units daily.

Most vitamins are manufactured by plants, but vitamin D is the exception. It is produced in human tissues. For this reason some nutritionists have asked that this vitamin be classified as a HORMONE rather than a vitamin. If vitamin D is taken in excess, it is stored in the liver for future use. Vitamin D is absolutely necessary for CALCIUM METABOLISM.

The risk in getting too much vitamin D is in disordering the calcium metabolism to the extent of causing hardening of the arteries. Also a retarded mentality in children has been associated with excessive levels of calcium in the blood. Calcium is absolutely essential to every HEARTBEAT. If for some reason your calcium supply becomes dangerously low, your heart will flutter or fibrillate or twitch, thereby sending out an SOS for more calcium. Vitamin D must be there before this calcium can be withdrawn from the bones to come to the aid of your heart. But if vitamin D is lacking, the heart is unable to complete this lifesaving maneuver. Without vitamin D our bodies would be open to all sorts of problems—from RICKETS in children, to OSTEOMALACIA in adults, to OSTEOPOROSIS in the elderly.

◆ *Synthetic Vitamin D_2*

Synthetic vitamin D_2 is an extremely dangerous drug. There are obvious reasons for this. Vitamin D_3 is partially responsible for CALCIUM METABOLISM. It is necessary for the absorption of calcium through the intestinal wall; it can increase the level of calcium in the blood serum; and it is partially responsible for the deposition of calcium into the bones. These functions can easily be overdone if the calcium involved is not accompanied by sufficient amounts of the minerals PHOSPHORUS and MAGNESIUM, both of which are indispensable to a proper regulation of calcium metabolism.

Synthetic Vitamin D_2 is unaccompanied by either the phosphorus or magnesium needed to regulate the calcium metabolism. Nevertheless some success has been achieved with it. One patient complained of low back pains and aching thighs for years. Samples of her bones showed a calcium deficiency. A normal diet was prepared with high vitamin D. But it had no real effect. When CALCIFEROL was given by muscular injection of 100,000 IU, the symptoms were promptly relieved. Calciferol (D_2) is a pure version of vitamin D prepared by the ultraviolet irradiation of ergosterol obtained from yeast. After 3 months of vitamin D_2 treatment, normal healthy bone was forming.

It is possible to get too much vitamin D, especially if you are taking the synthetic form which is not from fish liver oil. Under these circumstances your body does not use calcium properly any longer, and this is what causes the complaints regarding toxicity and harmful effects.

◆ *Vitamin D And Disease*

Babies are born with deformities due to the administration of excessive doses of synthetic vitamin D_2 during pregnancy. In nature vitamin D is always accompanied by vitamin A in liver oils. Vitamin D without vitamin A can lead to HYPERCALCEMIA, which means that calcium is drained from the bones and is deposited in the blood. It is thus capable of inducing reactions that are toxic because vitamin D is not in natural relationships with other necessary vitamins. Synthetic vitamin D also binds magnesium in milk, thereby making it unavailable.

RICKETS occurs either because there is insufficient calcium in the diet or because there is insufficient vitamin D to enable the child to absorb the calcium it has eaten. Another cause of this disease is insufficient phosphorus and magnesium in the diet, thereby preventing the proper disposition of the calcium into the bones and teeth. In Athens. Greece, 327 children under 1 year of age were given tests for a substance known to indicate rickets. 15% had rickets, and almost had clinical signs of the disease, meaning healed or inactive rickets. Breast-fed babies had only as great an incidence as those given formulas. The doctors gave those children with rickets vitamin D supplements, and all their symptoms disappeared. Greek women feel that their infants should be fully clothed at all times with just the head and upper arms exposed. This is just not enough exposure for the sunlight to work its magic upon the skin. A similar condition was discovered in the southern part of Israel where the babies clothing was to blame for the rickets.

On the other hand, when children are exposed too much to the elements with insufficient clothing, they can become chilled, and physical damage can occur. We are told that "keeping arms and shoulders uncovered has caused the lives of thousands of children and youth (2SM467). These children were martyrs to their parent's ignorance of the relation which food, dress and the air they breathe, sustain to health and life. MOTHERS in past ages should have been PHYSICIANS to their own children. God does not take pleasure in the sufferings and death of little children (2SM469).

More and more people are discovered who have PARATHYROID glands which are overactive. This gland, which removes calcium from the bones, can be countered only by consumption of additional amounts of calcium and vitamin D.

Regarding OSTEOPOROSIS in older people, many physicians believe that lack of calcium in the diet may play a part which results in pain, discomfort, and often broken bones. Some doctors believe that BROKEN HIPS which many older people experience are not the result of falls. but that the bone breaks first, causing the fall. There is evidence that vitamin D is often effective in relieving this condition. A study of 60 elderly women over 70 showed that those with the lowest vitamin D intake had the least dense bones, that is, the ones most likely to fracture. Although these women were apparently getting enough calcium and phosphorus, they did lack vitamin D to help them absorb these minerals.

Dr. Knapp a New York Ophthalmologist treats some EYE conditions of old people with massive doses of vitamin D. He believes that MYOPIA or shortsightedness is a manifestation of vitamin D deficiency. He gave a group of patients vitamin D and calcium supplements over periods of from 5 to 28 months, and found a decrease in the nearsightedness in more than, and a definite halt in the process in another 17%. Dr. Knapp also believes that lack of vitamin D and calcium may be related to the formation of CATARACTS. Laboratory animals kept on diets deficient in vitamin D and calcium invariably develop cataracts he says. In human beings there are some relevant facts linking vitamin D and calcium lack to cataracts. For example, DIABETICS often suffer from calcium imbalance. They develop cataracts more often than non-diabetics.

◆ *Deficiencies Of Vitamin D*

Any calcium deficiency disease can be caused by insufficient vitamin D as easily as by a lack of calcium. Children in England do not get sufficient vitamin D because of their limited exposure to sunlight. Negro children's skin resists the penetration of ultraviolet light. Hence, they do not receive enough vitamin D. That is why there are more negro children with RICKETS today. According to Dr. Lewis LIGHTER SKINNED PEOPLE moved from the tropics north to protect themselves from too much sun, and especially from the ultraviolet light. DARK SKINNED PEOPLE in the north would easily get rickets, so that they could not hunt or find other food. Hence, only the lighter skinned people among them survived. Eventually these people became the fair-skinned people of northern Europe and Scandinavia.

There is one exception to the general rule that all people need sunshine, and that is the ESKIMOS. Eskimos must wear thick heavy clothing which prevents the sun from getting to their skin. But rickets is unknown among them. The reason is that they eat the livers of fish and animals which are a dependable source of vitamin D.

Without calcium the BLOOD will not coagulate properly. A deficiency leads to widespread HEMORRHAGE lesions in the gastrointestinal tract, PARATHYROID enlargement, IRRITABILITY of NERVES, MUSCLES, and CRAMPS. Insufficient vitamin D may be the actual cause of all of these calcium deficiency diseases. CLOTHING and WINDOW GLASS shut out the ultraviolet rays which help develop vitamin D. Also winter sunshine has very little ultraviolet light, and with the addition of heavy clothing very little vitamin D is produced. The solution is to take FISH LIVER OIL.

◆ *Vitamin D And Aging*

Regarding older people there is good evidence that they continue to need vitamin D, as they still must absorb calcium and phosphorus for many different body functions. These minerals can be absorbed only if vitamin D is present.

Bones continue to need nourishment even in older people, since they lose minerals constantly which must be replaced. No one has ever been harmed taking vitamin D in recommended amounts to regulate the body's absorption of calcium and phosphorus.

As we age the skin is less efficient in making vitamin D. Furthermore, older people are less efficient at converting vitamin D from foods and supplements to a usable form. It is important for people 65 years and over to either drink two cups of fortified milk, or spend some time in the sun, or take a vitamin supplement which contains 200 to 400 IU of vitamin D.

Vitamin E

◆ *What Is Vitamin E*

Vitamin E was discovered in 1922 in wheat germ oil. Research has shown this vitamin to be in many foods, but in most of them in small quantities. Pure vitamin E was isolated in 1939. Soon afterwards synthetic vitamin E was made. Experimenters tried to produce the same effects with synthetic vitamin E as with wheat germ oil but they failed. So the consensus of opinion was that there is some substance in wheat germ oil, besides vitamin E which must be responsible for its significant effects. When new milling methods were introduced into the manufacture of wheat flour, permitting the complete stripping away of the highly perishable WHEAT GERM, the diet of Western man lost its only significant source of VITAMIN E in the diet. It was greatly reduced, and with the loss of this natural ANTITHROMBIN, CORONARY THROMBOSIS appeared on the scene. It doesn't seem to be a coincidence that HEART DISEASE MORTALITY, the number one killer in the U.S., has climbed steadily during the past 60 years since we have been eating bread from which the vitamin E has been removed. There is sufficient evidence to show that the refining of foods has worked this fatal mischief on our HEARTS, our JOINTS, and our MUSCLES.

Vitamin E occurs plentifully in natural food, but it is still difficult to obtain in adequate amounts without dietary supplements. This is one of the terrible results of food processing. It is abundant in whole grain, but it is stripped away in the process of flour making. It is abundant in raw nuts, but is destroyed by deep-fat-frying. It is important for one thing because our ability to reproduce depends upon it. If our food processors could succeed in stripping it completely from our diet, they might as well say good-bye to the human race.

◆ *Used In The Alphatocopherol form*

It is called a TOCOPHEROL which means "to carry oil." For most therapeutic purposes only the D-ALPHA TOCOPHEROL form is used. Whenever you see dl-alpha tocopherol, you should recognize this as the synthetic form. The synthetic form is only as potent as the natural form, and usually costs only as much. It is usually measured in international units (IU); but occasionally in milligrams (mg). 1 IU equals 1 mg. Alpha tocopherol, as an effective antithrombin, suffers none of the drawbacks of the ANTICOAGULANTS that are commonly used, and consequently may be used indefinitely without danger. What is tragic is that the medical profession, while feeling a distaste for the quack use of the vitamin, lost sight of the legitimate need for the vitamin and its valuable therapeutic use.

Dr. Shute mentions that the great value of alphatocopherol lies in the fact that it is CHEAP,

SELF-APPLICABLE, EASY TO USE, and can be WIDELY DISTRIBUTED when danger threatens. In a nuclear war, for example, the majority of injuries would be of the very kind which alphatocopherol handles best, namely BURNS, SCARS, OPEN WOUNDS, and ULCERATIONS.

◆ *Sources And Requirements Of Vitamin E*

Natural sources are unrefined WHEAT GERM, OLIVE, SOYBEAN oil, raw SEEDS, NUTS, GRAINS, GREEN LEAFY VEGETABLES, EGG YOLK, and WHOLE GRAIN CEREALS, WHOLE GRAIN OATMEAL, UNPOLISHED NATURAL BROWN RICE. A food highest in alphatocopherol is a food highest in usable vitamin E.

Butter and whole eggs contain about 3 mg of vitamin E per 100 gm. Green celery contains 2.6 mg of vitamin E per 100 gm. Peanuts contain about 30 mg per 100 gm. Wheatgerm oil contains as high as 420 mg per 100 gm.

The CORONARY PATIENTS are usually given a dosage of 800 IU alphatocopherol daily for 6 weeks. It usually takes 5 to 10 days to take effect and 4 to 6 weeks to diminish or relieve symptoms. If the patient is not improved very much, then the dosage is raised 200 IU per day to 1000 IU per day for the next 6 weeks period. Vitamin E is classified by the FDA as a nontoxic vitamin, not a drug. Except in extremely rare instances, vitamin E in normal dosages is absolutely without adverse side-effects.

Vitamin E daily requirement is 50 IU, but when taken in large doses such as 600 to 1000 IU, it increases OXYGENATION of the TISSUES by as much as 60%. Researchers have stated that vitamin E therapy is equivalent to being placed in an oxygen tent. It prevents unsaturated fatty acids from being destroyed in the body by oxygen. A deficiency may lead to STROKES, and REPRODUCTIVE DISORDER. There is a decline in the body's oxygen consumption as one grows older, leading to such ailments as HEART DISEASE, BODY WASTING, and other manifestations of OLD AGE.

◆ *The Need For Vitamin E*

Vitamin E is a fat and oil soluble vitamin that is highly concentrated in the ADRENAL GLANDS. The adrenals use it to regulate sodium and potassium in the blood, to produce SEX HORMONES, and to help the body respond to STRESS. It is also concentrated in the FATTY TISSUE, LIVER, and HEART.

Vitamin E is necessary for CONCEPTION, PREGNANCY, LACTATION, and the adequate absorption of IRON. It reduces the need for OXYGEN intake, and is therefore called an ANTIOXIDANT. In several experiments by Houchin and Mattill, it reduced the oxygen need in a heart muscle by from 50 to 250%. Its ability to thereby increase exercise tolerance has been demonstrated in many animals such as greyhounds and horses. By preventing premature oxidation of lipids (fats) in the bloodstream, it keeps available to the tissues a higher proportion of the oxygen taken into the blood. It is known also as an ANTITHROMBIN, which means that it has the ability to dissolve blood clots, as well as to prevent them from occurring. As a VASODILATOR it increases the blood supply to the heart by widening the arteries. Dr. Shute says that the average cardiologist can do nothing to help a damaged heart if he does not use vitamin E—except to treat symptoms and complications.

Vitamin E in the blood stream tends to bond itself with fatty acids and prevents their oxidation. The vitamin E is destroyed in this process which is the reason why there is a need of more vitamin E whenever there are POLYUNSATURATED FATS in the diet. Research indicates that the need for vitamin E is often increased six-fold if a person consumes large amounts of UNSATURATED FATS. In the early astronaut flights the men suffered a 20 to 30% loss of their RED BLOOD CELLS and therefore became anemic and fatigued. The reason was discovered to be a lack of vitamin E in their prepared foods. On later flights they took along the vitamin E, and there were no more breakdowns of the red blood cells.

Drs. O'Connor and Hodges of England concluded after 30 years experience in both medicine and surgery, that ALPHATOCOPHEROL treatment of cardiovascular and renal diseases as suggested by Drs. Shute and White is one of the greatest medical discoveries of the century. They also said that in the treatment of early GANGRENE, especially in DIABETIC patients, TOES and FEET, that formerly would have been amputated, may now be saved.

Dr. Beckmann of the University of Freiburg, Germany, found vitamin E particularly beneficial to the liver. He also found that a dose of 300 mg of vitamin E given to women at the start of DELIVERY reduces the incidence of BRAIN HEMORRHAGES in the child. He recommends large doses of vitamin E in SLOW GROWING CHILDREN.

◆ *Benefits of Vitamin E*

✓ PREVENTS ACCUMULATION OF CHOLESTEROL—Besides vitamin E, wheatgerm contains many other substances such as unsaturated fatty acids and other fatty substances which doctors claim prevent HARDENING of the ARTERIES as well as the accumulation of CHOLESTEROL. Vitamin E has been shown to prevent the HAIR LOSS of ADRIAMYCIN CHEMOTHERAPY.

✓ DOES AWAY WITH LEG CRAMPS—Vitamin E helps restore muscles to a healthy state after exercise. Vitamin E keeps the RED BLOOD CELLS from aging under stressful conditions, and increases their life span. In amounts of 400 to 800 IU per day, vitamin E can do away with LEG CRAMPS otherwise called INTERMITTENT CLAUDICATION. It protects against the damaging effect of many environmental POISONS in air, water, and food. It prevents SCAR TISSUE formation in BURNS, SORES, and POSTOPERATIVE HEALING. Both vitamins E and C are protective agents against the damaging effects of ASPIRIN.

Dr. Knut Haeger of Sweden extended the walking range of INTERMITTENT CLAUDICATION patients with 300 to 400 IU of VITAMIN E. Of a group of 95 patients who exercised and took vitamin E, there was need for one AMPUTATION, while among 104 patients who did not take the vitamin, there was a requirement of 11 amputations.

Postoperative patients who did not receive VITAMIN E and CALCIUM supplements had 200% more blood clots in the legs, 600% more in the lungs, and 900% more fatalities from PULMONARY EMBOLISM than the patients who received vitamin E and Calcium.

✓ INCREASES VITAMIN A AND C STORES—The stores of vitamin A and C are depleted in the livers of subjects deficient in vitamin E, and are increased when vitamin E is provided. Both of these vitamins are very sensitive to the presence of oxygen and may lose much of their value over time. But the presence of vitamin E protects them from oxidation. This indicates that with vitamin E less vitamin A and C are needed by the body. Vitamin E affords protection to the red blood cells in the presence of a blood-destroying agent like HYDROGEN PEROXIDE (H_2O_2). It helps to open up blocked channels, combats CHOLESTEROL within the blood system, and makes the arteries and veins more flexible and "clean" to permit normal passage of oxygen and blood.

✓ PREVENTS RANCIDITY—It prevents RANCIDITY when added to other substances. It DILATES the BLOOD VESSELS and improves the CIRCULATION. It retards the AGING process. It prevents leg ULCERS, and ANGINA PECTORIS. Vitamin E has a dramatic effect on the reproductive organs. It prevents MISCARRIAGE, increases male and female FERTILITY, and helps to restore male POTENCY. One study shows that it improves athletic performance.

✓ IMPROVES MUSCLE HEALTH—One researcher found that injections of vitamin E have been found to be powerful against muscle-wasting in LEPERS, and have been found to give satisfactory results in all cases. In everyone the volume of the muscles increased, the muscle tone and muscular movements of hands improved, and that partial or total functional recovery was obtained. In general it has been found that vitamin E is the MUSCLE VITAMIN, for it is essential for muscle health. Some researchers therefore say that MUSCULAR DYSTROPHY (MS) is a vitamin E deficiency disease.

Vitamin E makes it possible for the muscles to do their work with less oxygen, and consequently suffering less damage. Where there is a deficiency of vitamin E, Dr. Follis states that LESIONS appear in the muscles including the heart. This function has made vitamin E the food of champions. Many athletes and trainers have found that by permitting the muscles to do their work with less oxygen, vitamin E has increased the available energy, endurance, and performance levels.

✓ PREVENTS AND HELPS BLOOD CLOT-

TING—The story is told of a man who watched his weight and diet carefully, retained a trim figure free from any hint of obesity, exercised daily by taking a 2 to 3 mile walk every night, never smoked nor drank, went to bed early and slept 8 hours every night. He had a heart attack anyway. He was told that none of those measures can prevent a heart attack if the bloodstream is deficient in the ANTITHROMBIN content that should naturally be there.

An Italian medical journal tells of a patient who had a blood clotting time of 24 hours. This clotting time was normalized with vitamin E. After 10 days the clotting time was reduced to 2 hours. After 25 days it was reduced to 80 minutes, and finally to normal.

✓ IMPROVES RHEUMATIC FEVER—Rheumatic fever is now recognized as a chronic infection which is difficult to diagnose in its early stages. There is usually some damage to the heart, and no treatment currently used except the ALPHATOCOPHEROL treatment, has been shown to do anything to alter its inexorable course.

✓ HELPS RETARDED CHILDREN—Dr. Del Guidice of Buenos Aires has been giving two grams of vitamin E daily for many years to RETARDED CHILDREN and even MONGOLOIDS, and has achieved some amazingly beneficial effects, both mental and physical. He says that small doses simply will not work, for the results which he has seen occur only when the body of the patient is completely saturated with vitamin E.

✓ VITAMIN E'S ROLE SIMILAR TO EXERCISE—By proper exercise you increase your cardiovascular efficiency. As the training effect takes place you UTILIZE OXYGEN MORE EFFICIENTLY. This also helps you survive a heart attack. Both vitamin E and exercise encourage the establishment of additional blood vessels and DILATE SMALLER BLOOD VESSELS when there is an oxygen demand.

✓ VITAMIN E AND SELENIUM INCREASE ANTIBODIES—Dr. Spollholtz of Colorado State University has confirmed that VITAMIN E and SELENIUM together increase the body's production of antibodies to various invaders. Without them the body cannot defend itself against CARCINOGENS or WILD CELLS. With them the body cannot be damaged by them.

Drs. Lo and Black of Baylor University found that ANTIOXIDANT THERAPY with vitamins C, E, and selenium protected the body against sun-induced SKIN CANCER. They observed that after exposure to sunlight the CHOLESTEROL in the skin was oxidized to CHOLESTEROL ALPHA-OXIDE, a suspected carcinogen. They found that Vitamins C and E and selenium did prevent the formation of this compound, as well as did the antioxidant food preservatives BHA and BHT, and they all did it without causing any side effects.

✓ HAIR GROWTH AND VITAMIN E—Japanese researchers said that the administration of VITAMIN E was able to make hair grow 2.4 times faster than normal. The secret was that vitamin E increases the blood flow to the skin. It stimulates the circulation by OXYGENATING the blood.

✓ OTHER BENEFITS—It also increases the beneficial HDL cholesterol, protects against NITROSAMINES, neutralizes RADIATION EXPOSURE, it scavenges FREE RADICALS, inhibits the growth of CANCER CELLS, protects against the OXIDATION of POLYUNSATURATED ACIDS, is essential for the normal function of the RED BLOOD CELLS, is beneficial for FIBROCYSTIC BREAST DISEASE which affects 50% of all women, and it reduces LDL cholesterol levels and increases HDL cholesterol levels. 600 to 1200 IU of vitamin E daily prevents diabetic complications.

◆ *What Destroys Vitamin E*

✓ RANCID FATS AND OILS—Vitamin E is removed from wheat when flour is milled. When the flour is bleached, any vitamin E that might be left in the flour is destroyed by the bleach. Vitamin E is destroyed in the presence of RANCID FATS or OILS. MINERAL OIL also destroys it along with other fat-soluble vitamins in the digestive tract. Medicines that contain FERRIC CHLORIDE or other ferric or iron salts inactivate vitamin E in the body. DEEP-FAT-FRYING destroys 70–90% of the vitamin E, and BAKING PIES destroys from 25–75%.

Also CHLORINE or CHLORINATED WATER will destroy vitamin E. Chlorine is also an OXIDANT. Complications arise when pollutants react with chlorine to produce CARCINOGENS, thus requiring still more vitamin E.

✓ THE PROCESS OF PREVENTING OXIDATION—When oils are highly refined or hydrogenated, much of the vitamin E is sacrificed. Also 90% is lost in deep fat frying. Vitamin E in the bloodstream bonds with the fatty acids and prevents their oxidation. The vitamin E is destroyed in the course of this activity, which is why POLYUNSATURATES in any quantity create the need for proportionally more vitamin E. By this antioxidant activity, vitamin E prevents oxygen from being converted into TOXIC PEROXIDES.

◆ *Vitamin E And Disease*

✓ IT PREVENTS CANCER—A study of 21,172 men in Finland found that those who had high blood levels of vitamin E were less likely to develop CANCER than were those with low levels of vitamin E. A similar study with 15,093 women had the same result. Vitamin E is a protection against cancer.

New evidence indicates that vitamin E may have a therapeutic role in FIBROCYSTIC DISEASE of the BREAST which is a possible PRECURSOR to BREAST CANCER. It is suspected to also have such a role in INTERMITTENT CLAUDICATION, PREMENSTRUAL SYNDROME (PMS), and progressive MUSCULAR DISEASE in children.

✓ IT PREVENTS CATARACTS—Researchers found that people who took vitamin E were half as likely to develop CATARACTS as those not taking it. Exposure to ultraviolet light is thought to be a major cause of cataracts. It was found that people without cataracts had taken significantly more supplemental Vitamins E and C than those with cataracts. Those who took only vitamin E were half as likely to develop cataracts. Those who took both vitamin E and C had only a chance as those who took neither vitamin. About half of all people 75 years and over have cataracts.

✓ IT PREVENTS AND CURES HEART AND BLOOD VESSEL DISEASES—Vitamin E has achieved its greatest reputation in treating CIRCULATORY DISEASES. Its ability to help maintain a high level of oxygen in the blood has been a great boon to the economic action of the heart. Since blood which is rich in oxygen performs more efficiently on its trip through the body, less blood, and hence less pumping is required to do the same work.

In one study of 44 patients with VARICOSE VEINS complaints were treated with 300–500 IU of vitamin E daily for from 2 months to 3 years. 7 cases were healed completely, 9 cases showed improvement, and all of the others showed some improvement in relief of CONGESTION, PAIN, and EDEMA.

The amounts of vitamins E and C in the blood and blood vessels may be a factor in determining how rapidly one develops ATHEROSCLEROSIS. Many physicians are using it in the treatment of HEART and BLOOD VESSEL diseases. Heart disorders and disorders of the glands may result from MATERNAL MALNUTRITION. Nervous diseases and mental deficiency may be traced to the same source. One can disturb the normal development of the embryo by depriving the pregnant mother of certain essential nutritional elements. General starvation of the mother results in sterility, abortions, or stillbirths. Dr. H. Schmidt of England says that the person who eats a LOW CALORIE DIET, and takes large amounts of vitamin E is, for all practical purposes, immune from heart disease.

One patient with inflammation of the blood vessels, or BUERGER'S DISEASE, took 600 IU of vitamin E daily. There was slight improvement. Then he increased the dose to 2000 IU daily. At that point the ulcers began to respond dramatically, and the color of his legs began to normalize. This arrested the disease as well as his ANGINA. As a further bonus he found that he could reduce his medication for DIABETES and to eventually eliminate it entirely.

A doctor wanted to AMPUTATE the first three TOES of a woman's left foot after they became BLUE, ABSCESSED, and so PAINFUL that she was barely able to walk or sleep because of the pain. She had been taking 800 IU of vitamin E per day, but she increased it to 1600 IU, and gradually to

2400 IU a day along with LECITHIN GRANULES and 500 mg of vitamin C. In addition she massaged her foot and leg and got regular exercise. Within 3 days the pain was almost gone, and gradually her toes returned to their normal color. The International Record Of Medicine reports that 17 out of 18 patients with BUERGER'S DISEASE were cured with VITAMIN E.

A woman who had suffered a long time with PHLEBITIS, after the efforts of several doctors, engaged a new doctor who put her on 1500 units of Vitamin E a day, plus external application of vitamin E to the affected area. She said that it was like magic. The ULCERS healed, the SCAR TISSUE became pliable, and there was no further breakage. After 6 weeks she reduced the dose to 800 units per day for 3 months, then to 400 units a day. She says that she never felt better in her life.

A woman cured her 10 year old son's PLANTAR WARTS with 800 units of vitamin E per day. At the end of two weeks the warts were completely gone. Others have success with a single drop of MURIATIC ACID (HCL) placed on the wart once a day for 8 days. Others have success by applying to the wart the juice of MILKWEED, CELANDINE HERBS, or MARIGOLD.

✓ IT CURES MUSCULAR DYSTROPHY (MD)—In 1931 researchers found that VITAMIN E DEFICIENCY caused muscular dystrophy in RABBITS, HAMSTERS, and MONKEYS. It also caused FRAGILE BLOOD CELLS in all animals, thereby producing ANEMIA.

It has also produced some spectacular results in cases of DIABETES. In an article in the Associated Press it told of a girl who was made helpless by the muscle-wasting disease of MUSCULAR DYSTROPHY. Dr. Manville of the University of Oregon failed in his first attempt to cure human muscular dystrophy. But he later discovered that the purified wheat germ extract which was successful on rabbits did not work on humans. Then the brand of WHEATGERM OIL which retained all the natural vitamins and minerals was given to the girl, and she recovered from the disease. In 1937 vitamin E was synthesized, but it was not until 1962 that the synthetic product was proved to be only as powerful as the product derived from natural sources.

In another study researchers reported the treatment and improvement of 5 patients with MD. In this case the addition of vitamin B to vitamin E gave better results. This statement gives us a clue why doctors obtain conflicting results with vitamin E. One doctor might not pay any attention to a patient's diet. Another might make sure that the patient is getting all of the other vitamins necessary to good nutrition, and under these circumstances the addition of vitamin E in the diet might work wonders.

In the case of RATS on diets low in vitamin E, litters can be born, but the young rats often develop paralysis of the hind legs shortly after birth. This paralysis is much the same as muscular dystrophy in human beings. Vitamin E is closely related to healthy muscles, and we must not forget that the HEART is a muscle also.

In another study laboratory animals were kept on a vitamin E deficient diet and developed PARALYSIS due to lack of vitamin B_1, or THIAMIN, which was later found to be also deficient in the diet. Then giving the animals vitamin C of all things cured the paralysis. The close association between vitamins C and E is shown by the fact that GUINEA PIGS given MUSCULAR DYSTROPHY by diets deficient in vitamin E show far greater damage to muscles when there is a lack of vitamin C in their diets also. Vitamin E has been shown to slow the growth or to stop the growth of some cancer cells.

✓ IT DECREASES OXYGEN NEED IN THE BODY—The chief point of attack of TOCOPHEROLS in the body seems to be intimately connected with the UTILIZATION of OXYGEN and therefore with CELL RESPIRATION. OXYGEN is absolutely essential for every process that goes on inside our bodies, and it is believed that in many diseases one of the chief troubles is lack of enough oxygen in the cells.

Experiments with dogs showed that ESTROGEN induces THROMBOCYTOPENIC PURPURA (abnormal decrease in number of blood platelets), and that this HEMORRHAGIC disease, or easy bruising and easy bleeding, can be cured and prevented with vitamin E. Hence, it showed estrogen to be a vitamin E ANTAGONIST. Houchin also showed that in ANOXIC or oxygen deficient isolated heart muscle, the addition of alphatocopherol decreased oxygen need by some 50% or more.

The man who obtains a 250% decrease will never thereafter run out of oxygen, while the 50% man will be only partially helped.

✓ IT REDUCES HOSPITALIZATION TIME— Dr. Paul Dudley White and Samuel Levine were the first to demonstrate that bed rest in heart disease was undesirable. They favored hospitalization in an armchair for three weeks — The treatment to begin as soon as the initial chest pain was relieved. By this method they were able to demonstrate the reduction of the initial death rate to 9.9%, Instead of the expected 40 TO 60%. In other words, 4 out of 5 who would have died lived with intensive care and absolute bed rest in the ARMCHAIR TREATMENT.

✓ IT SPEEDS THE HEALING OF BURNS—Vitamin E is of maximum use in treating BURNS from the small domestic burns from hot iron or steam, to the most severe THIRD DEGREE burn. Its scars are so smooth, that they usually render skin grafting unnecessary. It has a very practical application in case of the common SUNBURN.

✓ IT IMPROVES CONCEPTION AND BIRTH RELATED PROBLEMS—Drs. Evans and Bishop noted that test subjects who were able to conceive but who could not carry to full term, when given LETTUCE, the fertility problem was corrected. When given UNBLEACHED WHEAT they became fertile and could conceive. It was noted that single daily drops of golden WHEAT GERM OIL proved remedial. Because this miracle substance enabled subjects to bear offspring, it was given the name TOCOPHEROL from TOCAS the Greek for CHILDBIRTH, and PHERO, the verb meaning TO BRING FORTH.

There are approximately 50 well-documented studies which demonstrate the value of vitamin E in producing HEALTHY OFFSPRING in previously BARREN COUPLES. There are also hundreds of animal studies which corroborate this observation in practically all mammalian species. This ability to produce healthy offspring has caused vitamin E to be tagged an ANTI-STERILITY VITAMIN, and this is still considered to be the vitamin's prime function by many medical authorities. From the oxygen standpoint Dr. Shute says that the fetus before birth is living of a mile above Mt. Everest.

Doctors, have attributed many MISCARRIAGES TO DEFICIENCIES in vitamin E. They attribute those failures which are classified as "of unknown origin" to an INSUFFICIENCY OF OXYGEN in the blood supply. Dr. Shute reported that by prescribing vitamin E for all his OBSTETRIC PATIENTS he has reduced the threatened miscarriage from 10% to 5%, and then with additional vitamin E therapy, has salvaged better than 80% of the remainder.

Dr. Strean states that in a normal birth the child born is already breathing. The doctor's spanking the baby to get the breathing started is necessary only because ANESTHETICS and PAIN-KILLING DRUGS used on the mother make it that much harder for the infant to breathe. A delay of even a minute or two before the newborn infant's breathing is started, can be enough to effect serious changes in the brain that has been starved for oxygen for that long. Here an ample supply of vitamin E can be all-important.

✓ IT PROTECTS AGAINST AGING—It does this by preventing oxygen from combining with essential fatty acids to form the AGE CAUSING PEROXIDES or RADICALS. It synthesizes ACETYLCHOLINE from CHOLINE and ACETATES. The body takes the substance and uses it to ease muscular weakness and wasting that is often symptomatic of advancing age.

Since aging is due to the process of OXIDATION, vitamin E as a natural ANTI-OXIDANT counteracts this process in the body. Oxidation forms high-reaction compounds which cause a breakdown and loss of function of PROTEINS. The debris from these destroyed proteins tends to pile up in cell membranes and accounts for the behaviors which are characteristic of aging. Vitamin E acts to prevent the formation of FREE RADICALS and serves as a built-in protection against accelerated aging. In normal cell cultures cells have a definite life span. Human embryonic LUNG CELLS will divide and reproduce about 50 times before they die. However, in a vitamin E enriched medium, cells have divided more than 120 times. Vitamin E increases the average life span of laboratory animals, but it does not increase the maximum life span.

The general conclusions are that a deficiency

of vitamin E will cause PREMATURE AGING. Vitamin E is more critical than other nutrients because it is involved in membrane protection; It is lacking in most diets, because it is processed out of many foods. It will protect the body against many POLLUTANTS and POISONS. It will PROTECT ALL MEMBRANES, AID CIRCULATION, and REDUCE CELL LOSS.

- ✓ IT CURES VARICOSE VEINS—A man with varicose veins took 2000 units of VITAMIN E a day, and then increased it to 3000 units. He also increased his VITAMIN C from 1000 mg to 2000 mg. Within two weeks the veins were back to normal. Before starting on vitamin E he was taking ORINASE for DIABETES. His doctor said that he would have to be on it for the rest of his life. But a short time after taking vitamin E, he was able to stop the use of the drug. His fasting blood sugar was now always between 85 and 95.
- ✓ SCAR TISSUE—It prevents the production of excessive scar tissue, speeds up the healing of wounds, and stimulates hair growth.
- ✓ IT DUPLICATES THE ACTION OF INSULIN—It does this by protecting against sugar imbalances that lead to problems such as DIABETES. It helps in the metabolization of sugar and spares the use of insulin.
- ✓ IT CURES "STIFF LAMB DISEASE"—A deprivation of vitamin E in sheep causes the "stiff lamb disease," which means that the lamb dies shortly after birth unless it receives vitamin E supplements immediately.
- ✓ ARTHRITIS—Arthritis patients were given 300–600 mg of vitamin E per day orally. After about 8 days PAIN was seen to decrease, and IN 3 OR 4 WEEKS, the calcium deposits ceased forming. Vitamin E was also used in HIP ARTHRITIS as a last resort before trying plastic surgery. Some severely inflamed hips responded so that they regained full motion with no further treatment necessary.
- ✓ NATURE'S OWN TRANQUILIZER—Very nervous horses were quieted down on vitamin E therapy, and their performance on the track was also greatly improved. This calming effect was first discovered by German researchers, who called vitamin E NATURE'S OWN TRANQUILIZER.
- ✓ SKIN DISEASES—Dr. Dam of Copenhagen found that the administration of large quantities of COD LIVER OIL to experimental animals resulted in severe disorders of the SKIN and other organs if the diet was devoid of vitamin E. All signs of illness disappeared in a rather short time after the supply of sufficient amounts of vitamin E. These diseases occurred because cod liver oil contains highly unsaturated fatty acids or vitamin F. Peroxides of fatty acids form in the arteries if there is not sufficient vitamin E in the diet.
- ✓ FIBROCYSTITIS—600 units of VITAMIN E improved the condition of FIBROCYSTITIS of 12 menstruating women. It relieved LUMPS, SORES, and TENDERNESS of the BREASTS WITHOUT HARMFUL SIDE EFFECTS. DOLOMITE will do the same also. Experts say that CALCIUM DEFICIENCY can produce swelling of the breasts as well as pain.
- ✓ EMPHYSEMA—is a disease in which the air sacs in the lungs are damaged by some oxidizing gases in the air such as OZONE, a corrosive form of oxygen, NITROGEN OXIDE from exhaust fumes, HOUSEHOLD SOLVENTS, and other TOXIC GASES. If laboratory rats are exposed to these fumes, they develop emphysema. The air sacs become inflamed and enlarged, and lose their ability to stretch when we breathe, like a balloon that has lost its elasticity. The ALVEOLAR FLUID bathes the air sacs. Lung tissue contains more vitamin E than most tissues. It helps us with emphysema and slows down the rate of its possible development.

◆ *Deficiencies Of Vitamin E*

The research of Dr. David Turner revealed why earlier spacemen up to and including the Borman flight, had suffered the loss of 20 to 30% of their red blood cells during flights, and thus became ANEMIC and FATIGUED. The REASON: A lack of vitamin E in the prepared foods carried by the astronauts. With the vitamin E in their food in later flights, they did not suffer any loss of red blood cells.

Deficiency signs of vitamin E are PIGMENTATION, ANEMIA, MUSCULAR DYSTROPHY as noted in animals, and BLOOD VESSEL DISORDERS. It has no known TOXICITY. People with OVERACTIVE THYROIDS, DIABETES, HIGH BLOOD PRESSURE, or RHEUMATIC HEARTS, should proceed cautiously, starting with 30 IU for a month, then increase by 30 IU's each month until a tolerance limit is reached. It is best absorbed when taken with meals, without any IRON compounds. Free iron in the same pill with vitamin E can destroy it. Strongly bound organic iron will not attack vitamin E, and the iron in food is usually organic iron.

MINERALS

The Body's Need Of Minerals

◆ *Organic And Inorganic Elements*

Chemical elements which are not combined with the carbon atom, or are not within carbon compounds, are called INORGANIC ELEMENTS. As such they participate in a number of physiological processes necessary for the maintenance of health. If they are part of carbon compounds and are combined with other elements, they are called ORGANIC ELEMENTS, because they originate from living substances. If they are required in amounts greater than 100 mg, they are called "minerals." If they are required in amounts less than 100 mg, the are called "trace minerals." Minerals are the elements or compounds of the elements of CALCIUM, MAGNESIUM, PHOSPHORUS, SODIUM, POTASSIUM, SULFUR, CHLORINE, and others.

The amount of minerals in plants depends to a large extent on the composition of the soil. If the soil contains a lot of minerals, so will the food which is grown on it. When there is a minimum of minerals in the soil, cattle will search out places which contain a lot of minerals which are called SALT LICKS. But salt licks do not merely refer to sodium chloride, but to salts of many other elements. We are as much in need of minerals as we are of vitamins. We have IRON in the blood, IODINE in the thyroid gland, CALCIUM in the bones, PHOSPHORUS in the brain. No symptom develops in the body without a foundation of disturbed tissue chemistry.

Every abnormal manifestation in the body is influenced by mineral imbalance. The vitamins represent the battery in your car; the minerals represent the gasoline. One cannot run the car without the spark from the battery. Vitamins will ignite the minerals to make them effective. We usually do not pay as much attention to minerals because we assume that we are getting a sufficient amount of them in the food we eat. It is true that they are not as easily lost as are vitamins, however, what we eat, how it is prepared. and how and where the food was grown has an effect on mineral intake. Without the basic minerals of CALCIUM, IRON, PHOSPHORUS, life is not possible, and without the trace minerals, major deficiencies will develop, and without an adequate amount of both, good health cannot be maintained. But when our food is PROCESSED, PRESERVED, CHEMICALIZED, and ARTIFICIALLY FERTILIZED, many minerals are lost in the process.

Inorganic chemicals, including drugs, for the most part cannot be very well utilized by the human body. Unless the body can eliminate the inorganic compounds, they settle in the tissues and often injure delicate cell structures. Many authorities now believe that such uneliminated foreign substances are responsible for many of the cancer cases today.

◆ *A Deficiency Of Minerals Causes Disease*

To make sure of an adequate supply of minerals, we should eat only unprocessed, naturally fertilized, organic foods. For example, the body requires about 4 gm of iron. More than one half of this is in the hemoglobin of the red blood cells. The utilization of iron cannot be accomplished without the trace minerals COPPER and COBALT. It is perfectly possible for you to develop IRON-DEFICIENCY ANEMIA if you aren't getting enough copper in your food, even though you are getting enough iron. A deficiency of iron means ANEMIA and without any iron at all we cannot live. Certain areas in Florida have only 20% of the normal amount. Iron deficient soils have now been reported in all of the 50 states. We can be fed into a disease through lack of minerals, and we can be fed out of it through remineralization.

Calcium (Ca)

◆ *Calcium Is Needed For Bones And Muscles*

- ✓ HELPS IN BLOOD CLOTTING—Calcium is one of the MACRONUTRIENTS which is needed in relatively large amounts. Calcium is in every cell of the body. About 99% of it is contained in BONES and TEETH. Calcium helps to maintain the acid-alkaline balance of the body and assists the blood in the CLOTTING PROCESS. If it were not for calcium, we would bleed to death at the slightest scratch. It transports NERVE IMPULSES from one part of the body to another. It is needed by muscles, for a lack of calcium will cause CRAMPS and CONVULSIONS, and MUSCLE PAIN. To relieve these conditions take either CALCIUM LACTATE or BONE MEAL. It is used by the immune system to strengthen the NERVE and MUSCLE NETWORKS and also to build and repair BONE and CARTILAGE.

- ✓ DEFICIENCY CAUSES SOFT BONES—A deficiency of calcium allows penetration of infectious agents that could trigger spontaneous cramping of the muscles and legs. It also causes SOFT BONES at the edges, joints to become irritated and not to be able to tolerate pressures, and SPURS may be formed on the joints.

- ✓ BED REST CAUSES CALCIUM LOSS—Calcium cannot be utilized properly by the body unless it is accompanied by magnesium, phosphorus, and vitamins A, C, and D. BED REST causes loss of calcium from the bones, and NITROGEN from the muscles. It is also better metabolized by the body if a person exercises regularly. ASTRONAUTS lost 200 mg of calcium per day, even with exercising. The absence of gravity in space makes walking impossible. DOLOMITE, a mineral consisting of both calcium and magnesium, is used as a calcium supplement. The magnesium makes the calcium soluble, so that the danger of KIDNEY STONES, which occurs with calcium alone, is eliminated.

- ✓ CALCIUM ABSORPTION NEEDS HYDROCHLORIC ACID—Calcium ABSORPTION depends partly on the presence of HYDROCHLORIC ACID in the stomach.

- ✓ DEFICIENCY CAUSES RICKETS AND OSTEOMALACIA—RICKETS is a childhood bone disease which is produced by improper nutrition. Deficiencies of calcium, phosphorus, and vitamin D may all be involved in producing rickets. OSTEOMALACIA, a bone disease of adults, is thought to be also due to a diet deficiency. Along with vitamin D, vitamins A and C are necessary in the diet to assure the proper use of calcium. Even though children play all day in the sunshine and soak up vitamin D, they may still be deficient in calcium, unless they are eating foods that are rich in vitamins A and C. For some reason Calcium must exist in the body in a proportion with phosphorus of 2:1, that is, there must be twice as much calcium as phosphorus. Green leafy vegetables are high in calcium and vitamins A and C, and seeds are high in phosphorus, hence, they seem to complement each other.

- ✓ AGING AND CALCIUM LOSS—Calcium loss becomes noticeable with age, in LOW BACK PAIN, SHORTER STATURE, and HUNCHED SHOULDERS. Substances that increase calcium loss are CAFFEINE, MEAT, ALCOHOL, and SMOKING. We only absorb about 35% of the calcium in our diet. Americans increased need for calcium seems to result from the EXCESS PHOSPHORUS in one's diet, which comes from the type of meal we eat. Soft drinks are another source of phosphorus. A diet with a calcium-to-phosphorus ratio of 1:1 is probably the best. Calcium combines with dietary fat and bile acids to form insoluble SOAPS. This is indirectly the same as removing cholesterol from your blood.

◆ *When In Need The Body Withdraws Calcium From The Bones*

- ✓ WITHDRAWAL OF CALCIUM CAUSES OSTEOPOROSIS—The body meets emergency needs for calcium by withdrawing it from the bones. This is especially true when a person's diet is OVERLY ACID, for then the body wants to neutralize the acid condition with calcium hydroxide which is an alkali This may tend to produce the condition of OSTEOPOROSIS, and such a condition may cause the bones to break. Fractures, such as that of the ribs, may then more easily occur through the bodily reactions of COUGHING, SNEEZING, AND VOMITING. WOMEN are twice as susceptible as MEN to bone fractures, primarily because of the hormonal changes of MENOPAUSE.

✓ NEGATIVE BALANCE METABOLISM—The two hormones involved are the PARATHYROID HORMONE (PTH), which releases calcium from the bone into the blood, and THYROCALCITONIN (TCT), which prevents calcium loss. When these hormones are out of balance one gets OSTEOPOROSIS. Tests taken prior to and after menopause revealed that women who had normal levels of calcium and phosphorus before their change of life lost these minerals from their bones and accumulated them in their blood and in their urine. This showed that their metabolism was in negative balance, and that they were headed for osteoporosis. The best way to fight osteoporosis is to prevent it from getting started — which means protecting yourself especially with foods from the CABBAGE FAMILY and with abundant vitamin D intake from sunshine and liver oils, and if necessary with supplements of BONE MEAL and DOLOMITE.

✓ VITAMIN D DEFICIENCY CAUSES CALCIUM DEFICIENCY—Such a deficiency should really be called a SUNSHINE DEFICIENCY. One can die from vitamin D deficiency at any age. Calcium works in each individual cell to keep it healthy and to regulate its growth. Absorption of any nutrient is less efficient when there is too much calcium. MELANIN is a body pigment which forms when excessive vitamin D is received by the skin, It also protects us from SKIN CANCER. An individual with weak THYROID and ADRENAL glands is unable to effectively utilize calcium.

◆ *The Heart Needs Calcium*

The heart is a muscle and calcium is the substance that regulates the rhythm of the HEART BEAT. The heart could not beat without it. However, no nutrient is self-sufficient. They all need assistance from other nutrients. An important partner for calcium for cardiovascular health is MAGNESIUM. It aids in the expansion and contraction of the muscle cells by providing a positive electrical charge which repels calcium thereby reversing contraction. The older one gets the more one needs calcium because one's ability to absorb it decreases with advancing years. The amount of calcium absorbed increases with the amount of calcium in the diet.

◆ *Calcium Requirements*

In order for you to meet you requirement of calcium, avoid refined sugar and flour foodstuffs. They are poor nutrients, which may be called NEGATIVE FOODS. They not only don't aid your nutrition, but they actually do harm. Not only do they provide you with no vitamins, no minerals, no enzymes, they will actually rob your body of these elements. For their digestion many extra vitamins and minerals must be brought into the body. It you eat a lot of cooked spinach and rhubarb, or are eating a lot of chocolate, you are eating foods which contain OXALIC ACID. Oxalic acid combines with calcium in the body to form CALCIUM OXALATE, which is a substance which the body cannot use, and which has been shown to contribute to the formation of KIDNEY and GALLSTONES.

The body uses calcium together with PHOSPHORUS to give rigidity to your bones. Hence, if the body is low in calcium much of your phosphorus is excreted.The phosphorus couldn't go to work because its partner was absent. Illness and disease can siphon off calcium from your diet. Patients with THYROID DISORDERS are particularly vulnerable. DRUGS tend to increase the body's need for calcium, while STEROIDS tend to depress calcium absorption. The very process of AGING calls for more calcium, and the lack of calcium hastens the process. Increased dietary calcium protects against HIP FRACTURE.

85% of women over 65 do not meet their daily requirement of calcium. The Recommended Daily Allowance (RDA) is 800 mg. In spite of the fact that milk and MILK PRODUCTS form a large part of the American diet, a USDA survey released in 1969 pointed out that of the general population 30% is CALCIUM DEFICIENT. The deficiency allowance is from 1000–1500 mg. Calcium supplements should be taken with meals. With the calcium also get 400 IU vitamin D. Soft drinks make soft bones. They contain PHOSPHORUS, which speeds up calcium depletion.

Studies have indicated that OLDER PERSONS absorb calcium at a slower rate than younger persons, but that they need more calcium to maintain a POSITIVE CALCIUM BALANCE. In fact, it is not necessarily the amount of calcium taken in that is significant, but rather a person's ability to absorb and utilize the calcium that is taken in.

◆ *Calcium-Rich Foods*

SOYBEANS are a very good source of calcium. Use them as a vegetable, use soy flour in everything you bake, use it as a thickener instead of white flour, and drink soy milk as a beverage. TAHINI or SESAME SEED BUTTER, is a good source of calcium. Tahini milk is an excellent substitute for cow's milk because of its high content of calcium. Use homemade HALVAH which is sesame meal mixed with honey into a consistency of dough. Cut it into squares or roll it into balls. It makes an excellent dessert snack. Other good sources of calcium are ALMONDS, FIGS, BEANS, OATS, MOLASSES, and most RAW VEGETABLES. A DEFICIENCY of Ca causes, besides RICKETS, DECAYED TEETH, FATIGUE, REDUCED DISEASE RESISTANCE, and a LACK of ADAPTABILITY.

◆ *Calcium For Pain Relief*

One doctor wrote that it should be common knowledge among doctors, that if one absorbs enough CALCIUM from day to day, if will do for the body what ANALGESICS, NARCOTICS, and SEDATIVES only seem to do. They are only half measures, but calcium is the real thing.

Phosphorus (P)

◆ *The Calcium-Phosphorus Balance*

The use of phosphorus in the body is closely interrelated with that of calcium. It is necessary for the proper absorption of calcium. The amount of phosphorus needed by the body is not as important as the relationship which exists between phosphorus and calcium. For perfect health the balance to be maintained between them is represented by the ratio of 2: 1, that is, there should be 2 times as much calcium as phosphorus in the body. MOTHER'S MILK has a ratio of 2: 1. It exists in bones and teeth along with calcium and other minerals, as well as in blood and cells. NIACIN (B_3), RIBOFLAVIN (B_2), CARBOHYDRATES, FATS, and PROTEINS cannot be digested properly unless phosphorus is present.

◆ *Dental Decay—A Phosphorus Deficiency*

The calcium-phosphorus balance can be most easily disturbed with WHITE SUGAR and WHITE FLOUR products. Dr. Melvin Page D.D.S. of Florida believes that diseases such as ARTHRITIS, POLIO, PYORRHEA, CANCER, and TOOTH DECAY, are brought about by disorders of the calcium-phosphorus balance. It means that if the proper balance is not maintained, these minerals will be drained out of the body without being used. The National Institute of Dental Research has gone on record with the opinion that DENTAL DECAY is fundamentally a PHOSPHORUS DEFICIENCY disease. In cases of DIARRHEA, for example, these mineral elements may be lost to the body. A sufficient amount of HYDROCHLORIC ACID must be present in the stomach for these minerals to be digested. Also VITAMIN D must be present. For this reason either a lack of calcium, phosphorus, or vitamin D can bring about RICKETS, for all three are necessary to prevent this disease.

◆ *Antacids Destroy The Calcium-Phosphorus Balance*

If you have ACID INDIGESTION, and for relief you take an ANTACID, containing ALUMINUM HYDROXIDE, MAGNESIUM HYDROXIDE or both, they will not be absorbed, for they are non-dietary in nature. They limit the gastrointestinal absorption of phosphorus by binding phosphorus. They decrease the nutrients of FOLATE, PHOSPHATE, CALCIUM, and COPPER. You may pay for such relief with cavities, lost teeth, and even with OSTEOMALACIA, the adult form of rickets. Why use an indigestible form of magnesium when the wholesome and digestible CALCIUM MAGNESIUM CARBONATE, as found in DOLOMITE tablets, will neutralize the acidity just as efficiently and will give you other health benefits. Furthermore, BONE MEAL tablets, consisting of calcium, phosphorus, and magnesium, are another good antacid.

◆ *Sources, Requirements, And Deficiency Symptoms*

The best SOURCES of calcium are most

RAW, DARK, LEAFY VEGETABLES, SESAME SEEDS, OATS, NAVY BEANS, ALMONDS, WALNUTS, MILLET and SUNFLOWER SEEDS. CALCIUM LACTATE is also a rich natural supplement. The recommended daily allowance (RDA) for adults is 800mg. For children or women during pregnancy and lactation 1000–1400 mg. A deficiency of phosphorus may result in POOR MINERALIZATION of BONES, RETARDED GROWTH, RICKETS, DECREASED NERVE and BRAIN FUNCTION, GENERAL WEAKNESS, and REDUCED SEXUAL POWER.

Magnesium (Mg)—The Miracle Mineral

◆ *Milk Is Low In Magnesium*

Mg is a protector of the KIDNEYS. One reason why the American people are Mg deficient is that they cook so much of their food. Mg salts in plants are so soluble that even blanching them will demineralize them. Mg is widely distributed in vegetables, and especially in the green chlorophyll. It is obvious that Mg, along with other minerals, is removed when grain is milled and refined into cereals, and WHEAT loses almost all of its Mg through the refining process. It is almost completely lacking in MILK. There seems to be some component of milk which interferes with the utilization of Mg. CALCIFEROL, the synthetic vitamin D, tends to bind Mg. Milk is loaded with it and therefore increases the problem. It is 10 times more potent in binding Mg than is the natural form as found in fish liver oils. They will not cause Mg depletion, but milk does. Hence one of the steps in treating Mg deficiency is to reduce milk consumption, especially in children, or to increase the Mg content foods. Not only are MEATS, EGGS, and DAIRY PRODUCTS low in Mg, but the more protein one consumes, the more Mg one needs to metabolize this protein. Mg is an important CATALYST in many enzyme reactions, especially those involved in energy production.

◆ *Artificial Fertilizers Cause Magnesium Deficiencies*

Poorness of soil in Mg can be caused by an excessive amount of chemical fertilizers which makes the soil rich in potash so that its excess has made it favorable for the development of CANCER. In this way one can explain the failure and at times harmful effect of the lacto-vegetarian diet which is that the Mg content is too low. CORN is the Mg food par excellence. Even if it grows in poor soil, corn always contains a relatively large amount of Mg.

The liberal use of POTASSIUM FERTILIZERS tends to cause a deficiency of Mg in plants and even lowers the calcium content. Cattle fed on such high potassium forage develop GRASS TETANY, a nerve condition.

◆ *The Refining Process Robs Food Of Magnesium*

Whenever researcher Schrumpf-Pierron found an excess of POTASH (Potassium carbonate) in the soil, there he discovered less Mg in the soil, but more human CANCER cases. Wherever he found a minimum of potash, he found a maximum of Mg and fewer cancer cases. Cancer in Egypt is that of Europe and the U.S. It is less in the country people than in the city people. That which characterizes the diet of the country people or FELLAHIN is its richness in the salts of Mg. The world is being robbed of Mg because of the refining of food. The fellahin obtains from 2.5 to 3 gm of Mg/day, while in Europe and Asia it is only gm/day. Theis and Bendikt have already found a higher amount of potash in cancerous tissue. It is the absence of Mg that allows potash to become toxic and carcinogenic. The older the individual, the easier the intoxication by potash. So Mg is also an ANTI-SENILITY mineral.

◆ *Magnesium Can Reduce High Blood Pressure*

Dr. Hans Selye allowed two groups of rats to undergo certain stresses which normally damaged their heart muscles and caused them to die. But when he gave them injections of Mg and K (Potassium), they always continued to live. A high Mg diet has prevented the development of ATHEROSCLEROSIS in rats. Over 100 patients suffering from CORONARY HEART DISEASE, were treated with intramuscular (injected) Magnesium sulfate ($MgSO_4$) with only one death compared to their findings the previous year when of 196 cases treated with routine anticoagulants, 60 died. Dr. Mildred Deelig said that there is a direct relationship between the amount of Mg in the diet and the ability to avoid HIGH BLOOD PRESSURE. She calculated that the average American diet falls short by 200 mg a day or more of the optimal amount of

Mg one should consume for good health. Mg is extremely sensitive to HEAT and is easily lost during the PROCESSING of food. People who eat RAW and unprocessed food should get enough. Someone has suggested that MAGNESIUM CHLORIDE ($MgCl_2$) in water should be in every household as a therapeutic treatment against POLIO.

◆ *Mineral Waters Neutralize Toxins*

Billard proved the power of MINERAL WATERS against various poisons, especially in $MgCl_2$ waters. These waters, such as at Sarasota Springs, will neutralize TETANY TOXIN and SNAKE VENOM. Guinea pigs injected with lethal doses of snake venom diluted in Chatel-Guyon water, containing $MgCl_2$, survived, as did a rabbit bitten by a poisonous snake when injected with 10cc of such water.

◆ *Magnesium Prevents Stone Formation*

Studies have shown that Mg protects against the accumulation of calcium deposits. In an experiment by Kohler and Uhle a 33 year old pregnant woman had passed at least 8 to 12 stones during each of her previous pregnancies. In this pregnancy she took from 500 to 1500 mg of Mg over a period of six weeks. It was the first pregnancy in which she did not pass any KIDNEY STONES. W. Cramer reported that the omission of Mg from the diet of laboratory rats induced extensive CALCIUM DEPOSITS in the kidneys. Before this another researcher had produced urinary stones in rats by feeding them a Mg deficient diet. After only a short time of taking one capsule of 250 mg of MAGNESIUM OXIDE (MgO) daily, a group of volunteers with a history of kidney stones had no more stones. Comatose DIABETIC patients and patients being treated with DIURETICS commonly develop Mg deficiency. CHRONIC ALCOHOLICS are also prime candidates because alcohol increases the urinary excretion of Mg.

Rodale found out that when eating cooked beets the stool was red, but not so when raw beets were eaten. When DOLOMITE, a calcium-magnesium supplement, was eaten for a while, then, after eating cooked beets the stool was not red anymore. It seems that Mg increases the intestinal flora so that it allows the body to absorb more nutrients from the food.

◆ *Magnesium Strengthens The Teeth*

For years it was believed that high intakes of calcium and phosphorus inhibited tooth decay by strengthening the enamel. Recent studies, however, indicate that the increase in these two minerals does not help much unless Mg is taken at the same time. It is the Mg and not the calcium, that forms the kind of hard enamel that resists decay. No matter how much calcium you take without Mg, it can form only soft enamel. And if too soft, the enamel will lack sufficient resistance to the acids of decay. It has been shown that dental structures can dissolve when additional amounts of these minerals diffuse through the enamel at different rates. Mg acts as an enzyme or CATALYST, which speeds up reactions, or as a glue that binds calcium and fluorine to build bone. Without Mg they cannot be used in the system. Thus MILK which is high in these two elements but poor in Mg, antagonizes Mg which is largely responsible for tooth decay prevention. Bacteria from sugar products produce LACTIC ACID which dissolves the calcium in the enamel layer of the teeth. Milk is recognized to be a greater producer of lactic acid than any other food.

Dr. Baronet made a study of the water supplies of Deaf Smith County and Dallas County in Texas to determine the effect of their mineral content on people's teeth. He determined that Deaf Smith County water had twice the Mg, the calcium, more iodine, and more fluorine than Dallas County water. As a result the people of Deaf Smith County had much better teeth than the people in Dallas County. He found that it is the extra Mg in the water of Deaf Smith County and not the fluorine that made the bones stronger in deaf Smith County. The high calcium content in Dallas county necessitated a greater supply of Mg than was available. Hence, he concluded that supplementing their diet with Mg would be a much better method than fluorides for decay prevention.

◆ *Magnesium And Disease*

Martin found that in a state of EPILEPSY there is a deficiency of Mg in the blood. Mg is an analgesic, and it is the only electrolyte found in higher concentrations in the spinal fluid than in the blood. The lower the blood level of Mg, the lower is the spinal fluid level. In a study with rats, a high Mg diet has prevented the development of ATH-

EROSCLEROSIS. It was shown that in many cases of coronary heart disease a dramatic improvement followed the injection of EPSOM SALTS ($MgSO_4$). $MgSO_4$ is known to produce a significant reduction in the serum cholesterol levels.

A 50 year old lady who had EPILEPSY heard about the benefit of Mg for this disease. As a result she started taking 2 DOLOMITE TABLETS a day with her regular medication, and as a result she has not had a PETITE MAL or a GRAND MAL. She also took BREWERS YEAST, DESSICATED LIVER, and VITAMINS C and E besides the dolomite. It has been found that VITAMIN B_6 can also control POLYNEURITIS and EPILEPSY.

Some hormones, such as CORTISONE, which claims to reduce inflammation from arthritis and allergies, has also been found to have the side effect of producing DIABETES, and has been shown to reduce Mg concentrations in the blood. The SODIUM FLUORIDE which is added to the community water supply, bonds with Mg in the blood so as to form INSOLUBLE MAGNESIUM FLUORIDE which cannot be assimilated, and can therefore lead to a Mg deficiency. TETRACYCLINE, an antibiotic, interferes with Mg metabolism by disrupting the chain of events in which energy is released in MITOCHONDRIA, which are the source of energy in the cell, and are involved in protein synthesis and fat metabolism.

◆ *Results Of Deficiencies*

Continuous deficiency of Mg will cause a loss of calcium and potassium, with consequent deficiencies of those minerals. Mg is essential for the health of the HEART, and for regulating the ACID-ALKALINE BALANCE in the system. It is also a natural TRANQUILIZER. Mg is a protector of the KIDNEYS.

When a person's Mg levels are subnormal, the nerves are unable to control such functions as MUSCLE MOVEMENT, RESPIRATION, and MENTAL PROCESSES. TWITCHING, IRRITABILITY, and NERVOUS FATIGUE are symptoms of what is frequently found to be Mg deficiency. Deficiency is simply the result of not obtaining adequate amounts of Mg from dietary sources such as GREEN VEGETABLES, SOYBEANS, WHEAT GERM, FIGS, APPLES, LEMONS, PEACHES, WHOLE GRAINS, SUNFLOWER SEEDS, SESAME SEEDS, ALMONDS, and BROWN RICE. Most natural foods have some Mg in them, but if the diet is too high in fats, one may need extra amounts of Mg, because one loses too much of Mg in the fats. The recommended daily allowance (RDA) of Mg is 350 mg, although therapeutic doses are up to 700 mg.

Potassium (K)

◆ *Needed For Proper Acid-Alkaline Balance*

When metallic elements in foods are oxidized in the body, they develop BASES which are ALKALINE. When SULFUR and PHOSPHORUS are oxidized, they give rise to acids such as SULFURIC and PHOSPHORIC. For ACIDOSIS it is recommended that one drink fresh-squeezed lemon juice in warm water before retiring. It restores the body's acid-alkaline balance.

Potassium (K) ranks as one of the body's most needed minerals. It is closely linked to the health of MUSCLES and NERVES. Your blood pressure as well as GLANDS and HORMONES, depend to some extent upon a sufficient amount of K in your body. It is also necessary for normal GROWTH, and as an alkalizing agent for keeping proper ACID-ALKALINE BALANCE in the blood and tissues. It also aids in retaining normal osmotic pressure of essential body fluids, and in using PROTEIN efficiently. The RED BLOOD CELLS need K in order to effectively carry carbon dioxide (CO_2) to the lungs to be exchanged for oxygen. It stimulates the excretion of water by the kidneys, thus ridding the body of poisonous waste materials. It also activates certain ENZYMES required in CARBOHYDRATE METABOLISM.

◆ *Potassium-Sodium Interaction*

Potassium (K) is concentrated mostly in the tissue cells of the body, whereas sodium (Na) is concentrated in the fluids around the cells. The action of K is closely related to the action of Na in the body. When there is too much sodium, the cell contains more water, and K is withdrawn from it and is excreted in the urine. When there is plenty of K, then Na and water are lost.

In case of MUSCULAR ACTIVITY the cells lose K and the Na moves in. The ratio between K and Na in the body should be approximately 2:1, that is, we should have twice as much K as Na in order to be healthy. The average daily diet intake of K in the American diet is from 1 to 6 gm. However, the average American gets from 8 to 15 gm of Na daily from all sources. This means that he may be getting up to 10 times as much Na as K which is 20 times as much as he should have.

◆ *Loss Of Potassium In Disease*

Potassium is lost when a person is taking HORMONES such as CORTISONE, ALDOSTERONE and so on. Na is retained and K is excreted. In DIABETIC patients, when blood sugar rises in the urine, K is lost. This is true also in the case of ULCERATIVE COLITIS. The level is also very low in LEUKEMIA and POLIO patients, but it is not known why. Giving K to patients with mild DIABETES causes a fall in blood pressure and also a fall in blood sugar. K is very closely related to the function of the glands that are disordered in diabetes. In a diabetic coma FRUIT JUICES and VEGETABLE BROTH are given because they contain so much K, and it is the K that apparently brings the patient out of a coma.

◆ *Loss Of Potassium From Food*

K is easily robbed from your foods before it can get to you. And what robs you of K are thieves which are disguised as friends. They appear as tasty SEASONINGS, delicious CANDY, helpful DRUGS, and so-called "advanced" AGRICULTURE. The most common robber is SODIUM which appears in the form of SODIUM CHLORIDE, and is called TABLE SALT. A little salt is needed in body chemistry, but in excess it upsets the acid-alkaline balance. The result is a TOXIC condition that fosters the formation of dead or dying tissue. While salt is found in nearly all foods, no addition to food is really needed, so that the complete elimination of table salt is generally advisable in order to preserve all possible K in your food. In an experiment it was found that 2000 mg of a K supplement lowered cholesterol by 20% after only 8 weeks.

◆ *Potassium Deficiency Caused By Sweating*

During a heat wave some people develop heat exhaustion which has been correlated to potassium exhaustion. In the sweating that then occurs, much sodium chloride and potassium is lost through the SWEAT. Sweat is composed of SODIUM CHLORIDE, POTASSIUM, AMMONIA, and UREA. When sweating continues, much of the potassium along with sodium chloride is lost. In one great heat wave 150 deaths were reported as resulting from "heat prostration" or "heat exhaustion." Upon investigation it was found that perspiration had been excessive in the days before collapse. Many who had cardiovascular disease had been taking salt which is known to encourage potassium loss, so that K depletion may have been an important cause of death in these cases. The use of SALT TABLETS also is not recommended, for it increases the exchange of Na for K in the kidneys, and promotes heavy kidney losses of potassium. When DIURETICS are taken, potassium is washed out with the sodium and the water.

DRUG DIURETICS are said to increase urinary output from the kidneys. Each kidney consists of about one million individual filters called NEPHRONS. The blood vessels from the nephrons permit fluid and dissolved particles from the blood to enter special tubules. As the fluid passes through the tubules, the body absorbs back some of the fluid and most of the nutrients that are also present in it. A drug diuretic works by crippling the kidneys' ability to carry on this reclamation process from the tubules. The result is that the volume of urine increases, but the quality of the urine becomes distinctly abnormal. The function of the kidneys is not only to remove waste matter, but also to conserve valuable nutrients. Drug diuretics damage the kidneys' ability to conserve nutrients. This can lead ultimately to kidney failure.

◆ *Signs Of Potassium Depletion*

Some signs of potassium depletion are: LISTLESSNESS, FATIGUE, WEAKNESS, CONSTIPATION, INSOMNIA, SLOW and IRREGULAR HEARTBEAT, ABSENT REFLEXES, MENTAL CONFUSION, and SOFT, FLABBY MUSCLES. When the body is low in potassium, water builds up in the tissues, which can indicate the start of kidney problems, of which SWOLLEN ANKLES are one of the symptoms.

Supplements that provide extra K are BONE MEAL, BREWERS YEAST, SUNFLOWER SEEDS, and WHEAT GERM. Fruits as well as vegetables have generous amounts of potassium such as POTATOES, AVOCADOS, BANANAS, CANTALOUPES, DATES, and PRUNES. Potatoes have almost twice the potassium content of bananas. A sufficiency of K is a preventative of cancer and many other kindred diseases. K is the salt of the tissues, and sodium (Na) is the salt of the fluids of the body.

Sodium (Na)

◆ *Stored In Stomach Walls And Joints*

Sodium (Na) in combination with Chlorine (Cl) gives us SODIUM CHLORIDE (NaCl), which is otherwise known as table salt, or simply as salt. Our word "salary" comes from the word "salt," for in ancient times salt had become so valuable that it was used as a means of exchange. There are records of wars fought for the possession of salt. In some nations even wives and children have been traded for salt. SALT LICKS often represent soils which contain more than the usual amount of POTASSIUM or MAGNESIUM SULFATE, and not necessarily common salt as is usually assumed. Sodium is in the INORGANIC FORM in salt. In the ORGANIC form in fruits and vegetables, it prevents the clotting of the blood, it helps to check fermentation, increases the peristaltic action of the bowels, and neutralizes acids.

The acid producing foods that we take in, sometimes in excess, may interfere with the proper functioning of the digestive juices, so that the ACID-ALKALINE BALANCE of the blood may be disturbed. Sodium as well as many other minerals are alkaline reacting. That is why they are called upon to neutralize the acids. Reserve supplies of sodium are stored in various organs of the body, but chiefly in the walls of the stomach. This makes the tissues of the stomach highly alkaline, as they should be in order to withstand the presence of the HYDROCHLORIC ACID which is normally in the stomach. The joints of the body have the next highest sodium-storing capacity. It is clear that if there is not enough sodium in the food we eat, this fact can be one of the causes of stomach ulcers.

◆ *It Neutralizes Acids*

Sodium is also the element which keeps CALCIUM in solution. When there is not enough sodium in the joints and tissues, calcium takes the place of the sodium. Then the joints may become rigid, and disorders such as neuritis, neuralgia, rheumatism, and arthritis follow. People usually take BICARBONATE OF SODA to neutralize the acids in the stomach and tissues. It will neutralize the acids it comes in contact with, but it is an inorganic substance which cannot be used by the body, and therefore acts as an irritant. Instead of using ALKALIZERS, one should use natural food alkalizers which are present in FRUIT AND VEGETABLE JUICES.

One doctor said: "If you ask me about RHEUMATISM I'll tell you that it is degeneration of the joint tissues due to nutritional deficiency, and that it is chiefly a CALCIUM, IODINE, and VITAMIN D deficiency.

◆ *Foods Containing Sodium*

RAW GOAT'S MILK is one of the foods highest in sodium. It is very beneficial in cases of stomach ulcers and in RHEUMATIC and ARTHRITIC conditions. Another sodium food is WHEY, the watery part of coagulated milk. The acids in green unripe fruits taste sour, but when they are allowed to mature, the sodium content gives them their sweet taste. Citrus fruits, when tree ripened are high in sodium. CABBAGE and STRAWBERRY JUICE are good sources of sodium. OKRA is one of our highest sodium containing foods, and is very soothing to the stomach walls, hence, it is very excellent for cases of ULCERS. Other foods that are high in sodium are CELERY, ROMAINE LETTUCE, CHARD, MUSTARD GREENS, SPINACH, CARROTS, APPLES, and APRICOTS.

Chlorine (Cl)

◆ *Chlorine Is A Strong Poisonous Substance*

Chlorine is essential for the production of HYDROCHLORIC ACID in the stomach. It is needed there for the proper DIGESTION of PROTEIN and for MINERAL ASSIMILATION. It is involved in the maintenance of proper fluid and electrolyte balance in the system. It also helps the liver in its activity of cleansing the body of poisonous substances. In its elemental form as a gas it is extremely poisonous. As inorganic compounds with other elements, in the form of chlorides, they represent powerful BLEACHES. As such they are also placed in our drinking water to help destroy the bacteria, but are not the best substances for us to swallow. In inorganic form chlorine destroys vitamin E and other vitamins in our system. It also destroys our intestinal flora which are the organisms that help us digest our food.

◆ *Chlorinated Water Causes Atherosclerosis*

Chlorinated water has given some people hives, asthma, and colitis. It has produced GASTROINTESTINAL as well as URINARY BLADDER CANCER. It has also produced ATHEROSCLEROSIS or hardening of the arteries. This was shown with two groups of chickens. One group was given pure water and the other chlorinated water. The chlorinated water group developed hardening of the arteries. Not so the plain water group. Irish farm workers, studied by Dr. Paul Dudly White, who drank their own well water, never developed coronary heart disease. Japan has a low incidence of heart attacks, but when Japanese move to Hawaii and drink chlorinated water, they develop atherosclerosis. During the Korean war, autopsies performed on American soldiers killed in battle, whose average age was 22 years, showed that over 75% had developed evidence of coronary arteriosclerosis. Soldiers who returned from Korea told that the water in Korea was so heavily chlorinated for sanitary reasons, that it was almost undrinkable.

◆ *Boil Chlorinated Water To Purify It*

If house plants are watered with chlorinated water, they will not thrive. Also guppies cannot live in such water very long. A study by Dr. Harry J. Johnson showed that chlorine destroys vitamin E in the system. Other studies have shown that a lack of vitamin E in the system causes heart disease. Dr. von Oettingen showed that severe exposure to chlorine causes CARDIAC INSUFFICIENCY. What we can do about the chlorine problem is to drink unchlorinated bottled SPRING WATER. If we must drink water from the tap, we can BOIL IT before we drink it. The heat will evaporate the chlorine. A DEFICIENCY causes impaired digestion of food. A deficiency of HYDROCHLORIC ACID results in a failure of the system to properly digest proteins, giving rise to high blood pressure. GRAPEFRUIT can at times substitute for reduced hydrochloric acid.

Chlorine foods are SEAWEED, WATER CRESS, CHARD, CABBAGE, KALE, CELERY, CUCUMBER, TOMATOES, ASPARAGUS, and OATS.

Sulfur (S)

◆ *Sulfur—The Beauty Mineral*

Sulfur is called "the beauty mineral," for it is vital for healthy hair, skin, and nails. Proteins contain sulfur, carbohydrates and fats do not. This means that proteins contain two substances— nitrogen and sulfur—whose waste products must be excreted by the kidneys. Carbohydrates and fats produce CARBON DIOXIDE as their waste product which is expelled by the lungs. Nitrogen and sulfur are acid-forming. Their waste products give an acid rather than an alkaline reaction in the urine. In contrast to this calcium, sodium, potassium, and magnesium have an alkaline reaction in the body.

◆ *Inorganic Sulfur Is Harmful*

When sulfur appears in plant or animal food, it is in organic form. When it does not appear in such food, it is in inorganic form, and as such it can be extremely harmful. It appears that nature always places elements in a package with other elements. Man seems to believe that he can take these packages apart and make use of the elements separated from the package. Elements outside of such packages can be very poisonous. We are living in the age of coal and petroleum and their products. The burning process has changed these substances and their products from nonpoisonous products to poisonous products as far as the human body is concerned. Coal smoke contains sulfur. The corrosive sulfuric acid is given off by chimneys, and it has been suspected of causing cancer. Sulfur is used on dried fruits to retain their color and some of their food value, but it is not best for the system. Buy unsulfured dried fruits. To avoid sulfur-containing insecticides, eat ORGANICALLY GROWN FOODS. Throw out of your medicine chest all of the COAL-TAR medicines, salves, ointments and pills that may contain sulfur as an ingredient, or may have been manufactured with the use of sulfuric acid.

◆ Sulfur Baths Are Beneficial To Health

Experiments have shown that mineral baths are better than plain water baths, although the experimenters have not found why this is so. It has been shown that ARTHRITIS PATIENTS are lacking in sulfur, and that mineral baths containing sulfur can make up this deficiency. In mineral baths the minerals are absorbed through the skin. Sulfur baths are used in the treatment of SKIN DISORDERS, NERVOUS CONDITIONS, NEURITIS, AND RHEUMATIC DISEASES. Drug stores carry ready made fluid preparations for sulfur baths.

Without a ready-made preparation use the following formula: take TWO OUNCES of POTASSIUM SULFIDE and dissolve it in 15 gallons of water, which is a little over tub full. CYSTINE is one of the essential amino acids which contains a lot of sulfur. It has been found that the cystine content of the fingernails increases after a sulfur bath.

◆ Sulfur Speeds Wound Healing

Sulfur in the diet is the key to the fast healing of wounds. Dr. M.B. Williamson reported that all wounds heal much more rapidly when the diet contains the SULFUR CONTAINING AMINO ACIDS. During the healing of a wound the sulfur containing amino acids accumulate in the body. It appears that during the stress reaction after wounding, tissue protein is being sacrificed to make these amino acids available for the healing process. Foods high in sulfur content are: RADISH, TURNIP, ONIONS, CABBAGE, CELERY, BRAN, BRUSSELS SPROUTS, STRING BEANS, KALE, SOYBEANS, NUTS, and EGG YOLK. One of the best brain and NERVE TONICS is egg yolk in black cherry juice. It contains iron, sulfur, cholesterol, and lecithin all in one. The cholesterol is kept in solution and is emulsified by the lecithin. This is similar to the grape juice and eggs Mrs. White prescribes in 2SM303 for a deficient diet.

The Need For Trace Minerals

◆ They Are Essential For Life

TRACE MINERALS or MICRONUTRIENTS are minerals which are needed in the body in very small amounts. They include IRON, IODINE, COPPER, MANGANESE, MOLYBDENUM, SELENIUM, CHROMIUM, and ZINC. Like the MACRONUTRIENTS they are essential for life. They are needed for TISSUE REPAIR, for GROWTH, for METABOLISM, and for SLOWING some of the DEGENERATIVE PROCESSES. Such foods as WHITE BREAD, NOODLES, WHITE RICE, SUGAR, SOFT DRINKS, ICE CREAM and so forth contain no trace minerals. It must again be emphasized that all of these minerals must be in ORGANIC FORM.

◆ Chromium (Cr)

Chromium occurs in almost all living matter. In man it appears in concentrations of 20 parts of chromium per 1 billion parts of blood. However, it has been estimated that diets with less than 100 parts per billion of chromium are deficient. It is present at birth in higher concentrations than at any other time of life. It plays an important role in the synthesis of FATTY ACIDS and CHOLESTEROL in the liver. According to Dr. Mertz of Hamburg, Germany, a deficiency of chromium impairs an animal's ability to handle SUGAR. Such inability in glucose metabolism, he said, could be prevented by adding BREWER'S YEAST to the diet.

Dr. Lane, an optometrist, says that the intake of sugar, along with other refined carbohydrates, may cause a depletion of the body's store of chromium. Sugar also forces the body to use up its supply of B-complex vitamins that are needed to regulate fluid pressure in the eye. Worsening NEARSIGHTEDNESS is also blamed on the large consumption of sugar. When 2 parts per million of chromium was added to the drinking water of rats, their glucose tolerance improved in a matter of days. Cr protects against CARDIOVASCULAR DISEASE and HIGH BLOOD PRESSURE.

Chromium works hand in hand with the hormone INSULIN in the body. Chromium deficiency is one of the factors which will upset the function of insulin. Chromium in the presence of insulin makes it easier for sugar to enter the tissue cells. Without chromium, cells become insensitive to insulin. With it, insulin becomes 100 times more efficient at converting glucose into energy. 100 micrograms (mcg) of chromium are required to metabolize 100 gm of white sugar. Physical damage and exercise also deplete chromium. It has also been determined that populations that consume the greatest amount of sugar have the lowest body levels of chromium.

The Recommended Daily Allowance (RDA) for chromium is set at 50 mcg/day. DIABETICS should get at least 200 mcg/day which will help normalize blood sugar levels. The refining of natural sources of carbohydrates is associated with a substantial loss of chromium as well as other minerals. This is indicated by comparing refined sugar with molasses, or white flour with whole grain flour. Chromium is normally present in natural highly mineralized water. The natural complex of the chromium, the GLUCOSE TOLERANCE FACTOR, is present in WHOLE GRAIN BREAD, MUSHROOMS, BREWER'S YEAST, RAW SUGAR, and CANE JUICE. A severe deficiency may be a contributing cause of DIABETES, HIGH or LOW BLOOD SUGAR, HARDENING OF THE ARTERIES, and HEART DISEASE.

◆ *Copper (Cu)*

The COPPER you would get into your system from cooking in copper kettles would be strictly INORGANIC COPPER, and as such it is TOXIC to your system. Copper works with iron to produce HEMOGLOBIN. It is involved in the oxidation of vitamin C in the body. Adults generally obtain the necessary 2mg per day of copper from their food. Copper deficiency can result in the weakening of the walls of blood vessels rendering them susceptible to ANEURYSMS and RUPTURE. Too little copper can also lead to OSTEOPOROSIS. Copper retards the development of cancers in animals as well as decreasing liver damage and cirrhosis from cancer causing chemicals. In the newborn infant the copper content is 5 to 10 times higher than in the adult. This is nature's way of insuring enough copper for the infant to help it through the nursing period. There is very little copper in milk. Copper is an ANTIOXIDANT, and it works against CANCER, ARTHRITIS, and CARDIOVASCULAR DISEASES.

COBALT is combined with other elements within vitamin B_{12}, and as such it helps to prevent and cure PERNICIOUS ANEMIA. The trace mineral IODINE is needed in the body only in parts per billion in order for it to do its work in helping to produce THYROXINE for the thyroid gland so as to prevent GOITER.

◆ *Iodine (I)*

The thyroid gland regulates BODY METABOLISM, that is, it is responsible for the rate at which you burn your food. If your metabolic rate is too rapid, you tend to be nervous and irritable. If it is too slow you may be sluggish, chubby, and lazy. SEA WATER is full of minerals including iodine. Studies have shown that plants absorb a greater proportion of the minerals deposited in the soil from sea water. In a test carrots which had been treated with sea water showed a mineral increase of 28% over the carrots which had been treated with ordinary water. In further tests carried out with ocean water treated CROPS, the yields were always higher with sea water.

GOITER is the visible manifestation of an iodine shortage. The enlargement of the thyroid gland represents an effort by the gland to manufacture more adequate amounts of THYROXIN, and can be avoided with proper iodine intake. An iodine lack in the soil is so evident through the incidence of goiter in the local population, that one can determine where the iodine supply is either sufficient or insufficient. In many so-called GOITER BELTS, extra iodine is introduced into the diet by way of IODIZED SALT. The danger here is that a person might be getting too much salt into his system. The same objective can be more healthfully obtained by putting POWDERED KELP into the salt shaker which will give us only the amount of salt, as well as many other minerals whose lack have been shown to cause disease. No set daily requirement of iodine has been established, but it is most likely from .04 to .10 mg. COD LIVER OIL has a good amount of iodine as well as its content of vitamins A and D. Other dietary sources of iodine are KELP, DULSE and other SEAWEEDS which are available in tablet form, SWISS CHARD, TURNIP GREENS, WATERCRESS, GARLIC, PINEAPPLES, and CITRUS FRUITS.

◆ *Iron*

IRON is a vital component of HEMOGLOBIN, the oxygen-carrying compound in the blood. We lose some iron every day by way of sweat, hair, and excretions. Drugs decrease iron absorption. Spinach is considered a good source of iron, but less than 2% of the iron is available to us. COFFEE and TEA can reduce the availability of iron in the body by 40 to 85%. Their TANNIN content is what binds the iron. Only 10% of the iron we obtain from food is absorbed. Orange juice increases iron absorption by 2 times, and it was shown that 60 mg of vitamin C tripled iron absorption. 80% of the iron in a WOMAN is in her blood, in her red blood cells. Loss of blood through MENSTRUATION also means a significant loss of iron.

IRON DEFICIENCY ANEMIA in children may be caused by an overemphasis on MILK and CEREALS. Milk has little iron, and cereals contains PHYTIC ACID which destroys iron in the digestive tract. This is avoided if sufficient iron containing foods are also eaten. Cooking in iron utensils adds a considerable amount of iron to the diet. Stainless steel gives you iron which leaches out of the pots and pans in small amounts each time you use them. Older people are often anemic in spite of having sufficient iron because they lack a sufficient amount of HYDROCHLORIC ACID in their stomach which is needed for proper assimilation of iron, besides being also needed for CALCIUM and PROTEIN metabolism. Anemia can also be caused by a reduction in the number of red blood cells, as well as by a lack of oxygen to the cells. SEEDS, NUTS, MOLASSES, and SOYBEANS, are all good sources of iron. We need from 10 to 20 mg of iron per day.

◆ *Manganese (Mn)*

Manganese is needed by the human body only in microscopic traces. It is necessary for the utilization of important B vitamins, and is essential for the transmission of impulses between NERVES and MUSCLES. Mn is a brain food.

It helps to develop the parenteral center of the brain, and is also necessary for a good MEMORY. A study by Everson and Shrader found that a lack of manganese can actually affect GLUCOSE TOLERANCE, which is the ability to remove excess sugar from the blood by oxidation or storage. They found that manganese deficient animals frequently produced babies with pancreatic abnormalities, or without a PANCREAS, which secretes the insulin necessary for the utilization of sugar. It has been suspected that metabolic or dietary manganese deficiency is one of several possible causes of DIABETES. In many countries plant extracts which are good sources of manganese have been used as home remedies for DIABETES MELLITUS such as extracts of BLUEBERRY, EUCALYPTUS LEAVES, ONION, CABBAGE, BAKER'S and BREWER'S YEAST. Plants are the chief source of manganese in the diet, but only if the soil is not deficient in the mineral and if an excess of lime is not applied to the soil.

When families of rats were raised on a manganese deficient diet, several animals of the second generation developed ATAXIA or DEFECTIVE MUSCULAR COORDINATION. A failure of muscular coordination is associated with the disease MYASTHENIA GRAVIS which means grave loss of muscle strength, and such loss in humans has also been linked to a manganese deficiency. Dr. Josephson reports remarkable recoveries from this disease in patients given a diet high in protein, vitamin E, all the B vitamins, and for a short period 50 mg of manganese at each meal.

Deficiencies of manganese may further cause RETARDED GROWTH, ABNORMAL BONE DEVELOPMENT, MALE and FEMALE STERILITY, POOR EQUILIBRIUM, and ASTHMA. Other natural sources of manganese are GREEN LEAFY VEGETABLES, BEETS, BRUSSELS SPROUTS, ORANGES, APRICOTS, BRAN, PEAS, KELP, SEEDS and NUTS, especially BLACK WALNUTS.

◆ *Zinc (Zn)*

ZINC is an ANTIOXIDANT. It maintains a HEALTHY IMMUNE SYSTEM, ACCELERATES WOUND HEALING, AND PREVENTS PROSTATE PROBLEMS. Zinc is essential for synthesis of BODY PROTEIN. It is needed in the construction of the INSULIN MOLECULE. As part of the insulin molecule it is involved in carbohydrate and energy metabolism. It helps the body to get rid of toxic carbon dioxide, and it also increases the rate of healing of burns and wounds. If a person is in doubt about getting enough of the trace minerals, then put powdered KELP in your salt shaker instead of salt, for kelp contains all the minerals and trace minerals that are in the sea, and there are over 60 of them. ALCOHOL flushes zinc out of the liver into the urine, and ORAL CONTRACEPTIVES do the same.

Frank Lloyd Wright, the famous architect, once said that when you build a house on a mountain, don't build it on a mountain, but make the house a part of the mountain. What he was actually saying is that we should move in the stream of NATURE, and not in opposition to it. Nature is an organic farmer and we must be the same.

Natural sources of zinc are WHEAT BRAN, WHEAT GERM, NUTS, GREEN LEAFY VEGETABLES, BREWER'S YEAST, MILK, EGGS, and ONIONS. It is not easily available in grains and seeds, because it is locked in by the PHYTIN, but it becomes unlocked by the fermentation process, as in sour dough bread, and by the sprouting of seeds.

Minerals And Other Poisonous Substances And Their Antidotes

◆ *Aluminum (Al)*

Aluminum is a very reactive metal. When food is cooked in aluminum pots, or is left to stand in it for a period of time, you will to a certain extent dine on aluminum. Aluminum reacts with various elements in the food, and such a combination can be the root cause of many ailments, especially digestive disturbances. Your saliva is alkaline. When it is swallowed along with the aluminum compounds in the pot, it produces gas in the stomach. You are getting the same chemical reaction in your stomach as you would get when you use an alum baking powder. Dr. Betts computes that the average person whose food is cooked in aluminum pots, and whose bread is baked with alum baking power consumes 4 to 5 grains of aluminum salts at each meal.

Some years ago a lady boiled two quarts of water for half an hour in an aluminum pot and the same quantity in a stainless steel pot as well as in a porcelain one. When the water cooled she placed some goldfish in each pot. Within six hours the goldfish in the aluminum pot were dead. The other fish kept on living. Trace minerals can be dangerous when they are consumed in amounts that are more than "traces," and when they are consumed in a form which is not natural, or not accompanied by its natural companions supplied by nature to work with them. Instead of aluminum pots, use STAINLESS STEEL and PORCELAIN ENAMEL for top-of-the-stove cooking and GLASS for oven use.

◆ *Carbon Monoxide (CO)*

Carbon monoxide is one of the most damaging constituents of polluted air. It interferes with the oxygenation of all the cells of your body by preventing oxygen to be absorbed by the lungs. It can cause RESPIRATORY DISORDERS, HEADACHES, LOSS OF MEMORY, SHORTNESS OF BREATH, ANGINA, EMPHYSEMA, ANEMIA, HEART DISEASE, AND CANCER. Use VITAMIN E which increases tissue oxygenation and decreases the body's oxygen need, by preventing the undesirable oxidation of lipids in the blood stream. Use a dose of 400 to 600 IU a day. VITAMIN A counteracts CO by increasing the permeability of blood capillaries, and thereby facilitating better delivery of oxygen to the cells. An oxygen lack weakens the lining of the artery, making it more susceptible to clogging.

◆ *Cadmium (Cd)*

A POISON may be said to be any substance capable of altering or destroying some or all of the functions necessary to life. Cadmium, although beneficial in minute amounts in natural form, is extremely toxic as an environmental pollutant. It is found in smoggy air produced mostly from AUTOMOBILE EXHAUSTS, for many brands of gasoline contain cadmium. It is also present in PHOSPHATE FERTILIZERS through which it pollutes the soil, and is taken up by vegetables and particularly by CEREAL GRAINS. It can also come to us through our water supply, which often contains considerable amounts of cadmium.

It has long been known that cardiovascular death rates are higher in soft water communities than in hard water communities. Autopsies have shown that people who die of cardiovascular disease have higher levels of cadmium in their bodies. Cadmium has been implicated as a causative factor in heart disease and death. Dr. Henry Schroeder believes that since soft water is more acid and corrosive than hard water and therefore collects cadmium from the water pipes in which cadmium has been used in the process of metal refining, tap water has more cadmium in it than ground water. This would explain why the HEART DISEASE RATE IS HIGHER IN SOFT WATER AREAS.

Cadmium poisoning can also be caused by the use of ENAMELED POTS AND PANS. Toxic cadmium is used to achieve the beautiful colors in the enamel, and this is dissolved by the acids in our foods and ends up in our bodies.

To counteract the effect of cadmium in our system, VITAMIN C is a specific protector against it. Use massive doses of up to 3000 mg per day, or in acute poisoning even more. Also use ZINC-RICH FOODS. Zinc and cadmium are chemical antagonists. If zinc is present in the body in abundance, it will displace cadmium. Avoid WHITE FLOUR, for in it 78% of the zinc in the wheat has been removed, while most of the cadmium remains.

◆ *DDT*

DDT is still widely used throughout the world, especially in developing countries. DDT is a cumulative poison, stored mainly in the fat tissues of the body. Pelicans north of the Polar Circle were found to have DDT in their tissues. It decomposes very slowly. Quick reducing programs, or a rapid loss of weight for any reason can be dangerous as the poisons from the dissolved fat can damage the whole system. When fasting for reducing purposes use FRUIT AND VEGETABLE JUICES which will minimize the danger.

VITAMIN C helps to neutralize all poisons, including DDT, and protects body tissues from its harmful effects. YOGURT and other soured milks neutralize DDT in the intestines and minimize its damaging effects. Research has discovered that LECITHIN binds up DDT so as to make it harmless.

◆ *Drugs*

All chemical drugs are toxic, more or less. They can all cause harmful side-effects. It has been conservatively estimated that 10% of all patients suffer from drug-caused diseases. Even such an "innocent" drug as aspirin, consumed in the U.S. at the rate of more than 30 tons a day, has caused many deaths and millions of serious injuries. It neutralizes vitamin C in the system, and also increases the rate of folic acid loss. Drugs also interfere with normal enzyme and vitamin action in the body, causing derangement in metabolism and vital body processes. They destroy vitamins and minerals, and also prevent their absorption. Many drugs damage the liver, kidneys, and can cause serious diseases, including IMPOTENCE, INFERTILITY, BIRTH DEFECTS, and CANCER. Only extreme emergencies warrant any use at all.

For protection take large doses of VITAMIN C, up to 10,000 mg. After treatment with antibiotics take high potency B-COMPLEX VITAMINS. Two to three teaspoons a day of LECITHIN. VITAMINS C AND E are of specific value against the damaging effects of ASPIRIN. Take YOGURT and WHEY or SOURED MILKS for a prolonged period to help establish a new flora of beneficial intestinal bacteria killed by antibiotics.

◆ *Lead (Pb)*

Lead is present in air, water and food. It is one of the most toxic metal contaminants, and can be fatal even in small amounts. It used to come largely from leaded gasolines from which the lead has now been taken out. It is found in ceramic glasses, lead-containing paint, and other industrial sources. Lead is a cumulative poison. Early symptoms are lack of appetite, fatigue, nervousness, and later developments damage the kidneys, liver, heart, and nervous system. MULTIPLE SCLEROSIS (MS) is believed by some researchers to be caused by lead poisoning. They have found a definite correlation between high-lead soil and areas of greater MS incidence. Children born to lead-poisoned mothers suffer growth retardation as well as mental and nervous disorders.

Protection: Extra amounts of calcium have both a preventive and curative effect by helping the body to safely excrete lead from the system. 1000 to 3000 mg of VITAMIN C helps in neutralizing the toxic effect of lead. VITAMIN A helps to activate enzymes which are involved in detoxifying lead poisons. ALGIN made from brown Pacific KELP, or SODIUM ALGINATE, has been shown to excrete lead from the body. Algin is a chelating agent, which means that it attaches itself to a metal so that it cannot react, and moves it through the intestinal tract without being absorbed. Powdered algin can be mixed with drinks and foods. Other antidotes are: SODIUM SULFATE (GLAUBER'S SALT), MAGNESIUM SULFATE (EPSOM SALT).

◆ *Mercury (Hg)*

Mercury is one of the most universally present poisons in our environment. It has contaminated our soil, our waters, and our food supply. It can damage the BRAIN and the CENTRAL NERVOUS SYSTEM. It interferes with ENZYME ACTIVITY, damages the KIDNEYS and LIVER, and causes PARALYSIS and BLINDNESS. Mercury is in ocean water but even more so in inland waters where industrial effluents have been dumped. METHYL MERCURY, a mercury compound is highly toxic. It has been dumped into water as a chemical by-product of the manufacture of chlorine.

When poisonous substances are dumped into water, they evidently get into the fish, and people eat the fish and get poisoned by it. In the dental office, the careless handling and spillage of mercury amalgam results in the rapid vaporization of the mercury at room temperature. Inhalation of these vapor fumes in sufficient quantities leads to illness characterized by depression, weakness, headaches, and tremors that render handwriting illegible. Also the mercury can gradually leach out of the FILLINGS and can cause similar problems. Mercury will leach out faster out of a filling if you chew gum, drink a hot drink, or put extra pressure on a filling such as grinding your teeth,

Some dentists have been able to reverse diseases such as HODGKINS DISEASE, and LEUKEMIA by removing the silver-mercury fillings from patients. Fillings have both positive and negative electrical currents. When both gold and silver are in the same mouth, the current is much higher than what the brain normally operates on. The bacteria in the digestive system take the mercury and convert it to METHYL MERCURY which is 100 times more toxic than mercury itself. It causes some bacteria to mutate to other bacteria with which food cannot be digested properly. If mercury ever becomes attached to the red blood cells at a point where oxygen is to be carried, they will not be able to carry oxygen again. The body will recognize them as foreigners and will proceed to destroy them. This loss of red blood cells will cause an IMMUNE DISEASE, for the immune system is now fooled into destroying its own cells. Examples of autoimmune diseases are DIABETES, MULTIPLE SCLEROSIS, LUPUS, and AIDS.

◆ *Protection Against Mercury*
- BREWER'S YEAST—contains SELENIUM, a trace mineral and an antioxidant that acts as an antidote, helping to destroy mercury in the body. Also eat organically grown foods, they contain traces of selenium.
- SPRING WATER—Instead of drinking tap water, drink unpolluted WELL or SPRING WATER, bottled if necessary. Eat large doses of VITAMINS A, C, E, and the B-complex.
- CALCIUM—helps to neutralize mercury and excrete it safely. Use up to 1000 mg per day.

◆ *X-rays*

X-rays have been used by doctors, hospitals, dentists, and chiropractors for decades. Sometimes they have been used indiscriminately while ignoring their potential danger. X-RAY EFFECTS ARE CUMULATIVE, so that even small amounts, such as those emitted from a color TV can be dangerous, as they add to the total amount received from all sources. Overexposure can cause LEUKEMIA, CANCER, BIRTH DEFECTS, and a later development of leukemia in a child born of a mother who received abdominal x-rays during pregnancy. Even the type of X-rays that are used diagnostically can cause cancer and leukemia. X-rays used to cure cancer themselves cause cancer. It has been estimated that the average life span of a radiologist is six years less than the average of the population, and that 2 years of life are lost for every roentgen absorbed.

◆ *X-Ray Protection*
- ✓ RUTIN, VITAMIN P, and BIOFLAVONOIDs—found in citrus fruits, strengthen the capillary walls and reduces hemorrhaging caused by X-rays. In animal tests rutin reduced the death rate caused by excessive X-rays by 800%.
- ✓ VITAMIN C—Large doses of VITAMIN C taken together with rutin strengthens the effect of rutin. Experiments in several hospitals show that patients can withstand heavier therapeutic radiation without damage to healthy tissue if given LEMON COMPOUND, LEMON, and LEMON PEEL, which contain large amounts of bioflavonoids. Bioflavonoids have antioxidant activity, and protect both VITAMIN C and ADRENALIN from oxidation by copper-containing enzymes.

✓ PANTOTHENIC ACID—found in brewer's yeast, prevents radiation injuries in doses of 5 to 15 mg for children and 25 to 50 mg for adults. In animal studies, the survival rate was increased by 200% by giving pantothenic acid before exposure.

The Use Of Salt

◆ *Salt And Inspiration*

Salt is a flavor enhancer. In the Old Testament, meat offerings were to be seasoned with salt (Lev. 2:13). The New Testament tells us that God's people are the salt of the earth (Matt. 5:13). This means that our actions are to enhance the life of the people with whom we come in contact. In that sense salt is good (Mk. 9:50). But if we are not carrying out our responsibility before God and our fellow men, then we have lost our savor, and are no longer a benefit in God's missionary endeavors.

◆ *Natural Food Contains Salt*

With the food of fruits, nuts, seeds, and vegetables which God gave to Adam and Eve, He did not also give them a salt shaker, so as to make the food flavorful. This means that natural food is sufficiently flavorful to the natural unperverted palate or taste buds. This is what people who turned to vegetarianism have always found. Once you turn to natural food, while at first it will taste flat, it will taste flavorful without any added salt, after you have gotten used to it. One can be perfectly happy without adding any salt to food, except for getting what is naturally contained in it. The need for extra salt represents an acquired appetite. Only GRAIN eating animals ever seek out salt licks.

◆ *The Body's Need For Salt*

SODIUM (Na) is a chemical element which when chemically combined with another chemical element called CHLORINE (Cl) produces the compound SODIUM CHLORIDE (NaCl), which is the formula for table salt. Salt is an INORGANIC COMPOUND. Inorganic means not related to, connected with, or derived from living substances. With a few exceptions, only substances originating from other nonpoisonous living substances belong in the body. Salt being an inorganic substance and not a food, is a dangerous substance in the body in too large a quantity.

The most dramatic case of salt injury occurred in a Binghamton, New York, hospital, where a number of babies died when salt was inadvertently used in their formula in place of sugar. An overdose of salt can kill a baby quickly. The body needs natural, organic sodium, rather than table salt which is an inorganic chemical. Natural sodium which nature provides in organic form can be obtained from BEETS, CELERY, CARROTS, POTATOES, TURNIPS, SEA VEGETATION such as KELP, WATERCRESS, and many other natural foods.

◆ *Some Salt Is Necessary*

A chemist who had studied the chemistry of salt gave the following explanation of its function. He said that we have to look for good natural salt. He said that salt, sodium chloride, is very essential to the body, but that almost all salt on the market today has been HEATED. That our blood is nearly 1% salt; that it has a vital part to play in the development of hydrochloric acid in the stomach; that it aids digestion; that it is very valuable in maintaining the balance which is necessary for osmosis which takes place in the cells; that it has a great influence over the fluids and weight of the body. He said that if your cell fluids are SODIUM CHLORIDE, you have a tendency to gain weight; if they are POTASSIUM CHLORIDE, you have a tendency to lose weight. This is controlled by the food you eat. During the bodily processes the sodium separates from the chlorine and recombines at the end as sodium chloride. Salt that has been heated is unable to perform this task. It does not separate during the bodily processes to the detriment of the body. All herbs have some salt in them, but this salt is in organic form, that is, it is combined with other elements so that it does not act as pure salt, so that basically, in most cases no added salt is necessary.

In 1869 Dr. R.T. Trall stated that "salt being a poison, should not be used at all." He did not realize at that time that a little salt was necessary. Mrs. White clarified the point when she said: "I use some salt, because salt, instead of being deleterious, is actually ESSENTIAL FOR THE BLOOD" (CD344). She said that "food should be prepared in as simple a manner as possible, free from condiments and spices, and even from an undue amount of salt" (CD340), She continued by saying: "In Michigan we get along better without SALT, SUGAR, and MILK, than can many who are situated in the far West or in the far East, where there is a scarcity of fruit. But there are few families in Battle Creek who do not use these articles upon their tables. We know that a free use of these things is positively injurious to health, and, in many cases, we think that if they were not used at all, a much better state of health would be enjoyed" (3T21).

Many groups of primitive people have remained healthy without even eating any salt at all. Explorers who wanted to imitate such people found it difficult for a week or so, but they gradually became accustomed to saltless food. After that they preferred their food without salt, and lived in good health without it.

◆ *Salt Binds Water*

Sodium is the prominent element in body fluids. Our BLOOD, SWEAT, and TEARS are all salty like SEAWATER. The chemical composition of SEAWATER is virtually identical to that of HUMAN BLOOD. Hence, seawater contains all the minerals and trace elements necessary to build and sustain health. In general salt has the tendency to attract or bind water in the body. It causes water retention. Every gram of salt binds or holds 50 to 70 gm of water. Dr. H.C. Sherman says that through overstimulating the digestive tract, salt may interfere with the absorption and utilization of the food. To protect its tissues against this poison—salt—the body automatically seeks to dilute it by accumulating water in these areas. As the tissues become waterlogged, the body tends to swell. The bad effects of accumulated fluid may be seen as the cause of many diseases. He also states that an excess of salt may disturb the OSMOTIC PRESSURE of tissues, involving almost every portion of the body. While some salt is needed to keep the TENSION of the BODY FLUIDS at a normal level, we get enough in our foods in their natural state to serve the purpose.

◆ *"Water Goes Where Salt Is"*

When an extra amount of salt enters the cellular fluid, it creates a higher concentrated salt solution. This extra solution increases the volume of the BLOOD PLASMA. If DIURETICS are taken to reduce water because of the tissue salt, then POTASSIUM, the needed cell mineral, is also washed out. In order to distribute the expanded blood, the heart must create additional pressure. It is therefore forced to pump harder, creating greater blood pressure. Salt may be the biggest reason why heart disease is our biggest killer. Hence, it is best to leave extra salt out of our diet, and in general there is no need to add extra salt to the food we eat, if we eat good natural food. Instead of salt use HERBS and LEMON JUICE. Use the salt shaker for garlic or onion powder.

◆ *Salt Creates Thirst*

The human organism can regulate the salt solution level in the body without outside help. For example, if an individual is not getting enough salt, the solution becomes weaker than it should be, and the body expels water to enrich the salt solution and brings the level up to par. It also reduces the amount of sodium passed through the sweat glands and kidneys.

On the other hand too much salt will make a person thirsty, and he will feel like taking in more fluids. Farmers like to give their cattle salt blocks to lick, for since salt attracts water, they believe that it will increase the production of milk.

◆ *The Function Of Salt In The Body*

We need only between 2 to 3 gm of salt in our diet per day. The average American gets up to 10 times this amount. The main functions of sodium and chlorine in the body are first, to control the VOLUME of fluid and the PRESSURE that exists between the wall of cells and the fluids that bathe them; and secondly, to regulate the ALKALINITY and ACIDITY of the body fluids. It works with the action of the kidneys which excrete sodium or chlorine as the occasion demands. Too high acidity excretes chlorine and retains sodium. If too alkaline, sodium is excreted and chlorine is retained.

◆ *The Effect Of Excess Salt*

✓ DEADENS TASTE BUDS—Salt tends to deaden the taste buds so that with time and age more and more salt needs to be used in order to taste it at all. No matter how much salt is put into the food in cooking, many people will still add more salt habitually without tasting the food first

- ✓ HYPERACIDITY—The production of hydrochloric acid (HCL) in the stomach depends upon the salt intake. Salt goes to make up part of this HCL. If too much salt is taken in, too much HCL is formed, and a condition of HYPERACIDITY is produced. This condition is often the cause of STOMACH ULCERS.

- ✓ MIGRAINE—and other headaches may be due to too much salt in the system, in which the extra water flows to the tiny blood vessels of the brain and puts pressure on the nerves. It could also be caused by FOOD ADDITIVES, LOW BLOOD SUGAR, THE PILL, and MSG. It can be cured by the FEVERFEW PLANT, HYSSOP, WALKING, RUNNING, or JOGGING. Comfort can be obtained with an ICEBAG on the forehead or on the back of the neck.

- ✓ PREVENTS USE OF CALCIUM—Table salt often interferes with the body's use of calcium. When most of it is eliminated from the diet, calcium metabolism is frequently restored to normal.

- ✓ SALT AS AN IRRITANT—We know how salt irritates an open wound, or salt water stings the eyes. In the same manner it irritates the delicate membranes throughout the body. We are told: "Do not eat largely of salt, avoid the use of pickles and spiced foods, eat an abundance of fruit, and the irritation that calls for so much drink at mealtime will largely disappear" (CD311). Spiced dishes "irritate and inflame the delicate coating of the stomach" (CD340).

- ✓ SALT AND WRINKLES—For people who are on the far side of 40, some dermatologists suggest that they not use any salt in their diet. They know that salt is especially difficult to eliminate, and that an excess can stay in the tissues to cause wrinkling.

- ✓ SODIUM-POTASSIUM BALANCE—Sodium and potassium exist in the body in a ratio of 1:2. Too much potassium in the diet results in the loss of sodium, and too much sodium results in a loss of potassium. Dr. Max Gerson attempted to build up the body's POTASSIUM content as an important part of his famous treatment for CANCER. Since salt is known to increase the body's loss of potassium, it seems to follow that salt might be an indirect cause of cancer by robbing the body of this vital element. This fact has been proven in experiments with cats and salted milk.

- ✓ SALT AS AN EMETIC—A tablespoon of salt in a cup of warm water is a quick EMETIC, or produces vomiting in case of poisoning.

- ✓ SALT AND HAIR—Dr. Foldes found that the reduction or elimination of salt, whether from the salt shaker or from processed foods, will help improve the GROWTH of HAIR. To put a shine on your hair, add the juice of a large LEMON to the final rinse water after your shampoo. The acid neutralizes the alkali that tends to dull the hair.

- ✓ SALT AND FREE RADICALS—Salt gives rise to free radicals that deposit toxic chemical fragments on healthy tissue. The salt-prompted free radicals then break down the primary genetic materials in your cells.

Salt And Disease

- ✓ CANCER—For a long time salt has been under suspicion as a cause of CANCER. Dr. Braithwaite of England found that the diameter of a tumor in one of his patients grew from 2 to 3 inches when the patient resumed the daily use of salt, even in small quantities. He says that it harms body tissues because it is a powerful stimulant to cell metabolism. F.T. Marwood, a layman, observed that in Denmark, where the consumption of salted fish is the highest in Europe, the cancer rate is also the highest in Europe. According to Dr. W.C. Daws' experiments, CANCER was developed in cats which were fed small quantities of salt in their milk. Other cats, subjected to the same environment and irritations, but without added salt in their milk, did not develop cancer.

- ✓ DEAFNESS—A woman who had been deaf for years was questioned by Dr. Murphy regarding her eating habits. She told him that she was a heavy consumer of salt. She was advised to stop taking it completely. After three weeks she returned to her doctor, who after testing her declared her hearing to be restored as good as ever.

- ✓ DROPSY—Doctors now believe that the cause of DROPSY is not too much water, but too much salt, which stimulates the body to hoard water in abnormal amounts, usually as a result of a heart or kidney ailment. An old aphorism says, "water goes where salt is."
- ✓ EDEMA—Salt attracts water to create edema. It deprives the tissues of oxygen, thereby creating a host of circulatory problems.
- ✓ HEART DISEASE—Of 35 cases of CONGESTED HEART FAILURE who were put on a low-salt diet, 22 received a definite benefit while 13 did not.
- ✓ HIGH BLOOD PRESSURE—Because salt clings to water, when an excessive amount enters the extra-cellular fluid, it carries extra liquid with it. This increases the volume of the plasma. In order to distribute the expanded blood, the heart must create additional pressure, and therefore pumps harder creating HBP.

  Dr. Frederick Allen introduced the low-salt diet for HBP in 1922 into the U.S., and has had consistently good results. He also conducted animal experiments which proved that with the feeding of salt, blood pressure increased causing hypertension. The Japanese suffer from the highest blood pressure in the world. They are also known as the highest salt consumers. The Danes have the second highest blood pressure, and they get it from eating a lot of salted fish. The Japanese get their sodium largely from the condiment MONOSODIUM GLUTAMATE, which they sprinkle on almost everything they eat, and as a result, they also have the HIGHEST STOMACH CANCER RATE in the world. The Danes have the second highest stomach cancer rate.
- ✓ INSOMNIA—A diet rich in salt will keep you awake at night. Salt is a stimulant. It stimulates the adrenal glands just as CAFFEINE does. In fact salt is a double insomnia offender, It leads to HBP which is itself an enemy of restful sleep. In a study of 100 people who had reported that they never salted their food at the table, only 1 had HBP. Among 100 people who added salt to taste, 8 had HBP. Among 100 people who added salt even before tasting their food, 10 had HBP.

  The amino acid TRYPTOPHAN has been shown to treat insomnia without side effects, when prescription drugs failed. It also helps to synthesize SEROTONIN, the neurotransmitter, which does not interfere with REM sleep. NIACINAMIDE (B_3) helps to reduce TENSION, FATIGUE, DEPRESSION, and INSOMNIA, and tends to increase REM sleep. It has been reported that insomnia may be caused by a deficiency of CALCIUM. Taking calcium and magnesium tablets may be helpful. MORNING SICKNESS may be caused in some cases by a vitamin B_6 deficiency.
- ✓ KIDNEY DISEASE—The kidneys can cope with eliminating up to 5 gm of salt per day. Salt hardens the tissues, that is why it is excluded from the diet in cases of heart, blood vessel, or kidney diseases. All the salt needed by the body is plentifully supplied by fruits and vegetables such as TOMATOES, CELERY, SPINACH, KALE, RADISHES, TURNIPS, CARROTS, LETTUCE, STRAWBERRIES ETC. When salt is omitted a person soon enjoys the flavor of the food more, even though it may taste flat at first.
- ✓ A MALARIA CURE—A quarter of a century ago an old Indian woman, who had a reputation for being a healer, gave a malaria cure to two young men who had malaria. She told them to SPRINKLE COMMON TABLE SALT INSIDE THEIR SHOES, and for them to wear thin white socks. This they did, and in one week's time, the malaria symptoms disappeared and never returned.
- ✓ OBESITY—Because of the water-holding properties of salt, in cases of obesity a drastic reduction of salt is advised. Fluid adds to the weight. Salt also excites thirst, producing a greater intake of water, and excites the appetite by increasing the flow of saliva.
- ✓ PREGNANCY—70 patients who were put on a salt-free diet in the latter stage of pregnancy showed a definite reduction in the length of labor, and in the severity of the pain as far as that could be determined. It is believed that the decreased salt intake brought about a removal of salt from the maternal tissues, bringing about a lessening of the excitability of the nerve centers and a definite sedative effect. ECLAMPSIA, or a toxemia of pregnancy, has been linked to a high sodium diet.

- ✓ SALT and CALCIUM—Salt will get into a battle with calcium in the body and win. The result is less than an adequate amount of calcium for the teeth and bones. Hence, the inclination toward tooth decay.

- ✓ SINUSITIS—When there is an excess of salt in the body tissues, the ears and the sinuses are effected. When free perspiration does not help to get rid of the excess, the kidneys force the salt into other organs or tissues. The salt collects water about it, and a waterlogged condition may result in the ears and sinuses.

- ✓ OTHER DISEASES—HIVES, EPILEPSY, NERVOUS TENSION, and RHEUMATIC SWELLING all respond to the restriction of salt intake. The following diseases can be caused by too high a salt intake: ARTHRITIS, CEREBRAL HEMORRHAGE, HBP, HEART DISEASE, and STROKES. There is a close relationship between salt intake and the level of CHOLESTEROL.

Salt In Food

- ✓ EXCESS SALT IN FOOD—Salt as well as sugar is added to almost any processed food, especially canned food. Since cooking takes some of the flavor out of natural food, salt is added to canned food in order to return some of the flavor to the food. Studies made during the last few years indicate that from year to year the amount of salt and sugar added to food has been on the increase, which might mean that the quality of the food we are eating has been on the decrease. One big way to cut down on salt is to limit processed foods, which account for about 75% of the salt in our food supply.

- ✓ BABIES AND SALT—If babies are given too much salt in their food or formulas, they have a tendency toward HYPERTENSION later on in life. Infants who are bottle fed with evaporated or whole cow's milk may be getting too much salt. A 5 month old infant drinking a quart of cow's milk a day will average 1 gm of salt. When 40 different jars of baby food were tested for salt content, it was found that they were getting the equivalent of the highest daily salt intake in adults who commonly develop hypertension. Due to the salt licks for the cows, the sodium content of cow's milk is nearly 4 times that of human milk. It is also poor in MAGNESIUM which is needed to assimilate calcium. Without magnesium, calcium deposits form upon the heart tissue and arteries. There is no need for putting salt in baby food. They enjoy it without salt. Some manufacturers have added salt to baby food in order to please the taste of the mother.

- ✓ SALT and SUGAR—If we add a sufficient amount of salt to the diet of rats, we will induce high blood pressure in them in 5 months. If we add sugar with the salt, the high blood pressure will develop in 1 month. So processed food which has both salt and sugar in it will develop HBP much faster.

Overcoming The Salt Habit

- ✓ BANANAS—are recommended in a low sodium diet because bananas are very low in salt content. 1 pound of bananas contains only mg of sodium.

- ✓ DIETING—Dr. Dahl found that simply reducing the weight of patients by diet did not produce a fall in their HBP. He needed to reduce their salt intake at the same time.

- ✓ KELP—The powder is one of the best substitutes for salt. It contains only 17% salt in organic form. Besides, it contains all of the trace elements necessary for health that are also in sea water.

- ✓ SEA SALT—is beneficial in supplying the trace minerals which are refined out of many of our foods. These missing trace elements are the ones that may, in their absence, cause DIABETES, GRAY HAIR, BALDNESS, MULTIPLE SCLEROSIS, MYASTHENIA GRAVIS, and other so-called deficiency diseases.

- ✓ SEA WATER and BLOOD TRANSFUSIONS—Sea water contains 60 or more of the many chemical elements in the earth. It especially contains many of the trace elements which have been refined out of our food. They are also essential to human health. In this respect it is in many respects like human blood in composition.

One doctor, who had given up blood transfusions 15 years before, began using only normal saline solutions for blood tranfusions. He said that he had never lost a case because of lack of blood. Even accident cases who had turned white because of lack of blood, never die from lack of blood. His reasoning was that taking on someone else's blood is at best dangerous because there is no such thing as absolute blood compatibility. There is only relative accommodative compatibility. So why not use transfusions of normal saline solution to start up the body's own blood making apparatus, so that the body manufactures its own compatible type of blood.

It has been shown that large doses of VITAMIN C, such as 7 gm/day, can eliminate HEPATITIS from blood transfusions.

✓ SUBSTITUTES for SALT—are CARAWAY SEED, GINGER, HORSERADISH, LEMON or LIME juice, MUSTARD SEED, PEPPERMINT, SAFFRON, and TARRAGON.

✓ SWEATING—The National Research Council has concluded that the average American gets enough salt in a day's food to make up for any losses in PERSPIRATION. Furthermore, salt accumulates in the tissues. The average person has an overabundance of salt in the tissues so that no extra salt needs to be taken on a day when there is profuse sweating.

✓ VEGETABLES—Dr. Dickey who studied the natives of Africa, found that by feeding them GREENS he could overcome their CRAVING FOR SALT. He mentioned that he wasn't implying that salt is not needed by the body, but he maintained that it should be gotten in the organic form found in fruits and vegetables.

Salt And Water Softeners

When water is artificially softened through a water softener, there is involved a transfer of two parts of SODIUM to the softened water for every one part of CALCIUM or MAGNESIUM removed. Some believe that the danger represented by the added sodium to the softened water far outweighs any convenience factors that might be present. People on a salt-free diet are counseled not to drink it. Excess sodium creates hardship for the KIDNEYS. Chronic kidney failure is common among the higher salt intake groups. Sodium intake is also closely related to HEART DISEASE, and commercially softened water means added sodium. Also, softened water will leach more vitamins out of food than hard water. In cooking, salt water will rob food of some of its vitamins and minerals.

In hospitals, through the softened water, patients may be placed unknowingly on a high salt diet, when the doctor has placed them on a low salt diet. The harder the water you use, the more sodium will be in it when it is softened. Such softened water will also have extracted some minerals out of the hard water.

Iodized Salt

The THYROID GLAND is of importance primarily in childhood. Its treatment with IODINE has not the same effect later in life. Children tolerate iodine much better than adults, and their iodine requirement is 3 times greater according to Monier-Williams, author of *Trace Elements in Food*. He pointed out that after iodine was introduced there was a marked increase of HYPERTHYROIDISM, or an overactivity of the thyroid gland in adults. The POTASSIUM IODIDE in table salt was not put there by nature. It is not accompanied by all of the substances that go along with iodine in foods. Also, it is not an organic combination with other factors in food substances.

He says that if we want a little salt on our food, we should get the iodine and the salt from some organic source such as KELP or SEAWEED. Powdered kelp would be the best possible salt substitute. So fill the salt shaker with powdered kelp, and you will get all the salt you need and the iodine also.

HEALING DISEASE BY NATURAL MEANS

How The Body Heals Disease

◆ *Healing depends upon Removal Of Cause*

All healing is the province of the internal laws and wisdom of the body which God has placed therein. Where medicine has beneficial value is in SETTING BROKEN BONES and REPAIRING INJURIES, so that the body's healing process can proceed more effectively. Healing takes place in spite of drugs, not because of them. Drugs and doctors ride to glory on the back of the healing power of the body. A true cure always remains a true cure, but it seems that the "cures" of yesterday are no longer cures. Physicians do not seem to learn anything from past failures. If they possessed any true knowledge, they would not fall for the new "cures" or drugs which are offered them by the drug companies. With so many cures, why should anyone ever remain sick or die of disease. Their ignorance leads them to ignore causes and to place their faith in "cures." Success of the body's effort at self-healing depends absolutely upon the removal of the cause of its ills. The BODY CURES ITSELF when the cause is removed. Healing is an inside job. All we have to do is to prepare the conditions that make healing possible.

Some time ago the New York Times printed an article about several North Dakota communities who tried to obtain a doctor, but without success. A survey by the health department of those communities revealed that their health condition was far above the national norm.

In Israel in 1973 the number of funerals dropped by nearly 50% since the doctors strike began, according to statistics released by the Jerusalem Burial Society. A similar drop was experienced 20 years before when the doctors last went on strike. So the physicians of Israel are saving the lives of their patients by staying away from their bedsides. Apparently the people of Israel did not learn from their first experience. When physicians struck in Toronto, Canada and in Holland a few years before this, there was a similar drop in death rates. A famous doctor lecturing in New York, once revealed a collection of AMA statistics to prove that if all hospitals, drug stores, and consulting offices were suddenly closed, and no one had any way to get any medical help or medicine or advice at all, the death rate in the country would very soon be cut in half.

◆ *The Drug Delusion*

The power of the drug delusion is protected by IGNORANCE, DEPRAVITY, and the wish for EASY DELIVERANCE from the effects of TRANSGRESSIONS. People need to learn that their sufferings are the results of flaunting the laws of life. Chemistry rather than the laws of biology are resorted to in order to solve the problems of disease. As soon as a drug is taken, the body's recuperative powers devote themselves to the task of expelling it. Medicine is endeavoring to cure CANCER, but it hasn't as yet found the cure for the common cold, and its methods indicate that it hasn't as yet determined what the meaning of a cold is.

◆ *The Purpose of Biological Therapies*

Biological therapies are directed at correcting the underlying causes of disease by ELIMINATING THESE CAUSES, by CLEANSING the body of various hindrances to its functioning, by STRENGTHENING the patient's resistance, stimulating and assisting the restorative and healing processes, and creating the most FAVORABLE CONDITIONS for the body's own healing forces to go into action. To accomplish this various natural substances and methods are utilized.

◆ *"Do The Patient No Harm"*

The first principle of healing. "Do The Patient No Harm," is probably violated in present day medical practice more often than in any other period of medical history. It is estimated that at least 10% of all patients suffer from doctor caused (iatrogenic) diseases. According to one doctor of Florida "adverse effects of nonprescription drugs as well as prescription drugs, are responsible for the hospitalization and death of a significant number of patients. Drug illnesses is the seventh most common cause of hospitalization in the U.S."

- ✓ VITAMINS, MINERALS, PROTEIN, and CALCIUM—When a wound occurs, the body draws on all of its reserves to move cells to the damaged tissue, produces new cells to replace those destroyed, and binds the new cells together into new tissue. Vitamins, minerals, protein, and calcium are called upon to join in these emergency repairs.
- ✓ PROTEIN—is absolutely essential for rebuilding body tissue. Your need for protein increases when you are recovering from a serious injury.
- ✓ VITAMIN C—An excess of vitamin C accelerates healing above the normal level. A deficiency impairs wound healing. Vitamin C regulates the formation of COLLAGEN, a protein that is the main structural ingredient of connective tissue. With 1000 mg of vitamin C the wound healed 40% faster according to Cheraskin and Ringsdorf. With 2000 mg of vitamin C, the wound healed 50% faster. An injury drains your body's supply of vitamin C. In one study it was found that the vitamin C levels in white blood cells of surgical patients had dropped by 42% 3 days after surgery. This may indicate that after surgery the vitamin C in the body migrates toward the healing site. Hence, it is wise after surgery to take 1 or 2 grams of vitamin C daily.

Wound healing requires the formation of connective tissue which, although made of protein, cannot be synthesized in the body without vitamin C. Hundreds of studies have shown that RESISTANCE TO INFECTION, SPEED OF RECOVERY, and STRENGTH OF NEW TISSUE, is dependent upon the amount of vitamin C obtained. Taking in addition to vitamin C 1000 to 3000 mg of BIOFLAVONOIDS per day increases the absorption and efficiency of vitamin C.

- ✓ VITAMIN A—works hand in hand with vitamin C in the healing process. Anti-inflammatory drugs, such as CORTISONE or even ASPIRIN retard the healing of open wounds, and increase the risk of their infection. DIABETICS often suffer from slow healing wounds, and are also prone to infections. A study showed that supplemental vitamin A was shown to increase wound strength in diabetic animals, and it is believed that it will also help fight infections by increasing the accumulation of collagen.
- ✓ ZINC—Zinc works as a teammate of vitamin A, without which the vitamin A stores could not be mobilized. It is a valuable coworker that is essential for the production of PROTEIN and COLLAGEN, and is necessary for normal growth and reproduction of cells.
- ✓ Vitamin E—is also a wound healer, and an unusual success has been reported in treating BEDSORES, DIABETIC ULCERS, and ULCERATED SURGICAL INCISIONS. One patient who had ulcers was treated with 800 IU of vitamin E twice a day by mouth, and vitamin E ointment was applied directly to the sores. In less than 4 months he was sent home. Dr. Wilfred E. Shute, the pioneer vitamin E researcher, says that vitamin E is the ideal treatment for BURNS, because of its ability to limit cell death to those cells that have been killed by the burning agent, and can even help reduce the old SCAR TISSUE when applied directly.

Natural IMMUNITY

- ✓ NATURAL—THE IMMUNE SYSTEM is essential for human survival. The WHITE BLOOD CELLS destroy all substances that are not naturally a part of the human body. The THYMUS GLAND is the master gland of the immune system. It is the staging ground for messenger cells, the T-cells, of the immune system. The T stands for thymus. The B-cells search out and identify the intruders. They are responsible for producing ANTIBODIES. Three types of white blood cells, T-cells, B-cells and K-cells have their home in the lymph system, and are therefore termed LYMPHOCYTES. VITAMIN C stimulates the production of all of the white blood cells. BROAD SPECTRUM ANTIBIOTICS destroy all bacteria, good and bad. They produce YEAST INFECTIONS. These can be destroyed by taking LACTOBACILLUS

ACIDOPHILUS. 15 women who had had at least 5 yeast infections per year were monitored for 6 months, and were found to average 3 infections each. Then the doctor asked them to eat a cup of ACIDOPHILUS YOGURT every day for 6 months. During this period their infections dropped to less than 1 per woman.

The health of the immune system depends on the harmonious interaction of all of the components which allow the body to recognize the presence of disease microorganisms, and to reject and destroy them. An imbalance or disruption of the immune system can result in a great number of diseases. CORRECT EATING HABITS, EXERCISE, ADEQUATE SLEEP, and other health practices can keep the immune system functioning well. Prominent herbs which boost the immune system are CHAPARRAL, PAU D'ARCO, ECHINACEA, and various Chinese herbal formulas. They have antiviral, antibacterial, as well as immunostimulating properties.

Food, Vitamins, And Mineral Therapies

✓ ALOES—Calvin Dence in his book *Your Heart's Desire,* tells of an 8 year old girl whose clothes caught on fire and burned large patches of flesh all over her body. He applied about 2 pints of FRESH ALOES all over her body. Within 8 to 10 days, she had all new flesh in the large burned areas. She experienced no more PAIN nor INFECTION. On small burns, he says, one may apply a paste of wet BAKING SODA. One should not break the blisters. He says that in the absence of aloes one could apply ICE or COLD WATER at first till the burning sensation stops. Some people have success with MASHED-UP ONIONS or KEROSENE applied to take away pain and to promote healing. Excellent results are also obtained by applying OLIVE OIL or WHEAT GERM OIL to the area until the new flesh comes. Cover area with a thin cloth to protect it, but allow the air to enter. The patient should also breathe deeply very often. A POULTICE of GRATED RAW POTATO also is a lot of help. MOIST SALT helps when it is applied immediately. So we see that there are many natural methods that can be used and applied to any one or many ailments.

✓ CHARCOAL—Lymphoid tissue contains two types of LYMPHOCYTES, B-CELLS and T-CELLS. Dr. Marjorie Baldwin of the Wildwood Sanitarium and Hospital, a private SDA institution, uses ACTIVATED CHARCOAL to promote healing. She says that any inflammation, any area that is RED, PAINFUL, SWOLLEN, and HOT, responds to charcoal. She applies charcoal as a poultice if the inflammation is on the outside of the body, or gives it by mouth if the inflammation is in the digestive tract. Dr. Baldwin tells of a young lady whose feet were damaged because she was diabetic, and she developed severe infections. ANTIBIOTICS didn't clear them up. The doctors at the hospital where she was suggested that one foot be amputated, but she refused and came to the Wildwood Sanitarium for treatment. Dr. Baldwin put the severely damaged foot in a plastic bag filled with a mixture of charcoal and water. It was kept in the bag around the clock, with the mixture being changed 4 times a day. This process restored her foot to normal, and she walked out of the sanitarium on both feet.

✓ COMFREY—Drinking strong comfrey tea and/or applying tea saturated cloths or a poultice of tea leaves is helpful. Comfrey contains ALLANTOIN, a cell proliferating substance that speeds healing.

✓ CUCUMBER—European folk healers apply ripe cucumber juice to small open wounds.

✓ SALIVA—Some doctors believe that when animals lick their wounds, that their saliva may aid healing by making the wounds knit faster. When the SALIVARY GLANDS were removed from animals, the wounds healed more slowly.

ACNE

Acne Is An Adolescent Problem

Most cases of acne have their beginning in adolescence, and most persons with acne are teenagers. It has been determined that three out of every four American teenagers have at least a mild case of acne. It is caused when the SEBACEOUS OIL GLAND in the skin is plugged up by dirt or the skin cells themselves. If the skin isn't cleaned frequently and some of the oil becomes trapped, bacteria multiply in the pit of the hair follicle, and the skin becomes inflamed. Each plug is called a COMEDOME. They turn into BLACKHEADS when the sebaceous fluid called SEBUM turns black because of oxidation. Blackheads may be contaminated by bacteria that can break down the walls of the surrounding skin cells. If this happens, the blackhead turns into a highly visible infection known as a PIMPLE.

The Causes Of Acne

One author states that ACNE is caused by BAD FOOD, a ZINC DEFICIENCY, VITAMIN A DEFICIENCY, and ALLERGIES. It may also be caused by too many refined STARCHES, FRIED FOODS, HIGH PROTEIN CONSUMPTION, DAIRY PRODUCTS, AND REFINED SUGAR. The skin is used to throw off excess waste which the kidneys and liver are unable to handle. Next to FAT, SUGAR is the most offending food. Once inside the body, sugar converts to TRIGLYCERIDES or FATTY ACIDS, which burden the blood and lymph, causing waste to accumulate in the tissues.

Acne is linked to an increase in the production of the male hormone TESTOSTERONE which makes the sebaceous gland larger. Everyone, both male and female, produces some male and female hormones, but males produce more testosterone, and they produce it more rapidly at puberty. Therefore they are more likely than females to have severe acne during adolescence. Some cases of acne do not begin until a person reaches the late twenties or early thirties. This kind of acne, known as ADULT ACNE, seems to target women more often than men. It often appears right before a woman's menstrual period when estrogen production slows, and clears up afterwards when it starts to rise again. We must remember that the skin is one of the main organs of elimination through which body impurities are expelled from the system, when it is convenient for the body to do so.

One aspect in the cause of acne is the contribution made by the condition of INTESTINAL TOXEMIA One study showed that 50 percent of patients with acne had increased blood level toxins which were absorbed from the intestines. In general it is said that acne is caused by CONSTIPATION, SWEETS, URIC ACID, and PUTREFACTIVE BACTERIA.

Food, Vitamin, And Mineral Therapies For Acne

◆ *Eliminate All Concentrated Carbohydrates*

Skin biopsies have shown that in acne the skin's glucose tolerance is impaired. In this sense one researcher called acne "skin diabetes." Since we know the immune suppressing effect of sugar and its role in the development of adult-onset diabetes, it is suggested that all refined and concentrated carbohydrates be eliminated. Foods containing TRANS-FATTY ACIDS, such as MILK, MILK PRODUCTS, MARGARINE, SHORTENING, and all other synthetically hydrogenated VEGETABLE OILS, or OXIDIZED FATTY ACIDS such as fried oils, should be avoided. Milk consumption, due to its high hormone content, should be limited.

✓ HIGH POLYUNSATURATED FATS AND LOW ANIMAL FATS—Dr. Gustav Hoehn, a dermatologist, believes that a diet high in polyunsaturated fats and very low in animal fats will cure acne. He says that WHOLE MILK is the biggest problem. He believes that the moles will disappear when you put people on SKIM MILK and eliminate hard fats. He also advises against FRIED FOODS.

✓ FRESH FRUIT JUICES—Extra iodine can aggravate acne, so the doctor advises patients to avoid IODIZED SALT. Many commercial soft drinks contain BROMINATED VEGETABLE OIL as stabilizers which may irritate the acne condition. Instead of such drinks people should drink FRESH FRUIT JUICES.

✓ ADDED ZINC—Foods rich in ZINC are WHEAT GERM, SESAME SEEDS, SOY BEANS, SUNFLOWER SEEDS, EGG YOLK, BREWERS YEAST, MOLASSES, OATS, CORN, BEANS, and AVOCADOS. In one experiment, zinc worked as well as the antibiotic TETRACYCLINE, and without any side-effects.

✓ VITAMIN A—RETINOLS, a form of vitamin A present in animal tissues, have been shown to reduce sebum production. They must be used in large quantities.

- ✓ VITAMIN E AND ZINC—Some doctors recommend 400IU of vitamin E and 50 mg of zinc daily.
- ✓ A RAW FOOD DIET—A natural raw food diet of either fruits or vegetables, lasting 5 to 10 days, has been recommended. FASTING with fresh raw fruit and vegetable juices for a few days, including CARROT, SPINACH, and GRAPEFRUIT juice, is very helpful. A GARLIC preparation called KYOLIC has helped people with acne. A NATURAL DIET, while avoiding refined sugar, saturated fats, fried foods, and chocolate, has eliminated acne in many cases.
- ✓ YEAST—Yeast has a beneficial effect on the skin, and has long been used as a remedy for pimples and acne. Vitamins in the yeast help the deranged liver to oxidize fats in the diet properly. It is the incompletely oxidized fats in the diet that clog the oil and sebaceous glands. A HIGH-CHROMIUM YEAST known to improve glucose tolerance and enhance insulin sensitivity, has been reported to produce rapid improvement in patients with acne.
- ✓ EPSOM SALTS—A hot Epsom salts bath, two or three times a week, will be extremely helpful in all cases of acne.

Herbs

◆ *Echinacea*

Echinacea is beneficial for skin eruptions of all kinds including acne. It can be used as a tea as well as an ointment. ECHINACIN ointment, which can be obtained in the health food store, was used in a trial of 4,598 patients with inflammatory skin conditions. It had a success rate of 85%. On the average the symptoms disappeared within four days. It is an ointment which is free of side-effects as compared with ointments containing steroids or antibiotics.

◆ *Goldenseal*

Goldenseal is indicated for acne due to its detoxifying and antibacterial properties. Its anti-microbial activity is due primarily to its major alkaloid BERBERINE, which is effective against bacteria, protozoa, and fungi. It kills toxic bacteria while not affecting the beneficial bacteria. Yogurt will do the same. Other herbal teas that are helpful are COMFREY ROOT, RED CLOVER, and DANDELION ROOT TEA.

◆ *Stinging Nettle Tea*

A useful treatment for ACNE has traditionally been sipping up to one quart daily of this tea. The reason being that disfiguring PIMPLES are often caused by sluggish KIDNEYS and a diet of CHOCOLATE, FATS, STRONG SPICES, SALTY and ACID FOODS. These foods should be omitted in order to give the kidneys the rest they need.

◆ *Calendula Flowers*

Apply a tea made from CALENDULA FLOWERS. Steep 2 tablespoons of calendula flowers in one cup of boiling water for 15 minutes, cool, and apply with a cotton ball. Calendula heals and soothes the skin through its antiseptic and anti-inflammatory properties. A skin-care product containing calendula can be purchased at a natural foods store.

◆ *Tea Tree Oil*

Tea tree oil is a broad spectrum FUNGICIDE and ANTISEPTIC that has been proven effective for a wide variety of skin problems, including ACNE. The oil is derived from the leaves of the MELALEUCA ALTERNEFOLIA, a tree that grows in New South Wales, Australia. It was nicknamed the "tea tree" by Captain Cook, who led a sailing expedition into the area in the 1770's, and used the leaves to make tea for his crew. It can be diluted with water or vegetable oil. With it one can treat ACNE, BOILS, STINGS and BITES, ATHLETES FOOT, WARTS, COLD SORES and BLISTERS, and SKIN RASHES. A cream has been developed with it which eliminates many cases of CANDIDA ALBICANS.

General Detoxification

According to Kushi, excess proteins and fats, are discharged also in the form of WARTS, MOLES, CALLOUSES, and TUMORS. BEAUTY SPOTS, FRECKLES, and BROWN MOLES may be the result of TOO MUCH SUGAR. When the body cannot process substances naturally, it will push them out through the SKIN.

A boy wrote to Dr. Hemermann, a naturalist, about how his mother helped him get rid of acne. He said that his mother made him stop eating all junk foods such as candy, potato chips, fries, shakes, colas, soft drinks, and ice-cream. He said that he about died when his mother told him this. But he could see a change for the better right away. Then she had him wash his face with PINE TAR SOAP. She also had him take 1500 mg of VITAMIN C daily, as well as a spoonful of WHEAT GERM OIL. In a couple of weeks his acne was 90% cleared up. If one takes as little as one teaspoonful of wheat germ oil, it is almost equivalent to getting under an oxygen tent.

AIDS

Nature Of The Disease

AIDS is an IMMUNE DEFICIENCY DISORDER which alters the body's ability to defend itself. The AIDS VIRUS invades the T-cells, a thymus derived white blood cell responsible for cell immunity, and multiplies, causing a breakdown of the body's immune system, which eventually leads to overwhelming infection and/or cancer. Many who die from AIDS have respiratory illnesses, usually PNEUMONIA, which the immune system is not able to fight.

The virus that causes AIDS is called HIV, which stands for HUMAN IMMUNODEFICIENCY VIRUS. Many people who are carriers of the HIV virus are not even aware that they have it. Between 1 and 2 million Americans are infected with the HIV virus but have no symptoms. They spread the virus primarily through sexual contact, or through the sharing of needles during intravenous drug use. AIDS patients may develop 3 cancers—ANAL, TONGUE, and KARPOSI SARCOMA, a cancer of multiple areas of cell proliferation. The exposure of skin and mucous membranes to contaminated blood may result in the transmission of the HIV virus. Dr. Robert Streker of California proved that the HIV virus got 50% of its genes from the BOVINE LEUKEMIA VIRUS and 50% from the SHEEP VISNA VIRUS.

Only 4% of those infected with the HIV virus will develop the disease within 3 years. After 5 years of exposure that figure climbs to 14%, and after 7 years exposure it jumps to 36%. People with the virus are more likely to contract AIDS if their immune system is severely suppressed. When the immune system is working properly, the virus is absorbed by the white blood cells and destroyed. When a person has full-blown AIDS, the virus is taken in, but the white cells can't kill it, and the virus reproduces itself unchecked. The AIDS virus uses human cells to perpetuate itself. It can lie dormant for many years, but when fully activated, it turns certain immune cells into virus factories. The AIDS virus can reside inside of people for up to 9 years without ever triggering production of the antibodies that doctors have relied upon as their chief evidence of aids infection.

AIDS is also passed from the mother with the virus to the child at birth. It is also possible for dentists and medical workers, who come into close contact with the bodily fluids of infected persons, to become infected. It takes 2 to 5 years or longer after infection for the symptoms of the aids virus to appear. When the virus becomes active some of the symptoms are FEVER, FATIGUE, SWOLLEN LYMPH NODES, DIARRHEA, SKIN DISORDERS, and ENLARGED LIVER and SPLEEN. 38% of those infected with the AIDS virus will develop AIDS in 5 or 6 years.

Causes Of AIDS

✓ PENICILLIN—There is some evidence that strongly suggests that penicillin and possibly other ANTIBIOTICS may be a co-factor in the development of AIDS. Penicillin does decrease the WHITE BLOOD CELLS. In toxic doses antibiotics, including penicillin, reduce the body's ability to defend itself against specific infection. Cancer patients receiving CHEMOTHERAPY, Patients with HEPATITIS, INFECTIOUS MONONEUCLEOSIS, and other diseases, show IMMUNE SUPPRESSION similar to that in AIDS patients. of all patients with AIDS either have or will develop a malignant cancer such as KAPOSI'S SARCOMA. Doctors know that the best defense against AIDS is a healthy immune system; hence, ironically, chemotherapy often injures the immune system.

Successful Natural Treatments Of AIDS

◆ *The Ozone Therapy*

Dr. Preuss of Stuttgard, Germany, uses OZONE THERAPY in combination with other factors to cure patients of AIDS. He said that he searched for a substance which is viricidal, fungicidal, and bactericidal all at the same time. He did this because he said that AIDS disease or diseases consist of VIRAL, FUNGAL, and BACTERIAL INFECTIONS. Ozone was to him the obvious solution, since it had been used for many decades for the elimination of microorganisms. It is a nonspecific therapy which covers all possible causes of AIDS. It is safe, effective, and nontoxic. He has documented case histories of 11 patients whom he has cured with this therapy. There is an immediate improvement of conditions in the AIDS patient. Other infections present at the same time such as HEPATITIS B or GASTROINTESTINAL CANDIDIASIS disappear automatically within 5 to 10 days.

There are 3000 doctors in Germany all of whom have announced that they have killed AIDS viruses with OZONE. They explain that the diseased cells have weaker enzymatic coatings, so that the free radical scavengers created by OZONATION DESTROY DISEASED CELLS ONLY. They state that to get them all they must give the patient repeated applications of ozone. The Medizone Company in the U.S. has a similar process with ozone which is under study by the FDA. At Syracuse, N.Y. University Hospital they have achieved a 100% kill ratio of AIDS viruses, both within and outside of the cells, and without damaging any lymphocytes.

◆ *A Garlic Treatment*

Dr. Abdullah of Panama City, Florida, treated 7 AIDS patients with a Garlic extract called KYOLIC which is a special garlic preparation manufactured in Japan and sold in health food stores. For the first six weeks they took 10 capsules a day, and 20 capsules for the last six weeks. All 7 patients showed a 3 to 14 fold increase in the activity of the key immune cells. All symptoms of diarrhea and genital herpes ceased. Some members of the medical team believed that some of the valuable constituents of the garlic may be lost if the cloves are cooked. That is why kyolic was chosen because it is a preparation which is not processed with heat.

◆ *Blue-Green Algae*

HIV-positive patients took a blue-green algae and reported more improvement than with the drug AZT which has many side-effects, but there were no side-effects with the algae. AZT is very toxic. It eliminates more than the AIDS virus. It leads to anemia by destroying normal bone marrow cells. After 18 to 24 months, HIV becomes resistant to AZT.

◆ *Compound Q*

Dr. Yeung of Hong Kong University asked Dr. McGrath of San Francisco General Hospital to add a protein called TRICHOSANTHIN or COMPOUND Q to a test tube of HIV infected cells. It killed all of the cells infected with the AIDS virus, but did not affect the cells which did not have the AIDS virus.

◆ *Herbs*

✓ ST. JOHN'S-WORT EXTRACT—was given to a group of mice in a National Academy of Science study. They were infected with viruses that cause LEUKEMIA, then given a single injection of the extract. It totally prevented the disease. Laboratory tests indicated similar action against the HIV virus.

✓ SILYMARIN—an extract of MILK THISTLE WEED, helps repair the liver, and cleanses the blood and lymph system of viral and bacterial infections. It acts as an antioxidant by protecting the liver cells from FREE RADICALS. It also stimulates the liver to produce increased amounts of SUPER OXIDE DISMUTASE (SOD), which is also a free radical scavenger. It also prevents the depletion of GLUTATHIONE in the liver cells, the amino acid the liver uses to excrete toxic chemicals.

✓ PAU D'ARCO—is a natural antibiotic that strengthens the immune system. RED CLOVER is also a good blood cleanser.

✓ KYO-GREEN—is excellent to take three times a day. It contains CHLOROPHYLL, PROTEIN, VITAMINS, MINERALS, and ENZYMES.

- ✓ OXIDATION—Oxidize the blood as much as possible through vigorous exercise. Eliminate all bad habits, and drink distilled water only.
- ✓ VITAMINS—At the Robert Koch Institute in Germany, a child born with the AIDS virus was given 2 years to live by the doctors. They felt, however, that a vitamin treatment would extend the life even further. The mother gave the child per day 2 KIWI FRUITS, 2 GRATED APPLES with LEMON JUICE, the JUICE OF 3 ORANGES, which produced an excess alkaline condition, with NATURAL VITAMINS. After some time the AIDS virus no longer showed up in the doctor's tests, and the child was considered cured.

  VITAMIN C does not cure AIDS but it works against AIDS by stimulating the IMMUNE SYSTEM: attacking FREE RADICALS; by acting against SECONDARY INFECTIONS; by reducing reactions to other MEDICINES.

◆ *Fruit And Vegetable Juices—*

Fresh fruits and vegetables and their juices are very helpful. Carrot and beet juices should be consumed with garlic and onion added.

ALLERGIES

What Are Allergies

An ALLERGY is an unusual sensitivity of the body's immune system to a substance that is not normally harmful. The immune system helps us to combat infection. It does this by identifying "foreign bodies," and mobilizing the white blood cells to fight them. It happens that at times the immune system wrongly identifies a nontoxic substance, and the white blood cells overreact, and consider the substance as a foreign body that should be eliminated. Then the allergic response becomes a disease itself and does damage to the system. When it does this, the body releases too much HISTAMINE, and it is too much histamine that causes those allergic symptoms. Allergic reactions can resemble the symptoms of almost any disease. They can affect how people feel, act, and even think. They are not just limited to physical ills, but they can also affect the mind. A severe allergic reaction is called ANAPHYLAXIS. This means that the body overreacts when it tries to protect itself from an allergen. The symptoms of anaphylaxis are a RASH, ITCHING, SWELLING in the THROAT to the extent that the airway is obstructed, and CIRCULATORY DIFFICULTIES.

There are over 40 million people in this country with allergies because of the processing of foods which contain thousands of chemicals. There are laws in many states requiring bread to be enriched. Some 20 natural vitamin and mineral elements are removed from the wheat, and only 4 or 5 are put back, including a little iron. But the vitamins which are put back into the flour are artificial rather than natural vitamins which often have a poisonous effect upon the tissues.

The Causes Of Allergies

The true causes of allergies are those factors which weaken the mucous membranes, making them hypersensitive to pollens and other substances. Were the mucous membranes in normal health, they would not be so overly sensitive to these common substances. ALLERGY, therefore, must be based upon a state of ENERVATION or nervous depletion, as well as TOXEMIA, the accumulation of the waste products of metabolism. When NERVE ENERGY drops below normal, the elimination of toxins, which are a normal product of metabolism, is largely stopped. The toxin is retained in the blood which fact brings on toxemia, which hygienists consider to be the only efficient cause of all disease. Enervation impedes normal elimination, and this in turn produces toxemia. When toxins are not eliminated as fast as they are generated, they irritate the mucous membranes to cause the symptoms of an allergy.
- ✓ POLLUTION—The increase in allergies throughout the world is due to the increase in levels of pollution. The pollutants are primarily TOBACCO SMOKE, NITROGEN DIOXIDE, OZONE, and SULFUR DIOXIDE.
- ✓ OTHER OFFENDING SUBSTANCES—Other offending chemicals may be HAIR, FEATHERS, COSMETICS, DRUGS, and HOUSE DUST. INHALED SUBSTANCES are considered the most frequent cause of allergy. Different persons are allergic to different substanc-

es. Leucretius of the first century B.C. said: "What is food for some may be poison for another."

NITROGEN TRICHLORIDE or AGENE, is a nerve poison. It is a BLEACHING AGENT for flour. It causes part of the wheat protein to be converted into a substance that is poisonous. It removes vitamins, and changes good protein into bad protein which causes nervous instability. Bleached flour is also blamed for some MENTAL DISEASES. CHLORINE DIOXIDE, another bleaching agent for flour, is also said to be toxic. It oxidizes the flour pigment.

✓ PROCESSED FOOD—Allergies from food are largely caused by FOOD ADDITIVES and FLAVORINGS. Of the foods the most common allergens are EGGS, WHEAT, WHITE POTATOES, MILK, and ORANGES in this order of frequency. Other foods that are allergens are PEANUTS, CITRUS FRUITS, CORN, PEAS, TOMATOES, and SUGAR.

With processed food we usually have no idea of what chemicals we are eating. Food chemicals react like drugs. With natural food if we are allergic to STRAWBERRIES, we stop eating them and that solves the problem. Additives can also combine with each other creating a whole new spectrum of allergens. It is said that of all chronic diseases in children under 17 are caused by allergies, and that allergies are the most common cause of DISABILITY among school children.

✓ COLORING ADDITIVES—Coloring additives in food such as "Yellow No. 5," known as TARTRAZINE, present in thousands of foods, has been reported to cause severe intractable ASTHMA. Manufacturers are usually "allergic" to labeling, so that all additives do not appear on the label.

Allergies From Various Substances

Substances that are TOXIC in moderate or large doses tend to cause allergy in smaller so-called "safe" doses.

✓ CHOCOLATE—Chocolate as an allergen can cause CHILLS, VOMITING, ITCHING, ABDOMINAL PAIN, COUGH, CLOGGED NOSE, ECZEMA, HIVES, and SORES AROUND THE MOUTH. BREAD is a common cause of HIVES, ECZEMA, and MIGRAINE HEADACHES, which latter can also be produced by an overuse of SUGAR products. One doctor says that most allergies are due to HYPOGLYCEMIA, OR LOW BLOOD SUGAR.

✓ COFFEE—Coffee will make the heart race, the blood pressure climb, nerves jangle, and the kidneys and heart work overtime. A recent study by Swedish researchers revealed that DECAFFEINATED COFFEE promotes the production of STOMACH ACID which could be damaging to people who have ulcers. It was earlier thought that the caffeine in regular coffee was the source of the stomach acid stimulation.

✓ MILK—Children who are nursed for at least the first year of life develop substantially fewer allergies. ANAPHYLACTIC SHOCK can be caused by the PENICILLIN in cow's milk. When this happens to little babies or children the blood pressure drops, the throat swells closed, and the individual collapses, and sometimes dies. The process of pasteurization has no effect on the penicillin in cow's milk.

Nature designed milk for babies. Adult animals don't drink milk. In many adult humans, nature has reduced LACTASE from the growing digestive tract, and it becomes very deficient in it. When such individuals drink milk, much undigested lactose pours into the colon, and bacteria multiply in it and ferment it, producing gas, cramps, and sometimes diarrhea.

✓ DRUGS—Allergic reactions to drugs are the unexpected reactions, besides the side-effects, which are the expected reactions.

✓ GLUTEN—Gluten is a vegetable ALBUMIN, a protein that is prepared from wheat and other grains. It has been implicated as a prime cause of wheat allergy. It is claimed that gluten will over a period of time form a plastic film in the small intestines which can seriously interfere with food assimilation. It gradually erodes the myelin sheath, the outer coating of the nerves, and eventually short-circuits them. It has caused

SKIN, RESPIRATORY, and DIGESTIVE ALLERGIES.

✓ POLLEN—HAY FEVER or ALLERGIC RHINITIS, represents a condition where the mucous membrane lining is sensitive to pollen and other airborne substances. It also effects the nose, eyes, and air passages. Symptoms include watery discharge from nose and eyes, sneezing, and nervous irritability. Hay fever has been eliminated by chopping a slice of onion, and putting it in one quart of distilled water, and then drinking cup every 4 hours.

✓ SACCHARIN—It is strongly suspected of causing CANCER. As a coal tar product it has caused allergies in some people.

✓ STRAWBERRIES—Some good foods, such as strawberries, produce allergic reactions because they have a strong tendency to purify the bloodstream. It means that they stir up poisonous substances which enter the bloodstream, and which the body endeavors to eliminate through the skin in the form of HIVES.

How To Prevent Allergies

✓ USE BETA-CAROTENE—Beta-Carotene strengthens the collagen in cells so that allergens are not able to penetrate the cells readily, thereby making them immune to the allergens.

✓ USE BIOFLAVONOIDS — Bioflavonoids strengthen the permeability of the capillaries so that they resist the invasion of allergens. Bioflavonoids are located in the peels and white pulp especially of citrus fruits.

✓ MULLEIN LEAF—This herb provides mucilaginous protection to mucous surfaces, thereby inhibiting the absorption of allergens through those membranes.

✓ THE PULSE TEST—First take your pulse before you get up. Then right before you eat. Eat just one food at a time. Then take your pulse 30 minutes later. Then 60 minutes later. If as a result of eating that food your pulse beats 20 points or more faster, then that food is a possible allergen. Foods with many ingredients can undo a nonallergenic diet.

How To Cure Allergies

◆ *Use Vitamins*

✓ VITAMINS A + C—Many types of allergies, such as HAY FEVER, POST-NASAL DRIP, CHRONIC RHINITIS, ASTHMA, and other infections involving the mucosa of the nasal passages and upper respiratory tract will respond favorably to megadoses, meaning large doses, of vitamins A and C.

✓ VITAMIN C—Take 1000 mg of VITAMIN C per day. Vitamin C acts as an antihistamine as well as a detoxifying agent. It aids in cementing body cells, strengthens the walls of blood vessels, stimulate the formation of white blood cells, forms new tissue, and regenerates existing tissue.

✓ VITAMIN E—possesses anti-allergic and antihistamine properties.

✓ PANTOTHENIC ACID—Under a doctor's supervision, high doses of this vitamin of 1000–1500 mg 4 times daily have been used to alleviate many allergies.

✓ WATERCRESS—Watercress will reduce allergy symptoms such as SNEEZING, WATERY EYES, and a STUFFY HEAD.

✓ YOGURT—The LACTOBACILLUS in yogurt also helps to reduce food allergy.

◆ *Fasting*

Fasting is an excellent way to remedy allergies. Repeated short juice fasts result in better tolerance of allergens. After juice fasting a raw vegetable or fruit diet of watermelon, carrots, grapes, or apples should be consumed for one week. After that add one other food a week until all real allergens can be spotted and eliminated from the diet. A familiar Spirit of Prophecy statement applies here also: "If they cannot at first enjoy plain food, they should fast until they can" (CD190). Fasting will cleanse the blood of impurities. ORGANICALLY PRODUCED FOOD that doesn't contain artificial manmade chemicals, will not develop allergies.

◆ *Garlic*

As an antitoxin garlic strengthens the body against all allergens by stabilizing the nasal MAST

CELLS. Mast cells are connective tissue cells that contain histamine in their granules.

How To Test For Food Allergens

Dr. Arthur F. Coca developed a method whereby a person can tell whether he is allergic to any food that he is eating. The principle behind this test is that any food to which you are allergic will INCREASE YOUR PULSE RATE. The test works as follows: When completely relaxed take your pulse rate at the wrist. Count the number of beats in a 60 second period. Then consume the food which you are testing for an allergic reaction. Wait 15 to 20 minutes. If your pulse rate increased more than 10 beats per minute, omit this food from your diet for a month and then test again. If the same effect occurs then you are allergic to that food and it is best to omit that food from your diet. The lifesaving principle behind this test is that it has been found that people who die young on the average have had a HIGH PULSE RATE.

ALZHEIMER'S DISEASE

Progressive Mental Deterioration

Alzheimer's disease represents a progressive MENTAL DETERIORATION, the LOSS of MEMORY and COGNITIVE FUNCTION, inability TO THINK CLEARLY, IRRATIONAL BEHAVIOR, DEMENTIA, and the INABILITY to carry out DAILY ACTIVITIES. It is characterized by the general destruction of nerve cells in several key areas of the brain devoted to mental functions. There is a shrinkage and atrophy of the brain, affecting the proteins of the nerve cells of the cerebral cortex. Alzheimer's disease strikes mainly elderly persons, and leads to a complete loss of mental functions usually within 5 years. It is always fatal.

Possible Causes

✓ ALUMINUM (AL)—Suspicions have been growing regarding a possible link between this disease and the accumulation of aluminum in the diet. Aluminum has been found in excessive amounts in the brains of Alzheimer's victims to the extent that the brain is poisoned by it. Aluminum has been under suspicion as a brain poison. It is not required by the body for any metabolic processes. The gradual accumulation of Al in the brain over a lifetime has been thought by many experts to be a contributory cause, for the brain tissue of people who died with Alzheimer's disease contains much higher levels of Al than the brain tissue of normal people. The AL collects in the center of every nerve cell. It inhibits the enzyme CHOLINESTERASE that is known to be responsible for maintaining normal functioning of the brain.

To reach the brain, aluminum must pass the blood-brain barrier that filters the blood before it reaches the vital organs. Elemental aluminum does not readily pass this barrier but those aluminum compounds found in processed foods do. Aluminum is more easily dissolved by acid-forming foods such as GREEN TEA, CABBAGE, CUCUMBER, TOMATOES, TURNIPS, SPINACH, and RADISH. Aluminum compounds are widely ADDED TO FOODS to adjust acidity, to make them lighter in texture, and to keep fruits and vegetables firm. A most common aluminum additive is SODIUM ALUMINUM PHOSPHATE, an ingredient in baking powder, cake mixes, and self-rising flours. Even salt may contain aluminum in the form of SODIUM ALUMINOSILICATE, which serves as a desiccant and anti-caking agent. Canned drinks in aluminum cans allow the acidic beverages to dissolve the aluminum during storage.

✓ IN CHEMICAL SUBSTANCES—Aluminum (Al) can get into the body from DRINKING WATER, BAKING POWDER, FLOUR, CAKE MIXES, TABLE SALT, SALAD DRESSINGS, FROZEN DOUGH, SELF-RISING FLOUR, PROCESSED CHEESE, some PICKLED CUCUMBERS, NON-DAIRY CREAMERS, BUFFERED ASPIRIN, ANTI-DIARRHEA PRODUCTS, ANTI-PERSPIRANTS, DOUCHES, DEODORANTS, SKIN CREAMS, LIPSTICKS, and HEMORRHOID CREAMS. The regular use of ANTACIDS, such as a normal dose of TUMS will give you 5 gm of ALUMINUM HYDROXIDE a day. This is several hundred times what is obtained from food sources.

- ✓ FLUORIDES—The FLUORIDE in municipal water supplies increases the aluminum leached from aluminum cookware, and absorbed in foods cooked in it. It has been found to increase the aluminum concentration by up to 1000 times more than cooking in water without fluorides. Most Americans routinely drink fluoridated water and use it in cooking, and many use aluminum cookware. There is evidence that FLUORIDES INTERFERE with the body's ability to get rid of aluminum.
- ✓ ALUMINUM SULFATE or ALUM—Commonly used by water systems during the water treatment process. It is added to the water as a coagulant to allow suspended solids to settle out of the liquid. Doctors have found that Al in water causes a rapidly developing SENILITY. The journal *Lancet* tells of a 40 year old man who received kidney dialysis in an area where the tap water had a high content of aluminum, He developed almost complete memory loss during the time of treatment. However, he became able to remember normally again after 259 mg of aluminum were removed from his body. ANTIPERSPIRANTS, such as sprays, sticks, and roll-ons, containing an aluminum compound are designed to be absorbed, temporarily POISON THE SWEAT GLANDS, thereby giving fairly long-lasting "dryness." For the same reason, presumably, aluminum is part of many feminine hygiene products. The body does not require aluminum for any metabolic processes. In fact, aluminum is increasingly under suspicion as a potent BRAIN POISON. In the mid-70's, patients undergoing DIALYSIS TREATMENT for kidney disease were found to develop symptoms of SENILITY. Doctors found that aluminum in the water used in the treatment caused it.
- ✓ ANIMALS—Animals fed Aluminum compounds for several months, eventually die with brain damage similar to that found in humans with Alzheimer's disease.
- ✓ LACK OF ACETYLCHOLINE—It is a NEUROTRANSMITTER that helps transmit nerve reactions in the brain. It is deficient in patients with Alzheimer's disease. It is known to play a vital role in memory and intelligence. Aluminum is known to lead to a decreased synthesis of other neurotransmitters also.
- ✓ CIGARETTE SMOKE—It is suspected of being a cause of Alzheimer's disease. It is known that smokers are 4 times as liable as non-smokers to get the disease. Other Aluminum containing substances are ANTACIDS, PROCESSED FOODS, UNDERARM DEODORANTS, and BENTONITE CLAY.

Healing Substances For Alzheimer's Disease

◆ *A Healthy Diet.—*

A healthy diet and megadoses, meaning large doses, of vitamins and some mineral supplements has brought increased vigor, restored memory, and stimulated better mental functions to 5 out of 8 persons with Alzheimer's disease. The blood stream needs to be cleansed by means of bowel cleansing, diet changes, chelation therapy to take out metals. Build up the blood with high IRON FOODS to raise the red blood count and pick up more oxygen. Also the patient should be given regular physical exercise. CHELATION is a process where a man-made amino acid latches onto a lot of unwanted toxic metallic substances such as LEAD, MERCURY, IRON, AS WELL AS CALCIUM, that have been deposited in the body and are then eliminated through the urine. It has been successfully used for conditions such as LEAD POISONING.

◆ *Use Of Acetylcholine*

Acetylcholine comes from CHOLINE, a B-Vitamin. The LECITHIN from soybeans is the richest source of choline which comes mainly from soybeans. Lecithin has been shown to improve the MEMORIES of a group of Alzheimer's patients as well as their ability to care for themselves. Acetylcholine also improves the memory of Alzheimer's patients. One researcher injected aluminum into the brains of lab animals, and specifically RABBITS. Here he had observed the same kind of NERVE FIBER TANGLES that Dr. Cropper had observed in his Alzheimer's patients autopsies. DEMENTIA patients were also shown to have brain concentrations of aluminum. Many psychiatric patients who experienced memory loss, were shown to have elevated blood levels of aluminum.

◆ *Lecithin*

According to a 1978 report in *Lancet*, a British medical journal, the early stages of Alzheimer's disease have responded to a daily dose of three tablespoons of LECITHIN granules. Lecithin increases the speed of nerve transmission, and it is needed to keep cholesterol in a semi-liquid state.

◆ *Vitamin B_{12}*

Vitamin B_{12} levels are low in Alzheimer's patients, which is also caused by insufficient blood and oxygen flow to the brain. It has also been found that long term use of ASPIRIN, ACETAMINOPHEN, CODEINE, ORAL CONTRACEPTIVES and NEOMYCIN can interfere with the body's absorption of vitamin B_{12} and cause a deficiency.

◆ *Ginkgo*

Gingko is a tree whose leaves are used as medicine. An extract of these leaves given the patient will increase the blood flow to the brain, resulting in an increase in oxygen and glucose utilization The extract also increases the rate at which information is transmitted at nerve cell level. Ginkgo is the best selling healing product in France and Germany for MEMORY LOSS and OLD AGE.

◆ *Antioxidants*

✓ HELP PRESERVE OXYGEN SUPPLY—Antioxidants are substances which prevent free radicals from causing damage to the cells of the body. They help preserve the oxygen supply for the beneficial oxidation processes in the body. Some of the dietary antioxidants are VITAMINS C and E, BETACAROTENE, SELENIUM, FLAVONOIDS, ZINC, and COENZYME Q.

✓ DESTROY FREE RADICALS—There is a decrease of oxygen to the brain when there is HEART INJURY, LUNG DISEASE, HEAD TRAUMA, or any condition leading to LOW BLOOD PRESSURE, HIGH BLOOD PRESSURE, or a STROKE. With decreased OXYGEN, free radicals multiply.

Some oxidations, except those that help burn food inside the body for energy, have a harmful effect. Butter turns rancid by oxidation, and sliced apples turn brown. These are the oxidations which we want to eliminate as much as possible. The antioxidants are substances which keep these processes from affecting our health. Oxidation in the body also forms molecularly unbalanced substances which are called FREE RADICALS. They have the ability to harm cells. A free radical is a wounded molecule that lacks an electron, and it therefore attacks other molecules to steal an electron so as to become balanced. The attacked molecule then itself becomes a free radical, which starts a chain reaction which can eventually destroy tissues and organs. Such damage can spread very rapidly, especially in FATS.

✓ CREATION OF FREE RADICALS—Free Radicals are created in the body by ULTRAVIOLET LIGHT, RADIATION, POLLUTION, SMOKE, CAR EXHAUSTS, and ALCOHOL. As a result they are suspected of causing ATHEROSCLEROSIS, CANCER, CATARACTS, and even AGING.

✓ ANTIOXIDANTS BRING RELIEF—They convert cellular oxidants to water and oxygen through the action of various enzymes. They also change free radicals to less harmful substances and rebuild the immune system. FRANKINCENSE and MYRRH of Bible fame, are both antioxidants and were used as preservatives thousands of years ago. Effective antioxidant spices are CLOVES, OREGANO, SAGE, ROSEMARY, and VANILLA.

✓ VITAMIN A—BETA-CAROTENE—Releases molecules that distribute phagocytes, stimulates T-cells, and dispatches NEUTROPHILS to digest foreign particles. Neutrophils are the shock troops of the immune system. They rush to the scene of a wound. LYMPHOCYTES are white blood cells that have been educated to attack specific targets. The various types of LYMPHOCYTES are the commissioned officers. They are the T-CELLS and the B-CELLS. They are born in the BONE MARROW. The T-cells carry chemical swords, while the B-cells hurl chemical spears. MACROPHAGES and NEUTROPHILS are the foot soldiers.

✓ VITAMIN C—ASCORBIC ACID—It penetrates a cell to cause a strengthening in the defense system, and thereby renders the body invulnerable to arthritis.

- ✓ VITAMIN E—It penetrates fat membranes and removes the dangerous impaired electron from an oxygen radical which reduces the free radical to a less toxic form.
- ✓ SELENIUM—It forms the anti-oxygen enzyme GLUTATHIONE, which minimizes the harm of free radical attack by pairing up the electrons to protect body cells. Sources are: CEREALS, BROCCOLI, CABBAGE, ONIONS, and WHOLE GRAIN BREAD.
- ✓ OLIVE OIL—2 to 3 tablespoons daily will increase the power of the immune system to prevent crippling arthritis.
- ✓ EDTA—The amino acid called EDTA, or ethylene diamine tetra-acetic acid, seems to help Alzheimer's patients regain lost skills, improve comprehension and memory, and live more normal lives. This fact somewhat disputes the conventional medical belief that the disease is incurable.

Things To Do And Not To Do To Avoid Alzheimer's

- ☛ Avoid foods containing aluminum
- ☛ Do not cook apples, tomatoes, or sauerkraut in aluminum pots, because these highly acidic foods leach out the aluminum from the cookware.
- ☛ Don't buy or drink carbonated beverages from aluminum cans
- ☛ Do not store acidic or salty foods in aluminum cans
- ☛ Drink three glasses of skim milk per day to help the body displace aluminum
- ☛ Do not use antacids that contain aluminum
- ☛ Avoid areas of known acid rain. Dr. Perl of Mount Sinai Hospital in New York suggests that acid rain leaches aluminum out of the soil into our drinking water, thereby increasing our exposure to aluminum.

ANEMIA

Nature Of The Disease

In ANEMIA the red blood cells that transport oxygen are deficient in size and number. The most common nutritional cause is a diet low in IRON. Iron is part of the HEMOGLOBIN, which is the red blood cell component which actually brings oxygen to the cells and tissues.

Causes Of Anemia

◆ *Bleeding*

Some cases of iron deficiency come from bleeding, the cause of which is not always easy to find. A bleeding gastric ulcer is usually obvious because of the associated indigestion and abdominal pain, but bleeding from cancer of the colon can be without symptoms until the tumor is far advanced. Iron-deficiency anemia can be caused by heavy menstrual bleeding in women who don't take enough iron to make up for it. In the tropics it can be caused by intestinal worms who absorb some of the person's blood.

Women of childbearing age lose blood each month at menstruation, and are therefore more likely than men to be deficient in hemoglobin. Women need 18 mg of iron a day. Men need only 10 mg.

◆ *Limited Production Of Red Cells*

Anemia can be due to a decreased production of the red cells, or to an increase in their rate of destruction. Every day, about 1% of our red blood cells wear out and are replaced by new ones, and anemia results when this balance is disturbed.

◆ *Other Diseases*

Any of a great number of diseases such as SYPHILIS, TUBERCULOSIS, MALARIA, THYROID TROUBLE, KIDNEY PROBLEMS, LEUKEMIA, POISONS, or dietary deficiencies can increase the destruction or decrease the production of the red blood cells.

◆ *Pica*

Iron deficiency can cause a condition called PICA, which is the compulsive eating of almost anything, including dirt, clay, starch, and ice. It represents an obsessive craving for the unconventional dietary experience. Pica usually responds quickly to an injection of iron.

◆ *Aluminum*

IRON-DEFICIENCY ANEMIA has been shown to also be caused by an accumulation of ALUMINUM, according to a report in *Lancet*. Apparently, aluminum accumulates in the bone marrow where the red blood cells are formed, and so combines with them that they are no longer able to absorb and utilize iron. Thus the iron can no longer be used for red blood cell production.

Dietary Considerations

◆ *Eat Raw Vegetables And Fruits*

The emphasis should be on raw fruits and vegetables which are rich in iron such as DARK GREEN LEAFY VEGETABLES, such as SPINACH, WATERCRESS, KALE, BROCCOLI, CHARD ETC. Iron-rich fruits are BANANAS, APPLES, DARK GRAPES, APRICOTS, PLUMS, RAISINS, and STRAWBERRIES. Bananas are particularly beneficial as they contain FOLIC ACID and VITAMIN B_{12} in addition to iron. Other iron-rich foods are: SUNFLOWER SEEDS, MOLASSES, SESAME SEEDS and HONEY. Besides containing the iron, HONEY is also rich in COPPER which helps in iron assimilation. Most grains are acid reacting. MILLET and RICE are on the alkaline side, and are therefore helpful in arthritis.

◆ *Iron-rich Foods Increase Iron Absorption*

It has been determined that iron-rich foods eaten with a meal such as cabbage or a glass of orange juice, will dramatically increase the iron absorption from foods. The adding of extra iron to an infant's formula has been found to encourage the growth of contaminant bacteria in the milk. Fortunately, the iron in mother's milk, unlike that in cow's milk, is bound to a special protein and is not available to bacteria.

Fruit And Vegetable Juices

Green vegetable juices should be freshly made in the juicer or blender from any available greens such as spinach, alfalfa, watercress, parsley etc. They can be mixed with carrot and red beet juice. Drink at least 2 glasses a day. Beneficial fruit juices are: red grape, blueberry, black currant, prune, and apricot.

Herbs

Beneficial herb teas are COMFREY, DANDELION, FENUGREEK, RASPBERRY LEAVES, and KELP.

ARTHRITIS

Nature Of The Disease

◆ *Inflammation And Pain In Joints*

ARTHRITIS is often traced to an imbalance of calcium and phosphorus. It is characterized by an inflammation and pain in a joint or joints such as in the knees, wrists, elbows, fingers, toes, hips, and shoulders. The symptoms of chronic arthritis are SWELLING, STIFFNESS, and DEFORMITY of one or more joints. It may appear suddenly or come on gradually. Moving a joint usually hurts, although there may only be stiffness. WOMEN tend to develop it in their FINGERS, while MEN tend to develop it in their HIPS. Generally, the joint on the dominant side of the body is affected first. 25% of people with OSTEOARTHRITIS have it in their knees, 60% in their hands, and 25% in their hips. Some may have it in more than one place.

The traditional treatments of arthritis such as SURGERY, RADIATION, and CHEMOTHERAPY, are often momentarily successful, but they do not free the body from the grip of arthritis permanently, because they do not change a person's lifestyle, and the risk of side-effects is very high.

◆ *Osteo And Rheumatoid Arthritis*

✓ OSTEOARTHRITIS—There are commonly two forms of arthritis, OSTEOARTHRITIS and RHEUMATOID ARTHRITIS. Osteoarthritis is related to the wear and tear of aging, and involves deterioration of the cartilage at the ends of the bones. It rarely develops before the age of forty. It typically runs in families.

✓ RHEUMATOID ARTHRITIS—Rheumatoid arthritis creates stiffness, swelling, fatigue, anemia, weight loss, fever, and often crippling pain. It attacks the SYNOVIAL MEMBRANES surrounding the lubricating fluid in the joints. The body must have ZINC and MAGNESIUM in order to produce the SYNOVIAL FLUID in the joints. The cartilage and tissues around the joints are destroyed. The body replaces the damaged tissue with scar tissue, causing the spaces between the joints to fuse together. The entire body is affected instead of just one joint as in osteoarthritis. It often occurs in people under 40 years of age, including young children. Twice as many women as men suffer from it. Six times as many girls are afflicted with juvenile rheumatoid arthritis as boys.

RHEUMATOID ARTHRITICS lose far more TRYPTOPHAN, the natural pain killer than non-arthritics. For this reason they create a deficiency of NIACINAMIDE (B_3). When they took more B_3, there was a greater retention of tryptophan, and more flexibility in the joints. Niacinamide mobilizes ARACHIDONIC ACID, a fatty acid, and stimulates the formation of PROSTAGLANDINS, which help to combat inflammation. NIACIN (B_3), from which niacinamide is derived, works as well as niacinamide, except that it causes a flushing of the skin. The recommendation is that from 50 mg to 100 mg of niacinamide will relieve much pain and stiffness. Tryptophan may work even better when B_6 is also added to it. Take 3 mg for every 2 lbs. of body weight. A 150 lb. person requires at least 200 mg daily.

An invigorating morning ARTHRITIS TONIC is composed of one cup of SKIM MILK, 4 tablespoons of WHEAT BRAN, and 2 pitted PEACHES blenderized and sipped slowly in the morning.

◆ *The Great Crippler*

Arthritis is the nation's greatest crippler. The blood of arthritics always has less than normal values of PANTOTHENIC ACID in it. The average level of pantothenic acid for arthritis patients is about 65% of that of well individuals. Dr. Bingham says: "No person who is in good nutritional health will develop either osteo or rheumatoid arthritis." The crippling of the arthritis patient is the logical outgrowth of a mode of LIVING that produces and maintains enervation; of a mode of EATING that maintains gastro-intestinal fermentation and putrefaction; and of a mode of TREATMENT that may be even worse than the mode of living that maintained the arthritis to begin with.

◆ *Gout*

GOUT is another form of arthritis. It occurs more often in overweight people and those who indulge regularly in rich foods and alcohol. People with gout seem to have a reduced ability to excrete URIC ACID, a by-product of the metabolism of PURINES, a substance in meat. It typically attacks the smaller joints of the feet and hands, generally affecting the big toe. It deposits crystallized uric acid in the joints where they break down into a substance called SODIUM URATE. This causes swelling, redness, a sensation of heat, and extreme pain. Four times as many men suffer from gout as women. Many MEDICATIONS that LOWER BLOOD PRESSURE also ELEVATE URIC ACID LEVELS.

A Fort Lauderdale woman had a husband who had GOUT for years and took medication for it that made him ill. She read about CHERRIES being good for gout, and she made him try them. She served him cherries every day and he never needed another dose of medicine. A lady who had swollen and tender fingers for months claimed that eating cherries helped relieve her symptoms in just 10 days. CANNED CHERRIES and CHERRY JUICE have worked as well as FRESH CHERRIES.

◆ *Side Effects Of Arthritic Drugs*

Arthritic drugs can have severe side effects such as ULCERS, STOMACH BLEEDING, RINGING in the EARS, LIGHTHEADEDNESS, SLURRED SPEECH, difficulty with CONCENTRATION, CONFUSION, MEMORY LOSS, HALLUCINATIONS, PARALYSIS, and even DEATH, according to "Geriatrics" magazine. It is reported that more than of all hospital admissions for BLEEDING ULCERS in British hospitals were directly linked to the use of ASPIRIN and IBUPROFEN. Elderly people as a group are 7 times more likely than the general population to experience adverse drug reactions.

The Causes Of Arthritis

◆ *The Basic Cause Is Diet*

The latest research has linked arthritis to DIET. It is the general opinion of biological doctors that the diet of arthritics has been deficient in vital nutritive elements for prolonged periods of time, which involved overcooked, canned, devitalized, and overrefined foods. Dr. J.B. Lust says that in arthritis there is a vitamin and mineral deficiency in the diet, with a preponderance of starches, sugars, fats, and a deficiency of B-vitamins.

◆ *Toxicity In The Bloodstream*

Most biological doctors also believe that arthritis, from the standpoint of the body's internal condition, is caused by TOXICITY in the bloodstream, and faulty removal of waste from the system. In general arthritics had lower levels of FOLIC ACID, PROTEIN, and ZINC in the system. The researchers also concluded that DRUGS brought about many biochemical changes in the body which created a need for those nutrients, such as vitamin C, which the drugs neutralized. Drugs palliate some of the symptoms of arthritis as long as the patient takes them; but they remove no cause, and they provide none of the conditions of health. If the drugs are discontinued, about 99% of the patients are right back where they were, and are most likely in a worse condition than they were in before. Persistence in IGNORING THE CAUSES of disease and the REFUSAL TO REMOVE THEM are the greatest evils of medical treatment. Dr. Walter C. Alvarez of the Mayo Clinic confesses that "the big difficulty is that the medicine can do much harm to some persons, and it can even cause death."

All bad habits lead to TOXEMIA, and it doesn't matter which habit or combination of habits has led to it. The symptoms of toxemia can vary in a 100 ways, and still toxemia remains the same. No one will develop rheumatism of any form without first having indigestion, and this must have maintained itself over a long enough period time to pervert nutrition and damage cell development. MUSCULAR RHEUMATISM represents a perverted state of nutrition where patients have eaten large quantities of starch, and produced a great deal of fermentation in the stomach. They complain of stiff joints, and find it difficult to get around early in the morning. Health can return and be maintained only when all enervating habits have been corrected.

Arthritis can be healed with a stronger immune system. The invaders causing the arthritis are BACTERIA, CELLULAR WASTE MATERIAL, FUNGI, PARASITES, PROTOZOA, and VIRUSES.

◆ *Overall Physical Malfunction*

Toxicity in the bloodstream is due to OVERALL PHYSICAL MALFUNCTION, which is due to POOR NUTRITION, INCOMPLETE ASSIMILATION OF FOOD, TOXINS, LACK OF EXERCISE, GENERAL FATIGUE, PHYSICAL AND EMOTIONAL STRESS, WORRY AND MENTAL STRAIN, and OVERWEIGHT which puts extra pressure on the joints. These health-destroying factors result in DIMINISHED VITALITY and RESISTANCE to DISEASE, LOWER GLANDULAR ACTIVITY, HORMONAL IMBALANCE, and AUTOINTOXICATION.

◆ *Milk Allergy*

Clinical evidence indicates that arthritis is largely the result of allergy as its major cause. ARTHRITICS have even become allergic to themselves. That is why rheumatoid arthritis is often called an AUTOIMMUNE DISEASE.

Some people who are allergic to milk develop arthritic pains from the consumption of milk. A 52 year old woman displayed symptoms of rheumatoid arthritis only when she drank milk. Doctors found this out by giving her milk powder capsules and non-milk powder capsules. In each instance, pain, stiffness, and swellings returned when she was given milk products even though she didn't know what she was given.

◆ *The Nightshade Plants*

The nightshade family of plants include EGGPLANT, PEPPERS, POTATOES, and TOMATOES. These are known to cause arthritis in some people. From 5% to 10% of the population are sensitive to them. These foods contain SOLANINE, a substance that penetrates the immune barrier and creates a painful reaction. They destroy the functions of the cells and deposit free radicals as wastes. This will trigger the arthritis reaction. The body reacts by making large amounts of an IMMUNOGLOBULIN ANTIBODY, and attacks the solanine microorganisms, and renders them harmless. Some people have been cured of arthritis on a no-nightshade diet. A man who was sensitive to nightshade plants eliminated them without showing any progress. However, he was secretly continuing to smoke, and TOBACCO is also a nightshade plant.

◆ *Chemical Additives*

Chemical additives such as PESTICIDES, HERBICIDES, and FUNGICIDES cause arthritis symptoms. Dr. Theron Randolph found that arthritis symptoms disappeared when patients skipped chemicalized foods and avoided ENVIRONMENTAL POLLUTANTS.

◆ *Stress*

Stress can cause arthritis in connection with a low level of VITAMIN C, PANTOTHENIC ACID, and VITAMIN B_6. An arthritis-like ailment was induced in rats by making them deficient in pantothenic acid, which condition depressed vitamin C.

Arthritis—An Acid Condition Of The Blood

◆ *Only A Small Amount Of Refined Sugar Can Be Assimilated*

The biological doctors say that arthritis is caused by a faulty diet, and that a natural diet can reverse it, if the disease hasn't progressed too far. That faulty diet is represented by a highly ACID BLOOD condition caused by eating too many acid reacting foods which cause destruction of the cartilage and bones. Such a condition must be counteracted with the aid of ALKALINE reacting foods.

1. SUGAR DISSOLVES CALCIUM—Sugar has an affinity for calcium. Dr. McCann demonstrated that the solubility of calcium in water is 1:1000, or one part of calcium in a 1000 parts of water. If sugar is added to the water, the ratio is 35:1000, or 35 parts of calcium to 1000 parts of the solution, or 35 times as much calcium can be dissolved. Dr. Katase of Japan proved that the human organism can accommodate a small amount of refined sugar with proper assimilation, less than 1 ounce or 20 gm per day. Any additional amount was immediately absorbed by osmosis into the circulation.

2. SUGAR ROBS THE BONES OF CALCIUM—In the blood stream sugar breaks up into CARBON DIOXIDE and WATER. Carbon dioxide then recombines with the water to produce CARBONIC ACID. This is what makes the blood highly acid. In order for the body to neutralize this acid, it will withdraw calcium from the bones in the form of CALCIUM HYDROXIDE, for calcium in solution is an ALKALI. This combination of an acid and an alkali will form a neutral salt which is CALCIUM CARBONATE. An excess of calcium carbonate is now precipitated into the tissues, the muscles, the blood vessels, and the joints, and causes the conditions of RHEUMATISM, ARTHRITIS, and ARTERIOSCLEROSIS. Under these conditions when the blood vessels are subjected to a relatively high blood pressure it can cause a BURSTING of a CAPILLARY in the BRAIN, which is a STROKE. In the heart it can cause a CORONARY OCCLUSION.

The story is told of a lady who had been on CORTICOSTEROID medication against arthritis for a number of years. One day she bumped her arm against a table and discovered that she had broken a bone. Her doctor told her that this substance weakens the bones by taking calcium from it.

Oxalic Acid

◆ *Oxalic Acid Causes Lime Starvation*

Another acid that is produced by sugar in the presence of proteins, such as meat, by means of the process of fermentation, is OXALIC ACID. The oxalic acid thus developed combines with the calcium in the blood to form insoluble OXALATE OF LIME, or CALCIUM OXALATE, thus causing a calcium or lime starvation in the body. This brings about diseases such as RICKETS, TOOTH DECAY, ADENOIDS, and INFLAMED TONSILS.

◆ *Inorganic Oxalic Acid Combines With Calcium*

The oxalic acid in raw foods, such a SPINACH and RHUBARB, is vital organic, and is replete with enzymes. As such it is a beneficial substance. It is one of the important substances needed to maintain and to stimulate PERISTALSIS. On the other hand, the oxalic acid in cooked and processed foods is inorganic, and is therefore destructive in the system.

Oxalic acid readily combines with calcium. If these are both organic, the result is a beneficial, constructive combination. When the oxalic acid has become inorganic by COOKING, then it becomes an interlocking compound with calcium which destroys the nutritional value of both. As an inorganic acid, it can form OXALIC ACID CRYSTALS in the kidneys.

◆ *Organic Foods Assimilate Minerals More Efficiently*

It is interesting to note in this connection, that a mineral such as IRON in organic form, cannot be readily assimilated if it has become inorganic through cooking. Such inorganic minerals often prevent the utilization of other elements through chemical action. Thus the iron in raw spinach juice is utilized 100% by the body, while only 20% or less of the iron in cooked spinach is utilized.

Uric Acid

Arthritis is often associated with URIC ACID POISONING. Carnivorous animals have the ability to secrete hydrochloric acid which is 12 times as strong as that of humans. They also have an enzyme called URICASE which breaks down the uric acid into the enzyme ALLANTOIN. Man does not have this enzyme, therefore the digestion of the uric acid in meat is difficult for him. Vegetable proteins contain enough carbohydrates to make this enzyme unnecessary. Beef contains about 14 grains of uric acid per pound. Hence, the meat eater is consuming a lot of this poisonous end product without having the means of breaking it down and eliminating it. It is, however, neutralized by body ALKALIS, and mostly by CALCIUM, which forms CALCIUM URATE SALTS or crystals which are deposited in the tissues of the joints where they accumulate along with other toxins and cause trouble there. In this process calcium is depleted from the bones, and the mineral deposits in these joints harden, and the final result is the fusion of the entire joint.

How to Restore Arthritics to Health By Natural Means

◆ *Recovery Is Possible*

Recovery is possible in almost all cases of arthritis. It is not possible by suppressing symptoms and "relieving" pains, but by removing the CAUSE. A period of REST for the recuperation of the power to function; a FAST of sufficient duration to free the body of its accumulated toxic load; a corrected MODE OF LIVING to prevent the development of enervation and toxemia; EXERCISE for the joints after they have been freed of inflammation; SUN-BATHS for healthful stimulation; and a PROPER DIET of fruits and vegetables for the essential nutrition.

◆ *An Alkaline Diet*

The best therapeutic diet for arthritics is a low protein diet with emphasis on raw, fresh vegetables and fruits, and with the exclusion of meat, fish, salt, white sugar, white flour, and everything made from them. Dr. Ersen of Sweden says that there is no question that arthritis can be cured. BIOLOGICAL METHODS are the only ones at present that can bring about the cure.
A diet of BEANS is important because beans are high in sulfur-bearing AMINO ACIDS that work toward strengthening the connective tissue in the joints.

◆ *Calcium*

Calcium is one of the most essential elements in the diet, but it must be in vital ORGANIC FORM. When any calcium containing food is cooked or processed, the calcium is automatically converted into inorganic form. As such it is not very soluble in water, and it therefore cannot furnish the nourishment which the cells in our body require for regeneration. Furthermore, enzymes are destroyed at 130 degrees Fahrenheit and above. The result is that such food literally clogs up the system resulting in conditions such as ARTHRITIS, DIABETES, VARICOSE VEINS, CORONARY HEART DISTURBANCES, HEMORRHOIDS, and GALL and KIDNEY STONES. These deposits of inorganic calcium increase cumulatively when nothing is done to rid the body of them. With the aid of ORGANIC SODIUM they can be dislodged, maintained in solution, and eliminated from the body.

Arthritic infections may be triggered when harmful fallout or pollution enters the body. This signals an erosion of the immune system, which paves the way for arthritis infection. Calcium is said to be protective against LEAD, MERCURY, and STRONTIUM 90.

◆ *Cherries*

Cherries and cherry juice are a good treatment for ARTHRITIS and GOUT. In the case of gout the patients have high URIC ACID levels, which is largely due to the eating of meat, and the drinking of alcoholic beverages. This is eliminated by means of ALLANTOIN, an oxidation product of uric acid. Carnivores have the ability to convert uric acid to allantoin, but humans do not have this ability because they do not possess the enzyme URICASE. Relief is obtained by eating either fresh black Bing varieties, or canned cherries, either sour, black, or Royal Anise. In one case the juice of canned cherries had the same good result.

In another case 12 GOUT patients were relieved of their disease by taking cherry juice. After this no attacks of GOUTY ARTHRITIS have occurred on a nonrestricted diet in all 12 cases as a result of eating about pounds of fresh or canned cherries a day. One arthritis patient just drank the juice from the can, and the curative powers were equally effective.

◆ *Cortisone*

CORTISONE is often given for arthritis. Since what is given is not the body's own cortisone, it doesn't have the same effect. Prolonged medication with cortisone tends to atrophy the ADRENAL CORTEX and make it waste away. Overriding the adrenal cortex makes it useless or superfluous for a substance which the body is supposed to produce itself. The same is true with INSULIN. If too much is given over an extended period of time, the insulin producing cells will begin to degenerate.

◆ *Flaxseed—Linseed Oil*

This is the only oil which contains both LINOLEIC and LINOLENIC ACIDS. They are valuable substances in the formation of prostaglandins.

◆ *Omega-3*

It helps to reduce the body's production of ARACHIDONIC ACID which is to blame for the inflammation of joints and other tissues. It has reduced tissue swelling in arthritis better than prescription drugs such as CORTISONE.

◆ *Eczema Helps The Pain Of Arthritis*

Since arthritis is caused by toxins in the body, and since the eczema symptoms indicate that the skin is acting as an eliminative organ, with the release of the toxins through the skin the arthritis pain is lessened. This also explains why ASTHMA gets better when there is an ECZEMA attack.

◆ *Raw Foods Neutralize An Acid Condition*

✓ POTATO JUICE—If the blood condition of an arthritic is highly acid, the logical conclusion is that this acid must be neutralized so as to eliminate the acid condition. A strict adherence to the natural diet which God gave to Adam and Eve in the Garden of Eden will eliminate this condition. An ALKALINE DIET is called for. One of these alkaline reacting foods is POTATOES raw or cooked. Also raw POTATO JUICE freshly made. Raw potatoes contain sugars which are easy to digest. This therapy has been used as a folk medicine for centuries. It consists of cutting a raw potato into thin slices with the skin on, placing them in a glass of cold water and letting it stand overnight. Drink the water in the morning on an empty stomach. It can be mixed with other juices such as carrot or pineapple juice to make it more palatable.

✓ VEGETABLE BROTH—is a highly alkaline, mineral-packed liquid, a wonder medicine for arthritics. It combats ACIDOSIS, a common condition in arthritis. Other alkaline reacting vegetables are WATERCRESS, CELERY, GARLIC, COMFREY, and ENDIVE. The most beneficial fruits are BANANAS, SOUR CHERRIES, PINEAPPLES, and SOUR APPLES. Good nutrition is much safer than aspirin, the most commonly used arthritis drug.

◆ *Raw Juice Therapy*

Rheumatic diseases are particularly responsive to JUICE THERAPY. The alkaline action of raw juices dissolves the accumulation of deposits around the joints. URIC ACID is dissolved by the juices and thrown into the blood stream. A temporary worsening of the condition may develop under these circumstances, depending upon how fast the purification process proceeds. When poisonous substances are thrown into the blood stream, the patient momentarily feels bad.

✓ BROMELAIN—Pineapple has been shown to have strong ANTI-INFLAMMATORY properties. An extract called BROMELAIN gives arthritics pain relief, and it is even an aid to

WEIGHT LOSS. DR. MATHIEU, a medical researcher, claims that bromelain will melt off 900 times its own weight in fat, and can help you lose as much as 7 lbs. in 2 days. Dr. Foxgord thinks that either pineapple or bromelain tablets will prevent swelling if a wrist or ankle is injured. Bromelain along with vitamins B_1 and B_6 will do an even better job in reducing arthritis pain. Arthritis patients experience near miraculous results when they eat a diet void of processed foods, and rich in natural foods. They usually have a deficiency in vitamins and minerals.

✓ GRAPE DIET—The grape diet consists of eating nothing but grapes for a month. It takes about 3 weeks for one to note a distinct improvement.

✓ BARLEY JUICE—from young barley shoots exerts a natural anti-inflammatory effect upon arthritis. According to a study this juice reduced the symptoms of arthritis in laboratory mice. One arthritic who used it said: "I have never seen or used anything so dynamic."

✓ TURMERIC—a member of the GINGER FAMILY, has shown anti-inflammatory capabilities. It achieves effects similar to the anti-inflammatory drugs HYDROCORTISONE ACETATE and PHENYLBUTAZONE without their serious side effects. Authorities recommend teaspoon of turmeric dissolved in fruit juice taken twice a day. It will also help the pain of CONTUSIONS, SPRAINS, and FRACTURES.

◆ *Royal Jelly*

Royal Jelly has been called "Nature's richest health food," and it has been known to help ease the pain and discomfort of arthritis in some people. It contains all of the AMINO ACIDS essential for human health, as well as 10 vitamins and 6 minerals.

◆ *Vitamin C*

Rheumatic diseases are COLLAGEN diseases, and vitamin C is essential for healthy collagen. These diseases rob the body of vitamin C directly, and the drugs used to combat them, such as CORTISONE also tend to drain the body of vitamin C. Hence, arthritics are usually low in vitamin C, and they must therefore take large amounts of it until the tissues are saturated with it. The excess will be eliminated in the urine. Vitamin C increases the production and utilization of the body's own CORTISONE. If possible the arthritic should EXERCISE so that the body can produce more of its own cortisone. He can exercise IN WATER where the pressure on the joints is greatly reduced. The arthritic should take from 1500 to 3000 mg of vitamin C from sources such as ROSE HIPS, ACEROLA BERRIES, and GREEN PEPPERS. Synthetic vitamin C does not have the same beneficial effect. According to some authorities FRESH GRAPEFRUIT JUICE daily has helped to dissolve the calcium deposits in the joints.

One reason why some arthritics are deficient in vitamin C is because they have been taking ASPIRIN PRODUCTS for pain, and aspirin uses up vitamin C in the system rapidly. When the BIOFLAVONOIDS are given with vitamin C, the response is even better than giving vitamin C only.

Vitamin C strengthens the immune system. A patient was asked by a nutritionist to add 2 tablespoons or about 2000 mg of a vitamin C powder to a fruit drink, and drink it daily. After 7 days he awakened with joint flexibility, and thereafter was free of arthritis pain. Vitamin C prompts the body to produce protective amounts of INTERFERON, a pain-fighting substance that alerts T-cells and B-cells to cast out arthritic-causing enemies from the body. The vitamin C drink also stimulates the production of PROSTAGLANDIN PGE_1, a hormone-like substance that is needed to produce T-cells. Former arthritis patients often state that "A glass of VITAMIN C a day will keep arthritis away."

◆ *Vitamin D*

In Oslo, Norway, researchers have found that RHEUMATOID ARTHRITIS seems to get worse during the winter months. They reasoned that this could be related to a lack of VITAMIN D as related to decreased SUN EXPOSURE. They found that vitamin D levels were significantly below normal in most of 143 arthritic women who were evaluated, even though calcium levels were normal. Most dietary vitamin D comes from fortified dairy products, whose use has been decreasing. The other primary source of vitamin D is the SUN. But with the scare of SKIN CANCER and the use of SUNSCREENS, it has also become a declining source. This "fear of the sun" has done more harm than good. Everyone with rheumatoid arthritis should get at least from 20 to 30 minutes of early morning or late afternoon sun every day without the sunscreen.

◆ *Vitamin E*

It also has the ability to relieve the pain of arthritis. It acts as an antiinflammatory agent.

◆ *Selenium*

Selenium is required for growth in human cells, and it helps protect against SWELLING and HEMORRHAGES. It stimulates the immune system in its work against the development of arthritis through its powerful antioxidant action. As a DETOXIFIER it helps to minimize the effect of toxic chemicals. Selenium is found in GARLIC, BREWERS YEAST, and BROWN RICE. Garlic is the richest source. It also contains the valuable mineral GERMANIUM, which works with selenium to protect against all invaders.

Herbs

✓ ALFALFA—A California man says that his doctor pooh-poohed the idea of ALFALFA as an arthritis treatment. He said "It won't do you any good but probably won't hurt you either." This man's wife had arthritis in her hands and wrists, and she found that the alfalfa tablets eased the pain and allowed her to use her hands again.

Another man reports that he had arthritis in his back for a number of years. He learned of a woman who had cured her arthritis by drinking ALFALFA TEA. He decided to try ALFALFA SEEDS. He ground up 3 tablespoons every day and mixed it with YOGURT or MILK as part of his lunch. This cleared the arthritis in his back.

A lady had suffered for 9 years with RHEUMATOID ARTHRITIS. She lived on ASPIRIN, CORTISONE, INDOCIN, and BUTAZOLIDIN, but not one of these drugs helped her. Then a friend recommended ALFALFA TEA, an ounce of alfalfa seed in hot but not boiling water, a little over half a quart. She simmered it for 30 minutes and drank it 4 or 5 times a day for about 3 months. After that she was able to live a normal life.

✓ CHAPPARRAL—Chaparral is also called CREOSOTE BUSH. It grows in the desert regions of the Southwest. It has ANTIBIOTIC and ANTISEPTIC properties. It also contains an ANTIOXIDANT and an ANTITUMOR AGENT, which makes it an ANTICANCER herb. It is also beneficial for arthritis and rheumatism. One lady took two 7 gm tablets three times a day and became pain free.

✓ ELDERBERRY—The gypsies called it "the healingest tree on earth." Hippocrates listed it among the prominent plants of his materia medica. The American Indians ate the cooked berries, and also prepared them as a drink for RHEUMATISM, SCIATICA, and BACK PAIN. Elderberry juice often banishes the pain of sciatica and neuralgia.

Other herb teas that are beneficial are PEPPERMINT, CHAMOMILE, BARLEY, ALFALFA, ROSEHIPS, and COMFREY.

✓ GINGER—People with arthritis reported significant relief of PAIN after taking less than a tablespoon of ginger every day for 3 months. The arthritis patients took ginger either in 5 grams of ginger root, or from gm to 1 gm of ginger powder. Ginger is now being studied as a possible arthritis medicine.

✓ KELP—Kelp or seaweed is very beneficial for arthritis sufferers. In Japan, where kelp is used extensively as an important part of the daily diet, arthritis is virtually nonexistent.

✓ PEONY AND ANGELICA ROOTS—According to a Japanese study a tea made from peony and angelica roots suppressed all symptoms of arthritis.

✓ YUCCA—Yucca is a plant which thrives in hot, dry climates. It is often called "The Lord's Candle." It contains a high concentration of SAPONINS, which are similar to steroids such as cortisone, and they act as a natural cortisone by REDUCING SWELLING, and ELIMINATING PAIN and JOINT STIFFNESS. The saponins are able to synthesize a natural cortisone that eliminates harmful free radicals. Yucca saponin extracts in tablet form relieve the swelling and pain of arthritis, and also have a beneficial effect on BURSITIS and RHEUMATISM. They also improve digestion and reduce the tendency to accumulate toxic wastes in the colon.

It keeps microorganisms which cause fermentation and toxins under control, and prevents these poisons from entering the bloodstream. It produces beneficial effects without side-effects.

Other Methods That Have Been Found Beneficial

- ✓ BEE STINGS—Bee stings contain two proteins called MELITTIN and APAMIN, which cause the pituitary and adrenal glands to produce more CORTISONE. Such cortisone produced naturally by the body itself does not have the strong side effects of artificial cortisone. It has brought arthritis relief to apiary workers.
- ✓ BLACK MISSION FIGS—The combination of BLACK MISSION FIGS and GOAT'S MILK has been found beneficial for arthritis. It is high in POTASSIUM and it acts as a purge to the intestinal tract, and helps to develop a toxin free body.
- ✓ BROMELAIN—It was demonstrated that the administration of 6–8 tablets a day of BROMELAIN, a pineapple enzyme, helped to reduce or eliminate swelling and inflammation in the soft tissues and the joints.
- ✓ EXERCISE—The SYNOVIAL FLUID is a lubricant that surrounds a joint or bursa and fills a tendon sheath. When you exercise, your metabolism speeds up the manufacture of synovial fluid. When it floods the aching joints, the free radicals are swept up and carried out. Exercise functions as an antioxidant when performed regularly. With exercise the body develops its own CORTISONE which aids in neutralizing calcium deposits. It is better than cortisone injected from without which at times also dissolves part of the bone.

  Doctors used to tell their arthritis patients not to exercise. However, new research shows that aerobic exercise, the kind that give the heart a workout, reduces joint pain. It is needed to keep joints flexible, to restore freedom of movement, improve the circulation, and increase mobility. Good general exercises are WALKING, HIKING, SWIMMING, and BICYCLING. Dr. James Rippe of the University of Massachusetts says that walking is just as beneficial as RUNNING or JOGGING—IT JUST TAKES LONGER. It makes bones stronger, denser, and less subject to bone-thinning OSTEOPOROSIS.
- ✓ FASTING—Studies in Japan have shown that arthritis sufferers placed on vegetable juice fasts, were relieved of many of the symptoms of arthritis. It is said to be one of the most curative measures in the treatment of arthritis. Dr. Shelton presents a case of a 44 year old Canadian lady whose arthritis had crippled her movements. Her physician could promise her nothing but temporary relief with aspirin or cortisone for the rest of her life. She came to the U.S. to undergo a fast. The fast lasted only 3 weeks, but it freed her of all pain and inflammation and restored normal movements to her joints.

  Fasting relieves the pains of arthritis more effectively than drugs, and does it without risk of harm. The fasting itself did nothing, but it provided the best condition for the body to repair itself. That is the purpose of the fast.
- ✓ GOAT'S MILK—Patients have been known to cure themselves of arthritis by drinking one quart of GOAT'S MILK per day. Goat's milk is known to have within it ANTI-ARTHRITIS and ANTI-CANCER factors.
- ✓ HEAT THERAPY—Heat is an excellent way to relieve pain, relax muscles, increase joint mobility, and decrease joint and tissue inflammation. A hot shower or bath in the morning can loosen stiffness which invades joints during sleep. Some people claim that sleeping in a sleeping bag reduces their morning stiffness, but no one is exactly sure why it does so. Heat can be applied by means of BATHS, SHOWERS, HOT PACKS, HOT WATER BOTTLES, HEAT LAMPS, ELECTRIC PADS and BLANKETS, HEATED WATER BEDS, WHIRLPOOLS, HOT SPRINGS, and SAUNAS. MOIST HEAT is usually preferable to dry heat.
- ✓ LOW FAT DIET—Doctors at Wayne State University found that people who followed a low-fat diet remained free of arthritis symptoms.
- ✓ PHENYLALANINE—Phenylalanine, one of the essential amino acids, has given pain relief in arthritis. It is an aspirin without side effects. It is nonaddictive and nontoxic. It is found largely in peanuts and peanut butter. It acts to extend the pain killing ability of naturally produced substances.

- ✓ ROYAL JELLY—Royal jelly, made from a substance that the honey bees produce for the queen bee, seems to help some sufferers of arthritis. It is a substance that contains PANTOTHENIC ACID or vitamin B_5. Some doctors have found it helpful in treating rheumatoid arthritis.
- ✓ VITAMIN B_6—A study at the University of Texas showed that one form of arthritis, namely CARPAL TUNNEL SYNDROME, was due to a deficiency of PYRIDOXINE or vitamin B_6.
- ✓ VITAMIN E—Two doctors in Israel found that vitamin E provided marked relief from pain in osteoarthritis.
- ✓ HONEY—A school teacher had long been afflicted with ARTHRITIS, and had reached the point where she felt that she just had to live with it. She moved to a boarding house where honey was served instead of sugar. Within a short time she found to her amazement, that her arthritis had disappeared.

A Swiss doctor reports the case of a man whose finger was smashed in a grinding machine. The bone at the tip of the finger was broken and hung by a flap of skin. After wrapping the finger in HONEY, the bone grew on and rapidly healed.

Steps To Strengthen The Immune System

- ✓ BREWER'S YEAST—Brewer's yeast is at most a perfect food with niacinamide, minerals, and protein needed to invigorate a sluggish immune system. Studies have shown that while blood cells need vitamin B_6 to produce antibodies, the thymus gland needs B_6 to command its legions of lymphocytes, or T-cells, so they can do their job. With 50 mg of B_6, an entire group of arthritic symptoms would vanish, including swellings.
- ✓ COMPRESSES—HOT AND COLD—Compresses increase sluggish circulation, and they will stimulate MACROPHAGES to destroy invading bacteria.
- ✓ CAFFEINE AVOIDANCE—Caffeine whips up your adrenal glands to send forth hormones that make you sensitive to pain.

  EXERCISE—30 minutes of daily exercise boosts resistance to arthritis and speeds up the healing process.

- ✓ INTERFERON—Interferon is a protein molecule secreted by the T-cells. It helps protect from pain as a natural pain reliever. But when the immune system is weak there is a reduction in the production of interferon, and arthritis pain builds up.
- ✓ VITAMIN B-COMPLEX—Specifically Vitamins B_2, B_6, and pantothenic acid help to produce important antibodies to fight off infectious invaders. Vitamin B_{12} produces T-cells and B-cells that seek out and destroy arthritic infections.
- ✓ VITAMIN C—It greatly enhances PHAGOCYTOSIS.
- ✓ VITAMIN E—Vitamin E enhances the production of both ANTIBODIES and PHAGOCYTES to boost the immune system.
- ✓ ZINC—Zinc is considered to be the most vital mineral for the immune system. Without it many of the lymph system tissues actually shrink including the THYMUS, where the crucial T-cells develop. It works with VITAMIN C to initiate the body's own production of INTERFERON which stops the arthritis virus from multiplying. For this reason zinc has been called a natural virus killer. Food sources are PUMPKIN SEEDS, BREWER'S YEAST, BROWN RICE, WHEAT BRAN, and WHEAT GERM.

ASTHMA

Nature Of The Disease

Asthma is an allergic nervous disorder affecting the breathing apparatus, and it can be brought on by a variety of constitutional causes, the chief of which is disturbance of the function of the digestive organs. It is characterized by intermittent attacks of shortness of breath, due to interference with the free flow of air through the small bronchial tubes. It involves spasms of the bronchial tubes and excessive excretion of a viscous mucus in the lungs that makes breathing difficult.

The stomach, bronchi, and the bronchial tubes are connected by the VAGUS NERVE, and by reflex action digestive disturbance affects the bronchial tubes, so that the passage of air through them is restricted, and an asthmatic attack precipitated. Contributing factors are a catarrhal condition, and a run-down condition of the organism.

Causes Of Asthma

◆ *Low Blood Sugar*

Tests show that asthmatics have a consistently LOW BLOOD SUGAR LEVEL, and have an excessive amount of POTASSIUM in their blood. DIABETICS who have a high blood sugar level, hardly ever have asthma. They become worse when they eat excessive amounts of table salt. Their attacks occur most frequently at night or in the early morning hours when the blood sugar level is at its lowest. Injections of GLUCOSE at this time relieves their attack, because it raises the blood sugar level, but it does not permanently help the asthma. The drugs used for asthma also temporarily normalize the blood, because they all raise the blood sugar level.

◆ *Food Allergy*

According to some doctors, FOOD ALLERGY causes most of the asthmas. Eating and drinking MUCUS-FORMING FOODS such as white bread, dairy products, cheese etc. may greatly contribute to it.

◆ *Intestinal Toxemia*

Some doctors say that most cases of asthma may be attributed to INTESTINAL TOXEMIA. Changing the intestinal flora and normal colon activity will accomplish permanent relief in the majority of cases. It is said that all acute diseases are attempts on the part of nature to rid itself of an overclogged system of toxic matter. What is needed is a thorough internal cleansing of the system.

◆ *Psychic Factors*

It may be due to mental-emotional factors such as the attitude of uncertainty, and an intense need for parental love, attention, and protection.

◆ *Physical Factors*

Some doctors believe that chronic allergy disorders are linked beyond a shadow of a doubt to AIR POLLUTION. It is also thought that ASPIRIN seems to induce asthma.

◆ *Milk*

Milk and milk products, as environmental allergens, can cause ASTHMA. When 22 asthma sufferers were taken off milk, 15 of them showed dramatic improvement.

◆ *Polyunsaturated Fatty Acids (PUFA's)*

PUFA's present in vegetable and nut oils can cause arthritis if they are refined, and do not have enough VITAMIN E in them. Without the vitamin E they can destroy cells including lung tissue. Also red blood cells tend to accumulate in arteries, and reduce or block BLOOD FLOW as well as OXYGEN delivery.

◆ *Monosodium Glutamate (MSG)*

MSG, the flavor enhancer, which is banned in some states and some nations, has been known to bring on an asthma attack.

◆ *Sulfites*

Sulfites, used to keep salad greens fresh and crisp in many salad bars, can also bring on an asthma attack. They are also used on dried fruits.

How Asthma Can Be Overcome

✓ A CLEANSING DIET—Eat plenty of RAW FRUITS and VEGETABLES and their JUICES, such as celery, pineapple, lime, lemon, orange, grapefruit, comfrey, garlic, and horse radish.

A lady who was a victim of childhood asthma was told that her case was hopeless, and that she would have to live with her breathing problem. A naturopathic physician said that an examination showed that her bronchial tubes were covered with long-accumulated glue-like wastes. She was told to go on a 2-day lemon juice fast, drinking up to 8 glasses of a warm lemon juice drink. By the middle of the second day she was able to breathe deeply with comfort, and by the end of the second day she had fully recovered. Thereafter she never again had an asthma attack.

✓ ICELAND MOSS—Iceland moss is a lichen native to the northern countries of Europe, especially Iceland, which is also found in the northern areas of North America. Decoctions or tablets are highly recommended for treating COLDS, HOARSENESS, BRONCHITIS, and EMPHYSEMA.

- ✓ HERBS—Whenever any herbal remedy for respiratory ailments is adopted, other good health practices, such as a proper diet, fresh air, sufficient rest should be maintained, so that a deficient lifestyle does not counteract the herbal treatment. The EPHEDRA plant has proved to be effective in the treatment of asthma and HAY FEVER. CHINESE SKULLCAP has confirmed ANTI-ARTHRITIC and ANTI-INFLAMMATORY actions. LICORICE has ANTI-INFLAMMATORY and ANTI-ALLERGY activities. Eight ounces of MULLEIN tea has cured asthma. It has long been used by herbalists for alleviating UPPER RESPIRATORY problems.

A man had asthma for 30 years. While chatting at a fence with a neighbor, he absentmindedly nibbled on a COMFREY LEAF. It made him feel better, and he had his first night of restful sleep in years. He now eats some comfrey every day and has not suffered from asthma since.

A friend suggested to a man that he drink 8 oz. of MULLEIN TEA daily for his asthma. He slowly began to improve and now feels great drinking mullein tea every day.

- ✓ GARLIC—Garlic is a miracle remedy that can help prevent or heal many respiratory ailments. In 1960 tons of garlic were used in Russia to bring to a halt a massive FLU epidemic. Researchers of Brigham Young University advise that if you feel a sore throat or cold coming on, for you to eat some garlic or onions. If you do it early enough you may not even get sick. Laboratory studies show that garlic extract can destroy human RHINOVIRUS, which causes colds, with almost 100% effectiveness. It kills on contact.

Some have, in a case of WHOOPING COUGH, suggested putting a poultice of garlic in the shoes without letting the garlic touch the skin. The garlic vapors will penetrate the skin and enter the blood stream. In about a minute the garlic can be smelled on the breath. A man's children who were subjected to this treatment laughed at the procedure, at the idea of treating the soles of the feet for a trouble in the chest. This seemed absurd to them. However, the children had a peaceful night, and in the morning the whooping cough was gone and didn't return.

Dr. Benjamin Lau tells the story of two sisters from Singapore who came to the U.S. for their college education. During their stay in Los Angeles they both developed HAY FEVER, with its symptoms of sneezing, nasal discharge, and watery itching eyes. The ANTIHISTAMINES prescribed by their doctor brought some relief but caused unpleasant side effects, including the inability to concentrate. Dr. Lau suggested KYOLIC 102, a garlic formula, of which they took 6 capsules every day. Within three weeks both were free of hay fever symptoms. One of the sisters who remained in Los Angeles takes these capsules whenever the smog becomes heavy. Kyolic 102 is a priceless formula, which is a harmless, odorless alternative to injections and drugs.

- ✓ FASTING—Begin with a fruit or vegetable juice fast of from 3 to 5 days. Then follow it with a restricted diet from 10 to 15 days, including baths, and hot Epsom salt baths. It should thereafter be followed by a natural diet of largely fresh fruits and vegetables.

- ✓ VITAMINS, FRUITS, and VEGETABLES—A New England farmer says that his grandmother used CRANBERRIES to stop his asthmatic wheezing. She mashed and strained them and added some warm water. It opened the bronchial tubes like adrenaline would.

A 4 year old boy was struck with a serious asthma attack which continued for 2 years. It finally turned into PNEUMONIA. His mother read that vitamin E increases the body's ability to utilize oxygen. He received 100 mg of ALPHA TOCOPHEROL daily. The attacks came to an end. Now, 11 years later, he takes 200 mg of vitamin E daily and has had no further problems. MAURICE MESSEQUE, the famous French herbalist, records the case of a Mr. Rauseau, an engineer from Paris, who was suffering from CHRONIC ASTHMA for over 30 years. The prime ingredient that cured him was GARLIC.

- ✓ COLD SHOWERS—Dr. Katsunuma of the National Children's Hospital in Tokyo has found a simple way of preventing asthma attacks in children. He gave each of 25 asthmatic children a cold-water shower every day. 20 buckets of 59° F water was poured over each child during a one minute period. 20 other patients received a similar shower of 86° F water. All in the cold-water group needed less or no medication at all. There was no change in the warm-water group.

CANCER—A DISEASE OF CIVILIZATION

The General Causes Of Cancer

◆ *Civilized People Have More Cancer*

Mr. Tobe of Canada lists the 20 most important causes of CANCER in the order of their importance as follows: a. Chemical additives in food, b. refined and fragmented food, c. Smoking, d. A heavy protein diet, e. Excessive use of dairy products, f. Commercial oils and fats, especially when heated and reheated, g. Diethylstilbestrol, h. Hormones and contraceptive pills and medicines, Hydrogenated oil, j. Refined sugar, k. Nitrates and nitrites, l. Drugs, m. Monosodium glutamate, n. Artificial sweeteners, o. Biopsies and other forms of surgery, p. pollutants, q. X-rays, r. Cosmetics, detergents and soaps, s. Chlorinated, fluoridated, and otherwise contaminated water, t. Aluminum.

✓ HEALTH-DESTROYING LIVING AND EATING HABITS—Prov. 26:2 says: "The curse causeless shall not come." This means that there is never an effect without a cause. This is also true of cancer. We say that cancer is a disease of civilization because it is not found to any great extent outside of civilization. Within civilization, cancer is the end-result of health-destroying living and eating habits, which result in a biochemical imbalance, and physical and chemical irritation of the tissues of the body. SDA's have only one half the overall national colorectal cancer rate, largely because they are vegetarians. They also avoid ALCOHOL, SMOKING, COFFEE, and TEA. Hence, their life expectancy is 7 years longer than that of the average non-SDA.

In 1945 1 out of 15 people died of cancer; in 1971 it was 1 in 6; in 1976 it was 1 in 5; now it is 1 in 4; if the world lasts that long, by 2008 it will be 1 in 3; by 2025 it will be 1 in 2. No known disease can really penetrate the strength of a healthy body. A low protein, low starch, low fat, high enzyme, high vitamin, highly alkaline, and a high mineral diet is the KEY. Anyone can restore health, if he makes the effort, by way of detoxification and the rebuilding of healthy cells so that the body can heal itself.

✓ INDUSTRIAL POLLUTION—The most advanced civilizations have the highest rates of cancer, because the people therein live a more artificial lifestyle, more remote from nature. Such a lifestyle involves more pollutants, and the more pollutants the more cancer is in evidence. Dr. Schneck of Germany says that "it is of the nature and essence of industrial civilization to be toxic in every sense. Poison is its hallmark, poison is its ineradicable brand." Another says that "The food we eat has in a few decades been so altered and contaminated with chemicals, that every mouthful we eat contains some traces of harmful substances."

✓ ADULTERATED AND DENATURED FOODS—It has been determined that the less developed and more primitive a nation, the less cancer there will be. Furthermore, primitive people which abandon the life of their ancestors, and adopt the ways of civilization, do develop a tendency toward cancer. The more civilization has advanced, the farther we have gotten away from a natural diet, and the more our diet consists of ADULTERATED and DENATURED foods. It becomes evident that man cannot stray too far from NATURE without impairing his health.

✓ POLLUTION OF OUR FOOD

◆ *Why Civilization Damages One's Health*

✓ IMPROPER LIVING AND FAULTY DIET—The basic environmental reasons why cancer is hardly found among primitive people is the fact that they are not subjected to DRUGS, X-RAYS, LAXATIVES, SMOG, COOKED FOOD, HOT FOODS or BEVERAGES, COFFEE, TEA, TOBACCO, CHEMICAL ADDITIVES, POLLUTION of our FOOD, AIR, and WATER, and the INGESTION of POISONS from them. The more civilization has advanced, the farther we have come away from a NATURAL DIET. Our present day diet consists largely of adulterated and denatured foods from which the most valuable essential factors have been removed by COLORING, BLEACHING, HEATING, PROCESSING, PRESERVING,

SEPARATION, EXTRACTION, and CHEMICALIZATION. Dr. Kollath says: "Respect for the natural product is an indispensable requirement in the field of nutrition. IMPROPER LIVING and a FAULTY DIET constitutes a lifelong preparation for CANCER."

✓ CANCER DEVELOPS IN THE WEAK SPOTS OF THE BODY—It is in the weak spots of our body that cancer develops. That is why we hear of a blow, as on the breast, or a frost bite, as causing cancer. The underlying tissue is either healthy or unhealthy; it is either cancer-liable or cancer resistant. When man resorts to synthetic remedies, he suppresses chronic disorders and produces disease. He then searches for remedies to cure the effects of remedies used to cure the original disease. For example, X-RAYS, RADIUM, and DRUGS are used to control cancer, but they themselves produce cancer.

✓ CHEMICAL SUBSTANCES, VIRUSES, AND RADIATION—Dr. Boyland said that most cancer in man, probably, is caused by CHEMICAL SUBSTANCES, the remainder being caused by VIRUSES and RADIATION. Drs. Spock and Wheeler have shown that civilized diets lead to poisonous substances in the bowels, and an undesirable intestinal flora. The more ROUGHAGE there is in the diet, the faster waste moves through the bowels, and the less chance there is of developing FREE RADICALS which can cause cancer. Over a 100 years ago, the disease called "cancer" was scarcely known. At that time the products of the soil were consumed just as they came from the land. Food was grown on soil that had been enriched by nature's own fertilizers, its own vegetation. With the introduction of the machine age, food began to be produced for profit, and many chemicals were added to it for purposes of preservation. NATURAL food became ARTIFICIAL so that it would keep longer.

◆ *How Refinement Of Food Affects The Blood*

✓ ELIMINATION OF FOOD SUBSTANCES—Chemicals in food are there for the profit of the food processors. Any service they might render to the consumer is strictly incidental. With the refinement of food, many vitamins, minerals, and enzymes were eliminated, and chemicals were added as preservatives. As a result, upon ingestion of such food, the blood was saturated with foreign matter so that it could not properly carry on the work of keeping the body in a healthful condition. It is well known that a few doses, or even a single dose of a CARCINOGENIC, or cancer causing chemical administered to a young animal can lead to the development of cancer in middle life or in old age. Such a condition is a perfect setup for the initiation of many diseases. Dr. Berglas lists the factors which allow the body's regulatory mechanism to fail as INJURIOUS INDUSTRIAL AGENTS, DENATURED NUTRITION, ARTIFICIAL FERTILIZERS, and the accumulation of INSECTICIDES IN FOODSTUFFS.

✓ POLLUTION OF THE BLOODSTREAM—When it comes to cancer, it has been shown that any tumor can turn into cancer if the blood remains sufficiently polluted for a long enough time. Toxins that are eliminated do not harm anyone. It is when they pile up in the bloodstream that trouble develops. The bloodstream can hold only so much impure matter after which it will deposit it at some point which is a weak point within the body. It develops what are called "rebel cells" which are then nourished from the blood's impurities which allow the cancer to grow.

◆ *Foreign Substances Cause Cancer*

✓ SUBSTANCES NOT ADAPTED TO THE BODY—A wound will often develop a cancer at its location, but the wound is not the cause of the cancer. It is the condition of the blood which allows impurities to be deposited there. Cancer does not overwhelm the body unawares, but rather does it develop from the abuse of the body. We are feeding the blood substances which are foreign to its nature, and which cannot be used to build healthy cells. Cancer can be developed from chemical irritants breathed into the lungs, absorbed through the skin, or taken in the foods we eat. The body's chemistry is unbalanced by the chemicals that enter through these channels.

Substances that are not adapted to the body and are foreign to it do not belong in it, and therefore become a hindrance to its proper functioning. The cells of the body can use nothing which does not conform to their nature. What they can use is substances which cleanse the body by eliminating waste products, maintain its normal functioning, and help to keep it in running order. "Our bodies are built up from the food we eat. There is a constant breaking down of the tissues of the body; every movement of every organ involves waste, and this waste is repaired from our food" (MH295).

The incidence of most cancer is due primarily to the cumulative effect during a lifetime of contact with various carcinogens — not just one cancer causing irritant, but the sum totals of all IRRITANTS which result from the incomplete burning of COAL, MANUFACTURED GASES, OILS, WOODS, TOBACCOS, and all other COMBUSTIBLES.

✓ THE BODY USES NONPOISONOUS ORGANIC SUBSTANCES—All cells are built up from organic substances, those which are compatible with the body's economy. It is largely only organic substances which the body can use. These have been prepared by plants which have the ability to change inorganic substances to organic substances. These organic substances, or plant vegetable matter, must also be nonpoisonous plants which do not act contrary to the body economy. Cancer can strike when the poisonous substances in the body are strong and prolonged, and when the body's defenses are low. Even the body's own METABOLIC WASTES become CARCINOGENS if they are chronically retained. Injecting certain substances into the body may produce cancer, while giving them by mouth may not. Substances which occur naturally may cause cancer when they are used OUT OF CONTEXT in other than NATURAL WAYS.

◆ *Present Methods Of Treating Cancer Themselves Cause Cancer*

The present methods of dealing with cancer have shown no improvement. They may even speed up the cancer since all of the orthodox methods of dealing with cancer, such as RADIATION, CHEMOTHERAPY, and OPERATIONS themselves cause cancer. Dr. Ewan Cameron of Scotland showed that TERMINAL CANCER PATIENTS lived 4 times longer when administered large doses of vitamin C. While doctors realize that a healthy immune system is the body's best defense against cancer, then why is cancer treated with CHEMOTHERAPY, which is injurious to the immune system?

It appears that the treatment for one form of cancer may cause another kind of cancer. Women who undergo CHEMOTHERAPY for OVARIAN CANCER have a higher risk than usual of developing LEUKEMIA later on says a report in the New England Journal of Medicine. Women are most likely to get leukemia 4 to 6 years after completing it, although the risk is still significant even 10 years later.

Dr. Dewey of the University of Michigan observed that in his 45 years of practice he has yet to see a single case of cancer, save a few semi-malignant cells, cured by SURGERY, X-RAYS, or RADIUM. With every facility for early diagnosis by the best experts, and early operations by the best surgeons, the cancer mortality rate among PHYSICIANS and SURGEONS is vastly higher than that among COAL MINERS, FARMERS, AGRICULTURAL LABORERS and many other occupations. Cancer is not the mysterious disease which can be fathomed only by eminent scientists. Cancer results from CHRONIC POISONING OF THE TISSUES of the body during decades. Kuhne proved that cancer is a curable disease, and that it is the final result of SELF-POISONING either from wrong nutrition alone, or from wrong nutrition and the use of drugs.

◆ *Cancer—A Nutritional Disease*

Sir Arbuthnot Lane, England's greatest surgeon, stated: "Cancer is essentially a nutritional disease, a disease of faulty feeding, plus the absorption of poisonous drugs. The foundation of cancer is laid in the kitchen and in the dining room, and women have it in their power to limit its ravages and even to eliminate it altogether." Scientists in Italy showed by interviewing 250 women with BREAST CANCER and 499 similar women without breast cancer, that those women with breast cancer reported higher consumption of WHOLE MILK, HIGH-FAT CHEESE, MEAT and EGGS. Those with the highest intake of SATURATED FAT or animal protein had 2 to 3 times the risk of those on a low-fat diet. With regard to breast cancer we are told that a woman who delivers her first child after the age of 35 has a 3-fold higher risk of developing breast cancer than a woman who bears her first child before the age of 18. Also if a woman has had an ABORTION in the first trimester of the first pregnancy, whether spontaneous or induced, she is 2 times more likely to develop BREAST CANCER. There is also an increased risk of breast cancer in those who are using ORAL CONTRACEPTIVES.

Some researchers estimate that 90% of all cancers are caused by ENVIRONMENTAL FACTORS. One of these factors is DIET, which some believe cause 30 to 60% of all human cancers.

Enzymes And Cancer

In the CANNING OF FOOD enzymes must be stopped in their tracts in any type of food preservation, because they bring food to maturity and will continue past that point to overripeness if they are not inactivated. In CANNING enzymes are permanently destroyed by heat at any point above 122 degrees Fahrenheit. Hence, a diet consisting exclusively of canned food is deficient in enzymes. Some years ago a woman doctor experimented with feeding canned food to mice and rats, and found them susceptible to cancer. Those animals fed on natural food were not found susceptible to cancer.

Vitamin C is destroyed by heating at low temperatures for long periods of time. Canned foods are sure to have lost of their vitamin C value. Several researchers have found that there is a pronounced vitamin C deficiency in the blood of cancer patients. It has been found that GUINEA PIGS suffering from SCURVY and given just enough vitamin C to stay alive are far more susceptible to cancer and get it sooner than healthy guinea pigs.

Reduced Respiration Of The Cells

Dr. R.A. Holman, a Welsh physician, believes that the answer to the cause of cancer lies in the RESPIRATION OF THE CELLS. When OXYGEN combines with some substances HYDROGEN PEROXIDE is produced, and it is a poison to living tissue. The enzyme CATALASE, which is an essential component of almost every cell, has the function of combining with hydrogen peroxide causing it to change to WATER and OXYGEN.

If more hydrogen peroxide is developed or not enough catalase available, permanent changes will take place which may result in cancer. Investigators have confirmed the theory by showing that those parts of the digestive tract where there is a smaller amount of catalase a higher incidence of cancer is found.

The Eating Of Meat And Cancer

◆ *Meat Eating And The Spirit Of Prophecy*

When man was created, he was created as a vegetarian and not as a meat eater. This can be seen by his physiological makeup, the type of teeth and colon that he has. For this reason we are told that "Flesh was never the best food; but its use is now doubly objectionable, since disease in animals is so rapidly increasing" (CD384). Among the various races of men, the CANCER INCIDENCE is highest among the meat eating people of the world. Highest of all is one section of Australia where per capita consumption of meat is the highest in the world. When we eat meat we take into our system the POISONS that are IN THE BLOOD of the animal. Also some of the processes of fattening animals for the market produce disease. It is in an excited state that the animals are killed and those who eat such meat are subject to many kinds of diseases. Science tells us that a carcinogen called MALONDIADEHYDE is formed immediately after an animal is slaughtered. It is also formed during the decomposition of polyunsaturated oils. But VITAMINS C and E, which are natural antioxidants, stop the breakdown.

Many naturopathic doctors believe that a FAULTY DIET is the basic cause of cancer. They believe from studies around the world, that the cancer incidence is in direct proportion to the amount of animal proteins in the diet. Hospital records show that the SDA's, MORMONS, and NAVAJO INDIANS, who eat little or no meat, suffer far less from cancer than the average meat eating Americans. Dr. Visek of Cornell University says that the high protein diet of Americans is linked to a high incidence of cancer. The villain according to Dr. Visek is AMMONIA, the carcinogenic by-product of meat-digestion. We are told that "the LIABILITY TO TAKE DISEASE is increased TEN FOLD by MEAT EATING" (CD386). In this connection

Dr. Robert A. Good, immunologist from the university of Minnesota, found that RATS and MICE are TEN times less likely to develop breast and blood cancers when he limited their protein intake. He found that chronic PROTEIN LIMITATION increases resistance TENFOLD.

Disease is transferred to those who eat the meat that contains disease. The quality of the blood is depreciated, and creates in the person acute attacks of disease and even sudden death. "Many die of diseases wholly due to meat eating" (CD391). As a result we are told that "CANCERS, TUMORS, and all INFLAMMATORY DISEASES are largely caused by meat eating. People are continually eating flesh that is filled with tuberculosis and cancerous germs. TUBERCULOSIS, CANCER, and other FATAL DISEASES are thus communicated" (CD388). As a result of understanding these facts we are told that "Among those who are waiting for the Lord, MEAT EATING will eventually be done away" (CD380). "The flesh of animals will no longer compose a part of our diet; and we shall look upon a butcher's shop with disgust" (CD407).

◆ *Why Meat Eating Causes Cancer*

Flesh food does not contain any fiber. Hence, such food causes cancer because it stays too long in the colon, and rots before elimination, and the putrefying residue is absorbed into the bloodstream from the colon, thereby poisoning the whole system. One of the waste products of meat digestion is AMMONIA, which is harmful to man. It destroys cells thus increasing cell turnover, and the chances that cells will become cancerous. Dr. Visek says that ammonia increases virus infections, and that VIRUSES are known to cause cancer in animals, and that they are suspected of doing the same in man. He says that in the U.S. intestinal cancer tends to increase as the amount of ammonia produced in digestion increases. We are also told that with a HIGH BEEF DIET the level of fecal BILE ACIDS is raised, and such a diet also increases the number of anaerobic bacteria called CLOSTRIDIA, which convert bile acids into CARCINOGENS.

According to Dr. J.H. Kellogg, INDOLE is a very destructive poison originating in the colon from the bacterial decomposition of TRYPTOPHAN, a constituent of protein which is especially abundant in the protein of animal flesh, that is, of LEAN BEEF, MUTTON, FOWL, FISH, OYSTERS and EGGS.

Dr. Robert Bell wrote: "The flesh of dead animals, when entering into the dietary, not only undergoes the most offensive form of decomposition, but gives rise to the most noxious TOXINS. It also favors the retention of these in the colon, and so favors their absorption." It also causes CONSTIPATION.

◆ *Cancer Among Meat Eating People*

Dr. H.M. Shelton says that cancers are found almost wholly among meat eating animals and people. Cancer never develops in healthy tissue. In tissues there is always more PRECANCER than cancer. If you CUT OUT the cancer, the precancer will develop into cancer if the lifestyle is not changed. Dr. B. Lust says that it is the excess ANIMAL ALBUMEN STUFFS such as meat, eggs, milk, and cheese, that produce terrible poisons during their decomposition. M.O. Garten, a naturopath, says: "Meat wears out the intestinal tract and kidneys prematurely by increasing the ACIDITY of the BLOOD, and by the accumulation of TOXINS in the tissues. High meat consumption favors the HARDENING OF VESSELS, HEART FAILURE, STROKE, KIDNEY DISEASE, and CANCER.

◆ *Overindulgence In Proteins Develops Tumors And Cancers*

Dr. Joseph Issels of Germany, considered to be the foremost cancer specialist in the world, said: "Excessive eating of meat and cholesterol rich foods not only contributes to ATHEROSCLEROSIS and consequent impaired BLOOD CIRCULATION and DIMINISHED OXYGENATION of cells, but also increases the risk of TUMOR DEVELOPMENT. Animal as well as human studies show that limiting the use of meat and ANIMAL FATS, including BUTTER, will diminish the risk of cancer." Americans eat more protein than any other people in the world. We also lead the world in cancer statistics. Most leading cancer researchers and nutritionally oriented doctors are convinced that OVERINDULGENCE in PROTEINS is one of the prime causes of cancer. Dr. McCollum of John Hopkins University discovered that he could induce CANCER and NEPHRITIS, or BRIGHT'S

DISEASE, in rats only on a high protein diet.

Dr. Good of the University of Minnesota found that rats and mice are 10 times less likely to develop experimental BREAST and BLOOD cancers when he limited their protein intake. According to Drs. LOPAGE and MIDLER, a high protein diet can cause blood and cells to become too richly supplied with protein. When this occurs, and the burden becomes too great for the body to handle, tumors are formed which are sealed off in order to protect the rest of the body from their contents. These tumors are therefore PROTEIN TRAPS.

VEGETARIANISM retards physical and sexual maturation. The average age of puberty in China is 17. In the U.S. it is 12. Animal protein produces fast maturation rates. It is the STEROIDS in animal protein which accelerate the growth rates.

Salt As A Cause Of Cancer

◆ *Excess Salt Produces Excess Hydrochloric Acid*

Most therapists agree that SALT is too freely used in the ordinary diet, and that it is suspected of playing a part in the cause of cancer. For this reason the diet of cancer patients is usually SALT-FREE. It is claimed that salt is often responsible for excessive HYDROCHLORIC ACID in the stomach which burns and injures the tissues, and gives rise to STOMACH ULCERS which may develop into cancer. Mrs. White says: "Do not eat largely of salt, avoid the use of pickles and spiced foods, eat an abundance of fruit, and the irritation that calls for so much drink at mealtime will largely disappear" (CD311). Dr. Froude wrote: "Salt is irritating and poisonous when taken to excess." Mr. Marwood made these observations, He said: "I have personally investigated over 100 cancer deaths, and in every instance excepting one, I have found that the victims have been abnormally fond of salt and SALTED FOODS, or had taken aperient (laxative) salts, which contain a proportion of salt, daily for many years."

◆ *The Average Person Takes In Too Much Salt*

The average person consumes about 12 gm of salt daily, when the recommended amount is only about 2 gm. This is 6 times as much salt as is necessary. Dr. Daws experimented with two groups of cats. He placed a small amount of salt in the milk of one group and none in the milk of the other group. A certain percent of the salt-group developed cancer, but the non-salt group developed no cancer. F.T. Marwood, a layman, made the interesting observation that in Denmark, where the consumption of SALTED FISH is the highest in Europe, the cancer rate is also the highest in Europe. Denmark has the second highest rate of stomach cancer, while Japan has the highest rate. They also eat a lot of salted fish, as well as using a lot of MONOSODIUM GLUTAMATE which is a SODIUM SALT.

◆ *Salt Overstimulates The Cells*

SALT, being an inorganic chemical and not a food, is dangerous in excess of need. It harms the body tissues, for it is a powerful STIMULANT TO CELL METABOLISM. Dr. Henry Sherman says that by overstimulating the digestive tract, salt may interfere with the ABSORPTION and UTILIZATION of FOOD. He says that an excess amount of salt may disturb the OSMOTIC PRESSURE of the tissues involving almost every portion of the body. Excess salt also causes EDEMA, a collection of water in the tissues. Every gram of salt binds 70 gm of water. The bad effects of this accumulated fluid may be seen as the cause of many diseases.

◆ *A Deficiency In Hydrochloric Acid (HCL)*

A deficiency of HCL can cause improper digestion as well as the loss of vitamins and minerals. Under these circumstances it is suggested that about 5 minutes before you eat, that you open a GOLDEN SEAL capsule and empty it into a little warm water and drink it. This will coat your stomach and help your body to make HYDROCHLORIC ACID.

Toxins Cause Cancer

◆ *A Toxic State Precedes Cancer*

Professor Boyland says: "Most cancer in man, probably, is caused by CHEMICAL SUBSTANCES the remainder being caused by VIRUSES and RADIATION. The most glaring examples of environmental pollution are EXCESSIVE SMOKING, ATMOSPHERIC POLLUTION, INDUSTRIAL CARCINOGENS, and FOOD ADDITIVES." Inorganic chemicals, including DRUGS, cannot be utilized by the human body. Unless the body finds a relatively fast way of eliminating them, they settle in the tissues and often injure the delicate cell structures, and become the source of cancer development. Cancer can develop from chemical irritants, breathed into the lungs, absorbed through the skin, or taken in the foods we eat. Through them the body's chemistry is unbalanced. Cancer is not generally of local or accidental origin, but it is constitutional. It may be caused by the gradual accumulation in the system of certain toxins which develop in decaying matter.

◆ *The Bloodstream Is Overloaded With Toxins*

The poisons are generated by certain germs in regions of the body where SCARS, MUSCLE SPASMS, or INJURIES prevent an adequate circulation of the blood, and where the body is therefore devoid of sufficient OXYGEN. Many hygienic experts have proven that cancer is a condition in which the bloodstream is overloaded with toxins. They have cured cancer by cleaning these toxins out. Dr. Bulkley says that the TOXINS produced by millions of microorganisms generated through INTESTINAL STASIS and FECAL PUTREFACTION is a real incidental cause of cancer. The reason why orthodox medicine cannot cure cancer is that its textbooks say that cancer is caused by a bug, which medical science has failed to discover over many centuries of trying. The MEDICAL PROFESSION has further handicapped itself by following its leaders in opposing successful natural methods which from their standpoint would do away with the huge profits from the use of RADIUM, X-RAYS, DRUGS, and OPERATIONS.

◆ *Medicine's Search For A Poison*

The search of medicine is for a poison that will poison cancer cells without injuring the normal cells of the body. It is looking for a poison that will kill germs without killing the patient. In the nature of things, a poison that will kill cancer cells will kill other cells also. It is an accepted fact that any drug that is powerful enough to kill cancer cells will also kill healthy cells. Many CANCER DRUGS have been proven to be themselves POSITIVE CAUSES OF CANCER."

◆ *Drugs And Cancer*

Many commonly used drugs are considered by many researchers to be possible carcinogens. The drugging system endeavors to make the sick well by administering poisons which make the well sick. The proper method, however, is the one which restores the sick to health by means which will also keep healthy persons well, or well persons healthy. The God-given nonpoisonous products of the earth can do this. Drug medication adds to the causes of cancer, by taking away the ACUTE SYMPTOMS of disease and changing them into CHRONIC DISEASE CONDITIONS. Persons who use drugs that inhibit the IMMUNE SYSTEM are many times as likely to develop cancer as persons not using drugs. The immune system can prevent cancer formation if it is in a healthy state. To attempt to cure cancer by adding to its causes is IRRATIONAL, and has no orderly relationship to maintaining the life of the patient. An axiom laid down by the medical profession is, "THERE IS NO HARMLESS DRUG."

When toxic drugs are poured into the bodies of dying cancer patients, the lowered immune system is decimated, and the victim falls prey to many other diseases, such as PNEUMONIA and HEART DISEASE, which are then given as the cause of death. By this means, the cancer statistics are improved. One school of thought is considering CANCER as a preventable metabolic disease. They have proven to their own satisfaction that cancer is a CHRONIC, SYSTEMIC, METABOLIC IMBALANCE. Deficiencies cause cells to malfunction and to neutralize normal body defenses. Dr. Pauling reports that a study indicates that BLADDER CANCER in cigar smokers often regresses if the patient takes 1000 mg of vitamin C or more daily. Certain cancers such as COLON, LUNG, MELANOMA, PANCREATIC, and STOMACH cancer do not respond to CHEMOTHERAPY.

◆ *Chemicals And Cancer*

✓ SODIUM FLUORIDE—According to Dr. Alfred Taylor of the University of Texas, even SODIUM FLUORIDE in fluoridated water, is linked to cancer growth.

✓ PESTICIDES—Many pesticides are carcinogens, such as DDT, which many countries in Europe have banned. In California it is still permitted on ALFALFA SEED CROPS, ONIONS, CITRUS FRUIT, and PEPPERS. Our AIR, our WATER, and our FOOD contain thousands of manmade chemicals, most of which are potential carcinogens. Any chemical preservative or additive will destroy ENZYMES.

- ✓ IMMUNOSUPPRESSANT DRUGS—It has been determined that kidney and heart TRANSPLANT patients, have to have their immune systems suppressed with IMMUNOSUPPRESSANT drugs, so that the donated organs will not be rejected by the body. These patients will develop CANCER 80 times more readily than the normal population.
- ✓ CYCLAMATES AND SACCHARIN—Artificial sweeteners can cause cancer in the stomach and other digestive organs. SACCHARIN has caused cancer of the BLADDER and UTERUS in animals.
- ✓ HEXACHLOROPHENE—As a BACTERICIDAL and BACTERIOSTATIC compound, it has caused cancer in the brain.
- ✓ AUTO EXHAUSTS—They contain three compounds closely linked to cancer. They are: BENZOPYRENE, ALDEHYDES, and HYDROCARBONS. Benzopyrene is also generated by TOBACCO SMOKE, as well as by POWER and INDUSTRIAL PLANTS. Cooks have one of the highest rates of cancer from benzopyrene due to the inhalation of the fumes and vapors of heated oils.
- ✓ CHLORINATED AND FLUORIDATED WATER—There is an association between RECTUM, COLON, and BLADDER cancer and CHLORINATED WATER. It is caused by cancer-producing chemicals formed by the action of chlorine on organic substances naturally present in surface water. WELL WATER lacks these substances. An EPA report showed a correlation between drinking chlorinated water and a higher risk of developing cancer. This is due to the destruction of VITAMIN E in the system. Most cases of cancer could be prevented, if the practice of putting harmful chemicals in our food was prohibited. Many chemical preservatives are CUMULATIVE, and they all destroy ENZYMES and beneficial body MICROORGANISMS. FOODS that do not contain their own enzymes, such as cooked foods, contribute to the destruction of the human organism.

A University of Texas researcher fed SODIUM FLUORIDE, the fluoride that is added to drinking water, to mice. His initial conclusion was that sodium fluoride definitely accelerates growth of breast cancer in female mice.

Acidity And Cancer

◆ *Acidity Brings Pain*

Alexis Carrol, a French scientist, kept a chicken heart alive for 28 years in an alkaline solution. In doing so he said that he had to make sure of two things: giving it the proper nutrition, and getting rid of waste products. Our body cells are surrounded by fluids which should be slightly alkaline in order to sustain life. Heavy exercise produces shortness of breath, tiredness, and muscle stiffness as a result of the accumulation of LACTIC ACID in the muscles resulting from the incomplete combustion of glucose. The body wasn't getting enough oxygen in order to metabolize the glucose. This produces a slightly ACID CONDITION OF THE BLOOD which manifests itself in proneness to catching a COLD etc. When the fluids become more acidic, manifestations of pain such as HEADACHES, CHEST PAIN, and STOMACH PAIN are felt. If an even greater acidic condition is developed, excess acid substances are deposited in some part of the body, so as to allow the blood to recoup an alkaline condition. ACIDOSIS is at the root of most of our bodily ailments. It is caused by the use of COOKED FOODS, MEAT, STARCH, WHITE BREAD and WHITE SUGAR.

◆ *Overconsumption Of Fats Causes Malignant Cells*

Some cells will die under these conditions, but others, instead of dying, adjust themselves to these conditions, and become ABNORMAL cells or MALIGNANT cells, or OXYGEN DEPRIVED cells for which no more external oxygen is required. They continue to exist through the process of FERMENTATION. One most common way of causing an acidic condition is by means of the overconsumption of fats. Fat clogs the arteries or capillaries and stops the supply of oxygen by stopping the nutrients from going through. This causes the death of cells at the end of the clogged capillaries, and the dead cells then turn into an acid substance. The acid debris accumulates to the point where resistance is broken down, and the body becomes susceptible to GERMS, FATIGUE, COLDS, and NERVE EXHAUSTION.

◆ *Acidity can cause Leukemia*

Dr. George W. Crile says: "There is no natural death. All deaths from so-called natural causes are merely the endpoint of progressive ACID SATURATION." Mary Hogle says: "Acidosis precedes and provokes disease." Acidity in the blood also causes an increase of WHITE BLOOD CELLS, and a decrease of RED BLOOD CELLS, which is the beginning of LEUKEMIA. Also acidity in the extracellular fluid kills nerve cells, and acidity in the intracellular fluid damages cell nuclei which control cellular growth. It has been determined that blood is more acid when it enters a malignant area than when it leaves such an area. This indicates that cancer cells thrive in an acid bloodstream. Under these conditions all acid foods, such as FATTY FOODS, PROTEIN RICH FOODS, and REFINED FOODS should be eliminated from the diet.

Aluminum And Cancer

Dr. Keens of London, England, has come to the conclusion that aluminum cooking utensils play an important role as a cause of cancer. It becomes toxic to organic tissues only when rendered soluble through interaction with certain elements and compounds. SODA, SULFUR, AND AMMONIA seem to have the property of bringing aluminum out of its normal compounds and rendering it free and soluble to interact with other elements to form compounds of a toxic nature. Aluminum cookware is positively known to contribute to the following conditions: ULCERS in the MOUTH, SPASMS of the ESOPHAGUS, STOMACH DISORDERS, GASTRIC ULCERS, and ULCERATIVE COLITIS, Many of these conditions can and do wind up as cancer.

Dr. Tomlinson tells us: "I have been a medical man for forty years, and I can state, without a shadow of a doubt, that the use of aluminum in the preparation of food and food products is one of the most harmful factors in modern civilization." In his book on aluminum Dr. Holder gives no less than 100 references indicting aluminum as a cause of disease, and states that aluminum compounds are classified as PROTOPLASMIC POISONS.

Lack Of Cell Oxygenation As The Basic Cause Of Cancer

◆ *A Lack Of Oxygen Causes Fermentation*

Cancer cells are ANAEROBIC, which means that they are able to function and thrive in an OXYGEN-FREE environment. Normal cells require oxygen in order to function properly. Unless there is sufficient energy generated within the cell through the oxidation process, the cell is forced into an ANAEROBIC METABOLISM, which is metabolism without oxygen. Whenever the cell is deprived of oxygen, it changes its mechanism from a process of oxidation to one of FERMENTATION. Fermentation is a process which needs no external oxygen. It thereby changes a normal cell to a cancerous cell, caused by the continuous deficiency of oxygen. Dr. Putney also explains the high incidence of cancer in the human race on the basis of poor or DIMINISHED OXYGEN CONSUMPTION. Oxygen is essential for the removal and destruction of many toxic agents in our cells. Other destroyers of the enzyme CATALASE, which is present in almost all cells, are the various forms of SULFUR in our air, AUTO EXHAUST, CIGARETTE and CIGAR SMOKE, and also the AEROSOL HAIR SPRAYS. The LIVER, where there is more catalase than in any other part of the body, is rarely the site of primary tumors among people who have adequate diets.

◆ *Poisonous Substances Keep Oxygen From The Cell*

Dr. Warburg of Germany, who twice received the Nobel Prize for his work in physiology, said that a LACK OF OXYGEN IS THE CAUSE OF CANCER. He said that he could make any cell cancerous by withholding oxygen from it. He then reversed the process and in turn destroyed the cancer cell with oxygen. He said that oxygen was replaced by an energy-yielding mechanism known as GLYCOSIS, which is the fermentation of GLUCOSE in the absence of oxygen. He adds that the cause of insufficient oxidation is MINERAL SHORTAGE in the vital fluids, and that in order to obtain normal oxidation the vital fluids must be normalized. Any CHEMICAL, DRUG, or VIRUS which has the ability to keep oxygen from the cell has the ability to make it cancerous. The WHITE BLOOD CELLS responsible for fighting infection and unwelcome microorganisms in the body, make hydrogen peroxide and use it to oxidize these organisms. The bubbling which occurs when hydrogen peroxide comes in contact with a wound indicates that oxygen is being released and bacteria are being destroyed. That is why HYDROGEN PEROXIDE, OZONE, and other OXYGEN THERAPIES have been effective in the treatment of cancer. Cancer cells cannot thrive in an adequately oxygenated environment.

The stools of persons in the U.S. and Great Britain, where the incidence of COLON CANCER is very high, have much higher counts of anaerobic bacteria, or non-oxygen using bacteria, than people in Uganda or South India, where the incidence of the disease is low. Dietary animal fat increases the number of ANAEROBIC BACTERIA, which produce carcinogens. Vegetarians have generally a high count of AEROBIC BACTERIA.

◆ *Cancer—A Type Of Yeast Growth.*

ANAEROBIC METABOLISM is synonymous with YEAST METABOLISM. This means that cancer is a type of yeast growth. Any body chemistry that supports yeast growth is also a likely candidate for the development of cancer. Yeast cells are unable to thrive in an oxygen environment. The POTASSIUM levels in the body are a good indication of the rate of oxygenation of the cells. This is the reason why Dr. Gerson had such great success in curing cancer with high potassium foods.

Cancer—A Deficiency Disease

◆ *Lack of Vitamins And Minerals Can Produce Cancer*

One author states that cancer should be considered a deficiency disease, for only by approaching it from that angle can we hope to conquer it. It can then be prevented and controlled by a suitable and BALANCED DIET, high in VITAMIN CONTENT.

Experimentation has determined that even a mild deficiency of CHOLINE will produce LIVER CANCER. Choline is a vitamin B-complex vitamin which is essential to the proper functioning of the liver. A VITAMIN E deficiency increases the risk of contracting cancer and leukemia. An IODINE deficient diet has resulted in THYROID cancer. Deficiencies of various B-VITAMINS result in liver damage which leads to various MALIGNANCIES. Serious deficiencies of ZINC may lead to cancer of the PROSTATE. VITAMIN A deficiencies break down the body's defenses against most carcinogens, and lead to TUMOR development. MAGNESIUM deficiency is also linked to cancer development. Dr. Forbes Ross showed that cancer is due to POTASSIUM deficiency, and that it improves when potassium is administered. He says that potassium is the salt of the TISSUES, and that sodium is the salt of the FLUIDS of the body. Examination of the botanical world indicates that potassium is also the salt of the chemical physiology of the VEGETABLE CELL. A malignant tumor will form where there is a deficiency of the pancreatic enzyme CHYMOTRYPSIN to digest food proteins. Since nutritional deficiencies are so widespread, they must constitute a large causative factor in cancer development.

It is known that cancer cells withdraw certain vital elements from the cells, namely POTASSIUM, CARBON, and others. Hence, in all forms of suspected cancer, the deficient elements have to be supplied in concentrated form. Among these IODINE, IRON, MAGNESIUM, and MANGANESE are essential, but of most importance is manganese.

◆ *Canned Food Can Produce Susceptibility To Cancer*

Vitamin C is destroyed by heat. In fact it has achieved a reputation for being the most destructive vitamin. Canned foods are heated in processing, and heated again before being served. By this time they have lost almost of their original vitamin C value. As a result researchers have found a pronounced vitamin C deficiency in the blood of cancer patients as compared to that of healthy persons. It has been found that GUINEA PIGS, who cannot produce their own vitamin C, who are suffering from SCURVY and given just enough vitamin C to keep them alive, are more susceptible to cancer and get it sooner than healthy guinea pigs.

ENZYMES are also destroyed by heat, such as in canning, at any point above 122 degrees Fahrenheit. Some years ago a woman doctor in Chicago experimented with feeding CANNED FOODS to mice and rats. As a result she found them susceptible to cancer. Those fed on natural food were not.

Heat, Fats, And Cancer

◆ *Heated Oil Can Cause Cancer*

It has been said that no food is ever nutritionally improved by heating. The best VEGETABLE OILS, when heated to a high temperature, 350 degrees or more, become CARCINOGENIC. Heated fats or oils are especially suspected of causing BREAST CANCER in women. Foods prepared in deep fat fryers, such as POTATO CHIPS, DOUGHNUTS, FRITTERS, FISH, and the PIES, CAKES, and PASTRIES must all be considered to be CARCINOGENIC FOODS. When VEGETABLE OIL is heated to any great degree, the fat molecule is broken down and changed into an entirely different chemical. In most cases this changed chemical cannot be absorbed through the digestive and metabolic processes. As a result superheated fats and oils act as irritants in the body, and become carcinogenic agents. SESAME OIL which had been heated to 350 degrees, caused cancer in laboratory animals. Non-vegetable oils do not usually change their chemistry at these cooking temperatures. This, however, should not be a reason for using them, for they contains lots of cholesterol. The basic principle should be not to heat vegetable fats. Such heated fats are what Mrs. White refers to as GREASE.

◆ *High Fat Diets Can Cause Cancer*

High fat diets have been shown to increase the incidence of BREAST, PROSTATE, lining of the UTERUS, and COLON cancer. There are population studies which show that people with high MEAT intake have higher incidences of cancer, which may be due to the intake of FAT, PROTEIN, lack of FIBER, or a combination of all of these factors. The Bible admonishes us not to eat flesh with the BLOOD (Gen. 9:4). It also tells us that of the flesh the FAT should not be eaten (Lev. 3:17; 7:23), so that we must assume that health reasons are implied in these directions.

The best foods get RANCID the quickest. This is particularly true in regard to natural, unprocessed, so-called health foods, such as WHEAT GERM, WHEAT GERM OIL, SUNFLOWER SEEDS, SESAME SEEDS, and WHOLE WHEAT FLOUR. They must be eaten absolutely fresh. The oxygen in the air makes these foods rancid very quickly. Rancidity develops harmful chemical substances, such as PEROXIDES.

BREAST, COLON, and PROSTATE cancers are rare where diets are low in fat. The reason is that to digest fat, the body produces substances called BILE ACIDS, which seem to encourage the growth of cancer. The less fat you eat the less bile acids are produced. Unlike complex carbohydrates, fat is easy to overeat because it does not contain stomach-filling bulk.

Fats that are exposed to intense heat will combine with proteins to form BENZOPYRENES, which are known CARCINOGENS. They are also found in cigarette smoke.

◆ *Heated Fats Neutralize Vitamin A.*

Experiments with local applications of heated fats have shown tumors to develop at the site of the application. COTTON SEED OIL heated to 220 degrees did not produce any cancerous tumors. This led to the conclusion that the dangers in fats vary in proportion to the heat applied. Even vegetable fats, once they are heated, may be causing cancer. In fact, polyunsaturated vegetable fats, from the standpoint of heat, are more dangerous than saturated fats, because they change their chemistry more than saturated fats. Many fats when heated develop an anti-vitamin A factor which destroys the biological activity of vitamin A.

◆ *High Heat Destroys Essential Vitamins*

In high heats the vitamins A, E, and K are utterly destroyed. In an experiment with rats, they were fed lard heated to 350 degrees and then cooled along with their rations. While the rats had normal offspring through 7 generations, with the heated lard it was necessary to feed the rats WHEAT GERM OIL and FRESH VEGETABLES before mating, because of the deficiencies in vitamins A and E caused by the heated fat. Beatrice Hunter says: "The essential fatty acids (EFA) are destroyed or changed into abnormal toxic fatty acid which are antagonistic to EFA. Such synthetic fat forms new molecular structures which makes it unacceptable to the human physiology."

Enzymes are destroyed at temperatures above 120 degrees Fahrenheit. 75% of the enzyme content of the average diet has been destroyed by heat. Hence, it goes as a corollary that the cooking process lowers the quality of food by also destroying vitamins and minerals to varying degrees.

◆ *Pasteurization Destroys Vitamins A And C*

Most reheated fats develop an anti-vitamin A factor which destroys part of the vitamin A activity of foods eaten at the same time. Much of the American diet consists of fried and deep-fried foods. The people who eat these foods seem to continually suffer from a deficiency, and such a deficiency is definitely known to be a factor in cancer. Even the low application of heat used in the PASTEURIZATION OF MILK will destroy much or most of the vitamins A and C. It has been proven that while CALCIUM is not lost in the presence of heat, it is nevertheless rendered less assimilable. Pasteurization reduces the proper utilization of the calcium in milk.

In a study of SDA's who drank 2 glasses of MILK a day, it was found that they had nearly double the risk of PROSTATE CANCER compared to those who drank only one glass. 3 glasses of milk a day raised the risk by 2 times. The main culprit in milk appears to be the fat. But there was no risk to drinking SKIM MILK.

◆ *Processed Fats*

Dr. Johanna Budwig, called Germany's premier biochemist, preaches against the use of what she calls "pseudo" or false fats. In order to extend the shelf life of their products, manufacturers use chemical processes that render their food products harmful to the body. These harmful fats go by a number of names including "hydrogenated," "partially hydrogenated," and artificial "polyunsaturated" fats. She says that the chemical processing of fats destroys the vital electron cloud within the fat. Once these electrons have been removed, these fats can no longer bind with oxygen, so that they often end up as fatty deposits on the heart muscle, and as carcinogens. They therefore end up blocking circulation, damaging heart action, inhibiting cell renewal, and impeding the free flow of blood and lymph fluids. To function efficiently cells require true polyunsaturated or monounsaturated, electron-rich fats that are present in natural oils, and especially in LINSEED or FLAXSEED oil.

◆ *Scorched Foods Can Cause Cancer*

Dr. John Weisburger in his research found that the BROWNING OF FOODS produces cancer-causing chemicals. The microwave oven, however, uses a cooking method which does not involve browning. TARS have been positively proven to be carcinogens. They are formed by high heat in any organic compound subjected to heat over a period of time. BREAD, POTATOES, SUGARS, CEREALS, and other foods which are TOASTED, ROASTED, BAKED, FRIED, or otherwise SCORCHED by heat until dark brown or black on the outside usually contain tar. COFFEE SUBSTITUTES derive most of their flavor from the TARS which form on the cereal grains when roasted. If you stick your nose into a jar of POSTUM, it will smell like tar. It is best to leave such drinks alone.

◆ *The Cooking Of Food*

In the cooking of food, both vitamins and minerals are destroyed in varying degrees by the heat of cooking. The same applies to milk where pasteurization will destroy most of the vitamins A and C. CALCIUM, while not lost in the presence of heat is rendered less assimilable by heat.

Hormones And Cancer

◆ *DES As A Cause Of Cancer*

Around 1940 it was brought to the attention of the scientific world that both men and women were suffering from hormonal deficiencies. Since medical researchers frequently try to circumvent nature, instead of correcting the diet of the affected individuals, they researched for drugs to correct the imbalance. They found the synthetic hormone DIETHYLSTILBESTROL, commonly known as DES. DES turned out to be one of the worst CANCER-CAUSING SUBSTANCES known. We know today that DES prescribed for pregnant women during the late 40's and 50's produced VAGINAL and other cancers in thousands of young women born of those mothers who had taken DES on their doctors advice. It was given to prevent MISCAR-

RIAGES. Later they found that those offspring were high VAGINAL cancer risks, which heretofore had almost never occurred in a young woman.

◆ *DES Is Toxic To Experimental Animals*

When millers refine the bran and the germ out of the wheat, they also refine out the essential MALE and FEMALE HORMONES of the wheat. Seven women whose mothers all took DES developed VAGINAL CANCER. Quantities of DES as small as 2 parts per billion are toxic in the diets of experimental mice. It can also cause LEUKEMIA and CYSTS in animal organs. In human beings it has produced BREAST CANCER, FIBROID TUMORS, STERILITY and IMPOTENCE in men, and ARRESTED GROWTH in children.

Dr. Rosalind Alfinslater of the University of California states that women who are taking the PILL should increase their vitamin intake or run the risk of becoming ANEMIC. They particularly need vitamin B_2. It appears that according to the best authorities on the subject more than 50 dangerous side-effects can result from taking BIRTH CONTROL pills. Dr. Royertz of the National Institute of Health said that long use of sex hormone drugs carries the danger of gradually inducing cancer of the BREAST, CERVIX, UTERUS, BLOOD CLOTS, DIABETES, and ARTERIOSCLEROSIS. Dr. Lewison finds that women over 45 who are on ESTROGEN THERAPY of some type are twice as likely to get breast cancer as those of the same age and marital status who do not take hormones. It is thought that ESTROGEN REPLACEMENT THERAPY (ERT) may increase the risk of BREAST CANCER, VAGINAL BLEEDING, LIVER DISEASE, HBP, and active THROMBOPHLEBITIS. On the other hand, estrogen therapy is said to prevent OSTEOPOROSIS, to ward off HEART DISEASE, and to raise HDL cholesterol and lower LDL cholesterol. Dr. Ratner has described the PILL as the most dangerous drug for use by the healthy in respect to lethality and major complications.

◆ *Hormones Included In Some Common Treatments*

It is virtually impossible to escape the ingestion of DES if one eats MEAT, POULTRY, takes DRUGS, uses the PILL, takes treatment for PROSTATE TROUBLE, for PREGNANCY, FEMININE HORMONAL DISORDERS, or MENOPAUSAL PROBLEMS. Meat as a part of the diet is suspect enough as a cause of cancer without the addition of DES. BREAST CANCER is 4 times as common in women who have used ORAL CONTRACEPTIVES for at least 6 years before they had reached the age of 25. This is especially true if the contraceptives contained large amounts of synthetic hormones known as PROGESTOGENS. SYNTHETIC ESTROGENS are a prime contributor to leukemia and cancer. Substances which occur naturally may cause cancer when they are used out of context, that is, in other than natural ways. When estrogen from an animal was injected into a human being, it became a carcinogen.

Monosodium Glutamate—MSG

◆ *MSG May Produce Stomach Cancer*

The food industries were no doubt happy when the flavor enhancer MONOSODIUM GLUTAMATE (MSG) was developed. Take note of the fact that it also contains a SODIUM atom. It has been said of it that it makes even the worst type of food taste good. MSG is the L-FORM OF GLUTAMIC ACID and is produced by the hydrolysis of vegetable proteins. It is added to a variety of foods to enhance their flavor. The Japanese hold two world records 1. the highest consumption per capita of MSG, and 2. males have the highest incidence of stomach cancer in the world and Japanese females have the second highest, and there is a strong indication that the second is caused by the first. Their stomach cancer rate is 7 times higher than that of the U.S. The Japanese use a lot of MSG in their food. There is always a shaker of MSG at hand in every Japanese restaurant, and they sprinkle it generously over practically all foods.

◆ *It Causes Various Diseases*

Evidence reveals that MSG contributes to BRAIN LESIONS, RETINAL DAMAGE, STERILITY, OBESITY, STUNTED GROWTH, FATTY LIVERS, EYE PROBLEMS, KIDNEY, BLADDER, SPINAL, PROSTATE, and PELVIC ABNORMALITIES, and that it is toxic to the CENTRAL NERVOUS SYSTEM. IN 1969 Worthington Foods expressed the company's stand on

MSG as follows: "MSG is a nutritional substance which possesses a certain flavor enhancing ability. It has been used for centuries in the Orient without deleterious effect. MSG occurs in substantial quantities in most proteins. It is a natural substance produced by natural processes. At present there is no scientific evidence indicating a need to limit the use of MSG in the adult diet. Because of political and emotional factors, Worthington Foods removed MSG from its food formulations." Actually, MSG is a processed product. It is the sodium salt of GLUTAMIC ACID which is a natural product, for it is actually metabolized in the brain. Apparently however, the brain doesn't seem to like the processed product. Any so-called food that requires chemical enhancing should not be called a food. We should use HERBS to improve flavor if needed.

◆ *It Makes Foods Taste Better*

The Chinese also use a lot of MSG. Some years ago the medical profession discovered a disturbance referred to as "Chinese Restaurant Syndrome." MSG was indicted as the guilty substance. It causes a dizziness when foods containing it are eaten. It makes even the most tasteless foods taste delicious. Glutamic acid is a NATURAL AMINO ACID. Since MSG is a chemical modification of a natural substance, it itself is not a natural substance. Researcher Tobe claims that it is not even a nutritional substance, and that its flavor enhancing quality comes from its ability to irritate and aggravate the taste buds to make you think the food tastes better.

Nitrates And Nitrites

◆ *They Prevent Botulism*

The nitrates and nitrites are added to many meat products as preventatives of BOTULISM. They also impart a pinkish color to all meats. Without them meats would be a dull grey-brown color, which is the true natural color of cooked meat. The nitrites also impart a SPECIAL FLAVOR. They also disguise and cover up RANCIDITY and INHIBIT BACTERIAL ACTION. They KILL ALL BACTERIA and MICROORGANISMS, but are NOT SELECTIVE. When the food is eaten, they start killing the body's microorganisms, good and bad. Therein lies the danger of preservatives. Since meat itself causes cancer, these substances add to the possibilities of getting cancer from meat eating.

◆ *They Produce The Carcinogen Nitrosamine*

While the nitrates in meat act as preventatives to botulism, they also tend to contribute to producing CANCER of the STOMACH through a chemical reaction, by combining with the AMINES in the stomach to produce NITROSAMINES which have been shown to be CARCINOGENS. They have been found to produce tumors in a wide range of organs and in every species of animal upon which they have been tested. Foods prepared by salt-curing or smoking should be avoided, for they give rise to nitrosamines.

◆ *Vitamin C Neutralizes Nitrosamines*

Nitrates and nitrites can also enter the body in DRINKING WATER which has been contaminated by agricultural nitrate-containing chemical FERTILIZERS. Some years ago the state of Minnesota Health Department reported 139 cases of INFANT POISONING in 2 years from nitrate salts contained in well water used in the babies formula. These salts got into the water from drainage of nitrate fertilizers which had been applied to the surrounding land. There were 14 deaths attributed to the poison. Dr. Mirvish of the University of Nebraska determined that VITAMIN C aids in neutralizing the formation of nitrosamine in the stomach.

Overeating And Cancer

◆ *Overweight Persons Have A greater Tendency Toward Cancer*

Most experts will agree that OBESITY is one of the main causes of the so-called degenerative diseases such as ARTHRITIS, DIABETES, CANCER, and HEART DISEASE. Obese people tend to have higher blood cholesterol and triglycerides, hence, they have a higher risk of coronary heart disease. Triglycerides are little known blood fats that are transported through the vascular system even more so than cholesterol. These waste-forming substances enter the body because of having ingested refined carbohydrates such as sugar and starches, or by having taken in hard animal source fats. They help to clog the arteries. The hard fats leave a thick sludge right on the MITOCHONDRIA within the cells, and the cells will be unable to receive enough OXYGEN to burn foodstuffs completely to energy-producing carbon dioxide and water. Metropolitan life statistics show that the prevalence of these diseases among the overweight is far greater than among those of normal weight. According to a study an older person had a 2-fold higher risk of death if he was only MODERATELY OVERWEIGHT. According to Dr. Issels, animal studies show that the animals which are allowed to eat as much as they wanted had 5.3 times more spontaneous cancer tumors than those animals who fasted every second day. The risk of BREAST CANCER increases 40% for every extra 1000 gm of FAT we eat a month. Scientists estimate that 35% of cancer deaths are caused by BAD DIET, 30% by SMOKING, 2% by a POLLUTED ENVIRONMENT, and 1% by FOOD ADDITIVES. This means that 68% of all cancer deaths are caused by things we do to ourselves.

The hunger years during and immediately after both World Wars resulted in a virtual disappearance of cancer, as well as most of the other degenerative diseases. When food rationing was abandoned, cancer statistics soared right back to the pre-war level. The National Cancer Institute acknowledges the relationship between overeating and cancer when it says, "There is statistical evidence from various insurance companies that overweight persons have a distinctly greater tendency for developing CANCER."

◆ *A Restricted Diet Prevents Cancer*

In an experiment on overeating, two groups of mice were kept on the same diet, but one group was allowed to eat all they wanted, which turned out to be about 3 gm a day. The other group was allowed only 2 gm per day.

The restricted mice had no cancerous growths. Of the unrestricted group, over half developed cancer after 90 weeks. NO TUMORS HAVE BEEN FOUND THAT DO NOT RESPOND TO A RESTRICTED DIET. One group of mice given 3.2 gm of food daily developed cancer growths in 54%, while another group given 2.3 gm developed cancer in 22%, and a third group given only 2 gm of food developed no tumors at all.

◆ *Excess Weight Hurts The Heart Most*

The overweight population of the U.S. dies from heart disease at three times the underweight population, and at twice the rate of those of normal weight. A person who is 30% overweight at age 45 can expect to die in 12 years. A 45 year old of normal weight has another 25 years of life. In men and women with a 40% or more than normal weight, the women were found to have a 55% greater risk, and the men a 33% greater risk of cancer than those of normal weight. Excess weight is a killer, and no part of the body is hurt more than the HEART.

Sunshine And Cancer

◆ *Skin Cancer Has A Low Mortality Rate*

It has been exclusively established by numerous studies that excessive and continuous exposure to the sun's ultraviolet rays can cause cancer of the skin in some people. Rimless eyeglasses, which concentrate the sun's reflections are particularly dangerous, and are responsible for many cases of cancer on the face. 85% of ultraviolet rays can penetrate the mist on overcast days. SKIN CANCER is more common among men than among women, simply because men work and take their recreation out of doors to a much greater extent than do women. Those who tan easily have plenty of pigment cells or MELANIN, the protective pigment that prevents burning. One out of every 3 new cancers are skin cancers. Some of them are MALIGNANT MELANOMA Skin cancer has a low mortality rate, and it is 95% curable.

◆ *Vitamins C And E Protect Against Skin Cancer*

Drs. Black and Low, two Texas researchers found that after skin is exposed to ultraviolet light, cholesterol in the skin oxidizes and forms by-products. One of the by-products of this oxidation process is CHOLESTEROL ALPHA-OXIDE, which is a known cancer-causing chemical. It was also found that the way to neutralize this carcinogen is with ANTIOXIDANTS such as VITAMINS C and E. The taking of these vitamins was found to increase their presence in the skin, and that as the antioxidant volume in the skin increased, the formation of cholesterol alpha-oxide decreased. This study shows that when supplemental antioxidants are consumed, they do get to the skin, and they do act as a deterrent to the formation of a carcinogen induced by ultraviolet light. Vitamins C and E have also been shown to have an effect on slowing and preventing CATARACTS.

◆ *PABA Is A Good Sunburn Lotion*

One of the most effective suntan lotions is the B-vitamin PARA-AMINOBENZOIC ACID or PABA for short. A 5% solution of PABA in alcohol is a highly effective lotion against sunburn. British researchers found that a preparation of 25,000 IU of vitamin A and 120 mg of CALCIUM CARBONATE in tablet form taken orally, is very useful in preventing sunburn. This calcium carbonate is in the form found in BONE MEAL supplements.

◆ *Vitamin D And Calcium Protect Against Cancer*

It has been shown that people who live in sunny climates and eat sufficient calcium have less cancer because they obtain more vitamin D through sunlight. People in the north of the U.S. have more cancer than people in the sunbelt. Outdoor workers such as lifeguards and farmers have no more skin cancer than indoor workers because the outdoor worker has a long period of gradually increasing exposure, while indoor workers may get a heavy dose in a short time. Hence, exposure to the sun should be built gradually. One report says that getting more vitamin D may help people living in areas of high air pollution avoid cancers of the breast and colon. Lower levels of vitamin D are linked to a five-fold increased risk of COLON CANCER and a doubled risk of BREAST CANCER.

◆ *Some Chemicals Create Photosensitive Skin*

There are many drugs and chemicals which are known as PHOTOSENSITIZING AGENTS. Among these agents are ANTIHISTAMINES, ANTIBIOTICS, DIURETICS, and ANTIDIABETIC DRUGS. These can increase our sensitivity to the sun to the extent where exposure that would normally cause only the slightest redness will produce a fiery agony. In addition photosensitization can be produced by antibacterial SOAPS, and a number of COSMETICS and lotions.

Sugar, Tars, And Cancer

◆ *Burnt Substances Are Carcinogenic*

TARS have been positively proven to be carcinogens. These tars are created by high heat. They form in any organic compound which is subjected to great heat a sufficient period of time. BREAD, POTATOES, EGGS, MEAT, SUGARS, COFFEE, CEREALS, and other foods which are TOASTED, ROASTED, BAKED, FRIED, or otherwise SCORCHED by heat until dark brown or black on the outside, usually contain tars.

COFFEE DRINKING may be related to cancer of the lower urinary tract, including the bladder. These rates are high in persons who drink more than 3 cups a day. CAFFEINE can cause DAMAGE TO GENETIC MATERIAL BY ALTERING THE DNA. It can act as a TERATOGEN, a substance which causes abnormal structures in an embryo resulting in a severely deformed fetus. Excessive coffee consumption by pregnant mothers can lead to LOWER INFANT BIRTH WEIGHT, ABORTION, PREMATURE BIRTH, and HEART DISEASE. One study indicated that coffee drinkers are more likely to develop BLADDER CANCER than abstainers.

Experiments have shown that COAL TAR, and coal tar products are known to be CARCINOGENIC AGENTS. COAL TAR DYES are used to produce artificial coloring substances, but they are still allowed to be used in FOODS, SOFT DRINKS, COSMETICS, MEDICINES etc. These agents act as irritants to body tissues and therefore can produce cancer. 90% of the vitamins sold in the drug stores, which are not natural, are made from coal tar. If ASPIRIN, which is a coal tar product, is applied to a raw place on a rabbit's ear, in six months time a cancer will develop at that spot

In 1938 Dakizawa, a researcher, created carcinoma in a mouse by prolonged subcutaneous injections of strong SUGAR SOLUTIONS. Nonaka, another researcher, produced carcinoma in rats after repeated injections of GLUCOSE solutions. It is not hard to understand that sugar is a POWERFUL CARCINOGEN, because it has been clearly established by reliable researchers that all BURNT SUBSTANCES are carcinogenic.

◆ Tumors Thrive On Sugar

In the making of sugar, sugar cane is boiled until it is pitch black, a charred sticky mass. Then with a host of chemical processes, dyes, and bleaches, this mass is turned into lily white sugar. Lalorde says that certain statistics seem to indicate that the increase of malignant tumors is in relation to the increased intake of sugar and other processed carbohydrates. Warburg has established that GLUCOSE is an excellent factor in the growth of malignancy. He indicates that from 100cc of blood, cancer borrows 70 mg of glucose, whereas only 2 to 16 mg is necessary for normal tissues. This indicates that cancerous tissues require lots of glucose to favor the growth of cancerous tumors.

Dr. Otto Meyerhoff of University of Pennsylvania and 1923 Nobel Laureate stated that possibly the growth of cancerous tissue might be stopped if biochemists could find a safe way to curb the appetite of TUMORS for sugar. Dr. Melvin Page of Florida said that he did not remember a single case of cancer who had a correct sugar level, yet in most non-cancer cases this is easily obtained by means of a sugar-free diet alone. He then describes a case of SKIN CANCER of the face which cleared up entirely within a few months when the patient gave up drinking daily 12 bottles of a widely distributed soft drink.

◆ Sugar Gives Us Only Calories

We must not lose sight of the fact that sugar contributes absolutely nothing to human nutrition but calories and harm. It is devoid of PROTEINS, VITAMINS, and MINERALS. It is an established scientific fact that in no way does the body require manufactured sugar in any form. Naturopaths say that commercial sugar is representative of the ultimate extreme in food degeneration. Merely to state that it is a starvation food is putting it mildly. That to call it a food is a misnomer. They would rather call it a habit-forming drug, and consider it to be the most injurious product in our national dietary with no exceptions and under every possible condition. Let us use a healthful, unrefined, natural sweet such as HONEY instead of sugar.

◆ Other Carcinogenic Compounds And Substances

✓ COAL TAR PRODUCTS—Practically all foods that have BLEACHING, PICKLING, PRESERVING, or other ARTIFICIAL INGREDIENTS added to them contain carcinogenic agents. MECHANICAL, PHYSICAL, or CHEMICAL IRRITATION can cause cancer, such as the smoker's pipe or the Taylor's needle, ill-fitting dentures, irritation of warts. SMOG which contains carcinogenic chemicals such as CARBON MONOXIDE, NITROGEN DIOXIDE, and other PHOTOCHEMICAL pollutants cause many health disorders, including CANCER of the LUNGS and RESPIRATORY ORGANS. SODIUM FLUORIDE, the fluorine put in drinking water, accelerates the growth of mammary or BREAST CANCER in female mice. 98% of all COLD REMEDIES, 90% of all COUGH SYRUPS, LAXATIVES, ALKALIZERS, are made from COAL TAR. HAIR DYES are made from coal tar products. The dye will be absorbed through the skin and thereby cause cancer. MINERAL OIL is made from coal tar. It produces RECTAL CANCER.

✓ POLLUTED AIR—The Sloan Kettering Institute For Cancer Research developed a machine that breathed in air from a down town New York street corner for six weeks. The TARS were collected and painted on the backs of MICE. 90% of the mice developed SKIN CANCER. LUNG CANCER among males went up 1900% from 1914 to 1950. This increase was reported to correspond exactly with the increase in gasoline consumption in the U.S. during those same years. It was also noted that lung cancer in males went down 35% from 1941–5, when gasoline consumption was reduced by exactly the same percentage because of World War II gas rationing. Gasoline vapor can cause cancer.

✓ ALLERGENS FROM KEEPING BIRDS IN THE HOUSE—Dutch researchers have discovered that people who keep BIRDS have almost 7 times more risk of developing LUNG CANCER than those who do not keep birds in the house. They think that it is because people with pet birds inhale large amounts of ALLERGENS and DUST particles which affect their lungs. Cancer and CANCER THERAPY are very stressful to the body, and those very stresses promote cancer growth.

Smallpox Vaccinations And Cancer

◆ *Mrs. White Was Vaccinated*

The Spirit of Prophecy doesn't have much to say about the process of vaccination because Mrs. White wasn't given any light on this subject. In the footnote of 2SM303, D.E. Robinson, for many years one of Mrs. White's secretaries, tells us that Mrs. White herself WAS VACCINATED when there was an epidemic of SMALLPOX, and that she urged her helpers to be vaccinated. Vaccination is a communal health measure, one which a governmental unit initiates on the basis of its responsibility to the community to keep from having an epidemic of disease, in this case smallpox, from breaking out. It seems to be a proper project where one cannot make the single individual take care of his own health, and where through transfer of an individual disease the community is in danger of acquiring such a disease from a single individual who unfortunately has acquired it. From the individual standpoint vaccination represents the pollution of the bloodstream with vaccines and serums as foreign substances which the body endeavors to eliminate as quickly as possible.

◆ *Mrs. White Would Enter Into Acceptable Communal Projects*

In the case of Mrs. White we must remember that she would go along with any worthy community project which did not interfere with her religion, and for which she had not been given any light to the contrary. On the other hand there are facts which have come to light regarding vaccination which tend toward a negative view of it. First of all, the SMALLPOX VACCINE is a standardized preparation of the living virus of VACCINIA, which is used to immunize against smallpox. As a living virus product it represents a foreign poisonous substance which as such does not belong in the body. It is no longer used since it is assumed that the disease of smallpox has been eradicated.

◆ *Vaccination As A Cause Of Cancer*

While vaccination was in vogue, some contemporary doctors had much to say about it. Dr. Robert Bell, a British cancer specialist said: "The chief if not the sole cause of the monstrous increase in cancer has been vaccinations." He said this because most INJECTIONS, SERUMS, TOXINS, INOCULATIONS, and VACCINATIONS add poisonous substances to the blood. It is always true that a TOXIC STATE exists before the cancer growth appears. Dr. W.B. Clark of Indianapolis said: "Cancer was practically unknown until cowpox vaccination began to be introduced. I have had to do with at least 200 cases of cancer, and I never saw a case of cancer in an unvaccinated person."

Dr. E.J. Post of Berlmont, Michigan said: "I have removed cancers from vaccinated arms exactly where the poison was applied." Dr. M. Laitie, former medical director of the Metropolitan Cancer Hospital of London said: "I am thoroughly convinced that persistent vaccination is an important contributing cause of cancer increase." Dr. Millard, President of the National League for the Prevention of Spinal Curvature said: "Abolish vaccination and you cut the cancer death rate in half." Dr. Glen Sawyer, president of the Canadian Cancer Society said: "It is startling to know that more children between the ages of 5 and 19 die of cancer than from the combined diseases of INFANTILE PARALYSIS, SCARLET FEVER, TYPHOID, and DIARRHEA, the ages when most school children are vaccinated."

Authorities on IRIDOLOGY, or eye diagnosis, claim that the eyes show signs of poisoning of the blood and glands immediately after vaccination. The whole process of vaccination seems to have been another example of giving a present assumed benefit for a future harm.

Emotions And Cancer

◆ *Happy People Have Less Cancer*

More and more valid research seems to indicate that personality traits play an important part in cancer development. J. Rodale claimed that "Happy people don't get cancer." Many researchers came up with similar findings that certain types of people, people with a lowered ability to deal with severe emotional stress and conflicts, are more predisposed to succumb to cancer. At a psychiatric meeting it was determined that "stress" merely meant "life." Human beings cannot live without stress. We must adjust ourselves to stressful situations, and if we remain healthy, they will not harm us. Dr. Kissen of the Southern General Hospital of Glasgow found that LUNG CANCER patients tended to have poor emotional outlets. People who had poor life situations and who DEPRESSED their feelings were more vulnerable to lung cancer than those who had good emotional outlets. An English research Council proved an earlier Swedish investigation that WOMEN who develop cancer are usually more EXTROVERTED, or OUTGOING in personality.

◆ *Emotional Control Produces Less Cancer*

A study of a group of 24 cancer patients by Bahnson and Bahnson showed that cancer patients very definitely show a massive denial of all that can be embarrassing or is viewed as socially undesirable. They were found to be socially conformists to such a degree, that even the mildest personality manifestation which they thought other people might frown upon, was unequivocally denied. They all had experienced a very close attachment to a parent or parent substitute early in life.

By the thirteenth century European physicians were noting that severe EMOTIONAL SHOCK, such as the DEATH of a LOVED ONE, contributed to a large extent to the onset and development of cancer. Cutter remarked that MENTAL DEPRESSION is often an element in cancer that is overlooked. He believes that the disease can be cured by diet combined with stimulating the patient's will to live. So we see that the cancer prone personality has feelings of ALIENATION, HOSTILITY, HOPELESSNESS, LACK of FOCUS or OBJECTIVE, that might be translated by the single word—DEPRESSION. It was found that depression doubles the risk of death from cancer.

Research has shown that cancer patients generally show a rise in CORTISOL, a hormone that depresses the immune system, a few months before they die. As long as the patient believes that there is hope, his cortisol production stays low. When he gives up hope, his cortisol production rises, his immune system is depressed, the cancer rages out of control and is soon followed by the death of the patient. When Dr. Pauling gave cancer patients vitamin C in large quantities, he also gave them hope, and as a result they kept on living much longer.

◆ *Cancer Caused By Low Bodily Resistance*

People with uncontrolled anxieties and worries, with low ability to deal with emotional problems, conflicts and stresses, with feelings of LONELINESS, INADEQUACY, HOPELESSNESS, and DESPERATION, who are generally unhappy, ARE MORE PREDISPOSED TO SUCCUMB TO CANCER, because such conditions increase the biochemical vulnerability and sets the stage for cancer growth. Hence, the ultimate cause of cancer is lowered resistance of the body's own defense mechanism against physical, chemical, emotional, and environmental stresses. Stress invites disease by assaulting the defenses of your immune system. It suggests that there is some link between disease and certain emotional states. Cancer is less likely to strike HAPPY PEOPLE. Louis Kuhne, who cured cancer by natural methods, maintained and proved that he could cure all diseases including cancer—but he was careful to add that he could not cure all patients.

A study by Dr. Le Shan found that the highest cancer rate was found among those who are WIDOWED, with the next highest rate among the DIVORCED, the lowest rate among SINGLE PEOPLE, with the married in between. RURAL FOLK had less cancer than CITY PEOPLE. Are Waerland of Sweden said: "We do not deal with diseases — only with mistakes in our way of living. Eliminate the mistakes, and diseases will disappear of their own accord."

◆ *Norman Cousin's Recovery From Cancer*

Norman Cousins in his recovery from cancer demonstrated the power of LAUGHTER to restore a person to health. He said that he had learned never to underestimate the capacity of the human mind and body to regenerate even when the prospects are most unfavorable. He took himself out of the hospital and OFF MEDICATION, and initiated his SELF-TREATMENT by taking large doses of VITAMIN C. He had a TERMINAL COLLAGEN DISEASE. After reading Hans Selye's *Stress Of Life,* he reasoned that if NEGATIVE EMOTIONS had a negative effect on the body, then POSITIVE EMOTIONS must have a positive effect. He watched funny movies and was read to from humorous books. He noticed that ten minutes of hearty laughter would leave him pain free for at least 2 hours and would allow him to sleep. He suffered from pain for over a year, but his pain eventually disappeared, and he made a full recovery.

There must be psychological reinforcement. The patient must believe in the power of the natural defense system, and must have faith that the natural bodily forces with God's help can cure him. ENKEPHALIN, another type of ENDORPHIN, increases the number of active T-lymphocytes that aggressively seek out and destroy cancer cells.

Radiation And Cancer

◆ *Diagnostic Radiation causes Cancer Also*

It has been scientifically proven that not only excessive X-RAYS, but even the kind that are used PROPHILACTICALLY or DIAGNOSTICALLY BY DOCTORS, DENTISTS, and CHIROPRACTORS, can cause CANCER and LEUKEMIA. Leukemia in children in later years is often caused by PRENATAL abdominal x-rays received by the mother during pregnancy. In every cancerous individual there is always more precancer. No radiation can ever hope to eliminate all of the precancer. Even if radiation could destroy all of the precancer, it could not restore health. It could not remove the causes of the precancer. It could not prevent the development of more precancer and finally of cancer.

◆ *Cancer Is Accepted As Being Incurable*

In radiation burns, the worst results are delayed, and death may occur many years later. One after another the pioneers of medical radiation have died of cancer caused by radiation burns, received as long as 20 to 40 years before. Madam Curie died of cancer at age 67. Her daughter, Irene Joliet-Curie died of cancer at age 59, all due to their work with radium. Radium will not cure cancer. It only destroys cancer tissue within a certain radius, but does not drive the disease from the blood. Medical doctors say: "Operations, radium, x-rays, and drugs are the recognized treatments for cancer." But they do not add that medicine also holds that cancer is INCURABLE.

RADIATION agents are most successful with superficial growths such as skin cancers. Mrs. White had some black spots on her forehead eliminated by means of x-rays, for which she was very thankful (2SM303). These were blemishes on the skin, which have a 95% success rate, and were not tumors in the deeper parts of her body.

◆ *Radioactive Fallout*

Such radioactive fallout substances as STRONTIUM 90 and IODINE 131, as a result of atomic tests and bomb explosions, are after many years still present on this earth. They cause LEUKEMIA, BONE CANCER and THYROID CANCER. They find their way into the human body through the food we eat, particularly through milk from the grass the cows eat.

Age And Cancer

It used to be that cancer was called a disease of the aged, of degeneration due to time. This is no longer the case, for the statistics of the Metropolitan Life Insurance Company have shown in recent years that the leading fatal disease in the 1 to 14 age group has been CANCER. It is said that LEUKEMIA claims approximately half of the total cancer mortality under age 15. This may to a large extent be true due to the past RADIATION of the FETUS of the mother during pregnancy. Cancer usually takes up to 20 years to develop from a healthy radiated cell.

Types Of Cancer

◆ *Bladder Cancer*

Dr. Lau of Loma Linda University cured BLADDER CANCER in a mouse with PARVUM VACCINE and GARLIC. Garlic is effective against INFECTIOUS MICROORGANISMS, PREVENTS OXIDATION of FATTY ACIDS, STOPS FREE RADICAL FORMATION, PROTECTS AGAINST HEAVY METALS, and BOOSTS the PRODUCTION of T-CELLS.

◆ *Breast Cancer*

✓ BREAST-FEEDING LOWERS INCIDENCE OF BREAST CANCER—It is known that breast-feeding mothers have a much lower incidence of BREAST CANCER than those mothers who do not breast-feed. Hormonal activity stimulated by the infant's sucking could promote the HEALTH of the mammary gland. Furthermore, nature provides a four day supply of a special fluid, COLOSTRUM, to get the newborn infant off to a good start. If the mother decides not to breast—feed her baby, her body is stuck with all that stockpile of colostrum. The baby does not get it, and the breast is not called upon to function as nature intended.

✓ NO TREATMENT AT ALL IS AS GOOD OR BETTER THAN TREATMENT—Careful consideration of all the evidence seems to indicate that if women with breast cancer do absolutely nothing from the time that they discover that they have breast cancer, their LIFE SPAN will be as long or longer than that of those who undergo radiation treatment or surgery. It has been shown that if the young of a cancer immune strain of mice are nursed by a female of a high cancer strain, they will develop cancer. When female mice of a cancer susceptible strain were sterilized, none developed cancer with the injection of a carcinogenic agent.

Human breast cancer is associated with a HIGH FAT DIET, particularly of animal fat. Among SDA's breast cancer mortality is to of the breast cancer mortality rate of the U.S. population in general. It has been shown that foods such as FRIED POTATOES, HARD FAT, ALL FRIED FOODS, SOME DAIRY PRODUCTS, and WHITE BREAD, are associated with breast cancer. All except white bread represent dietary fat.

✓ ESSENTIAL UNSATURATED FATTY ACIDS DEFICIENCY—One of the causes of breast cancer may be a deficiency of the ESSENTIAL UNSATURATED FATTY ACIDS or EUFA. These are found in abundance in all SEEDS such as WHEAT, BARLEY, RYE, OATS, FLAX, SESAME, MILLET, CORN, and RICE. It is in these EUFA that nature stores the hormones that the body needs for the prevention of cancer and other diseases, but they have been refined or MILLED OUT OF OUR FOODS such as BREADS or CEREALS. Breast cancer is 5 to 6 times higher in North America and Northern Europe than it is in most of Asia and Africa. Hence, it seems to be largely a disease of civilization.

✓ INCIDENCE OF BREAST CANCER—The highest breast cancer incidence is said to be in the GOITER BELTS. In the U.S. it is in the level of the Great Lakes States from New England to Washington. On the other hand, Japan and Iceland boost the world's lowest rates of goiter and breast cancer because of their IODINE-RICH environment. The mineral SELENIUM seems to have the same good effect. Selenium added to the drinking water of MICE susceptible to breast cancer, dropped the incidence of breast cancer from 82% to 10%. Women that have been VEGETARIANS most of their lives have the lowest rates of breast cancer.

✓ BREAST CANCER AND MILK—It is possible but not proven as yet, that a cancer-producing virus in COW's MILK may be passed along to humans who consume milk. Virus particles that can cause cancer have been found in human milk. In addition, one is exposed to the hormone DES in milk because it is used as a growth promoter in cattle. Furthermore, a high fat diet produces large amounts of STEROL CHEMICALS and BILE ACIDS in the intestines. Bacteria can alter these chemicals so as to produce certain carcinogenic ESTROGENS affecting the breast. Most strongly linked to increased rates of breast cancer were DAIRY PRODUCTS such as high-fat CHEESE and WHOLE MILK. Ranked just below dairy products were ANIMAL FATS and MEATS.

✓ HEATED FATS AND BREAST CANCER—HEATED POLYUNSATURATED FATS enhance breast cancer development by increasing the hormone called PROLACTIN. The woman who delivers her first child after the age of 35 has a 3-fold higher risk for breast cancer than a woman who bears her first child before the age of 18. A study of over 10,000 women worldwide showed a consistent relationship between high intake of saturated fat and higher breast cancer risk for postmenopausal women. Also a higher intake of VITAMIN C brought a lower breast cancer risk for all women.

✓ RELATIVES OF BREAST CANCER PATIENTS—There is evidence to indicate that the daughters and sisters of breast cancer patients are 2 to 3 times more likely to develop the disease than women not related to breast cancer patients. One out of every 14 women will develop the disease in her lifetime. There has been no change in the mortality rates in 50 years.

✓ ESTROGEN—Research indicates that long-term estrogen users had a 10% increase in breast cancer risk, and the risk jumped to 70% after 9 years of use. ESTRADIOL, a potent form of estrogen, was the most commonly prescribed, and it was a higher risk factor for breast cancer than ESTRIOLS, a less potent form of estrogen. Estrogen has a cancer-causing effect because it stimulates the growth of cells of the breast and UTERINE LINING.

✓ SUGAR—Eating and drinking foods with high sugar contents produces faster growing and more deadly tumors as shown in animal tests. Mice fed diets that were high in sugar were nearly 3 times more likely to die quickly than mice on low-sugar diets. Tumors seem to thrive on sugary diets. Countries with the lowest sugar consumption per person—such as Japan and Hong Kong—also have the lowest rates of death from breast cancer. Those countries with the biggest sugar hunger—such as the U.S. and Great Britain—have the highest rates of breast cancer deaths. The average person in the U.S. takes in 2 pounds of sugar per week. The average Japanese citizen eats 14 oz. of sugar per week. The death rate from breast cancer in Japan is about that of the U.S.

✓ SDA WOMEN—Scientists studied 24 Seventh-day Adventist women between the ages of 64 and 83, half of them vegetarians for more than a quarter of a century. The vegetarians ate more fiber and had significantly lower levels of ESTRADIOL and ESTRONE, two hormones that have been linked to cancerous tumor growth. Lower levels of these hormones translate into lower breast cancer risks. It is believed that steroid hormones stick to BRAN FIBER, OAT HULLS, CELLULOSE, and LIGNIN, and are removed from the body quickly. A French study showed that those women who ate the greatest amount of YOGURT had the lowest rate of breast cancer.

◆ Colon Cancer

A HIGH FAT DIET creates a favorable environment for ANAEROBIC BACTERIA who can live there without the need for oxygen. These bacteria are well adapted to change BILE ACIDS from the intestinal tract into CARCINOGENS such as DEOXYCHOLIC and LITHOCOLIC ACIDS. On the other hand, a LOW-FAT DIET encourages AEROBIC BACTERIA, those that live with oxygen, that are not cancer-causing, and have many other benefits. A study conducted in the U.S., Canada, and China found that the consumption of saturated fats was linked to a 4 to 7 times higher rate of colon cancer among Chinese-Americans than among their counterparts in China. The high-fiber low-fat diet reduces the transit time through the intestines. This fact also inhibits the creation of CARCINOGENS. The high-fat low-fiber American diet is highly conducive to the development of colon cancer, the second most common cancer in the U.S. On the other hand, the Finns who eat a high-fat and high-fiber diet have a low rate of colon cancer but a high rate of CORONARY HEART DISEASE. In other population studies those who eat only a 10% fat-calorie diet have virtually no cancer of the colon.

◆ Lung Cancer

In the United Staaes 1 out of 3 American men smoke, while in Japan 2 out of 3 Japanese men smoke. However, the rate of LUNG CANCER in Japan is the lowest in the industrialized world. The reason for this is suspected to be LOW LEVEL of FAT in the Japanese diet. HEART DISEASE is also very low in Japan, in spite of the high rate of smoking. It is interesting to note that VEGETARIAN SMOKERS in the U.S. also have lower rates of lung cancer.

A new study has demonstrated that a diet including CABBAGE and COLLARDS protects against the spread of BREAST CANCER to the LUNGS. This study indicated that the METASTASIS, or the spread of a tumor to a secondary site can be prevented. All the animals got injections of live breast cancer cells. Then researchers watched to see how many of these cells would travel to the lungs and develop cancer in them. After 2 months, the animals fed cabbages and collards had only half as many lung tumors as the rats fed a control diet without the two vegetables. But these two vegetables must be given them in the RAW STATE and must not be cooked.

◆ *Abortions*

It seems that ABORTIONS could be an important CONTRIBUTOR to breast cancer, because the moment impregnation occurs the body makes preparations for the ultimate birth. Abortion interferes with this process and creates a minor disaster for the normal function of the body. The study by M.C. Pike and colleagues showed that a first trimester abortion before the first full-term pregnancy causes a substantial increase in the risk of breast cancer.

◆ *The Pill*

✓ CONTRIBUTOR TO BREAST CANCER—Furthermore, the pill is a major contributor to breast cancer for the same reason. It interferes with the normal function of the female body. Dr. Rosalind Alfinslater stated that women who are taking the PILL should increase their VITAMIN INTAKE, or run the risk of becoming ANEMIC. They particularly need vitamin B_2. It appears that according to the best authorities on the subject, more than 50 dangerous side-effects can result from taking birth control pills. Dr. Roy Hertz of the National Institute of Health said that long use of the sex hormone drugs carries the danger of gradually inducing CANCER of the BREAST, CERVIX, UTERUS, BLOOD CLOTS, DIABETES, and ARTERIOSCLEROSIS. Dr. Lester B. Anderson of Los Angeles said that the Pill is essentially dangerous, and that he has never recommended that women go on it in the first place.

✓ ESTROGEN THERAPY—Dr. Lewison finds that women over 45 who are on ESTROGEN THERAPY of some type are twice as likely to get breast cancer as those of the same age and marital status who do not take hormones. Dr. Ratner has described the PILL as the most dangerous drug for use by the healthy in respect to lethality and major complications. It is certainly the most talented drug ever introduced in its ability to produce diverse and varied disease phenomena and systematic abnormalities in normal women.

Estrogens that are taken by mouth affect some cell divisions and may make them abnormal and cancerous. They increase the risk of cancer of the ENDOMETRIUM or of he LINING of the UTERUS. The use of estrogen in menopausal women to relieve menopausal symptoms seems to increase the risk of breast cancer. Oral contraceptives have been shown to cause an increase in breast cancer, although some studies show no increase in risk. Cruciferous vegetables are known to eliminate estrogens from the body.

✓ DES—PREGNANT WOMEN are still unknowingly taking DIESTHYLSTIBESTROL, known as DES, in the meat and poultry they eat. Implants of DES are permitted in cattle and chickens. DES is so powerful, that just 2 parts per billion is poisonous in the diet of mice. The argument used is that meat would cost a lot more if DES could not be used. It may be better to pay high prices than to pay the high cost of cancer treatments and deaths.

✓ CERVICAL CANCER—Those who use birth control pills have a higher risk of developing CERVICAL CANCER. Dr. Butterworth of the University of Alabama says that 10 mg per day of FOLIC ACID may arrest the precancerous HYPERPLASIA in pill users. Drugs such as BIRTH CONTROL PILLS, ASPIRIN, DIURETICS, ANTACIDS, and CHOLESTEROL LOWERING MEDICATION will cause a deficiency of folic acid. Folic acid can be obtained largely from BREWERS YEAST, SOY BEANS, ALFALFA, WHEAT GERM, and OAT MEAL. A study of 189 women with cervical cancer and 227 cancer-free women showed that the risk of cervical cancer was only half as great for those with high intakes of VITAMIN C, B, and BETA-CAROTENE.

◆ *Skin Cancer*

One lady heard that skin cancer could be eliminated with SOURGRASS. She went out and gathered a big bag full, juiced it, and dehydrated it to a thick consistency. She then applied it to the open cancer wound. In a week a great deal of pus discharged, and when the scab came off, the skin was as smooth and pink as a baby's. Another way to handle it is to pick the sourgrass when the "candles are standing upright. Rinse it and put through a juicer. Put the liquid in a glass container and leave it in the sun to turn to a tar-like consistency. Then put in a darkened glass container and put in the refrigerator. Apply to cancer and leave on 3 days. It causes some pain, but the cancer will come out by the roots. Another person had 40 skin cancers removed surgically, and then he discovered JOJOBA OIL. He found that when the jojoba oil is applied faithfully, the skin cancer disappears.

HEALING OF CANCER BY NATURAL METHODS

Methods Of Dealing With Cancer

◆ *Is There A Cure For Cancer?*

Dr. Barry Lynes says: "Finding a cure for cancer is not the problem. The cures for many cancers, if not most cancers, exist. But they are not offered to the patient who has cancer. Being legally permitted to use an ALTERNATE CANCER THERAPY is the problem." Dr. Robert C. Atkins says: "There is not one but many cures for cancer available, but they are all being systematically SUPPRESSED." The average cost of a cancer treatment is between 50 and 75 thousand dollars and rising. The financial incentives make a major change in cancer treatment for the nation almost impossible, unless determined leadership from other sources forces such a change. Cancer deaths have risen steadily in the past 30 years, and are climbing 4 to 5% annually since 1960. Some doctors admit that many PATIENTS DIE OF THE TREATMENT. One cancer specialist said: "If an inexpensive replacement for CHEMOTHERAPY were found tomorrow, all U.S. medical organizations would teeter on the verge of bankruptcy."

◆ *Cancer No Longer An Incurable Disease*

Cancer can NO LONGER be termed an INCURABLE DISEASE. Louis Kuhne, at the end of the 19th century, cured cases of cancer by naturopathic and hygienic methods. His slogan was: "ONLY CLEANLINESS HEALS." He proved that cancer is the final result of SELF-POISONING either from wrong nutrition, or from wrong nutrition plus the absorption of poisonous drugs. He also believed that all illnesses were an attempt on the part of nature to get rid of, or to burn up by means of a high fever, the poisons in the body. The BLOOD, when clean and healthy, will eliminate tumerous growths. Due to artificial foods most Americans are out of balance from the standpoint of vital elements such as minerals and vitamins, and they are in an irritated condition due to the addition of SYNTHETIC CHEMICALS to our foods. SIR ARBUTHNOT LANE SAID: "Everyone can avoid cancer who is prepared to keep internally clean by eating NATURAL FOODS and drinking plenty of water. I have never yet operated for cancer upon a healthy person." KOCH, LOFFLER, BLASS, and HOXSEY, have proven that cancer is a condition in which the bloodstream is overloaded with TOXINS. They have cured cancer by cleaning these toxins out.

◆ *Surgery Cannot Eliminate Cancer*

Dr. L. Duncan Bulkley, founder of the New York Skin and Cancer Hospital, and also the author of a book entitled *Cancer And Its Non-Surgical Treatment,* for many years treated cancer the SURGICAL WAY, until he felt that a mortality rate of 92% did not indicate a successful method. He then began studying the DIETETIC METHOD. The later records from Dr. Bulckley's work show that he had cured 60% of all cancer cases that came to him, including many who had been pronounced beyond help. His method is a VEGETARIAN DIET, avoiding all FLESH FOODS, and reducing the use of all DAIRY PRODUCTS to a minimum. By it CONSTIPATION was overcome, the MINERAL SALTS were supplied in abundance, and this change together with SUNBATHS corrected the FAULTY METABOLISM. Dr. Roger in *The Philosophy Of Science And Health,* said that the cancer must be starved out. The patient must "eat" the cancer, instead of the cancer eating him.

◆ *A Natural Cancer Treatment*

Arlin J. Brown, the director of a Cancer Information Center in Virginia, gives us what he considers to be a natural cancer treatment. He says that in treating cancer successfully, three things must be accomplished:

☛ The body must be detoxified

☛ The malignancy must be eliminated, and

☛ The body must be regenerated and the deficient nutrients replaced.

While many factors play a role in causing cancer, the primary cause is TOXEMIA. The toxins come from two sources — EXTERNAL and INTERNAL. The external poisons come from COOKED and REFINED FOODS, FOOD ADDITIVES, PRESERVATIVES, PESTICIDES, DRUGS, HORMONES, etc. The internal source of toxins in the body are the WASTE PRODUCTS of METABOLISM. Nature intended that these cellular wastes be continually cleansed from the body cells with raw fruits and vegetables, or their juices. In order to detoxify, one must internally clean out the body. This can be done slowly by changing to a diet of raw fruits and vegetables and their juices — or more quickly by also including DETOXIFYING HERBS, HERB ROOTS, PLANT ROOTS, SEA PLANTS, CHLOROPHYLL, VITAMINS A and E, and high doses of NIACIN and VITAMIN C

◆ *Patients Live Longer When Not Treated*

The present methods of dealing with cancer have been somewhat ineffective since they themselves have contributed to cancer growth. This means that we must look to other methods if this scourge is to be eliminated from the world. It may therefore surprise most of us but not all of us if we say that not treating cancer at all gives better results than treating cancer with the commonly accepted orthodox methods. Dr. Alan Levin said: "Most cancer patients in this country die of CHEMOTHERAPY, and they die faster with chemotherapy than without it."

◆ *A Five Year Survival Rate Is Not A Cure*

The great surgeon Benjamin Brodie, after operating upon nearly 600 patients with cancer of the BREAST, came to the conclusion that LIFE WAS SHORTENED rather than prolonged by his efforts in this direction. He decided never to remove another cancerous breast without first laying before the patient his experiences of its results. The promises that with early diagnosis and treatment with SURGERY, RADIUM, and X-RAYS, effective results in the treatment of cancer can be obtained, have been proven false. A 5 year SURVIVAL RATE does not represent anything close to a cancer cure. Finding the cancer earlier does allow more people to live 5 yrs. from the time of diagnosis. Of the nearly 1 million Americans diagnosed with cancer each year, only HALF will be alive in 5 years. In 1988 a Swedish study found that MAMMOGRAMS and EARLY DETECTION of breast cancer did not reduce death from cancer. Dr. John Gofman stated that about 94,000 cancer fatalities are caused by medical x-ray diagnosis each year in the U.S. X-rays given during pregnancy increase the cancer mortality in children.

Dr. Hardin B. Jones of the University of California Department of Medical Physics presents a startling and revealing finding after 7 years of study of cancer treatments. He says that his studies have shown that UNTREATED CANCER VICTIMS actually LIVE up to 4 TIMES LONGER than treated cases. People who develop cancer and refuse treatment live on an average of 12.5 more years, while people with cancer who submit to medical treatment live an average of only 3 more years. This means that the old war on cancer isn't winning many battles. Similarly, Dr. Stanley Remann of Philadelphia said that he had made a survey of cancer cases in Pennsylvania over a long period of time, and that he had found that those who received no treatment lived longer than those who received SURGERY, RADIUM, or X-RAYS. It also showed that much harm was done by these methods to the average cancer patient. X-rays themselves cause diseases of various kinds including cancer.

◆ *The Internal Power Of The Body Can Cure Cancer*

The new war on cancer is looking from the EXTERNAL AGENTS used against it to the INTERNAL POWER of the BODY to heal itself. This it does through strengthening every function, and especially the immune system, and with the help of those substances which help rather than hinder it in performing its duty. Instead of depending upon poisonous substances to heal, which they don't, we must depend upon bodily processes to heal by giving them an increased opportunity to heal the body.

So long as a malignant tumor is completely localized and in a place accessible to surgical attention, SURGERY will show good results. But if the tumor has METASTASIZED, and has been distributed to other parts of the body, then surgery is ineffective.

Dr. H. Packard of Boston University states that a vitality which is disease resistant is a protective immunity against cancer. It is a vitality that depends chiefly upon the minerals salts and vitamins found in nature. A.W. McCann says that there is a direct relationship between the known causes of CONSTIPATION and the suspected causes of cancer, a relation based upon the loss of CELLULOSE, MINERALS or FOOD ALKALIES, and VITAMINS in our modern dietary.

Hyperthermia—Fever

◆ *Fever Burns Bacteria And Impurities With Heat*

Fever is one of the body's own defense mechanism created and sustained for the deliberate purpose of restoring health. The high temperature of a fever speeds up METABOLISM, inhibits the growth of the invading virus or bacteria, literally burns them with heat and accelerates the healing process. Fever is an effective protective healing measure not only against colds and other simple infections, but also against serious diseases such as POLIO and CANCER.

In biological clinics in Europe OVERHEATING THERAPIES or ARTIFICIALLY INDUCED FEVER are used effectively in the treatment of acute INFECTIOUS diseases, ARTHRITIS and RHEUMATIC diseases, SKIN DISORDERS, INSOMNIA, MUSCULAR PAIN, and CANCER. Such giants of medical science as Drs. LWOFF, ZABEL, and ISSELS, recommend and use fever therapies extensively in their clinics. Most orthodox doctors try to suppress fever. Actually fever is a constructive health-promoting symptom, initiated by the body to fight infections. High temperature SPEEDS UP METABOLISM, INHIBITS THE GROWTH OF INVADING BACTERIA, and ACCELERATES THE HEALING PROCESS. In Europe artificially induced fevers in the form of OVERHEATING BATHS have been used successfully to treat RHEUMATIC DISEASE, SKIN DISORDERS, INSOMNIA, ARTHRITIS, and CANCER.

◆ *The Heat Of Fever Destroys Cancer*

The OVERHEATING BATH is named after an Austrian laywoman who in 1932 wrote a book entitled *So Are Cured Incurable Diseases*. Her method was scientifically tested and then incorporated into many hospitals. Fever has too long been a misunderstood symptom. It is often suppressed too much by orthodox doctors. In folk medicine in various parts of the world, fever has been used for centuries to heal disease. In the West Indies, natives afflicted with SYPHILIS or CANCER heal themselves by deliberately subjecting themselves to diseases which create fevers such as MALARIA and TYPHUS FEVER.

Cancer cells are more heat sensitive than normal cells. They cannot tolerate heat in excess of 107° F. In the U.S. artificial fever is developed with hyperthermic units which encase the body, and through which circulates water at 113° F which is gradually brought down to 107.5° F and held there for 2 hours.

Dr. Werner Zabel tells the following story: "Not far from Rome, Italy, there were huge swampy areas called the Pontine Swamps. They were breeding grounds for malaria mosquitoes, and the whole area was affected by MALARIA.

Then, by action of the government, the Pontine Swamps were drained and dried out. As a result malaria disappeared. But Italian medical researchers made a remarkable discovery. While earlier the whole malaria infected area was free from CANCER, now, one generation later, it had the same prevalence to cancer as the rest of Italy. The scientists concluded that the frequent fever attacks common in malaria stimulated the body's own defenses so that cancer could not develop. It has been reported that on the Island of Sardinia no case of cancer has ever been observed, and practically everyone is affected by malaria.

Dr. Issels cures cancer with artificially induced fever plus special diets of RAW FOODS, JUICES, and FERMENTED LACTIC ACID FOODS. He says: "Artificially induced fever has the greatest potential in the treatment of cancer."

Laetrile

◆ *An Effective Control Of Cancer*

Dr. Ernesto Contrares of Mexico, who is doing a great deal of work with Laetrile, admitted that it does not work on certain types of cancer, that it was an effective control of cancer, but not a cure for most types of cancer. Dr. Dean Burk, one of the best informed men in the U.S. on LAETRILE, AMYGDALINE, VITAMIN B_{17}, or NITRILO-

SIDES, all equivalent terms, said that it occurs in over 1000 species of plants, many of which are edible. In over 20 countries in the world well over 5000 cancer patients have been treated with no demonstrable contraindications. Dr. Dean Burk made it clear that there is little or no danger from the use of APRICOT KERNELS. He claims that adult mice can live indefinitely when their normal chow diet is made up to contain 50% defatted apricot nut flour. The best sources of nitrilosides are MUNG BEANS, LIMA BEANS, LENTILS, SHELL BEANS, CRANBERRIES, PEACHES, PLUMS, APRICOTS, CHERRIES, and APPLES. Apples should be eaten with seeds. SPROUTED SEEDS are excellent sources.

◆ *How Laetrile Works*

Ernst Krebs used the natural substance LAETRILE to replace the deficient pancreatic enzyme CHYMOTRYSIN. By combining with another enzyme called BETAGLUCORONIDASE, laetrile forms a compound called HYDROCYANIC ACID, which contains the poison CYANIDE. The cancer cell, which lacks the enzyme RHODANESE, cannot tolerate the cyanide and succumbs to it. Laetrile thereby destroys cancer cells but does not affect normal cells. Normal cells can tolerate the cyanide in small quantities, but cancer cells, being weaker cells, cannot.

◆ *Used In Many Countries In The World*

In many countries in the world but not in the U.S. Laetrile, developed by Drs. Ernst Krebs Sr. & Jr. of the U.S., is used to treat cancer with reported success. Treatment is available in Mexico and many European countries. Dr. Krebs maintains that Laetrile is to cancer what vitamin C is to scurvy; what vitamin B is to pellagra; what vitamin B_{12} is to pernicious anemia. He says that cancer is a chronic disease, and that no chronic disease has yet found therapeutic resolution except with food factors such as vitamins which are normal to the normal diet.

◆ *Natural Cyanide Is Not Dangerous*

Some of the controversy surrounding laetrile is due to the fact that when the apricot pits are crushed, a certain amount of cyanide is secreted. But according to McNaughton and the developers of laetrile, cyanide naturally occurring in food is not dangerous. Primitive people who eat only whole organic foods regularly ingest 250 to 500 mg of organic cyanide each day. This natural cyanide is locked in a sugar molecule, and is normal to our metabolism. When it is eaten and taken into normal cells, the enzyme RHODANESE detoxifies the cyanide and releases it into the urine.

Cancer cells are completely deficient in rhodanese, and are surrounded instead by another enzyme called BETA-GLUCOCINASE. It is secreted by the cancer cell, and releases the bound cyanide from the laetrile at the site of the malignancy, and the released cyanide destroys the cancer cell. Organic cyanide is therefore toxic only to the cancer cells and completely nontoxic to normal cells. Laetrile is also contained in apple seeds and almonds.

◆ *The Purpose Of Laetrile Use*

The purpose behind the use of laetrile is that in advanced cancer cases it has a palliative effect, improving the subjective conditions of the patient — he feels better and doesn't have pain. Objectively, his blood pressure improves, he gains weight, and frequently goes back to work, until eventually he dies of cancer because he is an advanced case.

Vitamins And Cancer

◆ *Vitamin A*

At the 116th AMA convention in Tokyo, Dr. Saffiotti of the National Cancer Institute announced a study indicating that vitamin A inhibits lung cancer induced in animals subjected to BENZOPYRENE, which is one of the CARCINOGENS in tobacco smoke. He pointed out that this discovery could possibly have a practical significance for the prevention of LUNG CANCER. This is interesting because for decades NATUROPATHS have pointed out that CARROT JUICE has been used both as a PREVENTATIVE and CURE of cancer.

Vitamin A is essential in maintaining the structural integrity of the cells. Animal studies have shown that vitamin A deficiency increases the risk of LUNG, STOMACH, PROSTATE, CERVIX, BLADDER, and COLON cancer, which are all cancers of EPITHELIAL TISSUE. Scientists at MIT reported an increased incidence of colon cancer in vitamin A-deficient rats exposed to cancer-causing chemicals.

In a ten year Japanese study of 122,261 men of ages 40 and above who reported a low intake of green and yellow vegetables, suffered death rates from PROSTATE CANCER more than twice as high as those men who ate plenty of vegetables. This effect was observed in every age group, every social class, and every region studied. Evidence has been found that vitamin A works against the development of cancer in all of the body's tissues. BETA-CAROTENE is the vegetable form of vitamin A. Once in the body this form is converted to vitamin A, the animal form. One needs the amount of beta-carotene equal to ONE CARROT A DAY in order to prevent cancer.

Beta Carotene not only helps to prevent cancer, but it also helps fight it. It has a direct toxic effect on TUMOR CELLS, for it reduces their proliferation. It also reduces pro-cancer FREE RADICAL activity, and it builds up ENZYME ACTIVITY to fight cancer. In the body beta carotene can change into RETINOIC ACID which is used in many countries to treat cancer with considerable success.

Studies show that if mice are inoculated with low doses of tumor cells, about 50% will develop tumors. However, if mice are pre-treated with beta-carotene supplements, only 10% develop tumors. Several forms of vitamin A called RETINOIDS have been effective against SKIN cancer. Some of the cancers returned when the treatment was stopped. This indicates that vitamin A in the form of daily vegetables is the way to lick the problem, for vitamin A foods should be eaten daily. In China VAGINAL SUPPOSITORIES containing a vitamin A derivative reversed precancer cervical changes in 26 out of 27 women. In one study low vitamin A and carotene levels were found in 50% of patients who had cancer. This seems to imply that vitamin A has a protective effect.

◆ *Vitamin B*

The person who studied the whole process of OXYGENATION with respect to its effects on cancer was professor Otto Warburg. He declared that the three B-vitamins RIBOFLAVIN (B_2), NIACIN (B_3), and PANTOTHENIC ACID, together form a powerful team to fight off cancer. They are prominent constituents of Brewer's yeast. He said that the thousands of secondary causes that stimulate and induce cancer are all reduced to a primary cause, namely, OXYGEN STARVATION.

As little as a 35% reduction in the oxygen available to the cell causes the cell, in its effort to stay alive, to make a fundamental change. It gives up trying to get its energy from the oxidation of food, and instead turns to securing energy by fermenting sugar, a process that requires no oxygen. It is this FERMENTATION PROCESS that provides the impetus for the growth of cancer cells. The above 3 B-vitamins act within our bodies as CO-ENZYMES, or enzyme activators, that are essential to the production of the respiratory enzymes within the individual cells. Hence, a basic reason for the development of cancerous cells may be that the particular tissues involved lack one or more of these B-vitamins, and thus are UNABLE TO BREATHE PROPERLY. Foods that do not contain their OWN ENZYMES contribute to the destruction of the body.

In their study of the apparent link between the HUMAN PAPILLOMAVIRUS (HPV) and CERVICAL CANCER they developed the idea that FOLIC ACID, a B-vitamin may help protect some women. They discovered at the University of Alabama that of 464 women subjects, those with medium or low levels of folic acid, and who also had HPV, were more likely to develop abnormal cervical cells, or DYSPLASIA, that can lead to cancer, than those with high levels of folic acid in their blood. Folate also seems to help prevent a virus that causes GENITAL WARTS FROM TURNING INTO CERVICAL CANCER. They also believe that folic acid deficiencies may contribute to neural tube birth defects such a SPINA BIFIDA, a deformation of the spine which leaves the spinal chord exposed. However, folic acid must be in the woman's system at conception because the defect is caused during the first month of pregnancy

Dr. Sugiura of the Sloan-Kettering Institute has shown that DESICCATED LIVER and BREWER'S YEAST both of which have a full complement of B-vitamins, have an ANTI-CANCER EFFECT on test animals. In his experiment 3 groups of rats were placed on a diet of butter yellow mixed with rice. Butter yellow is a chemical dye known to cause cancer. That is why it was banned many years ago. 3%, 6%, and 15% BREWER'S YEAST was added to the 3 groups respectively Within 150 days all of the rats in the first two groups had developed LIV-

ER CANCER. The third group which had received 15% brewer's yeast had normal healthy livers at the end of the 150 days. The 15% of brewer's yeast prevented the cancer from forming in spite of the presence of the carcinogen. This experiment proves that 15% brewer's yeast in the diet will prevent LIVER CANCER in rats. Furthermore, Dr. Bush of a West Coast research team identified NICOTINAMIDE or VITAMIN B_3, as a cancer inhibitor. He found B_3 to be consistently lacking in cancer cells, and consistently present in normal cells. It has also been shown to inhibit the cancer cell's abnormal protein synthesis.

One of the differences between a normal cell and a cancer cell is that the normal cell contains an inhibitor of a certain enzyme involved in protein synthesis and cell reproduction, while the cancer cell does not. This allows the cancer cell to be uncontrolled, hence, cell proliferation goes wild. The discovery that abnormal enzyme activity takes place when B_3 is added to cancer cell cultures suggests the possibility that an injectable ANTI-CANCER AGENT, which is NONPOISONOUS, could be a nutrient which the entire body uses and needs.

◆ *Vitamin C*

✓ NEEDED FOR COLLAGEN INTEGRITY—The possibility that Vitamin C deficiency may be causally related to cancer was a conclusion reached after years of study by Dr. W.J. McCormick. He believed that an injury, whether physical or chemical, could lead to cancer if the tissues affected were not properly cared for. He believed that precancerous tissues always showed a loss of connective tissue. He therefore claimed that cancer is a COLLAGEN DISEASE that results from a DEFICIENCY of VITAMIN C.

✓ DEFICIENCY OF VITAMIN C IN CANCER PATIENTS—The cement holding the cells together can be manufactured only if Vitamin C is present in ample quantity. EASY BRUISING, indicated by black and blue spots, BLEEDING GUMS, SLOW HEALING SORES, POISONOUS FUMES EXPOSURE, CATCHING COLD EASILY, show a deficiency of vitamin C which allows the COLLAGEN to disintegrate. Several researchers also found that there is a pronounced deficiency of vitamin C in the blood of cancer patients. It has been found that GUINEA PIGS suffering from scurvy, and given just enough vitamin C to be kept alive, are far more susceptible to cancer and get it sooner than healthy guinea pigs. The degree of malignancy is determined inversely by the degree of connective tissue resistance. Lack of vitamin C is perhaps the basic cause of the lack of such resistance.

✓ TERMINAL CASES LIVE LONGER WITH HIGH DOSES OF VITAMIN C—Rats that develop tumors produce, on a body weight basis, the equivalent of 16 gm of vitamin C in a 154 lb. man. Scientists believe that several cancers may be caused by viruses, and studies have shown that vitamin C also has an ANTIVIRAL and ANTIBACTERIAL effect. Dr. Pauling has predicted that an adequate intake of ascorbic acid might reduce cancer-related illnesses and death by some 10%, with a possible saving of some 15,000 to 20,000 lives a year. He also said that if people took from 1 to 10 mg of vitamin C daily, they would reduce their risk of cancer. Dr. Ewan Cameron of Scotland showed that TERMINAL CANCER PATIENTS lived 4 times longer when administered large *doses* of vitamin C

✓ VITAMIN C CAN BLOCK CANCERS—In animals vitamin C prevents or delays the growth of tumors triggered by excess doses of HORMONES. When vitamin C was given with the hormones only half of the animals tested got tumors. The upshot of one of several studies by Linus Pauling is that Vitamin C can block SKIN CANCER caused by ultraviolet light. The mice getting large doses of vitamin C had only 20% of the incidence of skin cancer compared with the mice who received no vitamin C. In another study at Mercyhurst College, the effect of vitamin C was even stronger if vitamin C was combined with vitamin B. A lot of conventional cancer therapies are so toxic that one cannot give a high enough dose to kill the cancer without extensively hurting the patient.

In a study by Dr. Frei blood fat was oxidized by cigarette smoke containing free radicals. As long as vitamin C was in the plasma, no oxidation took place. As soon as the vitamin C was used up, the oxygen damage to fats occurred.

◆ *Vitamin E*

HAMSTERS given a carcinogen and VITAMIN E developed no cancer, while those hamsters who didn't get the vitamin E did get cancer. A 10 year Finnish study of 21,000 men found that those with highest levels of vitamin E had a 36% lower risk of cancer than those with the lowest levels.

Vitamin E protects against most cancer causing chemicals, especially those that involve free radicals. Vitamin E blocks NITROSAMINES development in a manner similar to vitamin C, except that vitamin E works in fatty tissues because it is a fat. Vitamin E also strengthens the immune system, so that it contributes to cancer prevention indirectly also. Low blood levels of vitamin E and SELENIUM in women increase the risk of breast cancer 10 times more than normal. It is 2 times if only vitamin E is low.

Raw Foods Can Fight And Cure Cancer

◆ *Raw Vegetables Are Better Than Cooked Vegetables*

Raw vegetables are better than cooked vegetables for lowering the risk of digestive cancers, especially CABBAGE and BROCCOL They are much easier to digest in less than half the time of boiled vegetables, which leave more waste products, produce impure blood, and poisoned and impaired organs, whereas the raw food dissolves and excretes these poisons. The records show that people who live by natural means and on a RAW FOOD DIET DO NOT GET CANCER. Some doctors have said that "as yet no tumor has been found that does not respond to a restricted diet. The greatest damage done by a diet of processed foods is by the nutrition they lack, mainly ENZYME DEFICIENCIES. If the body is supplied with all the nutrients through enzymes in wholesome raw food, it can cope with cancer. Cancer can be produced in a mouse by feeding it nothing but CANNED FOOD, which is cooked food, and the same cancer can be eliminated by the feeding of RAW FOODS.

✓ CRUCIFEROUS VEGETABLES—The CRUCIFEROUS VEGETABLES, also called the CABBAGE FAMILY, include BROCCOLI, BRUSSELS SPROUTS, CABBAGE, CAULIFLOWER, COLLARD, KALE, KOHLRABI, and MUSTARD. Women with elevated ESTROGEN METABOLISM have lower risks of hormone dependent cancers such as BREAST, UTERINE, and ENDOMETRIAL cancer. The cruciferous vegetables immunize these cancers by managing ESTROGEN, speeding up its metabolism, and burning it up so less is available to feed the cancer. Specific INDOLES in these vegetables accelerate the elimination of estrogen from the body. Almost all FRUITS and VEGETABLES contain small amounts of ACIDS called PHENOLS, which stop cancer-causing agents from attacking healthy cells. POTATOES, GRAPES, and NUTS have especially high amounts.

✓ WHEAT BRAN—Eating wheat bran reduced ESTROGEN LEVELS in 62 pre-menopausal women 17% after 2 months. This effect was not achieved with OAT BRAN or CORN BRAN muffins. The main difference is that wheat bran fiber is highly insoluble, giving bacteria in the colon much to chew on, and causes less estrogen to be released back into the bloodstream. It is the only fiber which decreased the levels of ESTRADIOL, a steroid produced by the ovaries, which is thought to be the major villain in breast cancer.

✓ BEANS—Hispanic women average cups of beans 6 days a week. This compares with beans twice a week for white American women. Beans possess several anti-cancer compounds including PROTEASE INHIBITORS, and PHYTATES, according to Dr. Cohen of the American Health Foundation. Dr. Duke says that the ISOFLAVONES in SOYBEANS have the most promising potential for arresting BREAST CANCER. He has helped the cancer institutes to focus on the most potent of the 10,000 soybean varieties, but, he says drug companies don't want to know that plain old plants can cure disease.

◆ *A Completely Raw Vegetarian Diet Does Not Produce Cancer*

Dr. Bircher-Benner stated that raw vegetable food is the most potent healing factor that exists which is able to bring healing where all other curative measures have failed. He says that there is no healing force on earth as powerful as a RAW FOOD DIET. All degenerative diseases will yield to raw food including the most deadly and the most crippling, such as HEART DISEASE, ARTHRITIS, and CANCER. Dr. Robert Bell wrote that cancer is never found among two black races in Egypt, the BERKEVENES and the SUDANESE who live almost entirely on a vegetarian diet. If the body is supplied with all the nutrients through enzymes in wholesome food, it can cope with cancer. That is why RAW FOOD is the answer to cancer.

◆ *A High Fiber Diet*

It is now known that fiber plays a role in the regulation of BLOOD CHOLESTEROL, BLOOD SUGAR, and it even helps in WEIGHT CONTROL, and it is very likely that fiber can help to PREVENT CANCER. The types of fiber are:

- CHOLESTEROL—The supporting framework of plants
- HEMICELLULOSE—in whole grain foods
- LIGNIN—in grain, fruits, and vegetables
- PECTINS—in fruits and vegetables
- GUMS & MUCILAGES—in beans, oats, fruits, and vegetables.

The first 3 represent INSOLUBLE fiber, and the last two represent SOLUBLE fiber. Current research suggests that only the insoluble fibers help to prevent cancer. They create bulk in the digestive tract. Only plant foods contain fiber. Animal foods, such as flesh, fats, and oil contain no fiber.

Fiber reduces CHOLESTEROL in 2 ways: a. It binds dietary cholesterol, and b. it binds BILE ACIDS and eliminates them. The liver makes 85% of the cholesterol in your body. Some cholesterol is converted to bile acids which are necessary for good digestion. A low fiber diet is high in fat and sugar. But in the absence of fiber, sugar goes directly into the blood and raises your blood sugar level. Such absence also causes the body to raise BLOOD FAT, so that the liver makes more cholesterol to stabilize the extra blood fat.... the more cholesterol we then have in our blood, the greater the clogging of our arteries. So the objective is to keep cholesterol as low as possible. In 1988 the Surgeon General set the target level of 200 mg or less for blood cholesterol.

Dr. Denis Burkitt showed that many diseases of Western Civilization, including HEART DISEASE and BOWEL CANCER could be traced to a lack of fiber in the diet. He found that the East African natives were getting plenty of fiber. This is also indicated by the fact that they had no APPENDICITIS, OBESITY, DIABETES, HERNIA, or COLONIC POLYPS. This simply means that if we eat the diet that God arranged for us, we would get all the fiber that we need. The reason why we need to add fiber to our diet today is because the process of refining our food eliminates fiber from it. The American Diet contains from 10 to 20 gm of fiber per day. It should contain about 40 gm.

Scientists studied 24 SDA women between the ages of 64 and 83. Half of them were vegetarians for more than 25 years. The vegetarians ate more fiber and had lower levels of ESTRADIOL and ESTRONE, two hormones that have been linked to cancer. Lower levels of these hormones translate into lower cancer risks. They believe that these hormones stick to BRAN FIBER, OAT HULLS, CELLULOSE, and LIGNIN, and are quickly discarded from the body. It has been shown that people who eat a HIGH FIBER DIET have a low incidence of cancer, because fiber dilutes intestinal content and reduces the amount of time carcinogens spend in the intestines.

German researchers found that the immune system's WHITE BLOOD CELLS in VEGETARIANS are twice as deadly as those in MEAT EATERS. The scientists also found that the kidney reacts differently to a VEGETABLE PROTEIN than it does to MEAT PROTEIN, so that a vegetarian diet is a strong preventer of kidney diseases in people with DIABETES.

A Harvard University study showed that those who reported the highest consumption of CARROTS, SQUASH, TOMATOES, SALADS, DRIED FRUIT, STRAWBERRIES, MELONS, BROCCOLI, or BRUSSELS SPROUTS had a decreased risk of cancer. Scientists found that strawberries contain an acid, called ELLAGIC ACID, which can kill cancer-causing compounds. This acid is also found in GRAPES and BRAZIL NUTS.

Cancer Preventing Foods

✓ BEETS—Dr. Schmidt of Germany, has reported effective results with the use of BEET JUICE in the treatment of cancer. He found that in all cases of TUMOROUS DISEASES and LEUKEMIA, the juice of BETA VULGARIS (beets) produced favorable results. The juice of 2 lbs. of raw beets is taken daily before meals over the whole day. He says that the daily doses of beet juice will also reduce the toxic effects of ionizing radiation. Similar tests with animals have also proven successful.

✓ GARLIC—At the Kyoto University in Japan, researchers took tumor cells and treated them with an extract of freshly ground garlic, (ALLIUM SATIVUM) Mice injected with these tumor cells developed a strong immunity to them. Boiled garlic did not bring about immunity. The mice who got the tumor cells without the garlic all developed cancerous tumors.

In China researchers found that people who ate the greatest number of ALLIUM vegetables, such as ONION and GARLIC, had the fewest cases of stomach cancer. When at Harvard University an ONION EXTRACT was placed in a test tube with cancer cells, it stopped their growth. Several animal studies suggest that DIALLYL SULFIDE and other sulfide compounds in garlic fight the growth of cancerous tumors in the COLON, LUNGS, and ESOPHAGUS.

Feeding GARLIC to animals consistently blocks cancer. Those who eat more ONIONS and garlic are less prone to cancer. M. Wargovich of Houston's Anderson Cancer Center gave DIALLYL SULFIDE from garlic to some mice with other foods, followed by powerful carcinogens. These mice had 75% fewer COLON CANCERS. Dr. Milner of Penn State University blocked 70% of BREAST TUMORS in mice by feeding them fresh garlic.

✓ CARROTS—Dr. Kirschner cites a case of SPLENIC LEUKEMIA in a patient who was given RAW CARROT JUICE. Her weight increased from 65 to 135 lbs. She drank over a gallon a day. Her recovery was complete within 18 months, and there was no recurrence of the disease.

✓ ASPARAGUS—A man had a hopeless case of HODGKINS DISEASE, a cancer of the LYMPH NODES, and was completely incapacitated. He started an ASPARAGUS THERAPY, using 4 full tablespoons of a liquefied puree. Improvement was seen within 2 to 4 weeks. Within one year his doctors were unable to find any sign of the disease.

✓ TOMATOES—The RED PIGMENT that gives tomatoes their red color is called LYCOPENE. It has been found to be twice as powerful as BETA CAROTENE at destroying toxic oxygen molecules, or singlet oxygen which can trigger CANCER in cells. Lycopene is also highly concentrated in WATERMELON, and there is a bit of it in APRICOTS.

✓ LUTEIN—Lutein is an antioxidant in green vegetables which some scientists think is as potent as BETA CAROTENE in thwarting CANCER. Most of it is in the darkest green vegetables. The darker green they are, the more cancer inhibiting CAROTENOIDS they contain. It is not lost in cooking or freezing.

According to a Japanese study, drinking GREEN TEA is one of the most practical methods of CANCER PREVENTION available to the general public. It neutralizes the formation of NITROSAMINES.

✓ CITRUS FRUITS—One analysis of CITRUS FRUITS found that they contained 58 known anti-cancer chemicals, which is more than is contained in any other fruit. Some experts give fruits the credit for the dramatic decline in STOMACH CANCER in the U.S.

Recent research suggests that some natural substances, called LIMONOIDS may help to prevent certain types of cancer. When tested on rats the results showed that limonoids caused an increase in the secretion of an anti-cancer enzyme in the rat's stomachs, which gave them added protection against stomach tumors and cancers. Limonoids are the compounds that create the slightly bitter taste in some fruits, including ORANGES, LEMONS, LIMES, and GRAPEFRUIT.

✓ SOYBEANS—Soybeans possess at least 5 known anti-cancer agents. These have anti-estrogen activity that may thwart the development of hormone-related cancers, such as BREAST and PROSTATE cancer. Soybeans are the richest source of PROTEASE INHIBITORS which in animals hinder the development of COLON, ORAL, LUNG, LIVER, PANCREATIC, and ESOPHAGEAL cancer. Soybean compounds also block the formation of NITROSAMINES which can lead to LIVER cancer. In fact they have been shown to be better than vitamin C.

✓ OLIVE OIL—Evidence exists that OLIVE OIL type fats help deter cancer. FAT acts as a fuel to promote tumor growth. Without fat, cancer-prone cells might remain quiet. Fat also stimulates BILE ACIDS in the colon that drive cells toward cancer. Too much fat can also depress the system's TUMOR SURVEILLANCE MECHANISM.

Herbs That Fight Cancer

✓ CHAPARRAL—CREOSOTE BUSH—An octogenarian named Ernest Farr, of Mesa, Arizona, came down with MALIGNANT MELANOMA. His doctors said that there was little they could do. He made himself a tea of chaparral, also called creosote bush, which grows in the dry desert regions. He added 3 tablespoons to one quart of boiling water, and simmered it on low heat for 10 minutes, and then let it steep for an additional 10 to 12 hours. He drank 3 cups of the tea daily between meals. His melanoma soon disappeared, much to the amazement of his doctors. An Adventist herbalist by the name of Al. Wolfsen had a friend who was diagnosed as having STOMACH CANCER. One night this friend had a dream. In the dream an angel came to him and told him to go out into the desert and pick the leaves of the CREOSOTE BUSH, also called CHAPARRAL, take them home, make a tea out of them and drink the tea every day. In time he cured himself of the stomach cancer.

✓ GARLIC and SELENIUM—Dr. Benjamin Lau of Loma Linda Medical School did research relating garlic to cancer. He found that garlic stimulated the body's immune system, and allowed such disease fighters as MACROPHAGES and LYMPHOCYTES to be strengthened so as to have the power to destroy cancer cells. He used a liquid garlic extract, called KYOLIC, which produced for him the lowest incidence of bladder cancer. The evidence showed that garlic can help inhibit tumor growth, and that in general it can enhance the whole immune system. For patients he suggests 10 liquid-filled capsules daily. As a maintenance dose he suggests 2 to 3 capsules daily with meals.

Dr. Gerhard Schrauzer of the University of California states that garlic prevents cancer through the action of SELENIUM. He found that there were fewer cancer death rates where selenium intake was high. He believes that if every woman in America began taking selenium supplements, or followed a diet high in selenium, the breast cancer rate in this country would drastically decline. Dr. Schaumberger of Cleveland advises people to increase their intake of selenium to 200 micrograms (mcg), which is 200 millionth parts of a gram per day, in order to dramatically reduce the cancer rate. Dr. D. Frost of Dartmouth Medical School also says that selenium has anti-cancer value. The combination of selenium with YEAST has been found to be even more effective than selenium alone. Selenium is an antioxidant which protects against cancer by fighting FREE RADICALS in the body. Foods that contain selenium besides garlic are ONIONS, WHOLE GRAIN BREAD, WHOLE GRAIN CEREAL, RICE, and BRAZIL NUTS.

✓ GOLDENSEAL—Solomon Yoder of the Amish community in Sarasota, Florida, had developed stomach cancer four years before. He declined surgery but accepted limited CHEMOTHERAPY. He soon discovered that that didn't help. So he experimented with different herbs and found that powdered goldenseal root worked best of all. He took 3 capsules every morning for two weeks and then increased it to 4 capsules. He also took other capsules containing goldenseal. A medical exam several months later showed his tumor to be in remission

✓ PAU D'ARCO—TAHEEBO—A great protest was heard from the Brazilian Cancer Society when the Pau D'arco tea, also called Taheebo, cured half of the CANCER patients at the Santo Andre Municipal Hospital. They issued orders forbidding the doctors from using the herb. But since the city had to pay for the operation of the hospital, it was glad for the newfound cure for economic reasons, and this inner bark of the Pau D'arco tree was allowed to continue to be used. Many forms of cancer have been reported to have been healed with this bark in addition to patient's lifestyle changes. Pau D'arco is a strong tonic and a blood builder which increases the RED BLOOD CELL count as well as their HEMOGLOBIN content. It REVITALIZES the body and promotes new CELL GROWTH.

In 1960 an elderly gentleman was operated for PROSTATE CANCER. Further examination showed that the tumor had metastasized, and doctors gave him about 30 to 40 days to live. Later he went to the dentist to get a cavity filled. The dentist suggested that he drink some PAU D'ARCO TEA. He drank 4 cups of the tea every day on an empty stomach. After 15 days his pain left, and after 30 days he was able to move around quite well. After 7 years he was still in good health.

Dr. Orlando de Santi's brother lay dying from cancer, and he felt defeated because his medical skills were unable to help his brother back to health. Dr. Santi heard about a little girl who was cured of cancer with the bark of a tree called TAHEEBO or PAU D'ARCO. The Indians found that no moss or fungus or any disease could live on this tree. They wondered if the tea could cure any human diseases. They tried it and it worked for them. Dr. Santi tried the tea on his brother. His brother's pain quickly left him after he drank the tea, and after one month of drinking the tea, the cancer was gone.

✓ RED CLOVER—JETHRO KLOSS who wrote the book *Back To Eden*, became an HERBALIST by reading some of Mrs. White's books on health. On page 6 of his book he says: "I have been told that Mrs. White cured herself of CANCER by using RED CLOVER BLOSSOMS, and she used them all during her life as a beverage. She lived to the age of eighty-four years." On 2SM302 Mrs. White says: "I will show you the bag that contains my herb drink. I send to Michigan, across the mountain, and get the RED CLOVER TOP.... I have always used red clover top, as I stated to you." She doesn't say there that she had cancer, but red clover is reputed to be another ANTICANCER HERB besides CHAPARRAL, RED OAK BARK, GOLDENSEAL, PAU D'ARCO, and juices such as CARROT and GRAPE JUICE.

✓ ECHINACEA—A Dr. KING, a prominent medical practitioner of the last century, had a wife who had suffered from a virulent cancer for many years. He tried many remedies to relieve her symptoms but with little success. Finally, he resorted to Echinacea and found it to be her only relief. Whenever she stopped using it, her symptoms intensified. Until the day she died, she could not be without Echinacea. The early settlers learned of the uses of Echinacea from the Indians. It has been reported that the Indians used Echinacea for over 100 types of CANCER.

✓ ARTICHOKES, EGGPLANT, AND THISTLES—A medical team from the Medical School of Buenos Aires, Argentine, in the 1940's found that CANCER VIRUSES were spread around the body by EXCESS CHOLESTEROL; and that the excess cholesterol does not come so much from cholesterol-rich food as from a weakened or diseased LIVER. When weakened by poisonous substances, the liver undergoes a loss of control over the production of cholesterol, and therefore produces much more than the system can eliminate. The detoxification of the liver is possible by means of the substance CINEARIN, an active ingredient in THISTLES. Thistles are consumed instinctively by horses when needed. ARTICHOKES, a relative of the thistle, contains a good amount of cinearin. Patients suffering from high blood pressure (HBP) because of excess cholesterol, got almost instant relief from eating artichokes. This medical team found that EGGPLANT had an action similar to that of artichokes, so that they turned in a report suggesting that artichokes, eggplant, and even thistles be included in the diet of cancer patients.

The Prevention Of Cancer

◆ *Unorthodox Methods Not Allowed In U.S.*

Unorthodox methods of cancer treatments are not generally allowed in the U.S. U.S. Citizens usually go to Mexico to avail themselves of these. The European approach to cancer is a combined attack on all fronts, the total mobilization of all known anti-cancer factors. They consist of DETOXIFYING THE BODY, STIMULATING BODY ORGANS AND FUNCTIONS, IMPROVING GLANDULAR ACTIVITY, and INCREASING AND STRENGTHENING THE BODY'S OWN HEALING FORCES. Americans are generally drug oriented. This attitude is applied also toward cancer. Biological doctors are convinced that no drug or pill will be found that will cure cancer, just as there is no drug in existence that will cure any disease. A disease can be cured only by the body's own healing mechanism, its own DEFENSE MECHANISM. A TUMOR is nothing more than the body's effort to isolate the affected cells, in order to protect the rest of the body and extend life. Hence, an effective CURE for any disease can be accomplished only FROM WITHIN, by the BODY'S OWN HEALING FORCES. Therefore, the first principle of PREVENTIVE BIOLOGICAL MEDICINE is to create conditions most conducive to SELF-HEALING.

✓ THERE IS LITTLE PREVENTION ADVICE GIVEN BY DOCTORS—It has been estimated that 86% of all doctors do not give prevention advice to their patients. Taken together, diet and smoking account for 65% of the risk factors for cancer, and up to 80% of all cancers are preventable, and from the standpoint of the Christian doctor, 100% of all cancers should really be preventable. God's natural diet really does not cause any cancers, and harmful environmental conditions can be neutralized with natural substances. If many of the causes of cancer are considered officially to be unknown, then one cannot prevent a cause that is unknown. However, since some causes are known, such as smoking and drinking, still there is no prospective financial reward in the eyes of some doctors to tell the patient what to do in order not to have to visit the doctor anymore.

✓ HIGH FIBER DIETS—Cultures that have HIGH-FIBER diets of UNPOLISHED RICE, WHOLE WHEAT BREAD, AND UNPEELED ROOT VEGETABLES don't get COLORECTAL cancer. Fibers dilute intestinal content, and reduce the time carcinogens might spend in the intestines. B.H. Ershoff has shown that various poisons added to food can be neutralized if fiber-rich foods are eaten. Patients who have DIVERTICULAR DISEASE consume about 3.5 gm of fiber per day. If more dietary fiber is eaten, carcinogens pass out of the gut more quickly, and therefore have less of a chance to cause cancer. The average American eats 20 gm of fiber. It is suggested that they eat 30 to 40 gm/day. It is now known that fiber plays a role in the regulation of BLOOD CHOLESTEROL and BLOOD SUGAR.

✓ FIBER AND YEAST BREAD—Whole grains contain PHYTIC ACID as PHYTATE which can tie up minerals in the system. This will not be a problem with WHOLE GRAIN BREADS made with YEAST, for yeast destroys phytate. But it may be a problem among people eating a lot of UNLEAVENED BREAD. Studies show that people absorb 1% to 3% fewer calories when eating a HIGH FIBER DIET. It also helps WEIGHT CONTROL because high fiber foods take longer to chew. Studies also show that something in whole grains protects the teeth from DECAY-PRODUCING ACIDS in the mouth which are produced by bacteria.

✓ ONIONS AND GARLIC—Women who live in cultures that consume a lot of ONIONS and GARLIC have substantially lower rates of BREAST cancer.

✓ STRONG HERBS—In cultures that tend to have more spicy cuisines, such as the Indian, Mexican, and Chinese, there is far less incidence of PROSTATE and COLORECTAL cancers than in cultures with blander diets.

In those parts of the world, such as in the Indonesian islands, Philippines, and the West Indies, where the air is heavily scented with certain AROMATIC SPICES, such as cinnamon and nutmeg, there is virtually no lung cancer.

✓ CALCIUM—One study showed that the people who were cancer-free ate a diet richer in CALCIUM than those with COLON CANCER. It is thought that calcium may slow colon cancer development by binding with the FATS and BILE ACIDS that cause colon cancer.

✓ VITAMIN C—CATS, DOGS, COWS, SHEEP, and RABBITS all make about the same amount of vitamin C per pound of their body weight, or about 66 mg/lb. If we translated this into the equivalent for a 150 lb. person, it would average

10,000 mg or 10 gm. With such a large dose it is advisable to break it down into several smaller doses, so that more of it would be retained. For CANCER PREVENTION a dose of from 2000 mg to 5000 mg is recommended. Dr. Pauling dispenses from 6000 mg to 18,000 mg for cancer patients

◆ *Diet And Drainage*

Sir Arbuthnot Lane said in a lecture at John Hopkins Medical School: "Gentlemen, I shall never die of cancer, for I am taking measures to prevent it. It is caused by poisons created in our bodies by the food we eat. What we should do then, if we would avoid cancer, is to eat WHOLE WHEAT BREAD, RAW FRUITS and VEGETABLES and their JUICES; first, that we may be better nourished and, secondly, that we may more easily eliminate waste products. We have been studying disease when we should have been studying DIET and DRAINAGE. The world has been on the wrong track. No one need to have cancer who will take the trouble to avoid it."

Body tissues must be unhealthy for a long time before cancer develops out of them. This makes the prevention of cancer exceedingly simple. To prevent cancer prevent the tissues from becoming unhealthy. To do this it is important for a person in normal health to eat freely of natural foods. Mr. Tobe of Canada says that most of the cases of cancer could be prevented if the practice of putting HARMFUL CHEMICALS in our food was prohibited. Many of these chemicals accumulate in the body to cause trouble later on.

◆ *Raw Food Prevents Cancer*

Cooking food destroys their ENZYMES, and enzymes such as CATALASE play their part in preventing cancer. But foods in which the enzymes have been destroyed contribute to the development of diseases such as cancer. If therefore the body is supplied with all the nutrients including enzymes in wholesome food, it can cope with cancer. That is why wholesome RAW FOOD is the answer to cancer.

Many laboratory experiences have demonstrated in a most remarkable manner, the absolute controlling effect of DIET on the development of inoculated cancer in mice and rats. Their progress was inhibited almost entirely by a vegetable diet. The record also shows clearly that people who live by natural means, and on a raw food diet, do not get cancer. Experiments have shown that a great variety of diseases can be produced, prevented, and eliminated at will by regulating the DIET OF ANIMALS. It has also been demonstrated that HUMAN BEINGS are no exception to this rule.

The data of recent research suggests that DIET makes a difference in cancer. The scientists who developed the data now have become regular patrons of the salad bar. They were convinced by the fact that those who ate a lot of green and yellow vegetables and fruit reduce their risk of cancer. It has also been found that the DAMAGE done by bad habits is REVERSIBLE. They found that healthy people ate more vegetables.

Foods of the CABBAGE FAMILY of vegetables are said to be CANCER INHIBITORS. They include CABBAGE, CAULIFLOWER, BROCCOLI, and BRUSSELS SPROUTS and are all linked to reduced risk of STOMACH, COLON, and RECTAL cancer. The inhibitors in these foods are called INDOLES.

◆ *Beta-carotene Prevents Cancer*

What's in a CARROT seems to counteract cancer. It acts as a BUFFER against cancer. BETA-CAROTENE, the precursor of vitamin A, is said to be a SHOCK ABSORBER by protecting cells from damage caused by FREE RADICALS, which are by-products of fat metabolism, and can turn a normal cell into a cancerous cell. Cancer was found to have the highest rate in those who ate the least amount of beta-carotene. Research found that women with low beta-carotene intake had a 3-fold greater risk of developing CERVICAL cancer.

◆ *Rice Prevents Cancer*

Ehrlich has shown that mice living on a RICE DIET cannot be inoculated with cancer, while those living on a meal diet can be readily inoculated. Cancerous tumors develop quickly and continue to grow until the animal dies. He also found that when mice with cancerous tumors, the result of inoculation, were placed upon a rice diet, the tumors ceased to grow, and in many cases degenerated and disappeared. Such results are apparently also true with regard to humans. One researcher took an extensive trip through the far east. He visited many hospitals in different countries, and was repeatedly told by physicians, missionaries, civilian and military personnel, that there was no cancer among rice eating people.

Recent research has given us a possible explanation. The question which they tried to answer was, "Why do the Japanese get so little BOWEL CANCER when their diet is very low in FIBER?" The answer they found was STARCH. The Japanese eat a lot of starch-rich rice. They found that a certain amount of starch acts like insoluble fiber, and escapes digestion. That is why it has a positive effect on bowel cancer.

Dr. Hoffman says that one may keep himself immune from cancer if one refrains from OVERTAXING the ORGANS of DIGESTION and EXCRETION, and by moderate eating keeps the blood pure and resistance high through an abundance of VITAMINS and ALKALINE ELEMENTS in the diet, and if one periodically CLEANSES HIMSELF INTERNALLY by a modified FAST or ELIMINATIVE DIET.

Someone has said that the laws of EXTERNAL HYGIENE have been accepted and enforced, but the laws of INTERNAL HYGIENE have neither been accepted by the majority nor enforced.

◆ *Fasting And Cancer*

H. Carrington's book entitled *Vitality, Fasting And Nutrition*, gives references supporting the contention that cancer is due to OVEREATING, and should be curable by FASTING or a restriction of diet. Upton Sinclair quotes Dr. Haskell in *The Fasting Cure* as having cured several cases of CANCER by fasting. In one study 50% of fully fed mice developed cancers of one sort or another, but only 13% of the mice on restricted diets did. Other studies indicate that animals on restricted diets also have fewer CATARACTS, and less DRY SKIN, KIDNEY DISEASE, and HEART DISEASE. Dietary restrictions indicate that the IMMUNE SYSTEM is rejuvenated through a restricted diet.

◆ *Exercise Prevents Cancer*

One of the best preventive measures against cancer may be EXERCISE. Dr. Ernst Van Aaken of Germany checked 454 members of a club for older long-distance runners. He found that in the six year period of his study, only 4 of the runners got cancer, and they all recovered and are running again. He also kept records of a parallel group of 454 normal men who didn't run and found 29 cases of cancer during the same period, and 17 of the non-runners died of the disease. The reason the runners didn't get cancer is that they were constantly providing their bodies with more OXYGEN than they needed says Dr. Van Aaken.

In another study former ATHLETES were found to have only half the risk of cancer than non-athletes. The conclusion is that INACTIVE PEOPLE are at an increased risk of getting cancer. Special Chemicals are released by the body during periods of vigorous exercise, and these chemicals are responsible for the reversal of cancerous tumor growth. During exercise ENDORPHINS are released by the brain and continue to circulate throughout the body for hours. Higher demands for oxygen during physical activity causes blood vessels to expand throughout the body in order to deliver more OXYGENATED BLOOD. The metabolic processes are increased, and the incorporation of beneficial nutrients into body tissues is enhanced.

◆ *Negative Ions And Cancer*

Air charged with NEGATIVE IONS, such as the air at the ocean or at a waterfall, inhibits cancer growth and stimulates hormones to protect the body against stress factors.

An Anti-Cancer Diet

This may come as a surprise to many orthodox cancer specialists, but according to the leading biological cancer specialists of Europe, there is indeed such a thing as an ANTI-CANCER DIET — a diet that can help prevent cancer, as well help the body to cure cancer. Dr. Issels advises the following diet:

✓ ORGANICALLY GROWN FOODS—The diet must consist exclusively of ORGANICALLY GROWN FOODS, which are free from carcinogenic chemicals, such as toxic additives, insecticides, preservatives, and other manmade chemicals.

✓ NATURAL RAW STATE—Most foods must be eaten in the NATURAL RAW STATE. The diet doesn't have to be 100% raw, although it should be at least 80 TO 90% RAW. Certain foods such as BUCKWHEAT, SOYBEANS, MILLET, POTATOES, RICE, and some dried beans could be COOKED.

- ✓ FRUITS, VEGETABLES, NUTS, SPROUTED GRAINS, and SEEDS—The emphasis should be on RAW VEGETABLES, FRUITS, NUTS, SPROUTED GRAINS, and SEEDS. The best nuts are ALMONDS, WALNUTS, and FILBERTS. PEANUTS should be avoided by cancer patients. Although peanuts are an excellent food, they are often infected with a fungus called AFLATOXIN, which is carcinogenic. The best anti-cancer grains are: MILLET, BUCKWHEAT, BROWN RICE, and BARLEY.

- ✓ LACTIC ACID FOODS—An anti-cancer diet should include a generous amount of fermented LACTIC ACID foods, such as naturally fermented SAUERKRAUT, PICKLED VEGETABLES, POTATOES, SPROUTED SEEDS and GRAINS, NUTS and KVARK, which is raw, unheated, homemade COTTAGE CHEESE from high quality unpasteurized milk, FERMENTED GRAINS, and FERMENTED JUICES, according to Dr. Johannes Kuhl, originator of the lactic acid fermentation diet for cancer. Lactic acid has a beneficial ANTI-PUTREFACTIVE effect on the intestines, and keeps the digestive tract in good health. Fermented foods can be used as both food and medicine. They have a beneficial effect on metabolism, and a curative effect on disease. They destroy harmful bacteria in the intestines, and contribute to the better assimilation of nutrients even for people with a weak digestive system. They can be considered to be PREDIGESTED FOODS. To avoid commercial chemicals, it is best to make one's own HOMEMADE SAUERKRAUT, KEFIR, YOGURT, SOUR PICKLES, and LACTIC ACID VEGETABLES.

- ✓ VEGETABLE PROTEINS—A moderate amount of easily digested protein must be eaten. These should be mostly of vegetable origin, such as GREEN LEAFY VEGETABLES, POTATOES, SPROUTED SEEDS and GRAINS, and NUTS.

- ✓ AVOID ANIMAL PROTEINS—Avoid completely all other animal proteins: NO MEAT, FOWL, EGGS, or FISH. Some doctors advocate the use of RAW EGG YOLKS from fertile eggs. Egg yolks are ALKALINE FORMING. Egg white is almost 100% protein. It is ACID FORMING and hard to digest. So it is advisable to eat fertile eggs but yolks only.

- ✓ USE ACIDOPHILUS MILK PRODUCTS—Take no milk or milk products except the kvark and soured milks. The best forms of soured milks are: ACIDOPHILUS MILK, NATURAL BUTTERMILK, HOMEMADE SOURED MILK, CLABBERED MILK, preferably made from GOAT'S MILK. Goat's milk is better than cow's milk. Raw goat's milk of high quality contains ANTI-CANCER and ANTI-ARTHRITIC factors.

- ✓ AVOID ANIMAL FATS—AVOID saturated, cholesterol-rich ANIMAL FATS, including BUTTER, which the Spirit of Prophecy has told us is not best for health (CD352). These should be replaced with a moderate use of genuine, cold-pressed, VEGETABLE OILS, such as SUNFLOWER SEED OIL, FLAXSEED OIL, SOY BEAN OIL, and SAFFLOWER OIL. Oils should never be heated. Carcinogenic substances are produced in vegetable oils during prolonged healing.

- ✓ ELIMINATE PROCESSED AND DENATURED FOODS—Eliminate from the diet all processed and denatured foods, especially all REFINED CARBOHYDRATES, such as WHITE FLOUR and WHITE SUGAR, and all foods made with them.

- ✓ DEPEND UPON NATURE'S HEALING POWER—Dr. Bieler furthermore states: "There is no power on earth that can do what nature can do, and there is no healing power greater than a diet composed of raw vegetables, grains, fruits, and nuts. Nature knows NO INCURABLE DISEASES, and nature can easily defeat cancer, and the prevention of cancer is even easier." Dr. Bircher-Benner of Zurich, Switzerland, has stated: "Raw vegetable food is the most potent healing factor that exists. It is able to bring healing to every part of the body for many widely spread disorders of health and serious diseases, in quite astonishing fashion, where all other curative measures have failed."

- ✓ OXYGENATE THE TISSUES—Mrs. White says that fresh air is FOOD for the lungs. If according to Dr. Warburg a lack of oxygen is the cause of cancer, then the regaining of normal oxidation is the enemy of cancer growth. This also seems to be the cause of all other incurable ailments. It is maintained, however, that the cause of insufficient oxidation is MINERAL SHORTAGE IN THE VITAL FLUIDS.

- ✓ FAITH AND PROPER MENTAL ATTITUDE—Research has shown that cancer patients generally show a rise in CORTISOL, a hormone which depresses the immune system, a few months before they die. There is a mental factor that brings this about. It was found that as long as the patient believes that there is hope, the production of cortisol is very small. As soon as he gives up hope, his cortisol production rises, the immune system is depressed, and the cancer proceeds out of control. When the patient was told that he was getting large quantities of vitamin C, the cortisol level went down, because they exercised faith and developed hope, the hope of possible recovery. This improved mental attitude allowed the vitamin C to perform many beneficial bodily functions. That is why the Bible says: "According to your faith so be it unto you" (Matt. 9:29).

Natural Professional Cancer Treatments

◆ *Dr. Henry G. Bieler*

Dr. Bieler wrote the book *Food Is Your Best Medicine.* In it he shows clearly how food is related to health and disease. He treated both malignant and nonmalignant tumors with success using DIET only. He stated that one of the reasons for LEUKEMIA in children is related to the toxic condition of the mother at the time of conception. If the mother is very toxic, many poisons find their way into the fetus. He says that many childhood diseases are due to TOXEMIA, a kind of garbage upon which BACTERIA feed. The bacteria are not the cause of the disease, the WASTES are. To rid the body of bacteria does not get to the root of the problem, for it is the wastes that must be eliminated. Children who go through stages involving MUCOUS DISCHARGE, SKIN RASH, NAUSEA, VOMITING, and FEVER, are likely to be toxic. The body tries to rid itself of these by any avenue open to it, the LUNGS, the SKIN, the MOUTH, and the NASAL AREA. Ignoring the germs and clearing the waste is the answer.

Women who have MENSTRUAL problems in their early adult life are likely to have a toxic condition of the body that in turn uses the UTERUS as a garbage dump. The uterus is not designed to take this toxic load and becomes a sick organ, giving rise to all sorts of female complaints. Removing the uterus does not change the basic toxemia except that it removes an outlet of the toxins that now must escape by way of another route. The same thing occurs at the time of the MENOPAUSE. The escape route for toxins is now blocked and a wide variety of new ailments arise. These include HOT FLASHES, NERVOUS BREAKDOWN, HEADACHES, ARTHRITIS, NEURITIS, MENTAL DISEASE, ALIMENTARY PROBLEMS, VAGINAL DISCHARGE, PALPITATIONS of the HEART, and ultimately CANCER.

Dr. Hanley says that almost every culture uses plant medicinals to support women through menopause, and with good reason. Plants such as SOYBEANS, MEXICAN YAMS, and certain HERBS, are loaded with both estrogens and progesterones identical to those produced in a woman's body. Some simple plant-derived hormone creams work wonders without requiring women to take unnecessary health risks. Since the hormones are readily absorbed through the skin, topical creams are probably a good way to replace them.

If the uterus is still in tact, the poisons will gravitate into this organ, setting it up for cancer. If it has been removed, they gravitate elsewhere, and set up a cancer situation in another place or places. The woman with menstrual problems must detoxify and stay on a cancer prevention diet.

Dr. Bieler links both the over-intakes of protein and the use of cooked protein with cancer. The high protein craze in recent times damages the liver and sets up the individual for cancer. He also indicates that both animals and people are designed to use only RAW PROTEINS. Cooked proteins rot much quicker in the alimentary canal, thereby releasing large numbers of toxins.

He speaks of an experiment with cats. As long as cats were fed raw meat, they were well. When fed cooked meats, they developed PYORRHEA, LOSS of TEETH, LOSS of HAIR, DECALCIFICATION of BONES, ARTHRITIS, GASTRITIS, ATROPHY and CIRRHOSIS of the LIVER, and DEGENERATION of the BRAIN and SPINAL CHORD. Dr. Bieler reminds us that such common foods as PASTEURIZED MILK, and milk products made from pasteurized HEATED MILK or POWDERED MILK, CHEESE, and ICE CREAM, are all foods which are clearly dangerous.

If people did what Dr. Bieler suggests, the whole medical and pharmaceutical business would collapse. There would be no need for doctors except to take care of accident cases. Hospitals would close their doors. X-ray machines would be eliminated along with old cars and tires. People would throw out their cooking stoves and buy JUICE EXTRACTORS and BLENDERS. The whole processed food industry would collapse along with the supermarket. The GREENGROCERS would thrive and there would be one on every block.

◆ *Johanna Brandt — The Grape Cure*

Johanna Brandt was born in South Africa in 1876. Her family ate a great deal of meat, and as a result there was a lot of cancer in her family. She suspected that she had cancer also, and she decided that she would take no medicine, no drugs to relieve the pain, and no surgery. Instead she decided to FAST. She included WATER CURES, FRUIT JUICE CURES, SUN BATHING, DEEP BREATHING, SPINAL EXERCISES, CHEWED HER FOOD WELL, and SLEPT OUTSIDE. All this for 9 years, and was reduced to a walking skeleton.

Fasting checked the growth of the cancer, but when she broke the fast, the growth continued. She began to understand that cancer thrives on every kind of animal matter, the more impure the better. Finally, in 1925, she found the food that would not allow the tumor to regrow after a fast This was the use of grapes for a GRAPE CURE. The following are the directions for a grape cure:

A water fast for two or three days is recommended along with a lukewarm enema containing the juice of one lemon. The first day of breaking the fast, drink one or more glasses of pure cold water in the morning. Half an hour later the patient has his first meal. the grapes should be chewed well, swallowing only a few for roughage. Starting at 8 a.m. and every two hours thereafter, the patient has a grape meal, totaling 7 meals a day. This is continued from 2 weeks to 2 months and not longer. The grapes used can be of any variety.

The quantity of grapes used per meal will vary from a few ounces to half a pound. At least a pound should be used daily. The patient should not eat all the skins. Meals should be skipped if the patient really cannot tolerate the grapes. No other food should be used, but plenty of water should be taken. Loss of strength is due to poisons in the body. Once the poisons go, the patient regains strength and may even gain weight on the diet.

◆ *Dr. Max Gerson*

Dr. Gerson said that the cancer cells tend to live in an ANAEROBIC OXIDIZING SYSTEM rather than in an aerobic system. They do not require outside oxygen as do normal cells. In cancer the entire body is affected. The tumor is merely the outside sign. Those who live on natural foods such as fresh fruits and vegetables have no cancer, but they soon develop cancer when their diet is changed to canned foods. He says that the more the body is detoxified, the more the cancer is doomed. In countries where a great deal of GARLIC is used, such as Italy, Greece, and Yugoslavia, there is very little cancer. He saw 2 cancers of the breast disappear with the use of large amounts of FENUGREEK TEA in combination with a SALTLESS VEGETARIAN DIET. Dr. Schweitzer said of him: "I see in him one of the most eminent medical geniuses in the history of medicine."

His diet consisted of FRUIT, FRUIT JUICES, VEGETABLES, VEGETABLE SALADS, SPECIAL SOUPS, POTATOES, OATMEAL, and BREAD. He aimed therewith to detoxify the entire system, to restore the function of the liver and the metabolism. With his method he cured 50% of the terminal cancer cases sent to him by other doctors. He also received a citation from Congress for his greatly successful work with cancer patients.

◆ The Hoxsey Treatment

The Harry Hoxsey cancer treatment is based on a detoxification method which uses herbs such as RED CLOVER, which contains vitamin B_{17}, or LAETRILE, and BARKS and ROOTS, as well as certain chemicals including POTASSIUM IODIDE, and certain ZINC, SULFUR, and ARSENICAL compounds from which he made a tonic. The attorney for Morris Fischbein, former president of the AMA, said that Hoxsey's treatment did cure cancer.

◆ Dr. Joseph Issels

Dr. Issels treated some 8000 cancer patients for over 20 years, many of whom were terminal cases. He lost only 20% of his patients to cancer, The normal rate is an 80% loss. He said that infected teeth and tonsils had to be removed because they released poisons into the system which interfered with the body's resistance. He used DIET, FEVER THERAPY, and OXYGEN-OZONE THERAPY. He got cures with terminal cancer patients which were 8 times greater than the World Health Organization indicated was likely. He showed that cooked food is bad for people. He took two plots of land, one fertilized with the manure from animals fed raw food only, and he found that the soil became very fertile. The other was fertilized with the manure from animals fed only cooked food, but the soil remained infertile.

Dr. Issels said that the protein from SOURED MILK is the best and most wholesome of animal proteins. Sour milk is low in estrogens due to bacterial fermentation. It is preferred even to YOGURT because sour milk bacteria remain in the intestines keeping down putrefying bacteria, while yogurt bacteria are eliminated with the stool.

◆ Dr. William Kelley

Dr. William Kelley, a dentist, had cancer for more than three years. When he was examined he was told that he had less than one month to live. He says: "If I had not discovered God's laws concerning cancer and applied them diligently, I would not be here to tell about it." His method of treatment involves the use of PANCREATIC ENZYMES, as well as other methods taken from Dr. Gerson. Besides the pancreatic enzymes he used large amounts of VITAMIN C and BIOFLAVONOIDS or RUTIN, ORGANIC MINERALS and TRACE MINERALS, ALMONDS as a replacement for meat, and an AMINO ACID substance.

◆ Dr. C. Moerman

Dr. C. Moerman, a Dutch Physician, believed that cancer did not develop out of sound tissue, but out of sick tissue. He says that the POWER OF OXYGENATION is what protects the body from cancer, and reduced oxygenation of the body supports cancer. It is oxygen deficiency and certain toxic substances that block the oxidation process.

He utilized Vitamin A, C, and E to aid the oxidation process. With these he could cure persistent chronic LEG ULCERS. He indicated that there were two ways for the metabolism to be disturbed for cancer to develop. One was a deficiency of the helpful nutrients, and second was carcinogenic substances which would destroy the essential nutrients. He said: "If a healthy mouse was given a burn on the back, normal healing would occur. However, if a mouse was given carcinogens for a period of time and was then burned, a malignancy would occur at the site of the burn.

This means first of all that cancer cells will develop out of a SICK BODY. Secondly, they will develop at the site of the injury. Third, the rejuvenated cells are identical to embryonic cells. EMBRYONIC CELLS can undergo oxidation without oxygen, through FERMENTATION. This means that while degenerative cells in a healthy body do not develop into tumors, they do develop into tumors in a sick body. The deficiencies of one or more essential nutrients prevents injury to the MITOCHONDRIA that deal with the cell's use of oxygen. Whatever interferes with the function of the mitochondria will throw the cells' respiration into fermentation and tumor growth. Carcinogens will poison the mitochondria if they are not quickly removed.

Dr. Moerman is against RADIATION treatment, since it destroys normal cells as well as malignant cells, and inhibits the activity of vitamin C and the B-complex. Of 64 patients who had been given a little more than 2 months to live, he cured 27 of them (42%). He felt that if he had received them in earlier stages, his results would have been much better.

◆ *Dr. Christine Nolfi*

Dr. Nolfi of Denmark one day discovered a TUMOR IN HER BREAST. She decided to put herself on a completely raw food vegetable diet. On such a diet her pains quickly left her. She was taken to court for not using drugs, and she lost her medical license. She then took up the profession of running a Sanitarium where she fed people only raw foods, raw milk, sprouted grains as well as plenty of garlic. This she could do as a lay person, but not as a medical doctor. She did not cook any foods since she believed that cooked foods would rot in the alimentary canal, causing great increases in the white cell count of the blood, which to her suggested infection. She also believed that sweets would do the same. She agreed with Dr. Gerson that cancer is the final stage of an overly acid body, and if discovered early enough can be completely controlled through a raw food diet which is alkaline, and neutralizes the acid condition. If the cancer is discovered too late, the diet will relieve pain and lengthen life, but will not preserve it. She found that many other degenerative conditions responded well to this type of treatment, the basic reason being that raw foods cleansed the system of impurities.

◆ *Dr. Irwin Stone*

Most animals can produce their own vitamin C, but man cannot. Dr. Stone calculated that man should produce in his liver between 10 and 20 gm of vitamin C to keep him healthy, the equivalent of 500 oranges a day. In the GUINEA PIG, which also does not produce its own vitamin C, additional vitamin C was shown to offer protection from the effects of carcinogens. Some research papers showed that there is a precondition for cancer that involves a vitamin C deficiency. In 1943 it was shown that the carcinogens in tobacco smoke could be detoxified by vitamin C. Individuals with LEUKEMIA and SCURVY both tend to hemorrhage, and both have a deficiency of vitamin C. The white blood cells pick up the vitamin C, and remove it from the blood, thereby insuring that a leukemic person also has scurvy. To change this condition the white blood cells must be saturated with Vitamin C.

Dr. Stone states that 12 gm a day of vitamin C is the lowest amount that will help cancer. He recommends at least 50 gm a day. In 1973 a study by Cameron and Pauling showed that vitamin C inhibits an enzyme which cancer cells produce to destroy good cells in the environment so as to extend cancer.

◆ *Dr. Wong Hon Sun*

Dr. Sun, a naturopathic physician, wrote a book entitled *"How I Overcame Inoperable Cancer."* As a child he had a chronic sinus condition, and he always had a cold. He ate a lot of WHITE POLISHED RICE, WHITE BREAD, NOODLES, and DUMPLINGS which created mucous problems. His tonsils were removed. When he went on a fast his condition improved. Without it the old condition returned. He finally decided that he would treat himself without the use of drugs, for the drugs he had taken had not helped him. He again went on a fast. He figured that when animals are sick, they fast. Along with the fast he took nightly warm water enemas. He ate steamed liver extract and fresh pineapple juice which he sipped at four hour intervals. Gradually his strength returned.

To reduce the toxins he believed that he would have to use only PLANT FOODS, and that he would have to reduce his total food intake. He believed that one meal a day was all that was necessary for a cancer patient. He then decided on a LIVER diet which he ate almost raw. After three months of nutritional therapy, he started light exercise in the form of JOGGING. This was followed by a warm BATH and a brisk RUBDOWN. Gradually, the tumor at the back of the throat, near the entrance of his internal nostrils regressed. He could tell this by his ability to breathe through the nose. In addition to his nutritional regimen he took VITAMIN C, IRON, LECITHIN, BREWER'S YEAST, a PANCREATIC SUPPLEMENT, and WHEAT GERM. He also ate FISH LIVER for VITAMINS A and D. Eventually he was able to go on to a vegetable therapy. He hasn't had a recurrence of the cancer in 14 years.

◆ *Dr. Ann Wigmore*

Dr. Ann Wigmore, a naturopathic doctor, used the raw fresh juice pressed from SPROUTED WHEAT for many physical problems. She also applied the juice to cancer patients, and they were healed by it. She didn't know what caused the healing, but later a Dr. Virginia Livingston Wheeler discovered that it was ABSCISIC ACID, a powerful anti-cancer agent.

◆ Dr. Niehans

Dr. Niehans developed the method of CELLULAR THERAPY which represents the discovery that when one injects the cells of an animal that doesn't get cancer, such as SHEEP, into man, one injects also the power against cancer. He obtained results with most diseases that were nothing short of miraculous. He stated that almost none of his patients got cancer, and that all of his patients lived to be very old.

CANDIDA ALBICANS—CANDIDIASIS

Candida Albicans Is Present In Every Person

◆ Yeast Overgrowth Causes Candidiasis

The common yeast, CANDIDA ALBICANS, is present in every individual. Normally the yeast lives harmlessly in the GASTROINTESTINAL TRACT, MOUTH, THROAT, VAGINA, and especially in the MUCOUS MEMBRANES. It is controlled by the friendly bacteria which YOGURT aids in multiplying. However, occasionally the yeast will overgrow and lead to significant disease, weakening the immune system and causing an infection called CANDIDIASIS. Candida overgrowth is most often associated with chronic ANTIBIOTIC use. Antibiotics kill off the friendly bacteria which help keep candida in check. When this fungus infects the ORAL CAVITY it is called THRUSH. When it infects the VAGINA it is called VAGINITIS.

Candidiasis is a 20th century phenomenon caused by the introduction of ANTIBIOTICS, CORTISONE, and by the consumption of refined carbohydrates, mainly SUGAR, and the great use of BIRTH CONTROL PILLS. This fungus thrives in the presence of cortisone and the hormones of the pills. Refined carbohydrates are a favorite food of this fungus. They multiply readily in their presence.

◆ Foods Which Promote Yeast Growth

We must avoid foods which promote yeast growth, such as CHEESE, ICECREAM, SOFT DRINKS, AND SUGAR CONTAINING FOODS of all sorts. Also MOLDS, since most antibiotics are derived from molds. If in doubt avoid BREADS and BAKERY GOODS since they contain yeast. Because of the milk sugar LACTOSE, MILK promotes yeast growth. The PROGESTERONE COMPONENT of the PILL causes changes in the vaginal mucous membrane, which makes it easier for yeasts to multiply. Pure ESTROGEN pills do not encourage the growth of yeasts.

◆ Candidiasis Affects Men And Women

Candidiasis may affect both men and women; however, it is rarely transmitted sexually. An infected mother may pass the infection on to the newborn. Women diagnosed for a yeast infection should also be checked for DIABETES, because their vaginal environment is more conducive to the growth of yeast. Hence, they are at greater risk of contracting a yeast infection such as candidiasis.

Causes Of Yeast Infection

◆ Decreased Digestive Secretions

Digestive secretions such as HYDROCHLORIC ACID, PANCREATIC ENZYMES, and BILE normally prevent the overgrowth of candida and its penetration into the absorptive surfaces of the intestines. A lack of any of these will allow the yeast to overgrow.

◆ Impaired Immunity

When the immune system is impaired candida will overgrow rapidly. The things that will weaken the immune system are frequent ANTIBIOTIC USE, STEROIDS, ENVIRONMENTAL CHEMICALS, NUTRIENT DEFICIENCIES, CANCER, HYPOTHYROIDISM, AND STRESS. Yeasts aren't harmed by antibiotics, hence, their use makes them multiply more rapidly. Antibiotics destroy good germs while they are also destroying the bad ones, especially the broad spectrum antibiotics. Yeasts also release TOXINS.

Illness comes when the immune system cannot cope with a particular strain of candida. Dr. Crook blames ANTIBIOTICS and GROWTH HORMONES administered to cattle. Dr. Truss blames PENICILLIN, BIRTH CONTROL PILLS, ANTI-ULCER MEDICATIONS, CORTISONE, and childhood IMMUNIZATIONS, which suppress the immune system's ability to fight yeast infections.

◆ *Impaired Liver Function*

Impaired liver function promotes candida overgrowth in mice. Presumably the same phenomenon occurs in humans. The toxins of candida are filtered from the blood by the liver. Symptoms of chronic candidiasis occurring outside the gastrointestinal tract, are strong indications that the liver is not filtering the blood sufficiently.

How To Heal Candida

✓ LACTOBACILLUS SUPPLEMENTATION—LACTOBACILLUS ACIDOPHILUS is the type of bacteria found in natural YOGURT. It has been shown to retard the growth of candida in culture media. It can also control this fungus in the intestines.

✓ HONEY—Honey is a strong antifungal agent. It contains HYDROGEN PEROXIDE, which explains its ANTICANDIDIASIS and ANTIBACTERIAL activities.

✓ GARLIC—Garlic has demonstrated significant antifungal activity against a wide range of fungi. It is especially active against candida albicans, and is more potent than NYSTATIN, GENTIAN VIOLET, and other reputed antifungal agents. It can be controlled by the use of odorless GARLIC pills or liquid in a half glass of water.

✓ BARBERRY—The common barberry plant has been used as a valuable anti-infective agent in folk medicine. Its therapeutic action is due to its high content of the alkaloid BERBERINE. Its action on candida albicans prevents the overgrowth of yeast that commonly follows antibiotic use.

✓ RAW VEGETABLES—According to one therapist the consumption of fresh vegetables from the CABBAGE FAMILY helps resist candidiasis infection.

✓ CHAMOMILE—It is said to contain several compounds that destroy candida.

✓ PAU D'ARCO TEA—It can be controlled by drinking PAU D'ARCO TEA, two glasses every day.

CATARACTS

Nature of The Disease

◆ *Cataracts Are Not A Normal Consequence Of Aging*

Cataract is the clouding or OPACITY of the CRYSTALLINE LENS of the eye. It is the leading cause of impaired vision or BLINDNESS in the U.S. Many factors contribute to it including OCULAR DISEASES, INJURY, SYSTEMIC DISEASES such as DIABETES, DRUGS, GALACTOSEMIA, TOXINS, ULTRAVIOLET LIGHT, RADIATION and LIGHT EXPOSURE, and HEREDITY. It is related to the inability of the body to maintain normal concentrations of SODIUM, POTASSIUM, and CALCIUM within the lens. These abnormalities are apparently the result of the decreased CELLULAR PUMP which pumps sodium out and potassium into the cell. SENILE CATARACT was once considered to be a normal part of the aging process. Now it is considered to be the result of a lifetime of MARGINAL MALNUTRITION.

◆ *Galactose Speeds Development*

Incomplete absorption of the milk sugar GALACTOSE provokes or speeds up the development of cataracts in some individuals. Elevated BLOOD SUGAR combined with impaired vitamin C absorption due to lack of insulin is considered responsible for the high proportion of cataracts among DIABETICS. Cataract TRIGGERS include SUNLIGHT, DIABETES, and STEROIDS.

The Diet For Cataracts

◆ *The Need For Vitamins*

Deficiencies of VITAMINS A, B, C, and E, and/or CALCIUM may also contribute to the formation of cataracts. The suggested dosages are 50,000 to 200,000 IU of vitamin A, 500 to 15,000 mg of vitamin C, plus 100 to 1000 mg of BIOFLAVONOIDS which not only enhance the action of vitamin C, but actually prevent the formation of cataracts. VITAMIN C DEFICIENCY has been implicated in the formation of cataracts.

✓ VITAMIN C—Vitamin C Is often mentioned in

connection with CATARACTS. In experiments with laboratory animals upon whom cataracts had been induced, the growth of cataracts was inhibited by increasing vitamin C intake.

The concentration of vitamin C in the AQUEOUS HUMOR, the liquid in the anterior and posterior chambers of the eye, is 30 to 50 times that of the serum of the body. In a lens with cataract it is greatly reduced or entirely absent. Clinical studies have demonstrated that vitamin C does indeed halt cataract progression. In a study of 450 patients with cataracts, they were placed in a nutritional program that included 1000 mg of vitamin C per day. It resulted in a significant reduction in cataract development.

✓ VITAMIN B_2—RIBOFLAVIN—Almost 100% cures have been achieved with cataracts, using VITAMIN B_2 therapy. Healing occurred in 24 to 48 hours. The vision cleared, and the burning, itching, redness, and tearing were gone, using 15 mg in tablet form and nothing else. These results were reported by Dr. Sydenstricker of the University of Georgia. He tested 24 patients, 18 of them had a noticeable white coating on their eyes. All the others had advanced cataracts. Foods containing vitamin B_2 are BROCCOLI, COLLARDS, TURNIP TOPS, BEETS, WHEAT GERM, PEANUTS, BREWERS YEAST, NUTS, and BEANS.

◆ *Enzymes And Amino Acids Are Needed*

There may be a need for 1000 mg of CALCIUM, and up to 1000 IU of natural vitamin D daily. Insufficient or poorly assimilated calcium is believed to be indirectly involved. Vitamin D is necessary for calcium absorption. Vitamin E up to 600 IU daily. Vitamin E therapy has cleared cataracts from the eyes of children in 6 months, and with the addition of selenium has been equally successful with adults. Besides the vitamins the lens is dependent like many other tissues in the body on enzymes such as SUPEROXIDE DISMUTASE (SOD), CATALASE, and GLUTATHIONE. Glutathione, composed of three amino acids, namely GLYCINE, GLUTAMIC ACID, and CYSTEINE, is found at very high concentrations in the lens. It is a key protective factor against toxins. It exists in reduced amounts in all forms of cataracts. GLUTATHIONE with its three amino acids has been shown to be of some benefit in cataract treatment. Its activity is speeded up by the eating of CRUCIFEROUS VEGETABLES. They contain chemicals called INDOLES which help the body neutralize and excrete certain CARCINOGENS.

There exists also an ancient Chinese herbal formula which has been shown to increase glutathione levels in the lens.

◆ *Selenium*

✓ DEFICIENCY CAN PRODUCE CATARACTS—SELENIUM as an antioxidant is known to function synergistically with vitamin E. The glutathione in the human lens has been shown to be selenium dependent, thereby suggesting that a selenium deficiency would promote cataract formation. The fact is that the selenium content of the human eye lens is only 15% of the normal levels when a cataract is present, suggesting that selenium is strongly involved in cataract formation. A lack of selenium, particularly when accompanied by a lack of vitamin E, has been linked to all types of CATARACTS, including those of diabetics. The suggestion is the use of 150 to 200 mcg daily.

✓ SEAFOOD IS HIGH IN SELENIUM—Seafood is extra high in the trace mineral selenium, and the evidence suggests that people who skimp on selenium are more apt to suffer THE BLUES.

✓ BRAZIL NUTS—They are said to be the richest of all foods in selenium, and eating a single nut a day will guarantee that you are never deficient in it. They are grown in selenium-rich soil.

◆ *Natural Foods*

The diet should include GREEN VEGETABLES, FRUITS, WHOLE GRAINS, and POLYUNSATURATED OILS. Also 2 glasses of VEGETABLE JUICE, one of CARROTS, and the other made up of a combination of vegetable juices. Dr. Rinse suggests two teaspoons each of BREWER'S YEAST, LECITHIN GRANULES, and RAW WHEAT GERM, with teaspoon of BONE MEAL and 2 teaspoons of UNSATURATED OIL. Increase consumption of LEGUMES or high sulfur-containing AMINO ACIDS, YELLOW VEGETABLES for CAROTENE, and vitamin C and

E-rich foods such as fresh fruits and vegetables.

One man said that his eyes were very painful and that a film was gathering over them. He remembered reading about the medicinal value of OLIVE OIL. He applied it to his eyes on and under the eyelids. He claimed that after 2 or 3 days, his sight was completely restored.

In a U.S. Department of Agriculture (USDA) study, people who reported eating fewer than 1 servings of fruit or less than 2 servings of vegetables a day, were 3 times more likely to develop CATARACTS. There is a lower risk of cataracts among people who got more of the antioxidant VITAMINS C and E.

◆ *Antioxidants And Herbs*

Dr. Joseph M. Friedman, O.D. also says that cataract is caused by the oxidative damage of FREE RADICALS. Avoid rancid foods and other sources of free radicals. An adequate amount of ANTIOXIDANTS can undo them. Scientists don't know for sure why the vitamins prevent cloudy formations in aging eyes, but some believe that vitamins C and E as antioxidants, neutralize damaging lens proteins before they can clump together.

Use EYE DROPS of cooled, strained CHAMOMILE TEA each night and morning. Also the use of CHAPARRAL tea taken internally is helpful. Experiments with horses has shown that LIQUID HONEY placed in the corner of the eye at night has cured their cataracts. It has been discovered that BILBERRY is good for the EYES, VEINS, and NERVES. Pilots who flew at night reported that eating bilberry jam helped them to see better. People who can benefit from bilberry are STUDENTS, TRUCK DRIVERS, PILOTS, those who look at COMPUTER MONITORS for long periods of time, and those who work in very DIM LIGHT or very BRIGHT LIGHT. The diseases that can be treated are CATARACTS, diabetic-induced GLAUCOMA, and MYOPIA.

CIRCULATORY PROBLEMS

The Purification Of The Blood

◆ *Blood Is The Current Of Life*

"In order to have good health, we must have good blood; for blood is the current of life. It repairs waste and nourishes the body.... the more perfect the circulation, the better this work will be accomplished" (CD91). Lev. 17:11 tells us: "For the life of the flesh is in the blood." So blood in the Bible is equated with life. This principle can be applied both physically and spiritually. "The power of God is manifested in the beating of the heart, in the action of the lungs, and in the living currents that circulate through the thousand different channels of the body" (SD17).

◆ *Causes Of Impure Blood*

✓ LACK OF OXYGEN—"An insufficient supply of oxygen is received. The blood moves sluggishly. The waste, poisonous matter, which should be thrown off in the exhalations from the lungs, is retained, and the blood becomes impure."

✓ MEAT EATING—"The simple grains, fruits of the trees, vegetables, have all the nutritive properties necessary to make good blood. This a flesh diet cannot do." (CD322). "Few can be made to believe that it is the meat they have eaten which has poisoned their blood and caused their suffering" (CH115).

✓ IMPOVERISHED DIET—"Some are unable to obtain the most desirable foods, and instead of using such things as would best supply the lack, they adopt an impoverished diet. Their food does not supply the elements to make good blood" (MH318).

✓ DRUGS—"In our sanitariums, we advocate the use of simple remedies. We discourage the use of drugs, for they poison the current of the blood" (2SM280).

✓ OVEREATING—"Indulging in eating too frequently, and in too large quantities, overtaxes the digestive organs, and produces a feverish state of the system. The blood becomes impure, and then diseases of various kinds occur" (CD189).

✓ MILK-SUGAR—"Large quantities of milk and sugar eaten together are injurious. They impart impurities to the system" (2T369).

✓ FRUITS-VEGETABLES—"Fruits and vegetables taken at one meal produce acidity of the stomach; then impurity of the blood results"(CD113).

- ✓ CONDIMENTS and SPICES—"Condiments are injurious in their nature. MUSTARD, PEPPER, SPICES, PICKLES, and other things of like character, irritate the stomach and make the blood feverish and impure" (CD339). Also FLESH MEATS, BUTTER, CHEESE, and RICH PASTRY the blood-making organs cannot convert into good blood. (CH114). "Soon ordinary food does not satisfy the appetite. The system feels a want, a craving, for something more stimulating" (MH325).

◆ *Impure Blood And A Wrong Diet*

Impure blood is basically caused by a wrong diet. Eating wrong combinations of foods at the same meal causes fermentation. Often the very elements that would keep the blood pure are removed from especially the processed foods. Examples are the WHEAT GERM and BRAN from WHEAT, the PEELINGS of POTATOES, the BRAN of RICE, the HEART of the CORN taken out of the CORNMEAL. We are told that "If the physical heart is healthy, the blood that is sent from it through the system is also healthy, but if the fountain is impure, the whole organism becomes diseased by the poison of the vital fluid" (2T210).

◆ *Symptoms Of Impure Blood*

Symptoms of impure blood are complaints such as PIMPLES, BOILS, ACNE. SKIN DISCOLORATION, JAUNDICE, HEADACHES, DROWSINESS, WRINKLES, LOOKING OLD WHEN YOUNG, PREMATURE GRAY HAIR, STIFF JOINTS, and PAIN in various parts of the body. All of these symptoms will vanish to a great extent when the blood is purified.

How To Purify The Blood

◆ *Teas, Juices, And Other Methods For Purifying The Blood*

Herb teas for purifying the blood are:

- ☛ Make a combination tea by using cup of red clover, cup of alfalfa, cup of CHAPARRAL.
- ☛ ECHINACEA—This tea is a remedy for combating MORBIDITY of the blood, ABSCESSES, CARBUNCLES, and TOXEMIA. It is also regarded as a natural blood ANTITOXIN, whenever the bloodstream becomes impure.
- ☛ GINKGO TREE—The leaves of this tree have increased blood flow to the BRAIN, NERVE SIGNAL TRANSMISSION, FREE RADICAL SCAVENGING ACTIVITY, CELLULAR ENERGY PRODUCTION, PROTECTION AGAINST STROKE, PREMATURE AGING. Its use appears to improve MEMORY, IMMUNITY, CIRCULATORY ILLS, MENTAL ENERGY, and ATTENTIVENESS, INTERMITTENT CLAUDICATION, which is a spasm in the artery causing muscle cramping in the leg.
- ☛ DANDELION, ELDER, SASSAFRAS, SARSAPARILLA, and other teas.
- ☛ CARROT, BEET, and other vegetable and fruit juices
- ☛ Eliminate all harmful articles of FOOD and DRINK including all white flour products, all cane sugar products, the excess use of oil. Use an herbal laxative to cleanse the BOWELS.
- ☛ Drink plenty of pure WATER.
- ☛ EXERCISE outdoors with deep breathing.
- ☛ Get plenty of SLEEP in a room ventilated by fresh outdoor air.
- ☛ Keep the SKIN active with cold morning BATHS, and rub the skin vigorously with a towel or brush.
- ☛ Go on as FRUIT DIET for one week

◆ *How To Maintain Pure Blood*

Since the blood carries oxygen to all parts of the body, it is important that the lungs take in a constant supply of pure air. Such action assists the circulation of the blood and thereby "invigorates the whole system, excites the appetite, induces sound, sweet sleep, thus not only refreshing the body, but soothing and tranquilizing the mind" (Ed 198). It means that deep breathing must be engaged in, and where can this be done better than through EXERCISE in the OPEN AIR. We are told that "work performed in the open air is tenfold more beneficial to health than indoor labor.... vigorous exercise causes full, deep, strong inspirations and exhalations, which expand the lungs and purify the blood, sending the warm current of life bounding through arteries and veins" (FE73).

◆ *Bathing*

BATHING is an activity which should be engaged at least twice a week, for we are told that "Those who are not in health have IMPURITIES of the BLOOD, and the SKIN is not in a healthy condition.... The bath is a soother of the nerves. It promotes general perspiration, quickens the circulation, overcomes obstructions in the system, and acts beneficially on the KIDNEYS and URINARY organs" (3T70).

The Equalization Of The Blood

◆ *Health Demands Blood Equalization*

To have health the circulation of the blood must be equalized throughout the body. Speaking of ministers and teachers we are told: "The proper use of their physical strength, as well as of the mental powers, will equalize the circulation of the blood, and keep every organ of the living machinery in running order"(FE321). "By INDULGING the APPETITE in eating rich and highly seasoned foods.... The circulation of the blood is not equalized, and becomes impure. The whole system is deranged, and the demands of appetite become more unreasonable, craving exciting, hurtful things, until it is thoroughly depraved" (2SM420).

◆ *The Right And Left Sides Must Have Equal Blood Pressure*

In many people there is a wide difference between the blood pressure on the left side and the right side or the left arm and the right arm. That is why when blood pressure is measured, it should be measured on both arms to determine if there is a difference. Health depends upon both arms exhibiting the same pressure. In many people there is a wide difference between the blood pressure on the left side and on the right side. A healthy person has the same blood pressure in both arms and both legs. In some people the difference is as much as 30 points.

When Al. Wolfsen measured the blood pressure of different people, he found some men with equal blood pressure on both sides, but no women, even though he figured that women in general were healthier than men. One woman came into his office who had the same blood pressure on both arms and both legs. He asked her a straight forward personal embarrassing question which was, "What kind of underwear do you wear?" She blushed a bit and then said, "Well, I'll tell you, I wear a man's long-handled underwear." The reason he found fewer women with equalized blood pressure is because they expose their arms and legs more often to the outside cold air than men. Men wear trousers and women wear stockings, and even when they put on the overcoat, their lower legs are still somewhat exposed.

◆ *The Extremities Must Be Kept As Warm As Rest Of Body*

"Perfect health depends upon perfect circulation" (2T531). Special attention should be given to the extremities, that they may be as thoroughly clothed as the chest and the region over the heart, where is the greatest amount of heat. Parents who dress their children with the extremities naked, or nearly so, are sacrificing the health and lives of their children to fashion. If these parts are not so warm as the body, the circulation is not equalized.

When one is exposed to cold for extensive periods of time, the body will conserve its heat for the benefit of the vital organs, by reducing the BLOOD CIRCULATION to the extremities. This leaves the nose, fingers, ears, and toes exposed and vulnerable to FROSTBITE. The areas that are then affected will FEEL COLD, will ACHE and TINGLE, and may REDDEN. When the extremities which are remote from the vital organs, are not properly clad, the blood is driven to the head, causing headache or nosebleed; or there is a sense of fullness about the chest, producing cough or palpitation of the heart, on account of too much blood in that locality; or the stomach has too much blood, causing indigestion. "The limbs were not formed by our Creator to endure exposure, as was the face....

"Satan invented the fashions which leave the limbs exposed, chilling back the life current from its original course. And parents bow at the shrine of fashion and so clothe their children that the nerves and veins become contracted and do not answer the purpose that God designed they should. The result is habitually cold feet and hands. Those parents who follow fashion instead of reason will have an account to render to God for thus robbing their children of health. Even life is frequently sacrificed to the god of fashion" (2T531–2). People should not sit or walk around with cold feet. They should put on several pairs of socks if necessary. Some say that of the diseases that women suffer from are caused by cold arms and legs. Feel your ANKLES, WRISTS, and FOREHEAD. Ankles and wrists should be of the same temperature as your forehead. If they are not, then you have unequal distribution of blood.

◆ *Women Should Cover Their Limbs As Thoroughly As Men*

The solution to this problem of the extremities has been given us in (2SM479) where it says: "Whatever may be the length of the dress, females should clothe their limbs as thoroughly as the males. This may be done by wearing lined pants gathered into a band and fastened about the ankle, or made full and tapering at the bottom; and these should come down long enough to meet the shoe. The limbs and ankles thus clothed are protected against a current of air. If the limbs and feet are kept comfortable with warm clothing, the circulation will be equalized, and the blood will remain healthy and pure, because it is not chilled or hindered in its natural passage through the system." LAMBS WOOL UNDERWEAR is the best underwear. It is good against cold and heat. Eze. 34:3 says: "Ye clothe you with WOOL."

◆ *A Cold Shower Will Keep You Warm All Day*

People who worked on a major project outdoors in a cold climate were asked how they kept warm. They said that they were freezing all the time until they learned to take a COLD SHOWER EVERY MORNING. They said that it would keep them warm all day. Studies also show that taking massive amounts of vitamin C, at least 1500 mg for each 65 lbs. of body weight, will help the body maintain its normal temperature to prevent HYPOTHERMIA, the lowering of body temperature, and FROSTBITE.

◆ *Cayenne Pepper For Cold Feet*

For cold feet take red cayenne pepper, wet feet slightly and put cayenne pepper all over them before you put socks or stockings on. You will have warm feet all day. The CAYENNE PEPPER will not blister your feet.

COLDS AND FLU

The Nature Of The Diseases

◆ *They Represent A Body's Toxic Overload*

A natural practitioner regards COLDS and FLU as the means by which the body strives to rid itself of a toxic overload which it cannot get rid of in any other way. It is the result of inadequate habits of eating and living, strain and tension, while at the same time getting insufficient air, outdoor exercise, rest, and sleep. Eventually, the overworked eliminative channels such as the KIDNEYS, BOWELS, SKIN, and LUNGS are unable to cope with the situation, and a desperate cleaning process is set in motion in the form of a COLD or a bout of INFLUENZA. The difference between the two is that the flu has in addition to a cold also the symptoms of a FEVER and a HEADACHE. The reaction is set off when the person is CHILLED or OVERTIRED. Mrs. White says: "The more perfect our health, the more perfect will be our labor. When we overtax our strength, and become EXHAUSTED, we are liable to take cold, and at such times there is danger of disease assuming a dangerous form." (3T13)

◆ *A Cold Is Nature's Cleansing Agency*

The cold is nature's simplest and often-used CLEANSING AGENCY. It is a NATURAL ELIMINATIVE MEASURE. It is nature's way of removing toxic wastes from the system. Wastes attract germs because the wastes are food for the germs. If the viruses had nothing to feed on they would not produce any disease symptoms. Although it is true that a cold can be transmitted by means of viruses, it is only because individuals are in a food-clogged state, and are in need of systematic cleansing. When we cleanse the body of impurities through a diet of RAW VEGETABLES, FRUITS, and their JUICES, the cause of a cold is removed. When we remove IMPURITIES we also remove GERMS, because we remove the food which they feed and multiply on. Dr. J. H. Tilden said: "A cold is an elimination of toxins through the MUCOUS MEMBRANE." The COLD is responsible for more visits to the doctor than any other disease, and the HEADACHE is in 2nd place.

The Causes Of A Cold

◆ *Virus Containing Mucous Blocks The Passages*

Congestion and drainage is one of the first signs of a cold. When we take decongestant drugs, we are shrinking swollen blood vessels which decreases mucous production and makes it easier for us to breathe. But the blood flow is a part of the body's healing process which brings white blood cells to the site to help destroy the viruses. ANTIHISTAMINES are sometimes used for a cold. What they do is to dry up the secretions and the runny nose. However, the mucous secretion from the nose is the body's attempt to remove mucous and with it the viruses that cause the cold. Stopping this process only allows the viruses more time to increase their number. Hence, we should allow the mucous to flow freely out of the body in order to help eliminate the viruses that had a part in producing the condition in the first place. Blowing the nose gets rid of a lot of mucous. One may also use steam inhalation to which EUCALYPTUS, PEPPERMINT, or CAMPHOR have been added. This will open the passages and allow the individual to breathe.

◆ *Waste, not Viruses, are the Primary Cause Of a Cold*

The person who is perfectly clean inside through healthful living will not be able to "catch" a cold. Infection can only occur when one's body is in a toxic state. Viruses act as superficial agents, and they can only gain a foothold in the body when it is in a toxic condition. They represent SECONDARY AGENTS. They are scavengers which invade cells and live and multiply on WASTE PRODUCTS which are located there. It is the TOXIC "SOIL" which is the real cause of the cold, for it represents to the viruses their fertile soil upon which they can propagate themselves and remain in the body unless a body cleansing process can eliminate THE TOXINS, and with them the viruses.

◆ *Drugs Stop Natures Effort At House Cleaning*

DRUGS will stop nature's effort at house cleaning, and drive the poisons back into the tissues so as to later develop other more serious diseases. Nature gives us a warning in the form MUCOUS ELIMINATION. Mucous represents the secretion of too much accumulated waste. The body also does away with the viruses by rinsing them away, by sending extra amounts of BLOOD to the diseased area, by increasing body temperature thus producing a FEVER which burns waste matter more quickly. It sends WHITE BLOOD CELLS and ANTIBODIES to the area to capture the viruses and send them out of the system. We are told that "drug takers are never well. They are always taking cold, which causes extreme suffering, because of the poison all through their system" (4SGa 137–8). Furthermore, normal COLD REMEDIES give only symptomatic relief.

◆ *The Mucous Membranes Become Eliminative Organs*

It is said that 3 to 4 pounds of waste matter exudes through the pores of the skin of an adult every 24 hours. While the pores are closed, these exudations cannot pass through. But what causes the pores to close up? The normal temperature of the blood is said to be 98.6 degrees Fahrenheit. The question now is: "What keeps the blood at this temperature when the surrounding atmosphere varies all the time?" It is accomplished largely by the PORES of the skin. When the temperature of the blood begins to rise, the pores open in order to cool the blood. When the surrounding atmosphere begins to cool, the pores close in order to keep the blood from the cold environment. After the pores have closed, the wastes can no longer pass out through the pores, and must be sent elsewhere. Some may be sent to the lungs, and some to the kidneys for elimination. But if the amount is so great that these eliminating organs cannot take care of it all, the balance is deposited in the porous tissues and cavities of the body, principally in the THROAT, BRONCHIAL TUBES, and LUNGS. Now the mucous membranes become eliminative organs.

◆ *A Cold Results When Pores Stay Closed*

Mrs. White says about one lady who had limited the air in her room: "The surface of the skin is nearly dead because she has no air to breathe. Its million little mouths are closed, because they are clogged by the impurities of the system, and for want of air. The effects produced in living in close, ill-ventilated rooms are these: The system becomes weak and unhealthy, the circulation is depressed, the blood moves sluggishly through the system because it is not purified and vitalized by the pure invigorating air of heaven. The mind becomes depressed and gloomy, while the whole system is enervated; and fevers and other acute diseases are liable to be generated. The system is peculiarly sensitive to the influence of COLD" (1T701–3).

◆ *Open Pores With A Warm Bath*

The opening of the pores can be accomplished with a WARM BATH. We are told that "Scrupulous cleanliness is essential to both physical and mental health. Impurities are constantly being thrown off from the body through the skin. Its million of pores are quickly clogged unless kept clean by frequent bathing, and the impurities which should pass off through the skin become an additional burden to the other eliminating organs. A bath properly taken, fortifies against a cold, because it improves the circulation (MH276).

◆ *Overeating Causes Colds*

A cold is often initiated when a clogged system is suddenly shocked by a cold temperature. OVEREATING during the Christmas season causes more sickness than at any other time of the year. The liver and kidneys are overloaded. The thyroid gland comes to the rescue by helping to flush out poison through the mucous membranes, causing a runny nose. The most obvious way to remedy the situation is to relieve the strain by instituting a period of FASTING.

◆ *Why We Get A Cold Mainly In Cold Weather*

The reason a cold strikes mainly in winter is because there is less opportunity for vigorous exercise. Heavy clothing blocks the pores and keeps them from breathing effectively, and develops a poor functioning skin. Lack of exercise as well as the lack of heat keeps us from sweating. There is the tendency to eat more mucous-forming foods such as starches, sweets, milk, and ice-cream, and to drink less water. The inhalation of dust, smoke, and smog. More chronic constipation. Being cold or wet. An overacid blood. Getting chilled. "Leaving arms and limbs insufficiently protected could cause a cold, disease, and premature deaths" (2SM471). When the skin is chilled the pores close, ELIMINATION OF WASTE MATERIAL through the skin is STOPPED. As a result so many more impurities stay within the system, and decrease the resistance of the body in general.

◆ *The Flu*

The flu has two major types of viruses, namely A and B. B is the less virulent of the two. With the flu the trademark is a generally HIGH FEVER around 101° F or higher in young children. High fever is what the common cold usually lacks. Flu is also characterized by a sore throat, a dry cough, chills, weakness, loss of appetite, aching of the head, back, arms, and legs. We must make drastic changes in our diet in order to escape the effect of the flu virus. The herbs CAYENNE, GARLIC, GINGER, and THYME are antioxidants which are high in sulfur and copper. They help to reduce the severity of the flu.

How A Cold Can Be Cured.

◆ *Is A Cold Curable?*

Orthodox doctors say that a cold is incurable. If you take medicine for it, it will last about a week. If you take nothing for it, it will last about 7 days. There is no cure for the common cold, for the cold itself is the cure. The cold is cleansing the body to put it back into a healthy state. If you use drugs to treat the cold, it would be a suppressive method of treatment. Hygienists say that they have many cures for a cold. The development of a cold after exposure is determined to a large extent by the state of health of a person. If the body of a person is relatively internally clean, then for a cold he may experience nothing more than a sore throat. But if the pores of the skin are closed for extended periods he may get the FLU or even PNEUMONIA, and all this happens because the pores closed in order to protect the bloodstream.

◆ *The Use Of Herbs*

One doctor made a brew of teaspoon of CAYENNE PEPPER, the juice of one LEMON, one minced clove of GARLIC, and 1 gm of vitamin C to be sipped slowly as his recipe for a cold.

A person from Alaska said: "When our children get runny noses, coughs, nosebleeds, or just colds in general, I make GARLIC TEA and give it to them quite hot. The next day they have no stopped-up heads. This is also good for SINUS HEADACHES. I then repeat this every hour for sinus trouble or pneumonia. Smashed GARLIC in the vaporizer has proved successful for both chest and head congestion for children and adults as well."

A lady from New York said: "I awoke one morning with a fever. One gland in my neck was swollen, and my throat was so sore I could hardly swallow. I started taking GARLIC CAPSULES, three of them three times a day. By the next morning, the fever was gone, the gland was no longer swollen, and my sore throat was completely gone. Since then my children have used garlic in treatment of various virus or cold symptoms with excellent results, usually clearing problems within a day or two." GARLIC OIL combined with ONION JUICE, diluted with water and drunk several times a day, is effective against FLU, SORE THROAT, and RHINITIS.

For a sore throat — CAYENNE PEPPER; To increase sweating — BLUE VERVAIN TEA; For chest colds — SMARTWEED boiled in water and used in fomentations; for a cough — HOREHOUND TEA; For a fever — SAGE TEA.; for enhancing the immune system — ECHINACEA, HOREHOUND, GOLDENSEAL, ROSEHIPS, PEPPERMINT, and CHAMOMILE teas.

HOT FOOT BATH — increases the blood flow from the feet to the entire skin surface. It promotes decongestion in the head, chest, and is used to treat headaches.

◆ *Aromatherapy*

Aromatherapy will combat the unpleasant stuffiness that inevitably accompanies a cold. Add 3 drops of EUCALYPTUS, PINE, CLOVE, or THYME OIL to one quart of hot water. Hold a towel over your head to create a tent over the vapor and inhale for 10 minutes. Repeat as often as 3 times a day. A common vaporizer will do the trick also.

Thyme oil is 8 times stronger than PHENOL in its antiseptic action, and will not damage tissues as phenol does.

The Treatment Of A Cold And Flu

- Stay in bed and keep warm
- FAST; consume no solid foods until the fever is gone
- Take large doses of VITAMIN C, preferably in natural form. Doses of 500 mg to 1000 mg every hour will rapidly neutralize bacterial or viral toxins, and will bring the fever down within hours. Vitamin C has only a small value against colds in small amounts. The amount of protection increases with increased amounts, and becomes almost complete with 4 to 10 gm per day. If you increase your intake 10 fold, the concentration in the blood will become 10 times as great.
- Induce perspiration by drinking warm drinks made of CITRUS JUICES sweetened with honey.
- Take hot BATHS.
- Don't take fever suppressing drugs such as ASPIRIN. Aspirin has been shown to increase the number of viruses; to lower the body's production of INTERFERON, and to stop vitamin C from getting into the white blood cells which fight infection.

How To Prevent A Cold

◆ *Cod Liver Oil*

During a cold VITAMIN A levels in the body drop. This is a sign that vitamin A is used up at a faster rate. Mothers throughout the world have known that a daily spoonful of COD LIVER OIL, a rich source of vitamins A and D prevents colds. Vitamin A or beta-carotene has demonstrated significant immune enhancing action. Originally known as the "anti-infective" vitamin, it plays an essential role in maintaining the integrity of the lining of the respiratory tract and its secretions. It also demonstrates a potent virus killing activity.

◆ *Diet*

Dr. Pauling said: "I believe that most colds can be prevented or largely ameliorated by control of the diet without the use of any drugs." Mrs. White says: "I wish we were all HEALTH REFORMERS. I am opposed to the use of pastries. These mixtures are unhealthful; no one can have good digestive powers and a clear brain who will eat largely of sweet cookies and cream cake and all kinds of pies, and partake of a variety of food at one meal. When we do this and then take cold, the whole system is so clogged and enfeebled that it has no power of re-

Vitamin C

A dose of 100 to 1000 mg of vitamin C per day is recommended to prevent getting a cold. This enhances the WHITE BLOOD CELL production, increases INTERFERON levels, and increases the integrity of the CONNECTIVE TISSUE.

Dr. Ritzel made a study of school boys taking 1000 mg of VITAMIN C daily. He reported a decrease in the number of colds by 45%, and a decrease in the number of days of illness by 30%.

Dr. Pauling's studies indicate that individuals taking 70 to 200 mg of vitamin C daily averaged a decrease in illness per person of 31%, in comparison with PLACEBO SUBJECTS. Those taking more than 200 mg averaged 40% less illness.

Fresh Fruits And Vegetables

More fresh fruits and vegetables and their juices should be eaten during the winter months to prevent a cold from coming on. More attention must be paid to keeping the body clean, since normal conditions of cold, lack of exercise, lack of swimming, and heavy clothing, have more of an influence upon our bodily condition, so as to make it less likely for a cleansing action to be brought about.

CRAMPS

Causes Of Cramps

✓ LACK OF VITAMINS AND MINERALS—Cramps are usually due to vitamin and mineral deficiencies, particularly CALCIUM, POTASSIUM, MAGNESIUM, and VITAMINS D and B_6. The deficiency may also be due to the fact that while the diet may contain sufficient vitamins and minerals, for various reasons the body may be unable to assimilate these nutrients from the diet.

✓ OXYGEN DEFICIENCY—Cramps due to oxygen deficiency will be helped with VITAMINS C and E in large doses.

✓ SALT DEPLETION—Exercising in heat and humidity can cause cramps from a depletion of SALT.

✓ UNACCUSTOMED EXERCISE—MUSCULAR CONTRACTIONS and STIFFNESS caused by unaccustomed exercise can be prevented by taking 500 mg VITAMIN C before, each hour or so during, and immediately after the strenuous activity.

How To Heal Cramps

Muscle Spasms

Muscle spasms can be helped with extra POTASSIUM in the diet such as that from bananas. Nerve impulses are conducted by minerals. Hence, any deficiency or imbalance of CALCIUM, MAGNESIUM, PHOSPHORUS, POTASSIUM ETC. can cause muscle spasms. In general muscle spasms are believed to be due to vitamin and mineral deficiencies.

Menstrual Cycle Cramps

Cramps associated with the MENSTRUAL CYCLE and MENOPAUSE can be due to SEX HORMONE influence on calcium metabolism, as well as due to ENDOCRINE INSUFFICIENCY. It can be helped with extra vitamins E, B_{12}, B_6, and RIBONUCLEIC ACID. Also teas made of SARSAPARILLA and LICORICE are helpful, because they are natural sources of SEX HORMONES.

According to biochemists and orthomolecular physicians, most menstrual and menopausal difficulties are caused by nutritional deficiencies that can be corrected within a few months with NATURAL REMEDIES. Most women need to fortify their diet with additional iron, and extra vitamin C to absorb the iron and the B-complex vitamins to help build the blood. Additional amounts of vitamins B_6 and C are required when ORAL CONTRACEPTIVES are used. The amount of calcium in a woman's blood decreases before and during menstruation. Menstrual blood is 40 times higher in calcium than normal blood. The calcium and iron lost during menstruation must be replaced. CALCIUM DEFICIENCY is one of the causes of CRAMPS. Many menstrual difficulties are due to a shortage of MAGNESIUM which must be present in order for the body to utilize vitamin B_6 and calcium.

Leg Cramps

✓ RESTLESS LEG SYNDROME—Leg Cramps

are often relieved with VITAMIN B$_6$ and added CALCIUM. The RESTLESS LEG SYNDROME are nighttime leg cramps or jerking that can be relieved with supplements of CALCIUM and VITAMIN E, which usually resolve this problem in a matter of weeks, but additional vitamins and minerals may be necessary. NOCTURNAL LEG CRAMPS can also be due to LOW BLOOD SUGAR or HYPOGLYCEMIA.

✓ INTERMITTENT CLAUDICATION—The leg cramps suffered by women during PREGNANCY, MENSTRUATION, or MENOPAUSE can frequently be relieved by taking 1000 mg CALCIUM, 500 mg MAGNESIUM, 400 IU VITAMIN D, 400 to 800 IU of vitamin E, and 50 to 150 mg VITAMIN B$_6$. VITAMIN B-COMPLEX tablets or BREWERS YEAST are also helpful.

INTERMITTENT CLAUDICATION are LEG CRAMPS and PAIN that occur during walking but not while resting. It is caused by narrowed blood vessels providing insufficient oxygen-rich blood to the legs. Large amounts of VITAMIN E often correct this condition in a matter of months; particularly when VITAMIN C and LECITHIN are added. Some cases have improved after one month of taking 1600 IU of VITAMIN E daily. Taking 25 mcg of SELENIUM with each 200 IU of vitamin E is said to increase its effectiveness.

✓ BUERGER'S DISEASE—If left untreated, reduced circulation can result in BUERGER'S DISEASE, an inflammation of the blood vessels with clot formation. Even more vitamin E is then indicated, along with a week's bed rest to help dissolve the blood clots, and to prevent gangrene from setting in.

In general, for cramps avoid ANTACIDS, DIURETICS, TRANQUILIZERS, or other medications that can upset the mineral balance.

◆ *Other Diet Suggestions*

✓ SOURED MILK PRODUCTS—Eat green vegetables, fruits, and soured milk products, such as YOGURT, KEFIR, and CLABBERED milk.

✓ MILLET is the best cereal

✓ ALMOND and SESAME SEED MILK—One cup of almond nuts or sesame seeds, or cup of each, with 4 cups of water, one tablespoon of HONEY liquefied in the blender, becomes an excellent source of MINERALS and PROTEIN.

✓ SUPPLEMENTS—CALCIUM LACTATE TABLETS, COD LIVER OIL, 100 MG VITAMIN B$_6$, 400 to 1000 IU vitamin E.

✓ JUICES—GRAPE and PRUNE, CARROT, BEET, and CUCUMBER are especially beneficial for muscular health. APPLE and most other fruit juices improve the absorption of CALCIUM. A TIC or TWITCH may indicate POTASSIUM DEPLETION resulting from overingestion of sugar.

✓ HERBS—DANDELION, ALFALFA, CAYENNE, CATNIP, COMFREY, LICORICE, MINT, and PARSLEY

CRIB DEATH—SUDDEN INFANT DEATH SYNDROME (SIDS)

Crib Deaths Occur With Bottle-fed Babies

◆ *Due To A Magnesium Deficiency*

About of all crib deaths involve babies who are born prematurely. Yet when they die they have been gaining weight very rapidly and show no particular sign of weakness.

Most crib deaths, in fact almost all of them occur with babies who have been bottle fed and not breast-fed. Bottle fed babies are said to receive less usable magnesium than breast-fed babies. Hence, the theory is that crib deaths are due to a MAGNESIUM DEFICIENCY. Prematurely born infants are very low in magnesium, for the magnesium level rises sharply during the last period of gestation, and their subsequent rapid growth may exhaust their stores of magnesium, as the mineral is used up in the building up of protein. Magnesium deficiency cannot occur unless the mother is magnesium deficient. Animal studies show that when the maternal magnesium stores are borderline, the mother will retain what she needs and thereby shortchange the embryo.

With crib death magnesium deficiency is

blamed because such a deficiency triggers the liberation of HISTAMINE, which is the substance responsible for the swelling and irritation of delicate membranes of the respiratory tract in people suffering from hay fever or other allergies.

◆ *SIDS—A Biotin Deficiency*

A very common sign in the babies before they die is blueness of the skin, along with cold hands and feet, an indication of lack of oxygen, and difficulty in breathing. It is a form of ANAPHYLACTIC SHOCK, which means that the person subject to it is very allergic to a foreign protein or substance. It may also occur from a bee sting.

It is therefore suggested that SIDS may be a BIOTIN DEFICIENCY. It is also suggested that marginally chickens die when subjected even to mild stress. There are low levels of biotin in their livers, and supplementation with biotin eliminates the problem. It is said that a certain amount of BIOTIN is lost in the manufacture of infant formulas.

◆ *SIDS Occurs In Animals As Well As Humans*

The SIDS syndrome occurs in animals as well as in infants. A study of pigs in New Zealand gives an indication that crib deaths may be a DEFICIENCY SYNDROME. It was found that vitamin E deficiencies in young pigs will cause sudden death. This may also be true of infants. Very few babies, even partially breast-fed during the first five months of life are known to die in this manner. Breast-fed babies get plenty of vitamin E, while infants fed on cow's milk get very little. After vitamin E was given to the pigs the fatalities ceased.

SIDS Is An Allergic Reaction To Cow's Milk

◆ *Cow's Milk Protein Difficult To Digest*

Dr. Stowens of Louisville Medical School Children's Hospital, a coroner, came to the conclusion that crib deaths are due to an allergic reaction to cow's milk, or to an anaphylactic shock. The body produces antibodies to fight against the type of protein which it cannot absorb. It is these antibodies which produce a sudden shock reaction which results in death. Crib death never occurs in infants who are totally BREAST FED, and seldom even when they are partly breast fed and partly formula. It is because some infants do not digest the PROTEIN in COW'S MILK, but absorb it whole from the intestinal tract. This sensitizes them, causing kidney damage without any outward sign.

◆ *Due To Lack Of Vitamin E In Cow's Milk*

The critical point relates to a vitamin E level between human and cow's milk. Of 2500 crib death infants only 3 were raised on mother's milk. Human milk contains an average of 1.14 mg of vitamin E per quart, while cow's milk averages from .21 mg in early spring to a maximum of 1.06 mg per quart in mid fall. It is in the winter months when vitamin E levels in cow's milk are at their lowest that most crib deaths occur. The vital function of vitamin E is to combine with polyunsaturated-unsaturated fatty acids to prevent the formation of TOXIC PEROXIDES within the metabolism. Vitamin E keeps a greater oxygen supply in the system, by keeping other substances from combining with oxygen.

SIDS May Be Due To DPT Vaccinations

Dr. William Torch, of the University of Nevada, came to the conclusion that the DIPHTHERIA-PERTUSSIS-TETANUS shots, or DPT, may be the cause of SIDS. It was found that of 103 children who died of SIDS had been immunized with a DPT vaccine within 3 weeks before their deaths. There were many who died within a day after getting the shot. He believes that this was no mere coincidence, but that a causal relationship is indicated.

In 1983, the UCLA School of Medicine, reported a study of 145 SIDS deaths. It happened soon after DPT vaccinations had been given. It was found that 27 cases died within 28 days after being immunized; 17 died within a week and 6 within 24 hours after receiving the shot. Despite these happenings, DPT vaccinations are still continuing throughout the country.

DIABETES

Nature Of The Disease

◆ *An Imbalance Of Alpha And Beta Cells*

In DIABETES the alpha and beta cells of the ISLETS of LANGERHANS in the PANCREAS are out of balance. The beta cells secrete INSULIN, while the alpha cells secrete GLUCAGON which triggers the turning of GLYCOGEN in the liver into GLUCOSE for release into the bloodstream. The alpha and beta cells are supposed to check and balance each other. When too much sugar is absorbed, the pancreas become worn out and produce too little insulin. Insulin needs tiny amounts of CHROMIUM so as to lead glucose through the cell walls. Hence, a deficiency of chromium can lead to diabetes. This means that diabetes can be caused by eating a chromium impoverished diet which may be largely caused by the food refining process.

One adrenal gland hormone called EPINEPHRINE, which is released under stress, increases free fatty acids in the bloodstream, and shuts off the release of insulin, so that continued stress can invite diabetes. Similarly, OBESITY is a stress that also invites diabetes. There is then too much tissue for the insulin to service. When the body FAT competes with the MUSCLES for insulin, the fat usually wins. This means that carbohydrates are changed into still more fat.

◆ *Types Of Diabetes*

Diabetes is a disorder of CARBOHYDRATE, FAT, and PROTEIN metabolism. It is characterized by elevations of fasting glucose levels and a greatly increased risk of ATHEROSCLEROSIS, KIDNEY DISEASE, and a LOSS of NERVE FUNCTION. The SYMPTOMS of diabetes are INCREASED THIRST, ABNORMAL DISCHARGE of pale and watery URINE, WEAKNESS and DROWSINESS, and abnormal amounts of SUGAR in the URINE and BLOOD.

✓ TYPE I—JUVENILE DIABETES—due to a heredity viral attack which knocks out the PANCREAS which produces the INSULIN. Hence, such an individual is totally dependent on a supply of external insulin. Here one has to depend on extra insulin injections to get the blood sugar down to normal. This type of diabetes usually strikes at PUBERTY, hence the term "juvenile." It affects about 10% of all diabetics.

✓ TYPE II—ADULT ONSET DIABETES—is caused by a buildup of glucose outside the cells which cannot enter the cells. It is sometimes called SUGAR-DIABETES, for the URINE of such a person is sweet. This fact led to the discovery of diabetes, for it was found that the urine of diabetics attracted ants. 90% of 16 mil. diabetics in the U.S. have this type. This is half of all of the diabetics in the world. It is thought that largely excess FAT CONSUMPTION brings this about. This type can be controlled by DIET, WEIGHT CONTROL, and EXERCISE. It is said that NATURAL FOODS can reverse this disease in less than 2 months. SDA's have less than half the mortality rate from diabetes than have other Americans.

✓ INSULIN—Insulin acts as a bridge which allows the sugar in food to go from the bloodstream into the body cells where it is assimilated as energy for the body. If there is not enough insulin to accommodate all of the cells, or if the passage is partially obstructed, sugar accumulates and begins to form a bottleneck. SEDENTARY PERSONS require much more insulin than those who are ACTIVE. WHITE SUGAR does not have the raw materials required for the manufacture of insulin. With its extensive use insulin production may be greatly reduced or stopped altogether. Then DIABETES has arrived. This dreadful disease is prevalent in direct proportion to the intake of both REFINED SUGAR and FLOUR. Diabetes was unknown before the appearance of food refinement.

As long as excess insulin floats around in the system, the body cannot burn fat. One can't burn excess sugar that has been placed in storage as fat. This stored fat produces more cholesterol, and eventually cholesterol leads to DEGENERATIVE HEART DISEASE. This accelerated onset of coronary heart disease appears to be caused by the increased levels of insulin in the blood. Insulin is a growth promoter and speeds up the atherosclerotic process. If it is administered in high enough doses, it can bring down the glucose level in the blood, but it may also increase the risk of coronary heart disease.

◆ *Diabetes Is A Disease Of Physical Degeneration*

Diabetes is essentially a disease of PHYSICAL DEGENERATION, due to years of wrong diet and neglect of bodily functions, and due to the digestive tract functioning abnormally. It rarely develops in people under 40 years of age. One of the causes is an unbalanced diet consisting of DENATURED FOODS, highly refined. The SODA or SODIUM BICARBONATE in many denatured foods decrease the activity of the pancreatic juices which are used by the body to digest proteins, fats, and carbohydrates. Mrs. White told us: "The use of SODA or BAKING POWDER in bread making is harmful and unnecessary. Soda causes inflammation of the stomach and often poisons the entire system" (CD316).

The Causes Of Diabetes

◆ *Overeating And Overweight*

Diabetes is very closely related to OBESITY. Obesity causes diabetes by increasing the amount of INSULIN needed by the tissues to dispose of accumulated blood sugar. It is estimated that 90% of type II cases could be prevented if people would get to their ideal weight and stay there. People usually get diabetes from eating too much and gaining too much weight. 2 out of 3 diabetics are overweight. Five chemists and three physicians in the U.S. carried out an experiment on 4000 diabetics, and concluded that only 1% needed insulin. They recovered on correct nutrition alone.

Too much food paralyzes the normal activity of the PANCREAS. Diabetes is unknown in countries where people cannot afford to overeat. In many cases of diabetes, it is the increased intake of food which is at fault rather than a decrease in the production of insulin. Once the fat is gone, the insulin has a much better chance of clearing the blood of excess sugar. This is such an immediate and almost miraculous effect, that WEIGHT LOSS has become the basis of treatment for type II diabetes.

L-CARNITINE, a chemical that is important in metabolizing PALMITIC and STEARIC ACIDS, is found in BREWERS YEAST, ALFALFA, and WHEAT. It helps to burn off excess weight. An enzyme transports fat into the cell, but it can't get through unless carnitine is present. A shortage of carnitine can cause fat to circulate in the blood and be stored rather than burned. In this sense the reason for OBESITY and OVERWEIGHT is a deficiency of carnitine. It can be made by the body from LYSINE and METHIONINE, two essential amino acids, and VITAMIN C, B_6 (Pyridoxine) and B_3 (Niacin).

Most biological doctors agree that diabetes is a "prosperity" disease, primarily caused by systematic overeating and resultant obesity. Four out of five diabetics were overweight before diabetes was diagnosed. The chances of developing diabetes double with every 20% of excess weight. When weight is maintained at slightly below the "ideal" weight on the official charts, many diabetics have found that they needed no outside insulin additions to their own naturally produced insulin.

◆ *Sugar And Refined Foods*

Diabetes is prevalent in direct proportion to the intake of both WHITE SUGAR and WHITE FLOUR. Not only is the overeating of sugar and REFINED CARBOHYDRATES involved, but also ANIMAL PROTEIN and FATS, which are transformed into sugar if eaten in excess. With sugar eating, the long bones become longer, and there is also a decided softening of the bones. Healthy blood does not contain sugar for long, for by the sorting out process sugar will have been passed into the liver, or to the red blood corpuscles as hemoglobin, and can be doled out as required. Blood sugar should be below 110, which means 110 mg of sugar for every 100 milliliters of blood written as 110 mg%. Above this figure one is called a DIABETIC.

◆ *High Fat Levels*

Diabetics are dying from an excess of FAT, according to JAMA, the Journal of the American Medical Association. HEART and ARTERY DISEASE are the leading causes of death among diabetics. Instead of concentrating so much on carbohydrates as previous approaches to curing diabetes have done, it is now understood that FAT is a primary causative agent for type II diabetes. High fat levels in the diet and in the blood cause the insulin receptors on the cells to become relatively insensitive to insulin. In most diabetics a low-fat diet along with the elimination of excess weight, restores the sensitivity to insulin. With relatively normal glucose metabolism restored, insulin levels come down as well.

◆ *Drugs*

Prescription drugs used to lower high blood pressure may be the cause of diabetes in middle age men according to a report in the British Medical Journal. Men treated for HIGH BLOOD PRES-

SURE were more likely to develop diabetes than men with normal blood pressure who were not taking medication. Such treatment seemed to be more harmful to men who were predisposed to diabetes, that is men with high risk factors such as having an immediate relative with diabetes, having a low insulin index, or an extremely high blood pressure before the drug therapy.

Disease-Effects Of Diabetes

◆ *It Causes Cardiovascular Disease*

High blood sugar can damage the tiny capillaries that bring oxygen and nutrient-rich blood from the arteries to the rest of the body. One gets HEART DISEASE, STROKE, and CIRCULATORY PROBLEMS in arms and legs when neither oxygen nor nutrients can get through to the cells. Also the impaired circulation can lead to nerve damage that is itself ultimately responsible for 20,000 amputations per year. One out of every 10 diabetics undergoes FOOT AMPUTATION experts estimate. Others go BLIND. 25% of all new cases of blindness are blamed on diabetes, 25% of KIDNEY FAILURES, as are many cases of IMPOTENCE.

The incidence of diabetes increased by over 50% between 1965 and 1973, and is continuing to rise by about 6% per year. It is known that INSULIN brings about a DEGENERATION of the BLOOD VESSELS which causes diabetics to usually die of CARDIOVASCULAR-RENAL DISEASES.

◆ *It Can Cause Heart Disease*

The average diabetic spends $600/yr. on diabetic drugs. Long-term use of these drugs increases the CARDIOVASCULAR MORTALITY of these patients. A high animal protein diet is usually a high fat diet, which produces ATHEROSCLEROSIS, and promotes KIDNEY DISEASE. In fact diabetes is the nation's number one cause of KIDNEY DISEASE, BLINDNESS, and ULCERS, besides playing a part in HEART DISEASE, STROKE, and LOSS of LIMB. It is estimated that one out of ten Americans will become diabetic. When the muscles cannot get sugar to burn for energy, they will burn fat instead, and the resulting fatty acid residues leave deposits in the arteries, which may cause hardening of the arteries and heart disease.

Even with the best INSULIN SUPERVISION and DIETARY CONTROLS, 85% of all DIABETICS on long-term treatment of 15 years or more, develop other complicating diseases such as CORONARIES, CATARACTS, LEG GANGRENE, and ULCERS. DR. JOSLIN, coauthor of the book The Treatment Of Diabetes Mellitus, noted that as treatment with insulin progressed, so did deaths from vascular causes among insulin treated patients. For instance, between 1898–1914, before insulin, the death rate from vascular diseases of diabetics was only 17.5%, as compared with the period of 1915–48, when the vascular death rate of diabetics increased to 66.6%. Drs. Travia and Scapelato found that 80–90% of diabetics suffered from various forms of CARDIOVASCULAR DISEASES. Dr. Butturini of Bologna, Italy, discovered that vitamin E in doses averaging 300 IU was beneficial in most forms of cardiovascular diseases in diabetics, but that it also eliminated entirely the need for insulin in 50% of the patients, reduced the need in 30%, and was ineffective in only 20%.

◆ *It causes Gangrene*

People with diabetes are 50 times more likely to develop GANGRENE, for the impaired circulation can cut off the blood supply to any given area of the body. One of the insidious side effects is a threat of gangrene of the foot or lower leg. Dr. Wilfred Shute says that this can be corrected when the feet are already affected, with large doses of VITAMIN E taken internally. Diabetic RETINOGRAPHY or diabetic VISION PROBLEMS and gradual deterioration of eyesight, is one of the most common complications of diabetes. Oral doses of THYROID HORMONE EXTRACT. with large doses of B-COMPLEX VITAMINS, VITAMIN C, and DIGESTIVE ENZYMES, have been used successfully to treat it.

Curing Diabetes Naturally

Diet is very important with diabetics. What they should especially concentrate on is omitting all food and drink products that use refined sugar. They can drink orange and carrot juice with the natural sugars which they contain. They also need to avoid all foods which contain BAKING POWDER and SODA, all foods cooked or stored in ALUMINUM, as well as ALCOHOL and FOOD

PRESERVATIVES that might damage the liver.

The main dietary consideration for diabetics is a strict, low calorie, alkaline diet of high quality NATURAL FOODS. Plenty of WHOLE GRAINS, especially BUCKWHEAT, MILLET, and OATS, and RAW VEGETABLES, including ARTICHOKES, GREEN BEANS, and GARLIC. Also fresh fruits, especially GRAPEFRUITS and BANANAS. Contrary to popular opinion, fruits are beneficial in the diabetic diet. Fresh fruits contain FRUCTOSE which does not need INSULIN for its metabolism, and is therefore well tolerated by diabetics.

✓ RAW FOODS—The emphasis should be on RAW FOODS. Drastically increasing the amount of raw foods in the diet has succeeded in reducing the insulin requirement of some diabetics. Research has shown that CELERY, CUCUMBER, GREEN BEANS, GARLIC, ONIONS, and JERUSALEM ARTICHOKES contain NATURAL HORMONES that stimulate the pancreas and increase insulin production. About 80% of the diet should be raw foods. For protein, homemade COTTAGE CHEESE, and various forms of soured milks, such as YOGURT and KEFIR should be used. Diabetics have a tendency toward OVERACIDITY because of the slowed down protein and fat metabolism. Raw fruits and vegetables will reduce food consumption because of their FIBER. Besides, several raw vegetables contain insulin, especially JERUSALEM ARTICHOKES. Most vegetables contain in their raw state the precursor of insulin known as INULIN.

For a diet Dr. J.M. Douglas recommends RAW VEGETABLES, SEEDS, NUTS, BERRIES, MELONS, FRUITS, EGG YOLKS, HONEY, and GOAT'S MILK. He believes that the interaction of enzymes normally destroyed by cooking may be responsible for the raw diet's effect. An ALL-POTATO, ALL-RICE, or an ALL-OATMEAL diet is sometimes curative for diabetes.

Foods that contain CHROMIUM are WHOLE WHEAT, SEAWEEDS, BREWERS YEAST, FRUITS, VEGETABLES, HONEY, and MOLASSES. BEANS, PEAS, and LENTIL have the reputation of controlling diabetes. A cup a day of cooked NAVY or PINTO beans has slashed the need for insulin injections by 38% in one group of patients. Through such a diet, those whose insulin production has slowed down have eliminated the need for insulin shots altogether. Such a diet works because beans create a very slow rise in blood sugar, so that less insulin is needed. SOYBEANS are especially good for this.

✓ GARLIC—A startling fact is that diabetes has been cured with garlic alone. Garlic is said to be as effective as the drug ORINASE in clearing the bloodstream of excess glucose. Garlic has certain minerals that are of proven value in carbohydrate metabolism. Garlic is rich in POTASSIUM. In diabetes excess acidity, or ACIDOSIS, can rob the body of so much potassium that unconsciousness or DIABETIC COMA can result. LOW BLOOD SUGAR causes much potassium to be lost in the urine. At times taking POTASSIUM CHLORIDE brings about immediate relief and prevents blackouts. Garlic contains ZINC, which is found in concentrated form in the liver, spleen, and pancreas. It is a component of the insulin that is given to diabetics. It has been found that when insulin is given by injection, the addition of zinc to it prolongs its effect. Research has indicated that the zinc content of the pancreas of diabetic persons is only half that of normal persons.

✓ FRUIT AND VEGETABLE JUICES—The best fruit juices are the CITRUS juices. The natural juices of apples, grapes, pineapple, or prunes are not recommended as they may raise blood sugar levels too rapidly. One property of CHILI PEPPERS is their ability to LOWER BLOOD SUGAR LEVELS. This is good news for DIABETICS for which authorities suggest 3 capsules of CAPSAICIN daily. Some experts suggest 2 CAPSICUM capsules 3 times a day with a glass of apple juice.

✓ CUCUMBER—It contains a hormone needed by the cells of the pancreas to produce insulin. The natural hormones contained in ONIONS and GARLIC are also beneficial in diabetes.

✓ FIBER—Dr. James Anderson developed a diet that helps diabetics control their disease with minimum of outside help through the importance of fiber in the diet. A high CARBOHYDRATE, HIGH-FIBER DIET consistently REDUCES INSULIN REQUIREMENTS, IM-

PROVES BLOOD SUGAR CONTROL, and drives CHOLESTEROL and TRIGLYCERIDE levels down, which are results which benefit diabetics as well as non-diabetics.

Fiber may be the CURE-ALL of the decade. It helps in cases of HIGH CHOLESTEROL, DIABETES, CONSTIPATION, OVERWEIGHT, GASTROINTESTINAL PROBLEMS, GALLSTONES, and ULCERS. It may also prevent COLON and BREAST CANCER. Fiber causes sugar in the blood to be absorbed more slowly so as to give INSULIN a chance to keep the blood sugar on a more even keel.

The American Diabetes Association now advocates a high-fiber, complex carbohydrates, low-sodium, low-fat diet. Research has shown that the fiber in whole grains and many fruits and vegetables helps to stabilize blood sugar. It also reduces the diabetic's risk for heart disease, the leading cause of death. A study showed that the high fiber apple held off hunger longer than some other fruits while keeping blood sugar stable. APPLE JUICE left people feeling the hungriest, for it triggered twice the release of insulin causing a hypoglycemic effect as the sugar fell below normal. This experiment suggests that a FIBER-RICH DIET is ideal for DIABETICS since it reduces blood sugar as well as the need for insulin.

Studies in Britain found that FIBER and PECTIN improved glucose tolerance by delaying absorption of carbohydrates and reducing INSULIN REQUIREMENTS. SOYBEANS are particularly valuable as they contain more protein and fewer assimilable carbohydrates than other legumes. Taking two pectin capsules and/or a few teaspoons of unprocessed bran with meals provides both pectin and fiber.

Fibers help control Type II diabetes. One needs about 10 to 15 grams at every meal. This is obtained in a bowl of 100% BRAN CEREAL, or a couple of dried figs, cup of baked beans, or two slices of whole wheat bread. Replace finely ground flour with whole or cracked grains, or use coarsely milled flour. All of these are digested more slowly, and are less likely to increase blood sugar levels. Diets high in fiber-depleted starchy foods are an increased risk in diabetes. Hence, eat brown rice rather white rice.

The greater the amount of whole unmilled kernels in BREAD, the more slowly the bread digests. Hence, the less it causes glucose or blood sugar to rise. This helps in controlling diabetes. Too much milling pulverizes the essential parts of the kernel to substantially alter the speed with which they are digested.

A diet of HIGH-CARBOHYDRATE, LOW-CALORIE FOOD, with plenty of FIBER cured 20 diabetics with an average blood sugar count of 170 in 3 weeks. In addition patients walked for 30 minutes at normal speed, 3 times a day after meals.

✓ JERUSALEM ARTICHOKE—The Jerusalem Artichoke can give us the type of natural sugar which can supply our needs for a good natural sweetener. It is called FRUCTAN. It has two important benefits. It is low in calories, but since it has long molecules instead of short molecules found in most common sugars, the body cannot absorb fructan very well, so that not much of the sugar is absorbed. It also stabilizes blood sugar by not causing a drastic change in blood sugar levels. Eating carbohydrates usually raises blood glucose levels. But when fructan is used, the blood sugar levels are somewhat lowered instead of raised. Fructan also seems to reduce the body's NEED for INSULIN, which should be welcomed news for diabetics.

✓ VITAMINS—Dr. Klenner believes that all diabetics should be taking massive doses of VITAMIN C. He says lack of vitamin C is responsible for the slow healing of diabetic wounds. 60% of his diabetic patients can be controlled with only diet and vitamin C, as much as 10 gm daily. The other 40% need less insulin and less oral medication if they are taking massive doses of vitamin C.

BREWERS YEAST value in diabetes lies in its concentration of the trace mineral CHROMIUM. It aids in the metabolism of excess sugar. Many diabetics have normal amounts of insulin but somehow cannot utilize it properly. Dr. Mertz suggests that they are often simply suffering from a chromium deficiency. Tri-valent chromium is the biologically valuable form of this mineral, such as is found in brewers yeast. While GRAINS and SEEDS are a relatively good source of biologically valuable chromium, in WHEAT much of the chromium is concentrated in the GERM, which of course is eliminated in the refinement of flour. Two milligram of supplementary chromium can be given, preferably in combination with MANGANESE and other trace elements.

Some doctors emphasize the need for vitamin E for DIABETES MELLITUS. They say that the treatment of diabetes today requires 3 agents instead of 2. These are a BALANCED DIET, INSULIN, and VITAMIN E. Any one or two alone are not adequate.

✓ EXERCISE—Next to dietary restrictions, lots of exercise is the most important single thing that a diabetic can engage in to help himself. Exercise in the fresh air such as WALKING, JOGGING, SWIMMING, BICYCLING, will help to keep the fire of the metabolic processes burning fast. All such exercises diminish the need for insulin. They help muscle cells take up and use sugar. The best exercise is brisk walking. A daily 30 minute soak in a HOT BATH with some seaweed or sea salt is believed to help remove sugar and acid accumulations from the body. In a study at Duke University it was found that people who practiced RELAXATION TECHNIQUES after meals could handle 30% more sugar than they usually could before their blood sugar levels shot up.

✓ Exercise can control diabetes by a. lessening the amount of insulin secreted and improving the ability to use blood sugar properly; b. helping body cells get the most out of the available glucose; c. decreasing the negative influence of an occasional heavy intake of carbohydrates; d. contributing to loss of weight by normalizing it; e. increasing insulin receptors within the cells; f. increasing the effectiveness of insulin itself.

Herbal Teas

✓ BLUEBERRY LEAVES AND TEA—They have a long history of folk medicine use in the treatment of diabetes. Oral administration reduces glucose levels in dogs even without their pancreas, and even when glucose is injected at the same time.

It has been used for centuries in folk medicine for the treatment of sugar diabetes. There is a substance in blueberry leaves called MYRTILLIN, which reduces blood sugar as insulin does. One cup of this tea three times a day is the recommended dose. A lady with a mild case of diabetes was intent on curing herself if she possibly could. She used plenty of fresh fruits and vegetables, vitamins, and minerals. In addition she used BLUEBERRY LEAF TEA two or three times a day. When later the doctor took a blood test, he reported that the blood was perfectly normal.

✓ STRING BEAN POD TEA—It is an excellent natural substitute for insulin. The skins of the pods are very rich in SILICA and in certain hormones which are closely related to insulin. One cup of string bean skin tea is equal to at least one unit of insulin.

It has cleared up both diabetes as well as KIDNEY STONES in a man when he drank a quart a day.

✓ FENUGREEK SEEDS—They have demonstrated diabetic effects in experimental and clinical studies.

✓ CACTUS PODS—They are depined cactus leaves. It has been reported that they contain a huge amount of natural INSULIN.

Dr. Lamar And Fructose

Dr. Lamar of Cuba says that by using FRUCTOSE wisely in prescribed diets, he has revolutionized the treatment of diabetes. He says that fructose does not need insulin for its conversion into energy. The body cells obtain most of their necessary energy from it and less insulin is required. The fructose also makes the protein in the diabetic's diet go farther. Fructose is obtained from fruits, but fruits also contain glucose which demands insulin for its proper use by the body. So, Dr. Lamar says, a certain amount of glucose remains in the body, unburned, and passes into the blood and urine. But, he says, this does not cause the usual symptoms of diabetes, so long as enough of the fructose and of the glucose are properly utilized by the metabolic system. In other words, the diabetic who provides his digestive machinery with enough fructose can maintain a normal metabolism by bypassing the use of insulin entirely and thus avoid all the disturbances of FAT DIGESTION which, according to him, are the real cause of the symptoms of diabetes. Substituting OLIVE OIL for other fats, in one study, lowered GLUCOSE as well as TRIGLYCERIDES and LOW DENSITY (LDL) LIPOPROTEIN levels, while it raised the HIGH DENSITY (HDL) LIPOPROTEIN level.

All of his patients have needed less and less insulin as time went on, and some of them are taking no insulin at all, even though some had used it for more than 20 years. In his diet, he says, foods should be chosen in which there is more fructose than glucose, or at least as much. Such foods are fruits. For those who have no diabetes it seems the better part of wisdom to get your sugars from FRESH FRUITS to avoid ever getting diabetes.

DIARRHEA

Causes

✓ SYMPTOMS—Diarrhea is characterized by frequent and loose watery stools, and is often accompanied by severe vomiting. Symptoms include RUNNY STOOLS, CRAMPING, FREQUENT BOWEL MOVEMENTS, THIRST, and ABDOMINAL PAIN. Some people run a FEVER as well. Also caused by STRESS and ANXIETY.

✓ LOSS OF FLUIDS—Diarrhea is caused by INCOMPLETE DIGESTION OF FOOD, ALLERGIES. ANTIBIOTICS, BACTERIAL INFECTION such as AMEBIC DYSENTERY, EMOTIONAL STRESS, FATIGUE, FOOD POISONING, overuse of CHEMICAL LAXATIVES, DRUGS, PARASITES, FOODS OR CHEMICALS THE BODY CANNOT TOLERATE, GREEN FRUITS, and RANCID FOODS. Loss of fluids can lead to dehydration and loss of minerals. Drink plenty of liquids such as a hot CAROB drink, CARROT JUICE, and "GREEN DRINKS."

✓ FOOD MALABSORPTION—In diarrhea food passes through the body so rapidly that very few nutrients are assimilated. When irritated or inflamed, the mucus membrane within the bowels fails to absorb the liquid from food materials. This results in runny, frequent bowel movements. During bouts with diarrhea extra liquids should be taken throughout the day to compensate for the fluid losses in the watery stools. Death can result from excessive diarrhea in INFANTS who become dehydrated. It can be caused by difficulty in digesting GLUTEN or by CELIAC DISEASE.

✓ PELLAGRA—Pellagra is caused by lack of NIACIN (B_3). Such lack invites the 3-D's, DIARRHEA, DERMATITIS, and DEMENTIA.

✓ SORBITOL—This is an artificial sweetener. NATURAL SORBITOL is found in fruits, such as PRUNES, noted for their laxative effect.

✓ COLITIS—It is caused by unsanitary food and water generally from the E. Coli bacterium. It is also labeled "Montezuma's Revenge" by Americans who picked it up in Mexico.

✓ VITAMINS—It is also caused by VITAMINS B and C intakes, when the body is not used to them.

Preventing Diarrhea

✓ TRAVELERS DIARRHEA—Travelers diarrhea strikes 30% to 50% of the visitors of developing countries. The most prevalent cause is ESCHERICHIA COLI or E. COLI, which is responsible for at least half of all cases. To prevent travelers diarrhea, drink only bottled drinks, or drinks made with boiled water, or cooked foods, or fruits that are peeled. Avoid unpasteurized dairy products, tap water, and raw salads. To drink the local water, purify it by boiling it for 5 minutes, or adding IODINE or CHLORINE PREPARATIONS to it. When traveling in foreign countries choose CARBONATED WATER over plain water, because carbonation makes water acidic enough to kill most microorganisms including those that cause diarrhea.

✓ EAT YOGURT—YOGURT is the safest food you can eat to prevent diarrhea. The infectious bacteria die in yogurt, but they thrive in ordinary milk. So yogurt does not cause diarrhea, but milk can. YOGURT is recommended, especially if the diarrhea is caused by prescription of antibiotics such as PENICILLIN.

Curing Diarrhea

✓ ACIDOPHILUS CAPSULES—To avoid diarrhea in foreign countries with foreign food, take three acidophilus capsules during each meal.

- ✓ PECTIN and BRAN—Both absorb many times their own weight in liquid to help correct diarrhea. Pectin also absorbs and eliminates harmful organisms while promoting the growth of beneficial bacteria. CAROB is rich in pectin and therefore normalizes the bowels.

- ✓ APPLES and BANANAS—Bananas have proven even more effective than apples in recent tests, but both are rich in PECTIN and have long been favorite diarrhea remedies. They tighten up loose bowels, and supply MINERALS lost in diarrhea such as MAGNESIUM and POTASSIUM.

- ✓ GARLIC—Garlic taken regularly, can cure stomach and intestinal ailments. The ALLICIN in garlic stimulates the walls of the stomach and intestines to secrete digestive enzymes. It must be diluted or mixed with other foods. Garlic may even be used externally in poultices or FOOT- and HAND-BATHS. It is also successful in cases of FLATULENCE and COLIC, to expel gas from the stomach and intestines.

Dr. E. Weiss of Chicago gave GARLIC to a group of patients who had a history of intestinal disorders. During the treatment DIARRHEA, HEADACHES, and other symptoms of intestinal trouble vanished. There was a complete change in the intestinal flora. It was noted that the harmful bacteria were decreasing, while the beneficial ones were increasing. This is usually the case with natural medicines. Drugs would have destroyed both good and bad bacteria indiscriminately, but God's medicines do not harm the things that are good and beneficial, but rather promote them.

A laboratory assistant accidentally infected herself with a bacterium which causes DYSENTERY. She developed symptoms of no APPETITE, DIARRHEA, and BLOODY STOOLS. She became weak, exhausted and full of pain. She was given two grams of a GARLIC PREPARATION five times a day for six days. Almost at once, the vomiting stopped, and she found that she could eat again. The illness gradually subsided.

- ✓ ST. JOHNS WORT—In the early days European peasants assigned magical powers to ST. JOHN'S-WORT, and gathered it on St. John's Day for special cures. It was at times combined with BLACK RASPBERRY ROOT and was also drunk as a treatment for TUBERCULOSIS. Also BLUEBERRIES and HONEY are helpful. Also take 4 CHARCOAL tablets every hour with water until the diarrhea subsides. Take 5 tablets of KELP during the day in order to replace the lost minerals. For youngsters whole milk may be a cure, as well as SOYBEANS and SOY MILK.

- ✓ USE HIGH BULK FOODS—THE BRAT DIET—It is critical to continue to eat when you have diarrhea, and nature's medicines help to cure diarrhea. Shift to foods that will shorten the diarrhea such as HIGH BULK FOODS like *B*ANANAS, *R*ICE, *A*PPLESAUCE, and *T*OAST, which is called the *BRAT* diet. CARROT SOUP and TAPIOCA PUDDING work fine also.

- ✓ DON'T USE EXCESSIVE SUGAR—Solutions with excessive sugar have caused death in infants with diarrhea. That is why SWEET JUICES are bad choices for replacing the fluids lost in diarrhea. The best cures for diarrhea are STARCHY FLUIDS. Thick soups made from RICE, CORN, WHEAT, or POTATOES will work well. For ADULTS use teaspoon of FENUGREEK SEEDS 3 TIMES A DAY. Dried BLUEBERRIES and BLACK CURRANTS are rich in anti-diarrhea compounds.

- ✓ DIARRHEA FORMULA—Mix one pint of yogurt, 3 bananas, and one tablespoon of fiber.

FEMALE PROBLEMS

Breast Ailments

- ✓ CYSTIC BREAST DISEASE—It represents a premenstrual swelling of the breasts with nodes and pain. Help has been gained through the elimination of the METHYLXANTHINES such as CAFFEINE in coffee, THEOPHYLLINE in tea, and THEOBROMINE in chocolate. The elimination of these usually eliminates the lumps and pain.

- ✓ FIBROCYSTIC DISEASE—In order to make the hormone ESTROGEN, the body needs fat.

Reducing the fat reduces the estrogen levels, and therewith the possibility of developing fibrocystic disease. It can also be helped by adding 600 IU of VITAMIN E to the diet with added SELENIUM. Foods rich in vitamin E and selenium are WHEAT GERM, SUNFLOWER SEEDS, WHOLE WHEAT, WALNUTS, ALMONDS, CORN, and CABBAGE.

IODINE which is used to prevent GOITER has been successful not only in reducing the pain associated with FIBROCYSTIC BREAST DISEASE, but also in reducing the lumps as well.

Irregular Menstruation

✓ MENSTRUATION—THE MENSES—is a periodic monthly discharge of blood from the vagina, and the sloughing off of mucosal tissues. In really healthy women menstruation does not occur. The healthier the subject, the less pronounced the flow, and the shorter its duration. Nature, we might say, does not impose blood loss as part of her plan. It is characteristic of females with TOXIC BODIES. Many women who have adopted a completely healthy regimen, have been startled to find the cessation of menstruation to be a by-product. The body continually tries to rid itself of a toxic overload. But when such an overload collects faster than elimination can handle, then disease develops. To assist in the eliminative process, the uterus becomes an eliminative organ.

Normally, girls begin in the early teens and continue on until the late forties or early fifties except during pregnancy or when sick. A lady who hemorrhaged greatly with great pain, instead of taking ASPIRINS took 2 DOLOMITE TABLETS. Within 20 minutes the pain was gone, and the loss of blood was minimal. Dolomite contains CALCIUM and MAGNESIUM. A POOR DIET and a drastic loss of calcium during menstruation play havoc with a woman's body. BONE MEAL TABLETS seem to have the same result. Calcium can relieve both MENSTRUAL TENSION as well as MENSTRUAL CRAMPS. With calcium HOT FLASHES, NIGHT SWEATS, LEG CRAMPS, and MENTAL DEPRESSION will often disappear.

✓ MENOPAUSE—THE CHANGE OF LIFE—comes on anytime from the early forties to the late fifties. It is a normal event in life and need not be feared. 85% of women have no trouble at all. Some have a few HOT FLASHES that last a minute or two. The best years of life are often experienced after menopause. Menopause shuts down ESTROGEN production, and bone health is threatened with regard to OSTEOPOROSIS. Estrogen pills have been shown to cause fewer HIP FRACTURES, but they also have a potentiality for CANCER. WEIGHT-BEARING EXERCISES such as running, cycling, and lifting weights are the best exercises for your bones. A daily 45 minute walk may be all you need to keep from getting osteoporosis.

◆ *A Vitamin Deficiency*

AMENORRHEA or IRREGULAR MENSTRUATION, may be an indication of a vitamin deficiency that frequently responds to daily supplements of 200 mg of vitamin B_2, 50 to 150 mg of B_6, 400 to 800 mcg (micrograms) of FOLIC ACID, and up to 60 IU of vitamin E. A European formula for PREMENSTRUAL TENSION (PMT) is OIL of EVENING PRIMROSE, which is now available in American health food stores.

◆ *Unpleasant Symptoms Are Not Normal*

Many hormonal and metabolic changes occur before and during menstrual periods, which can cause unpleasant symptoms such as DEPRESSION, TENSIONS, CRAMPS, FAINTING SPELLS, TENDERNESS OF BREASTS, WATER RETENTION, BACKACHE, ETC. Although these symptoms are common, they are not normal. Healthy women living close to nature, and eating good diets of natural foods, such as women in Hunza, China, Russia, and Central American Indians, do not suffer from the monthly ordeal that women in Western countries do. Most menstrual symptoms are caused by nutritional deficiencies which lead to improper metabolism of female sex hormones which abound during the menstrual period. Deficiencies of VITAMIN E, B_6, as well as CALCIUM and IODINE are particularly involved.

Causes Of Excessive Bleeding

Factors contributing to excessive menstrual

bleeding are IRON DEFICIENCY, HYPOTHYROIDISM, VITAMIN A DEFICIENCY, and INTRAUTERINE DEVICES. As menstrual blood loss above 60 milliliter (ml) per period is associated with negative iron balance in most cases, it is a major cause of IRON DEFICIENCY ANEMIA.

Many premenstrual tension symptoms like stress, deplete the body's store of MAGNESIUM. At the same time these symptoms can be explained by a MAGNESIUM DEFICIENCY. It seems to be both cause and effect. The suggestion is to increase the intake of magnesium.

Premenstrual Syndrome (PMS)

PMS is a condition that occurs 1 to 2 weeks before the onset of menstruation. It is characterized by FATIGUE, TENSION, DEPRESSION, BREAST TENDERNESS, FLUID RETENTION, HEADACHES, ABDOMINAL PAIN, and WATER RETENTION which may be sufficient enough to cause EDEMA. An improper diet seems to play a major role in it. SALTY FOODS cause water retention; SUGAR and CAFFEINE put stress on the nervous system; and FATTY FOODS contribute to HORMONAL IMBALANCE.

- ✓ FOODS TO EAT—The B-complex-rich foods such as WHOLE GRAINS, BEANS, SEEDS, and NUTS. Calcium-rich foods such as DARK LEAFY GREENS, BROCCOLI, SESAME SEEDS, and TOFU.
- ✓ SKULLCAP—relaxes the nervous system and will ease premenstrual tension. Take 30 drops of skullcap tincture 3 times a day in a small amount of warm water.
- ✓ DANDELION LEAF—is a safe and effective DIURETIC. Make a tea by pouring 2 cups of boiling water over 1 heaping tablespoon of the herb and steep in a covered pot for 20 minutes. Drink 3 cups a day.
- ✓ CRAMP BARK—an antispasmodic, will relieve menstrual cramps. Make a tea by simmering 2 teaspoons of the dried bark in 1 cup of water for 15 minutes. Drink 3 cups of warm cramp tea 3 times a day.

How To Cure Menstrual Problems

- ✓ A NATURAL DIET—A good diet is proteins from RAW, UNPASTEURIZED MILK if possible, and soured milks such as YOGURT, KEFIR, and CLABBERED MILK, plus homemade COTTAGE CHEESE daily.

  The diet should be low in animal fats, and high in LINOLEIC and LINOLENIC ACIDS from vegetable oil sources. GREEN LEAFY VEGETABLES and other sources of VITAMIN K should be eaten freely.
  WHOLE GRAINS and SEEDS, especially in SPROUTED form, should form the basis of the diet. ALMONDS, BUCKWHEAT, MILLET, OATS, SESAME SEEDS, SUNFLOWER SEEDS, will supply high quality proteins, essential minerals, as well as the all-important VITAMINS E and B-COMPLEX.
  Plenty of RAW VEGETABLES and FRUITS, particularly GRAPES, APRICOTS, RED BEETS, MOLASSES, and VITAMIN C.
- ✓ JUICES—The best juices are RED BEET, GRAPE, CHERRY, PRUNE, BLACK CURRANT, and the GREEN VEGETABLE JUICES.
- ✓ HERBS—To decrease flow use SORREL, UVA URSI, YARROW, WITCH HAZEL, PLANTAIN, and BAYBERRY BARK. Dr. Airola suggests the following herbs for menstrual difficulties: LADY'S MANTLE and AMARANTH for excessive menstruation, LIFE ROOT for suppressed menstruation, BLACK COHOSH for obstructed menstruation, BLUE COHOSH and YARROW for menstrual difficulties, MOTHERWORT to promote menstrual flow, WORMWOOD and PENNYROYAL in painful menstruation, GARLIC also encourages the menstrual flow, DESERT TEA (EPHREDA VIRIDIS) for delayed or difficult menstruation.
- ✓ RELEAF—A herbal product, is used for PREMENSTRUAL SYNDROME (PMS). It contains no aspirin, acetaminophen, caffeine, sugar, starch, artificial colors, flavors, or preservatives. It does not cause drowsiness. It is sold in capsules of 365 mg. It is composed of WOOD BETONY, BAYBERRY BARK, UVA URSI, CAPSICUM, and HAWTHORNE. It can be obtained in a health food store.

- ✓ KELP—A THYROID DEFICIENCY can cause irregular and/or profuse menstruation. KELP is of specific importance in such a condition.
- ✓ AGNUS CASTUS or CHASTE TREE—It grows along the shores of the Mediterranean. Many medical herbalists regard it as nature's alternative to chemical drugs for the hormone imbalance of PMS, MENSTRUAL TROUBLES, and MENOPAUSE. It alleviates HOT FLASHES, CRAMPS, and EXCESSIVE BLEEDING. It has the power to correct the hormone imbalance through its influence on the PITUITARY GLAND. Agnus castus tablets can be obtained in a health food store.

  One lady said: "I went to one gynecologist after another for years on end. I had a terrible discharge. The last doctor I went to suggested having a HYSTERECTOMY, since the pills and suppositories didn't seem to be helping at all. Instead, I started drinking a cup of YARROW TEA every day. I picked the yarrow myself while the sun was shining, and six weeks later I was cured of this unpleasant condition."
- ✓ VITAMINS AND MINERALS—PREMENSTRUAL EDEMA, SWELLINGS, and SORENESS are often relieved by the administration of VITAMIN B_6, 50 to 150 mg a day, especially during the 10 days preceding menstruation.

  PREMENSTRUAL TENSION SYMPTOMS are also believed by scientists to respond to treatment with VITAMIN E, ZINC, and IRON. They believe that monthly hormonal changes cause deficiencies in some nutrients, and that these deficiencies may be the cause of many premenstrual symptoms.
  VITAMIN B_{12} is helpful in restoring the normal menstrual cycle. 25 to 100 mcg daily is recommended
  MENORRHAGIA or excessive bleeding, has been shown to reduce supplementation with VITAMIN C and BIOFLAVONOIDS in 14 out of 16 patients. Vitamin C is known to increase IRON ABSORPTION significantly from 3 to 6-fold. The vitamin C foods must be eaten with the iron foods. They work only when eaten together. In grandmother's time, the iron that leached from iron pots into the food and pans acted as a kind of unintentional fortification. In one study spaghetti sauce simmered in an iron pot for about 20 minutes increased its iron content 9-fold.

The Uterus

- ✓ HEMORRHAGE—For hemorrhage apply ICE to the nipples. Also take some CAYENNE powder in water and drink it.
- ✓ PAIN—For pain put on warm clothes on arms and legs. One of the greatest causes of female disease is unhealthful dress. Mrs. White has told us that "it is impossible for women to have habitual, chilled limbs and cold feet, without some of the internal organs being congested. The many extra coverings over the chest and back and lower part of the body, induce blood to these parts and the animal heat thus retained, weakens and debilitates the delicate organs, and congestion and inflammation result" (HL551). "She should not call vitality unnecessarily to the surface to supply the want of sufficient clothing" (2T382). "Half of the diseases of women are caused by unhealthful dress" (HL544). "More die as a result of following fashion than from all other causes" (HL275).
- ✓ VAGINAL INFECTION—A lady after reading that GARLIC acts as an antibiotic cured herself of vaginal infection by taking fresh garlic, and later on garlic pills. They are a lot cheaper than ANTIBIOTICS, and there are no side effects.

Dr. Holman tells us that BARBITURATE PILLS and various drugs for bringing down fevers have been cited as possible cancer causers. ANTIBIOTICS are very potent respiratory poisons contained in much of our food such as MILK, CHEESE, BUTTER, and MEAT, because the animals involved have been fed antibiotics. FRESH PRODUCE and POULTRY are also soaked in antibiotics to preserve them.

FEVERS

Fever And Inspiration

◆ *Fever—A Symptom Of Disease*

Fever is a symptom of disease rather than a disease. It indicates that something in the body is out of line, and out of order. "Fever is nature's effort to correct unhealthful conditions in the body" (MH235). The body has been misused usually by the overuse of foods of all kinds. "It is possible to eat immoderately, even of wholesome food" (CH119). There is a penalty attached to every transgression (CD124). "A wrong course of eating and drinking destroys health.... Thousands, by indulging a perverted appetite, have brought on fever or some other acute disease, which has resulted in death" (CH114–5). "Nature bears abuse as long as she can without resisting; then she arouses and makes a mighty effort to rid herself of the encumbrances and evil treatment she has suffered. You have to suffer the penalty of Nature's violated laws" (CD124). "Then come HEADACHES, CHILLS, FEVERS, NERVOUSNESS, PARALYSIS, and other evils too numerous to mention" (CD125).

◆ *Cooling The Fever*

When you have a fever, your body is BURNING ENERGY MORE QUICKLY. Theoretically, you need more calories than normal. But it is hard to eat when you have a cold because the sensitivity of your sense of taste is reduced, which is linked to your ability to smell the food you eat. Under these circumstances it is best to rely on liquids and liquid food to carry you along. The liquids will also keep the mucous membranes in your nose moist making it easier for you to clear your nose and cough up mucous from your throat. Temperatures of over 104 degrees should be lowered immediately by cooling the body in a TUB OF COOL WATER, RUBBING it with WARM WATER, or by wrapping the body in a WET SHEET, cooling the forehead and neck with a cold towel or ice bag. Also a cool ENEMA of catnip tea, strawberry leaf tea, or plain water will bring down the temperature

◆ *Mrs. White's Experience With Fever*

Her attention was called to a man whose daughter was ill with a fever. He had already buried his wife and a son and a daughter, and this daughter was all he had left. He related to the doctor that his son was first attacked with a fever. The doctor gave him a powerful medicine which broke the fever, but the son grew worse. Twice more the doctor gave him the powerful medicine, but he obtained no relief. The fever left him, but he did not rally. He sank rapidly and died. The wife grew ill from her son's death, and a second physician gave her a liberal dose of OPIUM. The opium stupefied her and she could not be aroused. She grew more feeble and died without ever awakening. The first daughter was given many medicines when she grew ill with a fever. She lived a few years with her limbs crippled by the powerful poisons, and died in much agony. The physician who was now attending to the second daughter after hearing the family history, said that the three family members need not have died if they had not been so DRUGGED. He gave the second daughter no medicine, but a few healthful directions, and after a time she recovered. The father said that his wife, son and daughter need not have died; that they were sacrificed while in the hands of physicians by their poisonous drugs. (2SM443–8).

◆ *Fever Should Not Be Brought Down With Drugs*

Nobel Prize winner Dr. Lwoff of France said: "High temperature during an infection helps to combat the growth of virus. Therefore, fever should not be brought down with drugs." The Spirit of Prophecy also tells us that poisonous drugs are not the proper treatment for fever (5T195). There is no need for ASPIRIN, which reduces fever by acting on the heat regulating center in the brain rather than acting on the underlying cause of the fever.

What Fever Accomplishes In Disease

◆ *It Burns Up Waste Matter*

A FEVER is nature's attempt to burn up or incinerate WASTE MATTER in the system. When there is no waste matter and the body cells are properly nourished, there is then no need for fever.

Parmenides said 2500 years ago: "Give me a chance to create a FEVER and I will cure any disease." Fever is a defensive process as well as a healing process. The high temperature SPEEDS UP METABOLISM, INHIBITS THE GROWTH OF VIRUSES AND BACTERIA, and burns GERMS AND TOXINS with HEAT. It helps to contain an infection by preventing its spread throughout the body. For each 1 degree rise in centigrade temperature, the body's metabolic rate of the HEART, RESPIRATION, and all other metabolic functions are increased about 10 percent. Fever mobilizes the body's immunological defenses against infectious organisms. It was shown that animals such as FISH, LIZARDS, RABBITS, and DOGS are more likely to survive disease if they are allowed to raise their body's temperature. Body temperature goes up during VIGOROUS EXERCISE, producing a fever. This fever remains elevated for several hours after the exercise is over.

◆ *It Combats Viral Infection*

Fever also combats viral infections by triggering production of the virus-fighting substance of INTERFERON by the infected cells. LYSOSOMES—are cellular "suicide bodies" which are also stimulated by fever. They help fight viral infections and also destroy TUMOR CELLS, which are more sensitive to heat than normal cells. FEVER BLISTERS are caused by the virus herpes simplex. The ACIDOPHILUS bacillus inactivates but does not destroy the herpes virus. Eating acidophilus YOGURT is very helpful especially if the sores are inside the mouth.

◆ *The Hypothalamus Regulates Body Temperature.*

Nerve messages, originating in the HYPOTHALAMUS, that regulate body temperature, trigger rapid muscle contractions, or SHIVERING, WHICH PRODUCES HEAT. The MACROPHAGE, which is a cleanup cell in the blood, releases a hormone called ENDOGENOUS PYROGEN, or EP, which stimulates the production of PROSTAGLANDINS to act on the HYPOTHALAMUS to raise the body temperature. A moderate fever is beneficial, while a high fever is dangerous. Dr. Mackowiak says that we may be doing patients a disservice by giving them anti-fever medication at the same time that we are treating the infection, because research shows that antibiotic induced destruction of bacteria is increased at fever temperatures. Dr. Kluge of the University of Michigan Medical School infected adult rabbits with bacteria. All those who received an ASPIRIN-LIKE substance to lower their fever died. But 70% of the infected rabbits who maintained a fever survived.

The Causes Of Fever

◆ *Impurities In The System*

Fever is often associated with animal protein, which if it doesn't move fast enough through the intestines will putrefy, and thereby attract bacteria as scavengers. Fever then starts to burn up the putrefying matter as well as the bacteria. Interrupting this process of cleansing with drugs sets the stage for more complicated infections later on. The Spirit of Prophecy tells us that "With many, their first error is with making a god of their appetite, subsisting mostly on highly-seasoned ANIMAL FOOD which produces a feverish state of the system, especially if pork is used freely. The blood becomes impure. The circulation is not equalized. Chills and fever follow. The appetite fails" (4SGa126).

◆ *An Interrupted Infection Leaves Debris*

The development of RYE'S SYNDROME in children with the administration of ASPIRIN emphasizes this point. Each interrupted infection leaves debris in the body. This also indicates why people become sicker with age, for subsequent illnesses have more debris to clean up, which housecleaning job was not completed previously, so that the body has become overloaded with debris.

How To Cure A Fever

◆ *The Use Of Water*

In all cases of fever, a few days of a liquid diet will lessen the severity, and give the stomach a much needed rest. Drink plenty of water as it dilutes and carries away toxins through the kidneys. "Pure water is one of heaven's choicest blessings…. (it) assists nature to resist disease…. Water can be used in many ways to relieve suffering…. thousands have died for want of pure water and pure air who might have lived…. If in their fevered state, water had been given them to drink freely, and applications had also been made externally, long days and nights of suffering would have been saved and many precious lives spared" (CD419). All fevers need a FASTING TREATMENT for their real cure.

◆ *Fruit Juices*

Fruit juices of all kinds are beneficial and especially orange juice, but the juices must be given without extra CANE SUGAR, for cane sugar will increase the fever, and produce ACID BLOOD. If necessary sweeten drinks with honey, and use fresh fruit juices wherever possible. When the fever subsides eat light and nourishing food such as SOYBEAN MILK, POTASSIUM BROTH, BROWN RICE, or BANANAS very ripe. "In cases of severe fever, abstinence from food for a short time will lessen the fever, and make the use of water more effectual" (2T384).

◆ *The Use Of Herbs*

The herbs that are commonly used against fever in form of tea are CHAMOMILE, CATNIP, CAYENNE, RASPBERRY LEAF, SLIPPERY ELM, GINGER, SAGE, ROSE HIPS, and RED CLOVER. These teas can be flavored with lemon juice and honey.

- ✓ FEVERFEW—The herbalist Eleanor Sinclair Rhode said that feverfew was used as our forefather's aspirin, and she added that it was a good deal less harmful than aspirin.
- ✓ BAYBERRY—The Indian tribe of Choctaws boiled the leaves and stem of the bayberry plant and drank the tea as a fever remedy.
- ✓ DOGWOOD—Several Indian tribes used the bark of the flowering dogwood by making a tea out of it for reducing fever.

Hay Fever

Congestion due to hay fever can be cleared up in 20 minutes with herb teas of FENUGREEK, ANISE, HOREHOUND, as well as with a concoction of GARLIC OIL in water. The vapors of EUCALYPTUS will do it also. One person had no problem with hay fever when he drank RAW MILK on a farm. But when he moved to the city and started drinking PASTEURIZED milk, he had allergy problems. When he started drinking GOAT'S MILK his allergies left him. In Vermont, HONEY is used for treating hay fever. Chewing on HONEY -COMB is recommended. In one case the hay fever vanished in seconds. Each time it occurred, the same remedy eliminated it. It is reported that people have gotten complete relief from hay fever by eating two 6 inch COMFREY LEAVES a day throughout the hay fever season. Comfrey can also be taken in the form of a tea.

◆ *Vitamins*

- ✓ VITAMIN C—Use lemon, orange, and grapefruit juice. Also CHAMOMILE, COLTSFOOT, and CHINCHONA BARK tea. Vitamin C acts as a natural ANTIHISTAMINE by reducing the swelling and inflammation. For many people large doses of vitamin C will break up an allergic reaction. Take from 150 to 1000 mg of Vitamin C every hour, then 2000 mg daily until healed. Applying vitamin C powder on the sores often causes them to dry up within hours.
- ✓ VITAMIN B—The STRESS of fever increases the need for B-vitamins. Taking a B-complex tablet daily, and 500 to 1000 mg of vitamin C, plus a CALCIUM tablet each hour often accomplishes a rapid lowering of temperature by destroying bacteria and viruses. Vitamin B_6 does away with FEVER BLISTERS or COLD SORES.
- ✓ Steam Baths

According to Al. Wolfsen who has practiced this method in the mission field, have a steam bath ready and hot when a MALARIAL FEVER attack is expected. While in the chill give a steam bath before the fever starts. If done properly there is no more malaria unless you get a mosquito bite again. If you are too late with the heat, get it at the next chill.

Rheumatic Fever

- ✓ SEAWEED—Eat a good natural diet with the emphasis on eating SEAWEED daily.
- ✓ CHARCOAL—Mrs. White tells the story of a young woman who had contracted a fever. The physician could not help her any further and he asked Mrs. White for a suggestion. She suggested that they send for PULVERIZED CHARCOAL, make a poultice of it, and lay it over her stomach and sides. A half hour after doing so relief came, and the girl had a natural sleep for the first time in days. (2SM295)

GALLBLADDER DISEASE

Nature Of The Disease

Bile is a secretion of the liver that passes from the BILE DUCT of the liver into the common bile duct, and then into the DUODENUM as needed. The bile from the liver is colored like straw, while that from the gallbladder varies from yellow to brown and green. BILE is a blend of ACIDS, CHOLESTEROL, LECITHIN, MINERALS, PIGMENTS and WATER. Their job is to work on digested FATS, CAROTENE, and the fat soluble VITAMINS A, D, E, and K, so that they can pass through the intestinal wall into the blood. When not enough bile is produced, fats melted at body temperature cover carbohydrates and proteins, thereby making it difficult for enzymes to continue the digestion process, so that bacteria attack this partially digested mass, causing MALNUTRITION.

The gallbladder serves as a reservoir for BILE not required for use by the liver. CHOLESTEROL is a vital ingredient in the bile which is secreted by the liver, and stored and concentrated in the gallbladder. From the gallbladder bile pours into the intestines to help digest FATTY FOODS. BILE ACIDS are the major FAT EMULSIFIERS of the body. Little bile is produced when the diet is low in PROTEIN or is excessively high in SUGAR and REFINED CARBOHYDRATES.

The Cause Of Gallstones

◆ *Why Gallstones Form*

The predisposing factors to the development of gallstones are OBESITY, DIABETES, INFECTIONS, and long periods of INACTIVITY or bed rest. It was found that being 20% OVERWEIGHT doubles a person's susceptibility to gallstones. A person who weighs 300 pounds produces twice the amount of cholesterol of a person of half that weight. Women taking ORAL CONTRACEPTIVES are twice as susceptible as those who are not taking them. Many studies indict excess SUGAR and a deficiency of FIBER. Also the cause of gallstones can be found in the eating of GREASE and FATTY FOODS, BUTTER, RICH FOODS, TOO MUCH STARCH, MILK, EGGS, CHEESE, SODA DRINKS, and in a lack of WATER.

Fewer than 30% of persons with gallstones ever develop symptoms. In most cases such a condition can be left alone unless there is an attack. But a low fat diet can work. Otherwise, the FAT you eat causes the small intestine to send a message to the gallbladder for more BILE.

◆ *Caused By Diet Of Fatty Foods*

A high fat cholesterol diet causes gallstones. Experimental animals fed a diet deficient in VITAMIN E developed gallstones. With sufficient vitamin E they formed no gallstones.

At times cholesterol begins to crystallize out of solution to form STONES. Often a patient with gallstones has no symptoms. But when a stone blocks the bile passage, NAUSEA, VOMITING, and severe PAIN occur. These symptoms often arise after the patient has eaten fried or fatty foods. Gallstones can occur at any age, but are more frequent in middle age. They develop in four times as many women as men, and appear to run in families.

◆ *Obesity*

According to a Harvard study OBESE WOMEN were 6 times as prone to gallstones as women of normal weight. What is surprising is that women who were only 10 pounds overweight had nearly twice the chance of developing gallstones. A Greek study showed that people who ate lots of animal fat were more apt to develop gallstones. On the other hand, people who ate lots of OLIVE OIL actually discouraged the formation of gallstones.

◆ *The Incomplete Digestion Of Fat*

An excess of fatty, rich foods in the diet can injure the gall bladder, and increase the chances of forming gallstones. They may consist of different substances, but the most common ones are composed of CHOLESTEROL, and these, the herbalists say, have the greatest possibility of being dissolved. COOKED FATS and FRIED FOODS are the most common cause of a disorganized gall bladder function. The incomplete digestion of fats, and excessive fermentation in the system, cause improper secretion and flow of bile from the liver. GALLSTONES and GRAVEL represent the accumulation of INORGANIC CALCIUM due to the inability of the system to assimilate it.

◆ *The High Fat/Low Fiber Diet*

Gallstones are almost unknown among primitive people eating unrefined foods. The prevalence of gallstones in the U.S. has been related to the HIGH FAT/LOW FIBER diet consumed by the majority of Americans. The consumption of fiber-depleted refined foods as the MAIN CAUSE of gallstones has a great deal of support. Since the solubility of cholesterol is dependent upon the BILE ACID content of the bile, when bile acid levels are low, cholesterol-rich gallstones form. In one experiment, Dr. Ginter gave guinea pigs a diet deficient in VITAMIN C. As a result their level of bile acids was greatly reduced. Also a deficiency of VITAMIN E has been shown to cause gallstones in experimental animals. Associated with increased incidence of gallstones are some of the DRUGS used to lower body cholesterol. The theory with the most circumstantial evidence is that the stones are precipitated by a decrease in the ratio of lecithin to cholesterol.

Dr. Burkitt showed that people who ate high fiber foods didn't have gallstones. People who eat a lot of FAT need more cholesterol in their intestines as well as in their blood. When the cholesterol in the bile duct gets too high, it forms small cholesterol crystals which can grow in size as large as golf balls. With lots of fiber in the diet, it would be low in fat, so the bile wouldn't be full of cholesterol. Gallstones are almost pure cholesterol.

Women are thought to be predisposed to gallstones possibly because of the SUPPRESSION OF BILE ACID SYNTHESIS by ESTROGENS. Women who use BIRTH CONTROL PILLS are 2 times more likely to develop gallstones, and those who take estrogen are 2 times as likely to develop them.

◆ *Symptoms Of Gallstones*

The symptom of the presence of gallstones is the fact that at times the SKIN TURNS YELLOW. Also there is excruciating PAIN when a stone attempts to pass through the gall duct. Such pain can stop suddenly after a few minutes, or it can last for a few days. It develops on the upper part on the right side of the abdomen.

DIMINISHED BILE FLOW is caused by the presence of GALLSTONES, STEROIDAL HORMONES, DRUGS, HYPERTHYROIDISM, and VIRAL HEPATITIS.

The Treatment Of Gallstones

✓ FRESH VEGETABLES—To cure gallstones, meals should be low in fat and rich in all kinds of FRESH VEGETABLES, especially ARTICHOKES, which have a long-standing reputation in treating many liver ailments, DANDELION GREENS, RED BEETS, CUCUMBERS, SWISS CHARD, and BEET GREENS. Low fat YOGURT is also beneficial.

A vegetarian diet has been shown to be protective against gallstone formation.
ANIMAL PROTEIN has been shown to increase the formation of gallstones, while SOY PROTEIN was shown to be preventive against gallstone formation. It was also shown to dissolve gallstones in hamsters.

A Harvard study of 88,000 middle aged persons of normal weight found that women with the highest intake of vegetables were only 60% to 70% as likely to have gallstone symptoms as women who ate the least vegetables. Women who ate the most NUTS, BEANS, LENTILS, PEAS, LIMA BEANS, and ORANGES were largely resistant to gallbladder attacks. The gallstone fighting ingredient is probably FIBER, but also most likely VEGETABLE PROTEIN such as is in SOYBEANS. It seems that soybean proteins block gallstones by reducing the saturation of cholesterol in the bile. According to animal studies, when soybeans were fed to hamsters, they caused small gallstones in the hamsters to dissolve.

✓ VITAMINS AND MINERALS—Supplements of VITAMINS A, C, the B-COMPLEX, plus MINERALS and AMINO ACIDS are helpful. BREWER'S YEAST, SOY FLOUR, and WHEAT GERM, can be used to add PROTEIN to the diet without extra fat. PEARS are believed to have a specific healing effect on the GALL BLADDER.

✓ OLIVE OIL—Give a tablespoonful of olive oil and a teaspoonful of LEMON JUICE every hour till relieved. GRAPEFRUIT juice can be used in place of lemon juice. Lemon juice itself is a powerful purge for the empty gallbladder when taken before breakfast. Olive oil stimulates the production of BILE and the fat-digesting enzyme LIPASE.

One person drank a half gallon of APPLE JUICE every day for three days. After three days he drank 4 ounces of OLIVE OIL and 4 ounces of LEMON JUICE and got rid of a dozen stones.

In another case, for 2 days a person drank ORGANIC APPLE JUICE. On the third day he drank a half cup of olive oil with a cup of apple juice. On the 4rth day the gallstones passed.

One person discharged several dozen waxy stones after drinking six ounces of olive oil. She lay on her right side all night while waiting for the oil to work.

Take one or two tablespoons of olive oil before each meal. It starts the flow of BILE before the rest of the food enters the stomach. Another method for passing gallstones is fasting for two days while drinking APPLE JUICE at two hour intervals.

The reason the olive oil cure for the elimination of gallstones works is because it stimulates the secretion of the bile, which then carries the small and medium stones with it. According to Richard Lucas, herbalist, olive oil causes strong contractions of the gallbladder, and seems to melt the stones. When gallstones were immersed in pure olive oil, they lost 68% of their weight.

✓ HEAT—Applying heat to the sore place will often dislodge the stone and give speedy relief.

✓ LECITHIN—A PHOSPHOLIPID, can prevent gallstones by holding cholesterol in suspension so that it does not precipitate out of the bile to form gallstones. Giving gallstone patients two tablespoons of lecithin a day immediately results in increased PHOSPHOLIPID concentration in the bile which helps to keep cholesterol dispersed, and prevents the formation of gallstones.

✓ SKIPPING BREAKFAST—One study has determined that people who skip breakfast have a greater incidence of gallstones than those who don't. One cardiologist found that skipping breakfast nearly triples a person's clot-forming potential, leaving one more vulnerable to heart attacks and strokes. Blood platelets stickiness is lowest overnight, then it climbs rapidly when you wake up. But for some mysterious reason, eating breakfast seems to unstick the platelets.

✓ HERB TEAS—If you have any kind of gallbladder disease or complaint, give yourself a treatment with NETTLE TEA, drinking up to four cups a day for several weeks. Drink the tea slowly, one sip at a time. For another treatment drink one mouthful of CALAMUS ROOT tea before and after each meal, for a total of 6 mouthfuls a day, which equals one cup. Also COMFREY, PARSLEY, DANDELION ROOT, PEPPERMINT, and FENNEL tea are helpful. CELANDINE is an herb which has cured many gallbladder problems. Three cups of SMART WEED tea a day have dissolved gallstones. ROSE PETALS contain MALIC and TARTARIC acids which are of great value in dissolving gallstones and GRAVEL from the urinary organs. The dried petals and leaves are often used as a tea substitute with peppermint, lemon peel, and linden leaves. CHAMOMILE tea has long been known to dissolve gallstones. When two gallstones were placed in a glass of CHAMOMILE tea, they were completely dissolved in 10 days.

The Prevention Of Gallstones

✓ SOYBEAN LECITHIN—Gallstones can be prevented with SOYBEAN LECITHIN, according to Dr. R.K. Tompkins of Ohio State University. It liquifies the cholesterol.

✓ FIBER—Fiber helps prevent gallstones by stimulating BILE flow, and preventing the reabsorption of bile. Dr. Ben Ershoff of the University of Southern California proved that fiber would make a toxic diet safe. He also showed that SOLUBLE FIBERS are better at detoxifying than INSOLUBLE FIBERS. He proved that the soluble fibers of ALFALFA and PSYLLIUM are better than the insoluble fiber of WHEAT BRAN. Wheat bran improves regularity but it doesn't lower CHOLESTEROL. OAT BRAN and OATMEAL lower cholesterol better than they improve regularity. WHEAT BRAN also reduces POLYPS, which are tumors found in vascular organs such as NOSE, UTERUS, and RECTUM. OATMEAL is a good source of SOLUBLE GUMS which are excellent for removing BILE ACIDS, which is practically the same as removing cholesterol from the blood. BEANS will do the same.

GASTROINTESTINAL COMPLAINTS

Stomach Problems

◆ *Acid Stomach*

The stomach's digestive juices, such as the HYDROCHLORIC ACID and the enzyme PEPSIN slosh into the lowest part of the esophagus and cause irritating sensations and pressure beneath the breast bone. Such sensations are sometimes taken for a heart attack. CHOCOLATE and chocolate cookies can bring on HEART BURN through the THEOBROMINE which might enter into the opening of the SPHINCTER MUSCLE at the end of the esophagus to cause irritation. CAFFEINE and THEOPHYLLINE will do the same. CHOCOLATE MILK is a threat to heart burn because it contains caffeine, theobromine, theophylline, and fat, which will allow stomach acid to escape up the esophagus to cause heartburn.

To avoid heartburn, cut down on FATTY FOODS. They are twice as likely to cause it as is chocolate. For an acid stomach use cup of COOKED RICE as an antacid, for it ties up excess stomach acid. Other studies found that BEANS, CORN, and TOFU were good at combating stomach acid.

◆ *Stomach Cramps*

For STOMACH CRAMPS—you can use GINGER ROOT from the grocery store, either chew it, make it into a tea, or take it as a tincture. You can also take CATNIP and FENNEL tinctures. If the cramp is strong, use CRAMP BARK, or ANTISPASMODIC tincture. This is a tincture that contains SKULLCAP, LOBELIA, CAYENNE, VALERIAN, SKUNK-CABBAGE, GUM MYRRH, and BLACK COHOSH.

◆ *Stomach Pain*

For STOMACH PAIN—stop eating between meals. The stomach needs REST. Use PEPPERMINT tea. "HOP poultices over the stomach will relieve pain" (2SM287). Research found that healthy people were most likely to react with stomach pain by eating MAYONNAISE, CABBAGE, and FRIED and SALTED FOODS.

◆ *Upset Stomach*

For an UPSET STOMACH—BANANAS are the longtime folk remedy.

◆ *Colic*

If a newborn infant has COLIC, one should suspect COW'S MILK. Studies have shown that about 70% of colicky infants have an aversion to cow's milk. The infants with the cow's milk formula usually quickly recovered when SOY MILK is substituted for the cow's milk. It is also important that the mothers themselves cut out cow's milk because some of the elements that cause colic in the infant can still get into the mothers milk.

Intestinal Problems

◆ *Constipation*

BOWEL MOVEMENTS SHOULD OCCUR AT REGULAR INTERVALS—During digestion, fluids and nutrients are absorbed in the small intestines, thereby leaving a good deal of indigestible material to be disposed of by the large intestine. PERISTALSIS involves the contraction and relaxation of the muscles lining the walls of the intestines. These actions can be quite irregular in the large intestines. For any given person, bowel movements should normally occur at the same regular interval. Any variance from that pattern could result in constipation, which is intestinal sluggishness resulting in delayed action, and in few or incomplete bowel movements.

Retaining WASTE MATERIAL can result in APPENDICITIS, CANCER, DIVERTICULOSIS, and HEMORRHOIDS.

✓ LACK OF FIBER AN IMPORTANT CAUSE — Most constipation results from either LACK OF FIBER and FLUID in the diet, or a DELAYED RESPONSE to nature's call. EMOTIONAL STRESS can cause it. So can IRREGULAR EATING HABITS and LACK OF EXERCISE. The use of ANTACIDS or DRUGS such as ACTH, CORTISONE, CODEINE, which slow nerve reactions, or DIURETICS which deplete the body of liquids, may also be responsible. Most chronic constipation can be corrected by increasing the proportion of BULKY, FIBROUS FOODS in the diet. Refined SUGAR and FLOUR products cause constipation because they lack fiber.

In constipation, waste matter is left too long in the body due to LACK OF MUSCULAR TONE in the bowels, IMPROPER MASTICATION of food, a MEAT diet, too many VARIETIES of food at one meal, eating food that is too CONCENTRATED, and not enough BODILY ACTIVITY.

THE SYMPTOMS OF CONSTIPATION—Some of the symptoms of constipation are a COATED TONGUE, FOUL BREATH, BACKACHE, HEADACHE, INSOMNIA, LOSS OF APPETITE, and VARIOUS PAINS. Children become irritable and cross when bowels are irregular.

HOW CONSTIPATION CAN BE CURED—Many cases of chronic constipation can be corrected by increasing the daily intake of fruits and vegetables.

- YOGURT and KEFIR—is effective for some. Some require the addition of BRAN for a return to regularity.
- VITAMINS and MINERALS—As supplementary materials have proven of benefit to many people.
- FIGS and PRUNES—because of their fiber content, are natural bowel relievers. Figs have been recommended in a one day program of figs only.
- BANANAS—as an addition to the diet are often helpful.
- WATER—an addition of more water to the diet has often relieved long-standing sufferers. A glass of water before orange juice and cereal at breakfast, and also an extra glass of water before bedtime is recommended.

TREATMENT—Take an ENEMA or HERBAL LAXATIVE. Eat your food as dry as possible. If it is thoroughly saturated with saliva, it will lubricate the bowels, make the system ALKALINE, and will greatly increase the rapidity of digestion. Do your drinking one hour before or three hours after eating. Practice DEEP BREATHING just before and right after eating, or take a slow WALK after eating. The extra oxygen thus acquired is one of the greatest factors in helping digest your food, and in making red blood.

One of the mildest laxatives is OLIVE OIL. Take one tablespoon at bedtime. In enema form it is often used to relieve FECAL IMPACTION.

CASCARA SAGRADA BARK—is one of the most effective, gentle, and nonhabituating LAXATIVES available. It is also an aid in restoring the natural tone of the colon. Its action is mild, unaccompanied by discomfort, and can restore habitual constipation to normal. Also use FENUGREEK SEEDS and BLACKSTRAP MOLASSES.

◆ *How To Avoid Constipation*

- FIBER—Use enough fiber in the diet.
- ALLERGENS—Eliminate all food allergens.
- YOGURT—Eat a cup of yogurt daily
- FOLIC ACID—Take at least 60 mg of folic acid daily.
- EXERCISE—Get at least hour of vigorous exercise daily.

◆ *Piles*

Use DANDELION, BURDOCK, and YELLOW DOCK root teas. For INFLAMMATION—FENUGREEK seed tea is used internally for inflamed conditions of the STOMACH, BOWELS, and INTESTINES. It helps to clear the body of excessive mucus. It is also used in DIVERTICULOSIS and COLITIS. FENULIN TABLETS is a preparation of fenugreek seeds, which can be obtained from the health food store.

◆ *Other Gastrointestinal Ailments*

✓ COLITIS—A patient complained that he had suffered from GAS DYSPEPSIA and COLITIS for 17 years. He was given 2 gm of a Garlic Preparation, two or three times a day. In 2 months the patient considered himself cured.

✓ GAS PRODUCERS—FLATULENCE—Gas producers are foods such as DRIED BEANS, CABBAGE, CAULIFLOWER, ONIONS, UNRIPE APPLES, FRESH BREAD, CHOCOLATE, FRIED FOODS, PEANUTS, RADISHES etc. Refined carbohydrates such as sugar and refined flour contribute to it. SUGAR alone irritates the lining of the digestive tract to cause GAS, INDIGESTION and FLATULENCE.

One author says that DAIRY PRODUCTS, and not beans, are perhaps the number one cause of flatulence in the country due to the varying degrees of LACTOSE INTOLERANCE. Lactose is a gas producer for people who are deficient in the enzyme LACTASE, which is needed to digest the milk sugar LACTOSE. Drinking 2 cups of milk boosted gas release by 8 times in those persons who were lactose intolerant. One can have from mild to severe lactose intolerance and not even know it. But YOGURT is exempt. It does not produce gas.

In one test drinking a quart of APPLE JUICE increased gas output 4 times. At times starchy foods can be gaseous, but the least starchy gaseous food is RICE. Bacteria are normally present in the digestive tract. When they work on the undigested parts of a big meal, one by-product is a mixture of gases, including HYDROGEN SULFIDE, with the familiar rotten egg odor, as well as residues of fatty acids.

✓ GAS ABSORBERS—All of the MINTS, including PEPPERMINT, SPEARMINT, and PENNYROYAL make good CARMINATIVE, or gas destroying teas. Peppermint tea is a GASTRIC STIMULANT, TONIC, ANTISEPTIC, and an ANODYNE, or pain reliever. It is a popular beverage for INDIGESTION, and resulting DISTRESSES. It stimulates the flow of gastric digestive juices, and also relieves BLOATING. HEATHER is a tea which quiets many a stomach problem. "EXERCISE will aid the work of digestion…. The diseased stomach will find relief by exercise" (HL697)

GOLDENSEAL ROOT as well as LICORICE ROOT tea will eliminate the development of gas. Also take CHARCOAL for gas. Foods which prevent flatulence are: BEETS, ENDIVE, GARLIC, JERUSALEM ARTICHOKES, OLIVES or OLIVE OIL, PAPAYA, and PINEAPPLE. Also DIGESTIVE ENZYME tablets.

✓ HEMORRHOIDS—PAPAYA contains an enzyme PAPAIN. It can be obtained in the form of enzyme tablets. It is helpful in coping with INDIGESTION. It is also helpful in HEMORRHOIDS, and is also useful as an ANTHELMINTIC, or against intestinal worms.

✓ BAD BREATH—We are told that "If more food is eaten than can be digested and appropriated, a decaying mass accumulates in the stomach, causing an offensive breath, and a bad taste in the mouth" (HL399).

✓ DYSPEPSIA—SUGAR that is not completely absorbed by the digestive tract is consumed by bacteria and fermented. The bacteria produce hydrogen, causing a wide array of gastrointestinal problems, including GAS, BLOATING, AND CRAMPS. When HIGH-FAT FOODS are consumed, the gall bladder secretes greater quantities of BILE ACIDS, which are used by the liver to digest fat. The increased bile acids disrupt digestion and cause a variety of painful side effects, from HEARTBURN to ULCERS.

Diet For Gastrointestinal Problems

✓ WHOLE GRAINS AND FRESH VEGETABLES—Use these as sources of FIBER. Fiber has been shown to decrease all forms of stomach and digestive problems, including severe disorders, such as DIVERTICULAR DISEASE and ULCERS.

✓ LACTOBACILLUS—Foods containing lactobacillus, such as YOGURT, MISO, and homemade PICKLES and SAUERKRAUT.

✓ HERBS—CHAMOMILE or PEPPERMINT will effectively settle an upset stomach. Pour 1 cup of boiling water over 1 heaping teaspoon of either herb and steep for 10 minutes in a covered pot. ANISE or FENNEL SEEDS relieve intestinal gas. Pour a cup of boiling water over 2 teaspoons of slightly crushed seeds and steep for 10 minutes. Drink a cup hour before meals. Herbal bitters improve digestion by stimulating the production digestive fluids and enzymes.

GLAUCOMA

Nature Of The Disease

◆ *Pressure In The Eyeball*

Glaucoma is the second leading cause of blindness in the U.S. There are approximately 7 million known cases today. It usually affects people over forty, and is generally more common in women than in men. It is characterized by an INCREASE in PRESSURE of the FLUID within the EYEBALL, and a hardening of the surface of the eyeball which may lead to blindness. Symptoms of GLAUCOMA include EYE PAIN or DISCOMFORT mainly in the morning, BLURRED VISION, HALOS around LIGHT, INABILITY of the PUPILS to adjust to a DARK ROOM, and PERIPHERAL VISION LOSS.

◆ *A Blocked Drainage Canal*

The watery substance of the AQUEOUS HUMOR is constantly produced, and flows through it to nourish the CORNEA, and then drains through a minute natural canal. This DRAINAGE CANAL may become blocked for reasons not clearly understood. The pressure within the eyeball builds up. This pressure is transmitted to the retina which contains sensitive nerve cells and fibers that relay light stimuli through the optic nerve to the brain. This pressure can cause destruction of these cells, and with each cell destroyed, a portion of the field of vision is lost. Eventually all sight will be gone. GLAUCOMA begins with the loss of peripheral vision, then slowly closes in until only straight-ahead vision is left, and then none at all.

The Causes Of Glaucoma

◆ *Stress And Nutritional Factors*

Glaucoma has many causes, but it is most often related to STRESS and NUTRITIONAL FACTORS. Whenever stress is a major factor, the injection of the VITAMIN B-COMPLEX appears to have good results. Some of the other possible causes are errors in COLLAGEN METABOLISM which are often associated with eye complications such as GLAUCOMA, MYOPIA, RETINAL DETACHMENT, DISLOCATED LENS, BLUE SCLERA, and CORTICOSTEROIDS which induce glaucoma by destroying collagen structures in the eye. Their use should be abandoned.

◆ *Danger Signals For Glaucoma*

There is a chance that glaucoma is in the process of developing if one or more of the following symptoms are in evidence: RAINBOW-COLORED RINGS, or HALOS around lights; narrowing of the VISUAL FIELD; frequent changes in EYEGLASS PRESCRIPTIONS; poor vision in DIM LIGHT; BLURRED VISION which may come and go; EYE ACHES after watching TV in darkened rooms; WATERING of eyes; any change of EYE COLOR.

The Cure Of Glaucoma

◆ *A Vitamin C-Rich Diet*

It is generally believed that restoration of vision already lost due to nerve degeneration, caused by increased intraocular pressure, cannot occur. However, certain dietary factors have proven effective in controlling the condition and preserving the remaining vision. The DIET should emphasize RAW VITAMIN C-RICH FOODS, that is, fresh fruits and vegetables.

Take megadoses of vitamin C. Allow 60 to 250 mg per pound of body weight per day. That means that a 150 lb. person should take about 7 gm of vitamin C, 3 to 5 times a day. It has been demonstrated in studies in Rome, Italy, that the intraocular pressure in glaucoma-affected eyes can be dramatically reduced by the oral application of megadoses of vitamin C.

Some people will respond to as little as 2 gm of vitamin C per day, while others will respond only to extremely high doses up to 35 gm/day. The mechanism by which vitamin C lowers the eye pressure is by diminished production of eye fluid, and improved fluid outflow. In the light of recent research, its role in collagen formation may be the key to its action.

◆ *What To Avoid*

✓ CAFFEINE—should be avoided, for it causes an elevation of blood pressure, and an increasing blood flow to the eye. Caffeine causes stimulation of the VASOCONSTRICTORS, elevating the blood pressure.

✓ STRESS—Glaucoma is considered a STRESS DISEASE, so avoid emotional stresses. Avoid prolonged eye stresses such as long TV WATCHING. and EXCESSIVE READING.

◆ *Herbs*

Use EYEBRIGHT and GOLDENSEAL in capsule or tea form.

◆ *Juices*

Use LEMON, GRAPEFRUIT, ORANGE, CARROT, and RED BEET Juices.

◆ Carrots

A 60 year old man's eyesight was so bad he could see only shadows. On a friend's advice, he began to eat 3 carrots a day boiled in a quart of water. He also drank all the water and used no seasoning. After using this procedure for two months, he now can see SHAPES and COLORS.

◆ Applied Experiences

✓ VARIETY of VITAMINS—Dr. Stanley C. Evans found that good nutrition can often prevent and cure some cases of glaucoma. He gives patients large daily doses of VITAMINS A, B, C, and E. In most cases, he says, the pressure within the eye was reduced to normal limits in a week. He says that he found IMPROVED NUTRITION to be much better for glaucoma than drugs, which he had also used in the past. Today he rarely uses drugs. Many researchers believe that there is a connection between it and a lack of VITAMINS A, B, and C.

A 36 year old lady had glaucoma. Her eye pressure was up to 36 in one eye and 32 in the other. EYE DROPS did not help. She decided to try vitamins. She used 2000 to 3000 mg of vitamin C with ROSE HIPS plus 150 mg RUTIN twice a day for three months. After that the pressures were a normal 20.

✓ FILTERED LIGHT—Letting bright sunlight filter through closed eyelids while slowly turning the head for two minutes several times each day has been of benefit during the early stages of glaucoma.

✓ EXERCISE—Researchers found that the fluid pressure in the eye dropped when people exercised 45 minutes 3 times a week.

✓ DIET—TESTIMONIAL—A woman of around 70 years of age with GLAUCOMA went to an ophthalmologist who gave her drugs to be dropped into her eyes 3 times a day. She followed those directions rather spasmodically and then discontinued them. Then she started on a short fast and made a radical change in her lifestyle, especially in her eating habits. Her Glaucoma cleared up. A few months later she returned to her doctor, who, upon examination, found no trace of glaucoma. Her vision was much better and so was her health, and he called her a very "lucky woman." He didn't think that her changed lifestyle and diet had anything to do with her fortune. He didn't think that food had anything to do with it. An intelligent man, on the other hand, who was not subject to medical blinders, would recognize that eyes are parts of the body, that eye-health is the product of the same factors that produce and maintain general health, and that eye-disease grows out of the same causes that impair health in general. If food affects the health of the body as a whole, there is no reason why it will not affect the health of the eyes.

HARDENING OF THE ARTERIES— ARTERIOSCLEROSIS—ATHEROSCLEROSIS

Nature Of The Disease

ARTERIOSCLEROSIS is the clogging or filling up of the arteries by deposits of CHOLESTEROL, FAT, and/or MINERALS. Clogged and hardened arteries bring on HEART ATTACKS. It is the low density LIPOPROTEIN (LDL), that causes problems, while the high density lipoprotein (HDL) protects against arteriosclerosis. Cholesterol is necessary for the body and has many different functions. It is now believed that the ratio of "good" HDL to "bad" LDL cholesterol is more important than the total amount of cholesterol.

Arteriosclerosis involves the buildup of CALCIUM DEPOSITS on the inside of the artery walls, which cause thickening and hardening of the arteries. If the deposits are FATTY substances, the condition is referred to as ATHEROSCLEROSIS. Both conditions have about the same effect on the circulation. Such conditions cause STROKES, VERTIGO or DIZZINESS, A PARTIAL LOSS of HEARING, RINGING in the EARS, LEG PAIN, CRAMPS, or TIREDNESS in the LEGS, CORONARY DISEASE (angina), and HIGH BLOOD PRESSURE. High blood pressure can also in turn cause arteriosclerosis. The calcium or fatty deposits usually form in areas of the arteries that have been weakened by high blood pressure. As the arteries become less pliable, CELL STARVATION or ISCHEMIA results due to insufficient circulation in the cells. When one of the coronary arteries becomes completely obstructed by accumulated deposits, a HEART ATTACK occurs which is also referred to as a MYOCARDIAL INFARCTION or a CORONARY OCCLUSION. A STROKE occurs when one of the arteries of the brain is closed.

Causes Of Arteriosclerosis

✓ REFINED FOODS—It has been demonstrated that excessive consumption of WHITE SUGAR and REFINED FOODS is one of the prime causes of hardening of the arteries. Also a deficiency of VITAMINS B, C, E, and CHROMIUM, other MINERALS, as well as a LACK of FIBER in the foods eaten.

✓ VITAMIN C DEFICIENCY—A very significant factor in human arteriosclerosis is a DEFICIENCY in VITAMIN C. It could in part be described as a DEFICIENCY DISEASE, which is preventable and treatable by a VITAMIN C THERAPY. It can be induced in GUINEA PIGS by giving them a vitamin C-free diet.

Dr. Constance Spittle of England believes that hardening of the arteries is a VITAMIN C deficiency disease. On a diet of only fresh fruit and vegetables, she found that the levels of cholesterol in her blood declined from 240 mg/% to 160 mg/%. (% means per 100 cc of blood). When she boiled all of the fruits and vegetables thoroughly before eating them, the cholesterol levels began to climb again.

✓ FATS and CHOLESTEROL—The disease is induced in animals by feeding them a diet inordinately high in FATS and CHOLESTEROL. The FRAMINGHAM STUDY determined that cholesterol levels above 300 created 10 times more heart disease than cholesterol levels of less than 200. One cannot develop ATHEROSCLEROSIS unless one has a cholesterol level of above 160. SKIM MILK is recommended in preference to WHOLE MILK. There is mounting evidence that high cholesterol is an EFFECT, and not a CAUSE, and that the "CIVILIZED DIET" of white sugar, white flour, and processed foods results in hardening of the arteries and atherosclerosis. There is evidence that it is the TRIGLYCERIDES rather than the CHOLESTEROL which are manufactured from sugar in the body, which appear to contribute to the development of atherosclerosis.

✓ OBESITY—Obese men have 5 times more cardiovascular disease than normal weight men. When it comes to OVEREATING one can trust one's INSTINCT only as long as one uses NATURAL FOODS. It becomes confused if the food eaten is overprocessed, and adulterated with artificial flavors and colorings. We are told that "We must be satisfied with pure simple food, prepared in a simple manner. This should be the diet of high and low. ADULTERATED SUBSTANCES are to be avoided" (CD85).

✓ CHLORINATED WATER—has been shown to contribute to ARTERIOSCLEROSIS.

✓ INORGANIC CALCIUM—Arteriosclerosis represents a DEFICIENCY of ORGANIC CALCIUM and an excess of INORGANIC CALCIUM in the diet, causing the blood vessels to lose elasticity, and causing the blood to coagulate in the veins. Hence, it is sometimes called "arthritis of the eye."

✓ COFFEE—A strong association exists between coffee consumption and MYOCARDIAL INFARCTION.

How To Heal Arteriosclerosis

✓ FIBER—Laboratory tests have shown that high fiber diets reduce the formation of fatty deposits in the arteries and increase the excretion of cholesterol. All ROOT VEGETABLES, DRIED LEGUMES, and WHOLE GRAINS are rich in fiber, but unprocessed OAT and WHEAT BRAN are the most concentrated. They are also rich in minerals. The PECTIN in fruits such as APPLES, limits the amount of cholesterol the body absorbs. Eating nothing but CHERRIES for several days is a folk remedy for clearing accumulated debris from the arteries.

✓ GARLIC—It dilates the blood vessels and reduces cholesterol levels, as well as do eggplant and onions. It is rich in SELENIUM and GERMANIUM along with sulfur compounds, which are especially beneficial to cardiovascular physiology. Dr. Hans Reuter of Cologne, Germany, found that garlic helps clear fat from the blood vessels of people who like to eat rich foods, thereby reducing the risk of HEART ATTACKS and STROKES. He says that in some cases it is more effective than PENICILLIN and other ANTIBIOTICS. He also points out that in countries such as JAPAN, RUSSIA, KOREA, GREECE, and INDIA, where garlic is commonly consumed, there are fewer cases of ATHEROSCLEROSIS, STROKES, and other manifestations of hardening of the arteries.

✓ RAW POTATOES—Eating grated raw potatoes in salads or cereal is a Russian method of avoiding arteriosclerosis.

✓ YOGURT—Hospital tests have shown that yogurt lowers blood cholesterol by as much as 22 points when three cups are eaten daily.

✓ CALCIUM—If you don't take in enough calcium, your body will dissolve calcium from the bones into the bloodstream to prevent muscle cramps, maintain normal heartbeat, facilitate nerve conduction, and even aid in blood coagulation. Taking 1000 to 2000 mg of calcium daily for a year resulted in an average drop of 25% in cholesterol for the volunteers who were tested.

✓ EXERCISE—Plenty of outdoor exercise is needed. A sedentary life is one of the major contributing causes. It is known that exercise increases the "good" HDL levels.

✓ HERBS—Those that are most helpful are GARLIC, COMFREY, CAYENNE, GOLDENSEAL, HAWTHORN BERRIES, GINGER, GINSENG, ONION, SAGE, SLIPPERY ELM, TARRAGON, and YARROW.

The term GINSENG means "man-like." It is a general physical restorative which improves the work of the BRAIN CELLS, has a mild stabilizing effect on the BLOOD PRESSURE, whether high or low, relieves ATHEROSCLEROSIS, strengthens the body's DEFENSE SYSTEM, increases PHYSICAL endurance and stamina, reduces blood cholesterol, stimulates the function of the ENDOCRINE GLANDS, and in general increases the RESISTANCE of the organism.

✓ SYSTEMATIC UNDEREATING—It is recommended that one practice systematic UNDEREATING. It represents the number one health and longevity secret. OVEREATING on the other hand, even of health foods, is one of the main causes of disease and premature AGING. Studies of centenarians around the world show that they are moderate eaters throughout their lives. You will never see an obese centenarian. Studies in Russia and in the U.S. show that overeating is one of the prime causes of most DEGENERATIVE DISEASES. Food eaten in excess of body needs act in the system as a POISON. It INTERFERES with PROPER DIGESTION, causes INTERNAL SLUGGISHNESS, GAS, INCOMPLETE ASSIMILATION of NUTRIENTS, PUTREFACTION in the BOWELS, and ACTUALLY POISONS the WHOLE SYSTEM. Overindulgence in protein is particularly harmful. It is especially dangerous for older people who are less active and have a slowed-down metabolism. The unbelievable truth is that the less you eat, the less hungry you will feel, because the food will be more efficiently digested and better utilized. Good eating habits and LIFESTYLE more than GENETICS produce longevity.

✓ JUICES—All fresh fruit and vegetable juices are considered beneficial, with BEET, CARROT, CELERY, GRAPEFRUIT, LEMON, PARSLEY, PINEAPPLE, and SPINACH heading the list. Up to two glasses daily of any combination is recommended. PINEAPPLES, especially their enzyme BROMELAIN, inhibit PLATELET AGGREGATION, reduce ANGINA PAIN, reduce BLOOD PRESSURE, and break down ATHEROSCLEROTIC PLAQUES.

✓ LECITHIN—Use 1 to 5 tablespoons daily. In worldwide studies lecithin has proven effective for maintaining low LDL cholesterol levels with a normal diet. Lecithin helps to prevent cholesterol and other fats from accumulating in the walls of the arteries, and it helps any deposits that may be there which may lead to PHLEBITIS, STROKE, CORONARY THROMBOSIS, PULMONARY EMBOLISM, and ATHEROSCLEROSIS. If enough lecithin is eaten, ATHEROSCLEROSIS does not occur regardless of how much cholesterol is eaten. Even if far advanced, health can be restored if enough lecithin is in the diet.

✓ VITAMINS and MINERALS—Large amounts of VITAMIN A, 10,000 to 25,000 units daily, decrease cholesterol levels and increase the proportion of lecithin in the blood. BREWERS

YEAST and CHROMIUM also reduce cholesterol. 400 TO 1200 IU of VITAMIN E daily, increases HDL levels while reducing total serum cholesterol, elevates blood lecithin, and helps dissolve arterial scars so that atherosclerotic deposits will not form. It also protects the essential fatty acids from being destroyed within the body. Insufficient VITAMIN B_6 produces pathological changes in the arteries and other connective tissues which eventually cause arteriosclerosis. 80% of those who suffer heart attacks have NORMAL CHOLESTEROL levels.

HEART DISEASE

Nature Of The Disease

◆ *Heart Disease Is Based On Lifestyle*

HEART DISEASE is a disease caused by years of wrong eating, lack of exercising, and years of changes occurring within the most remote corners of your body. CHOLESTEROL, FAT, and CALCIUM collect in clumps until a clogged vessel blocks blood and oxygen needed by the heart. Then occurs a heart attack. Today doctors believe that heart disease is not only treatable but also preventable. It can often be avoided by a change in lifestyle, and one of the most important lifestyle changes is DIET, the food you choose to put on your table. Dr. L.G. Morgan of Columbia University says that foods can be used to cure most major diseases, but that they can be very important in preventing a wide range of major diseases.

The high fat diet can put you at high risk for CANCER and heart disease, while a diet which is low in saturated fats will reduce your risk of heart disease significantly. Saturated fat raises your cholesterol more than anything else you can eat. Eating right can even reverse ATHEROSCLEROSIS, one of the main causes of heart disease. Heart attacks are 2 times more likely to occur on Mondays than on Fridays. It is the PATTERN OF LIVING over the weekend, such as keeping later hours, going to parties, getting less sleep, that can bring about "problems" on Mondays. Death rates from heart disease are 4 to 7 times higher among people with HOSTILE ATTITUDES according to Dr. R. Williams.

◆ *Arteriosclerosis Is Largely Responsible For Heart Attacks*

HEART DISEASE is the leading health problem in the Western World. It is the number one cause of death in the U.S., claiming more than one million lives annually, which is over 50% of all deaths. When the heart's blood vessels narrow, insufficient amounts of oxygen reach the heart, causing the chest pain called ANGINA. When these vessels close entirely a HEART ATTACK or MYOCARDIAL INFARCTION can occur, resulting in damage to the heart muscle. ARTERIOSCLEROSIS is the most common cause of obstruction, and is responsible for most of the deaths resulting from heart attacks. BLOOD CLOTS also result in heart attacks, and HIGH BLOOD PRESSURE is a precursor to heart problems.

Cardiologists have urged people to sharply reduce CHOLESTEROL LEVELS by reducing saturated animal fats and increasing the consumption of polyunsaturated fats. Many have responded with changes in their diets but the heart attack rate continues to rise year by year. Dr. Ancel Keys of the University of Minnesota compared the MORTALITY RATE of men from ITALY, YUGOSLAVIA, GREECE, FINLAND, the NETHERLANDS, the U.S., and JAPAN. He found that men from countries with highest FAT intake, namely the U.S. and Finland, also had the highest death rate from HEART DISEASE.

◆ *God Forbade The Eating Of Animal Fat*

God had expressly forbidden the use of the fat of animals when He said: "It shall be a perpetual statute for your generations throughout all your dwellings, that ye eat neither FAT nor BLOOD" (Lev. 3:17; 2T61). As a scientific principle this was to apply to us today also. He told us that the vegetable oil in the olive is far better than the second hand animal fat, because animal fat would make the blood diseased. (CD359–60; 393–04).

The Prevention Of Heart Disease

◆ *Cholesterol Must Be Kept Below 160.*

CALCIUM and MAGNESIUM—Dr. H.A. Schroeder determined that in a town in West Texas which has water which is high in the minerals CAL-

CIUM (Ca) and MAGNESIUM (Mg), heart disease was consistently low. Besides these two, POTASSIUM, CHROMIUM, AND SELENIUM also guard against heart disease. If cholesterol is kept below 160, one can reverse coronary heart disease. HOT PEPPERS, GARLIC, and ONIONS have beneficial effects on factors associated with cardiovascular disease. Hot peppers dissolve BLOOD CLOTS, and so do garlic and onions. A University of California study found that detrimental LDL cholesterol rose by 6% in 181 healthy men with normal cholesterol, when they switched from regular coffee to DECAFFEINATED COFFEE. Decaffeinated coffee is not the answer to the coffee habit. The process that is used to take out the caffeine in coffee concentrates the oil known as CAFFEOL, which gives coffee its AROMA and FLAVOR. Caffeol is known as a carcinogen which irritates the stomach, liver, kidneys, and bladder, and causes BLADDER CANCER. It does so by restricting the size of the capillaries which carry oxygen to the cells. The reduced oxygen uptake allows the cells to become cancerous.

◆ *Monounsaturated Oils*

✓ OLIVE OIL—is better than any POLYUNSATURATED OIL in that it doesn't reduce the HDL or high density lipoprotein cholesterol, while it is driving down the LDL cholesterol level. People around the Mediterranean are only about as likely to die of heart disease as Americans. Such diet is not low fat but it is high in olive oil. Hence, olive oil is sometimes called the "LONGEVITY DIET."

Olive oil reduces the risk of ATHEROSCLEROSIS. This disease begins as "scratches" on the inside of your arteries. This is similar to rubbing coarse sandpaper on the inside of a plastic pipe. These "scratches" are a good place for cholesterol to attach itself to. They can be caused by the OXIDATION of the LDL cholesterol in the blood. Olive oil reduces the chance of the "scratches" forming and thereby lowers the risk of heart disease.

✓ OMEGA-3 FATTY ACID—FISH OIL—It significantly reduces cholesterol and triglycerides levels. Also SOYBEAN OIL, FLAXSEED, CANOLA OIL, ENGLISH WALNUT OIL are all high in omega-3 oil. Fish oils were also shown to significantly reduce the incidence of CANCER in laboratory animals. An increased consumption of fish oils and LINOLENIC ACID, and a decreased consumption of SATURATED FATS and ARACHIDONIC ACID, will significantly reduce PLATELET AGGREGATION, and hence atherosclerosis. Seafood eaters worldwide, have less heart disease. A Dutch study found that eating one ounce of FISH a day cut the chances of a fatal heart disease in half. A 25 year study of 17,000 men found that fatal heart attacks dropped the more fish they ate. If you suffer a heart attack, your odds of having another one go down more if you eat fish twice a week and lots of fruits and vegetables, than if you simply cut down on fat in your diet.

Fish bodies function at cold temperatures. They don't solidify until a temperature of minus 103° F, and the colder the water the more oil the fish has.

✓ EXERCISE—A University of Pittsburg study found that a mailman who walked an average of five miles a day had higher than average blood levels of HDL, the good cholesterol.

✓ VITAMIN B—A deficiency causes BERIBERI. If prolonged, it damages the heart. A Lack of any essential vitamin or mineral could damage the heart.

✓ VITAMIN C—Vitamin C has the ability to drastically lower the amount of cholesterol in the blood, and prevent atherosclerosis directly through its role in cholesterol and fat metabolism. No heart or blood vessel can be maintained in healthy condition without vitamin C.

✓ VITAMIN E—Vitamin E has been shown to prevent ATHEROSCLEROSIS through its inhibition of the platelet-releasing reaction, its action as a free-radical scavenger, its inhibition of platelet aggregation, and its elevation of HDL levels. In one study it was shown that the risk of a heart attack is inversely related to the vitamin E level in the blood.

✓ SOLUBLE FIBER—It increases the output of BILE. The liver then has to make more bile, and is therewith using up more cholesterol. Dr. Denis Burkitt says that serum cholesterol rises when fiber is removed from the diet.

- ✓ OXYGEN—The heart revolts against an abnormally low oxygen supply.
- ✓ WHOLE GRAIN—Dr. Helden of Austria has statistics which show that in countries where people eat whole-grain bread and whole-grain cereals, they are relatively free of ISCHEMIC HEART DISEASE. Because of their better utilization of oxygen, they help to prevent arteriosclerosis and heart disease due to their rich supply of vitamins B and E. We are getting less OXYGEN into our tissues because air pollution is interfering with oxygen absorption.
- ✓ GARLIC—KYOLIC—a Japanese developed garlic extract, is recommended for preventing HEART DISEASE and ATHEROSCLEROSIS, for maintaining CHOLESTEROL LEVELS in normal range, and for improving the body's IMMUNE SYSTEM. It has no unpleasant side effects. Added benefits are the LOWERING of BLOOD SUGAR in DIABETES, and the RAISING of BLOOD SUGAR in HYPOGLYCEMIA.
- ✓ HAWTHORN BERRY—It is not for cutting short ANGINA attacks, as does NITROGLYCERIN. Instead, it is safe for long-term use. In France it was believed to be the tree from which Christ's crown of thorns was made. Its RED BERRIES are classed as a CARDIAC, TONIC, ANTISPASMODIC, and a SEDATIVE. It is used in case of a WEAK HEART MUSCLE, IRREGULAR HEARTBEAT, NERVOUS HEART PROBLEMS, HIGH BLOOD PRESSURE, and ATHEROSCLEROSIS. Dr. Eric Powell calls it the finest general heart tonic ever discovered. It helps to clear deposits from artery walls.
- ✓ BETA CAROTENE—A Harvard 6 year study of 333 male physicians with heart disease, who took a 50 mg BETA CAROTENE supplement every other day, had a 50% lower rate of HEART ATTACK and STROKE. It is believed that the beta carotene neutralizes the plaque from the "bad" LDL cholesterol on the walls of the arteries. It must be realized that we must always use beta carotene in its natural form. Beta carotene is also made synthetically from petroleum derivatives. Synthetic beta carotene does not provide the ALPHA factor that natural beta carotene has. Natural carotene was found to be almost 8 times as potent as synthetic beta carotene.
- ✓ NUTS—Dr. Gary Fraser of Loma Linda University found in a study of 31,208 Seventh-day Adventists, that NUTS stood out as the number one food among those who did not suffer a heart attack. Nuts are rich in FIBER and monounsaturated olive oil type fats known to counteract heart disease. They are also packed with antioxidants including VITAMIN E, SELENIUM, and ELLAGIC ACID, that guard against the ravages of cholesterol.
- ✓ SELENIUM—Selenium is required for our health, but too much of it can be deadly. The recommended daily allowance (RDA) is 70 mcg. Whenever a person is deficient in both selenium and vitamin E, LIVER DEGENERATION develops, showing how 2 nutrients work together. Selenium is a protector mineral that works well with vitamin E. Dr. Ip showed again that a high fat diet promotes cancer, and that therefore such a diet requires more vitamin E and selenium.

Symptoms Of Heart Disease

- ☞ Some of the symptoms of heart disease are:
- ☞ SHORTNESS OF BREATH—after a slight exertion
- ☞ PAIN AND TIGHTNESS OF CHEST—often running down the left arm
- ☞ SWELLING—of ANKLES or ABDOMEN
- ☞ BREATHING—bent forward
- ☞ SLEEP—needing several extra pillows to sleep.

The Causes Of Heart Disease

◆ *The Framingham Heart Study*

The basic causes of heart disease can be found in faulty eating and living habits, and various mental and physical ENVIRONMENTAL STRESSES. The famous Framingham Heart Study identified the following risk factors in coronary heart disease.

- ☞ ELEVATED BLOOD LEVELS of CHOLESTEROL, TRIGLYCERIDES, and other FATTY substances.

- ☛ ELEVATED BLOOD PRESSURE
- ☛ ELEVATED BLOOD URIC ACID LEVELS, mainly caused by a high ANIMAL PROTEIN diet.
- ☛ METABOLIC DISORDERS, notably DIABETES.
- ☛ OBESITY
- ☛ SMOKING
- ☛ Lack of PHYSICAL EXERCISE

The successful treatment of heart disease is contingent on the elimination of all the above, mostly dietary, risk factors, which are the underlying causes of the disease. Dr. Pritikin cites a 5-year study of 8000 men which evaluated drugs given to coronary patients. It indicated that the patients would have been better off if they had taken PLACEBOS.

◆ *Dietary Considerations*

✓ CHLORINATED WATER—The reason for not drinking chlorinated water is that chlorine destroys Vitamin E in the body, which is absolutely essential to the health of the heart.

✓ FAULTY NUTRITION—OBESITY—It is one factor that is causing the OXYGEN DEFICIENCY in the tissues. The key is in the kitchen. It starts with overeating especially of refined sugar and refined flour, from which WHEAT GERM and VITAMIN E have been removed. Also too much MEAT, MILK, and MILK PRODUCTS. The death rate is 50% greater among the overweight. "The thin men bury the fat men." One overly FATTY or SALTY meal can bring on an ANGINA attack because it raises your BLOOD PRESSURE suddenly.

When a person overeats, the fatty materials in the blood, the TRIGLYCERIDES, increase, and this is more of a factor in heart disease than is CHOLESTEROL. Men with average cholesterol readings of 260 mg % are 3 times as likely to have a heart attack as compared with those men of 195 mg %. The average male level of cholesterol in the U.S. is 210–220 mg/dl, which most researchers consider as being too high. Dr. Yudkin shows that a person eating 4 oz. of refined SUGAR daily, has 5 times the chance of having heart disease than someone eating only 2 oz. of sugar.

✓ FISH—are high in SELENIUM and FATTY ACIDS which protect against heart disease.

✓ IMPURITIES—can cause heart disease by clogging up the blood vessels which in turn place an excessive strain on the heart.

✓ MILK—Its consumption is related to heart disease because it lowers the amount of MAGNESIUM in the system. Magnesium increases HDL levels, decreases platelet aggregation, and prolongs clotting time.

✓ NAKED EXTREMITIES—When the limbs are not properly covered, the circulation is not equalized, producing PALPITATION of the heart, on account of too much blood in that locality (HL773).

✓ OXYGEN DEFICIENCY—A middle-aged man who is frequently out of breath may be a prime candidate for a heart attack. In a British study, nearly 4 out of every 10 men who had breathlessness but no sign of heart disease at their initial exam developed ANGINA, suffered a HEART ATTACK, or DIED within 5 years. On the other hand, only 1 out of every 12 men without breathlessness developed heart problems in the following 5 years.

Dr. Sandler claims that heart attacks are caused by an OXYGEN DEFICIENCY in the tissues caused by LOW BLOOD SUGAR which is caused by the OVERCONSUMPTION of SUGAR and STARCHES. Refined and processed foods must be eliminated. ANGINA is an artery-clogged heart crying out for oxygen. Smoking is probably the worst thing that brought it on, for smoke increases the levels of CARBON MONOXIDE which displaces oxygen, and produces an oxygen shortage. It also makes the blood platelets stick together, thereby decreasing the opening of the arteries. It has been found by some researchers that CALCIUM tablets enhance vitamin E's effect.

✓ SALT—It is one of the most CARDIO-TOXIC substances. With respect to it one can easily see why heart disease is the number one killer. While the body needs only 1 to 2 gm of salt daily, which can be largely obtained from fresh fruits and vegetables, the average American takes in from 8 to 10 gm daily. We all get more salt when we eat CANNED FOODS, for extra salt has been added to them. Canned foods are also usually COOKED FOODS. Cooking the food with increased sodium eliminates the POTASSIUM in the food. When there is more potassium much of the sodium is eliminated. Hence, with extra salted foods the body needs extra potassium to keep the balance intact. FRUIT and VEGETABLES are among the best sources of potassium, and with an abundance of these in the diet, the potassium-sodium balance is maintained in the proper ratio of 2:1 approximately.

✓ SUGAR & COFFEE—They have definitely been proven to be contributing causes to heart disease. Dr. Yudkin demonstrated that excessive consumption of SUGAR, even more so than fat, is associated with heart attacks. Table sugar promotes increased concentrations of PLASMA CHOLESTEROL, TRIGLYCERIDES, URIC ACID, and increased PLATELET AGGREGATION, all of which are known to be involved in the development of ATHEROSCLEROSIS. The ETHIOPIANS, who have one of the world's lowest sugar intakes, have practically no heart disease, regardless whether their blood cholesterol levels are high or low.

The Healing Of Heart Disease

✓ 1. EXERCISE—The heart is unstrained when it works on a level plane. It is suggested that all exercises be done in a horizontal position. Lie on your chest or back and make-believe that you are a swimmer. Vigorous exercises in the standing position force the heart to pump the blood upward against gravity.

✓ 2. VITAMIN E—Any vitamin or mineral deficiency may directly or indirectly lead to heart disease. The most important vitamin for lowering the INCIDENCE of HEART DISEASE is VITAMIN E; it may also be the MOST DEFICIENT in our diet, since it is refined out of many foods. A patient with heart disease was out of the hospital 2 days when she contracted DIGITALIS POISONING. She was taken back into the hospital and was released 4 months later. She then quit all drugs and went on a Vitamin E therapy. She has been fine ever since. Vitamin E oxygenates the tissues and reduces the need for oxygen. Researchers in vitamin E believe that the so-called "normal" person can ward off a potential manifestation of cardiovascular disease by taking 100 IU per day as a start, and then building up to an average of 400–600 IU for women and 600–800 IU for men. Dr. Passwater ranks the nutrients that help heart disease in the following order: Vitamin E first in importance, followed by SELENIUM, VITAMIN C, VITAMIN B_6, and MAGNESIUM.

✓ 2. DR. RINSE'S FORMULA—For heart disease it is a mixture of one tablespoon each of GRANULATED SOYBEANS, BREWER'S YEAST, RAW WHEAT GERM, and BONE MEAL POWDER. A man was having difficulty getting the proper words out during conversation, and his memory was bad. He had an enlarged heart causing him to pant like an old dog, in his words. He read about Dr. Rinse's formula and began taking it. Now, he says, he has no more of those problems.

✓ VITAMIN A and D—The great amount of vitamin A and D in the livers of FISH, SEALS, and BEARS, may account for the mystery of the resistance of the fat-eating Eskimos to heart problems. Biochemists have discovered that FISH LIVER OILS contain a substance with qualities similar to ASPIRIN, that may avert strokes by making blood platelets less sticky, and less likely to clot, without any of aspirin's side effects.

✓ NIACIN—A doctor of the Royal Infirmary of Edinburgh found that patients who have had a MYOCARDIAL INFARCTION always had raised levels of FREE FATTY ACIDS in their blood. These raised levels come from body fat tissues. It is known that niacin controls the release of fats, so they found that the level of fatty substances began to fall after the niacin was given. It must be given every two hours, and it must be given in large doses of 200 mg.

✓ RELIGION—In a Journal of Cardiology a study of 500 men and women found that devout Jews had lower heart attack rates than non-practicing Jews. A strong belief in a Supreme Being and prayer was said to lower one's risk of heart disease.

✓ VEGETARIAN DIET—A vegetarian, low-sodium, low-calorie diet of high quality natural organic foods will greatly reduce heart disease. Also such a diet is rich in protective factors such as FIBER, ESSENTIAL FATTY ACIDS, VITAMINS, and MINERALS.

- ✓ VEGETABLE OIL—Small amounts of vegetable oil of highest quality, cold-pressed and unrefined, such as OLIVE, FLAXSEED, SAFFLOWER, or SESAME OIL, are beneficial, even essential if supplemented with vitamin E.

- ✓ FISH CONSUMPTION—It has been demonstrated in population studies that FISH consumption is protective against mortality from heart disease, while MEAT consumption is causative. Death due to heart disease is 50% lower among those who consume an average of 30 gm or 1 ounce of fish per day compared to those who eat meat daily. Meat eaters have a 300% increase in risk for heart disease. The JAPANESE have the highest rate of cigarette smoking, a high average blood pressure, a stressful lifestyle, but heart disease is very limited, and is less than ours. The reason is that they eat a large amount of fish, and fresh ocean vegetables. Meat and dairy products are scarce. Only 15% of their total calories are from fat.

- ✓ MOLASSES—Cyril Scott mentions the case of a man who had a CARDIO THROMBOSIS or BLOOD CLOT. He was a railroad worker who had to give up his job for life because of his condition. He was induced to try the MOLASSES TREATMENT. This treatment consists of dissolving one teaspoon of molasses in a half cup of hot water, and then filling it up with cold water. The result was that he was able to go back to work. The POTASSIUM and MINERAL SALTS in the molasses had dispersed the blood clot. Cyril Scott tells the story of another man who was completely paralyzed on one side of his body. He tried the molasses therapy. With it he recovered the use of all his limbs, and became completely fit, much to the astonishment of his doctors and friends.

- ✓ MAGNESIUM—It has been indicated that the incidence of heart disease is inversely proportional to the amount of MAGNESIUM in the water supply. It is said that the low incidence of heart disease in ESKIMOS is, besides other factors, also attributable to their high levels of SERUM MAGNESIUM in their blood.

- ✓ LECITHIN—Adele Davis in her book *Let's Get Well*, reports that within three months, the blood cholesterol level of patients who had suffered HEART ATTACKS dropped markedly after they took 4 to 6 tablespoons of LECITHIN daily. Lecithin has also caused ANGINA PAINS to disappear, and has been especially beneficial to elderly patients who have suffered a STROKE, or who have CEREBRAL ATHEROSCLEROSIS. Usually a dose of 1 to 2 tablespoons of lecithin per day was sufficient to maintain a normal cholesterol level.

Dr. Morrison says that lecithin is especially valuable against HARDENING of the ARTERIES, and all the complications of HEART, BRAIN, and KIDNEY FUNCTIONS that follow.

- ✓ TAURINE—is an amino acid which is most abundant in the heart, lowers blood pressure and relieves congestive heart failure because it removes SODIUM from the cells. It also controls HEART RHYTHM IRREGULARITIES, and is a treatment for EPILEPSY.

- ✓ APPLIED EXPERIENCES—A man of 85 had high blood pressure in the range of 160/100 to 180/110. He began to take multiple vitamins such as VITAMIN E, LECITHIN, BONE MEAL, B-COMPLEX, A, D, and others, and in a short time noticed improvements in his condition. His doctor said that vitamin E has been tried and found to be useless, but if you want to spend your money to keep the vitamin factories running, it's your money. His doctor dropped dead from a heart attack before he reached 60.

PAPAYA contains an enzyme called CARPAIN which is extremely valuable to the heart. A 30 year old lady had been suffering the excruciating pain of ANGINA PECTORIS. She was advised to eat nothing but MANGOES and PAPAYA. In a short time her pains were completely gone, and her heart beat was normal again.

HIGH BLOOD PRESSURE — HYPERTENSION (HBP)

Nature Of The Disease

High blood pressure (HBP) is not a disease in and of itself, but it is a symptom of the body's defensive mechanism initiated to cope with various adverse disease conditions. From the NATURAL PHILOSOPHY standpoint the objective is not simply to lower the pressure, but to eliminate the causes for the high pressure. When these are removed, the blood pressure will go down to normal by itself. When we lower HBP with drugs, we are not getting at the reasons behind the HBP, the causes of the condition. The higher the blood pressure, the more likely you are to die before your time. High blood pressure damages the NERVOUS SYSTEM, OVERWORKS THE HEART, SPEEDS UP ATHEROSCLEROSIS, and kills 250,000 or more people in the U.S. every year. HBP is extremely dangerous because it will almost always lead to HEART, VEIN, and ARTERY trouble in the form of a STROKE, a HEMORRHAGE, KIDNEY FAILURE, HEART FAILURE, or SUDDEN DEATH.

The general way to remove high blood pressure is to eat the natural diet of fresh fruits, vegetables, nuts, and seeds, and this without spices. VEGETARIANS have less heart disease because they get more fiber in their diet, and consequently have a lower blood pressure. Those vegetarians, the VEGANS, who eat no animal products, not even eggs and milk, have the lowest blood pressure of all. HBP is not normal with age. It is a disease of civilization. Primitive tribes existing on natural eating habits do not have HBP. HBP affects 1 of 4 Americans, and half the population over 65. It has been shown that stroking a dog or a cat will lower blood pressure.

Symptoms Of High Blood Pressure

The symptoms of HBP may be HEADACHE, IRRITABILITY, DIZZINESS, LOSS OF MEMORY, LOSS OF POWER OF CONCENTRATION, SHORTNESS OF BREATH, INDIGESTION, and various HEART symptoms.

The Causes Of High Blood Pressure

◆ *General Disease Conditions*

Some of the conditions which cause HBP are GENERAL TOXEMIA, IMPAIRED KIDNEY FUNCTION, DEFECTIVE CALCIUM METABOLISM, ARTERIOSCLEROSIS or HARDENING OF THE ARTERIES, OVERWEIGHT, EMOTIONAL DISFUNCTIONS, HIGH SALT CONSUMPTION, HIGH SUGAR CONSUMPTION, UNDER-OXYGENATION OF THE BLOOD DUE TO POOR VENTILATION, INADEQUATE BREATHING, EMOTIONAL INSTABILITY, DEPRESSED THINKING, LACK OF EXERCISE, NUTRIENT-POOR DIETS, CONTRACEPTIVES, DRUGS, STRESS, and ALCOHOL. This indicates that a great many disease conditions will raise the blood pressure, but the most common of all is said to be the hardening of the arteries. People with uncontrolled HBP have 7 times more STROKES, 4 times as much CONGESTIVE HEART FAILURE, and 3 times as much CORONARY HEART DISEASE as people with normal blood pressure.

The accumulation of TOXIC WASTES is a key factor in erratic and runaway readings of blood pressure. Consuming synthetic substances; artificial ingredients; excessive fat; and irritating stimulants such as coffee, tea, and soft drinks, all cause the deposition of these toxic wastes on the vital segments of the cardiovascular system.

◆ *Salt*

Salt is a specific cause of HBP. Among primitive people who add no salt to their food, there is no rise in blood pressure with age. There are a large number of communities and populations around the world that show no increase in blood pressure with age. Aging Americans can point to excess poundage and bad health habits as triggers for blood pressure problems. Naturopathic doctors do not consider such a rise in blood pressure as being normal. It is merely due to lowered health conditions. While a normal blood pressure is considered to be 120 systolic over 80 diastolic, Dr. Harvey Kellogg had a blood pressure of 118/80 at age 72, which is that of a young man.

Some people are so sensitive to salt, that even a small amount can greatly raise their BLOOD PRESSURE. For others an excess of salt will cause people to retain excess body fluid, which can raise the blood pressure.

The average American gets about 3 gm of salt naturally from his food. Another 4 to 6 gm is added to the food from commercial processing, and 3 gm is added by the cook and at the table, which adds up to 10 to 12 gm of salt a day. At the same time the processed salt has depleted the potassium in the food.

The Japanese males have the highest incidence of STOMACH CANCER, and the females have the second highest incidence in the world. It is 7 times higher than in the U.S. The reason is their excessive use of MONOSODIUM GLUTAMATE (MSG). They use it in their food as a condiment, and sprinkle it generously over all of their food. They use synthetic MSG rather than the natural form which is made from seaweed. Instead of using salt, season your food with HERBS. Use GARLIC POWDER, DILL SEED, POPPY SEED, CHILI-PEPPER, OREGANO, PARSLEY, EXTRACTS, PAPRIKA, RED PEPPER, and SAVORY. Also use LEMON JUICE, FRUIT PEELS, EXTRACTS, UNSALTED NUTS, SUNFLOWER SEEDS, and SESAME SEEDS to add flavor to your meals.

◆ *An Inadequate Diet*

HBP can be the result of impurities in the blood vessels caused by deposits in the blood stream of INORGANIC SUBSTANCES accumulating from cooked and processed foods, particularly the concentrated starches and sugars; by the retention of WASTE in the eliminative organs and channels, and by the retention of DRUGS in the system. A contributing cause is the lack of proper and sufficient rest. It is said that 85% of people's high blood pressure can be eliminated by an improvement in the DIET.

In our society it is considered "normal" for a person's BLOOD PRESSURE to RISE WITH AGE, but this does not occur in societies that avoid a high-fat, high-salt diet, such as the people of New Guinea, Botswana, and the Yanomamo of Brazil and Venezuela, whose blood pressure stays relatively the same throughout life.

◆ *Overweight*

A Minnesota study showed that blood pressure can be lowered by losing weight and reducing salt intake. The craving for salt is a learned behavior, an acquired taste, for salt craving is created by a high salt diet. Getting used to a low salt diet makes former foods taste too salty. It takes three months to lose the craving for salt. Most people find that once they get over the initial craving for salt, they don't miss it. Dr. Dahl remarks that after you have drastically reduced your salt intake, you will find that you really never tasted the real food before. What you tasted was the salt. From then on you will feel a revival of interest in your meals when for the first time you enjoy a baked potato without salt. Reducing salt intake to 500 mg per day will lower blood pressure in most people. For every extra pound of weight above normal, the heart must pump blood through an added mile of capillaries. Studies have shown that up to of overweight hypertensives can substantially lower their blood pressure by losing their excess weight.

◆ *Potassium Deficiency*

Evidence suggests from a number of studies that a diet low in potassium may lead to HBP, while a high potassium intake leads to the lowering of CHOLESTEROL. Foods high in potassium are BANANAS, POTATOES, BROCCOLI, TOMATOES, and ORANGE JUICE.

◆ *Stress*

Stress makes BLOOD PRESSURE rise, ADRENAL glands engorge, and the THYMUS and LYMPH glands shrink.

◆ *Creatinine*

CREATININE is a waste product of metabolic processes in muscle cells, like the smoke from a fire. Normally, the kidneys filter creatinine out of the blood. For this reason high levels of creatinine in the blood may indicate kidney problems. Those with high creatinine levels in the blood usually die of HEART DISEASE and STROKE, which seems to indicate that creatinine should be recognized as a risk marker for HEART ATTACKS and STROKE.

◆ *Insulin*

Studies have shown that INSULIN in some cases contributes to the HARDENING of the ARTERIES by helping the body produce excessive CHOLESTEROL. It also encourages the body to retain SALT in the kidneys. Men in the study had higher levels of insulin, which may indicate that the body adapts itself to a low-salt diet by producing more insulin.

◆ *Other Causes*

Home WATER SOFTENERS increase both

the sodium and cadmium content, both of which increase blood pressure. NITRATES in the water can cause HBP. ESTROGEN is a salt retainer, hence, it can cause HBP. The salt as well as the sugar content of processed foods has increased in the last few years. It has been determined that while salt raises the blood pressure, when salt is combined with SUGAR, it raises the blood pressure much more than does the salt alone. So why is that combination in processed PEANUT BUTTER? Sugar seems to lower the amount of salt excreted by the body. About a third of people have lower blood pressure when they are at home or on the job than when they are in the DOCTOR'S OFFICE. To avoid this have your blood pressure measured by a nurse instead of the doctor. It may make a difference. When communication is a problem in families everybody's blood pressure goes up. One study shows that LISTENING, rather than TALKING, lowers blood pressure. Most people experience a rise in blood pressure when they speak. The louder and faster a person talks, the higher the blood pressure.

Results Of High Blood Pressure—Strokes

◆ *Symptoms Of Strokes*

HBP is present in 40 to 70% of people who have strokes as a result of a BLOCKAGE or a RUPTURE of arteries in the brain. The blockage is caused by the accumulation of cholesterol. 70% of all strokes occur in those 65 or older. Men have more strokes than women, and blacks have more than whites. In Japan, where there is a high level of the use of salt in the diet, as well as a high level of smoking, there is a high level of HYPERTENSION. This has lead to the condition of INTRACEREBRAL HEMORRHAGE, which is a form of stroke which is a major cause of death in Japan. Our chance of a stroke doubles with each decade after age 55. One must keep one's blood cholesterol below 200 in order to prevent a stroke. Untreated hypertension can also lead to HEART DISEASE, KIDNEY FAILURE, and even BLINDNESS. Because of the fact that it leads to other diseases, it is rarely listed on death certificates as the cause of death.
- ✓ DIABETICS—are at a greater risk for strokes, because diabetes allows arteries to collect fatty deposits.
- ✓ HEADACHES—may be symptoms of an oncoming stroke.
- ✓ ORAL CONTRACEPTIVES—increase stroke possibilities.
- ✓ OVERWEIGHT PEOPLE—are at a greater risk for strokes.
- ✓ SALT—HBP is not a problem in countries where little salt is produced.
- ✓ SNORERS—a University of Helsinki study showed that snorers are at a higher risk for strokes.

◆ *Prevention Of Strokes*
- ☞ FRUITS AND VEGETABLES—Researchers at the University of Cambridge discovered that eating FRUITS and VEGETABLES prevented strokes and diminished the damage that occurred. A Norwegian study found that men who ate the most vegetables had a 45% lower risk of strokes. It also found that women who ate lots of fruit were less likely to have a stroke. Eating CARROTS 5 times a week or more was found to slash the risk of strokes by, compared with eating carrots but once a month, according to a Harvard study of 50,000 women nurses over a period of 8 years. SPINACH was also found to be a powerful stroke deterrent. This is probably due to their antioxidant activity, which inhibits cholesterol from becoming toxic, and from forming clots and plaques in the arteries.

A study in Southern California determined that an extra serving of a POTASSIUM-rich food every day would reduce the risk of a stroke by 40% according to an experiment with 859 men and women over the age of 50. Nobody with the highest intake of potassium, or more than 3500 mg a day, died of a stroke. Those who ate less than 1950 mg per day had a much higher fatal stroke rate than all the others. Extra potassium kept artery walls elastic and functioning normally, thereby keeping the blood vessels from being damaged by high blood pressure.
When it comes to potassium, what is important is the ratio of sodium to potassium. In our culture food processing reduces the sources of potassium in our diet, and sodium is generally added to our food as a preservative. This fact oversupplies the sodium at the expense of the potassium. What will increase our potassium every day is a glass of orange juice, a raw

vegetable salad, and a rice and fruit diet.

Studies in Japan show that heavy FISH EATERS are less apt to die if they have a stroke. Another Japanese study found that women who drank at least 5 cups of GREEN TEA every day were only half as likely to suffer a stroke compared to those who drank less. Green tea prevents strokes because another study showed that it REDUCES BLOOD PRESSURE.

Ways To Restore Normal Blood Pressure

✓ A NATURAL DIET—HBP should be treated with nutrition rather than drugs, because faulty nutrition is largely responsible for it. Natural foods generally have enough salt in them so that no salt needs to be added. The basic reason why we add salt to our food is that the TASTE BUDS have been perverted by having to come in contact with processed food from which the natural flavor has been destroyed in the processing. In order to put some of the flavor back into it, the processors add a lot of salt to the food to make it palatable. That is also the reason for the use of monosodium glutamate as a flavor enhancer, which itself has sodium in it.

✓ FASTING—Dr. Buchinger of Germany, a fasting expert, says: "High blood pressure is one ailment for which fasting practically never fails to bring about a complete cure."

✓ FIBER—People who eat lots of fiber tend to have lower blood pressure than those who have little fiber in their diet. 7 gm of supplemental fiber a day, the amount in a single bowl of bran cereal, reduced the systolic pressure by 10 points, while the diastolic pressure fell by 5 points. The cholesterol level also fell by 5 points over a 3 month period. In a test SDA women who ate only fiber-rich vegetables had an average blood pressure of 98/65, while their Mormon counterparts, who ate meat, had an average blood pressure of 103/73.

✓ FRUITS, VEGETABLES AND THEIR JUICES—Since fruits and vegetables are among the best sources of potassium, they act as a natural blood pressure preventive. JUICE FASTING is one of the most effective treatments for HBP. The very helpful juices are CITRUS, GRAPES, CRANBERRIES, and BLACK CURRENTS.

Most NATUROPATHS and some PHYSICIANS recommend juice fasts from two to four days out of alternate weeks for six months. Take three or four cups of herb teas and two 8 oz. glasses of raw vegetable juice, and one glass of fresh fruit juice. It normalizes and corrects most other disturbances which contribute to the elevated pressure. The recommended vegetable juices are CARROTS, SPINACH, BEET, COMFREY, singly or in combination with small amounts of onion or garlic juice added to them.

A 62 year old man ate 2 stalks of CELERY every day for a week. His blood pressure dropped from a high of 158/96 to a normal of 118/82. Dr. Elliot says that the active blood pressure lowering compound is found in rather high concentrations in celery, and not in many other vegetables. He speculates that the compound lowers blood pressure by reducing the blood concentrations of STRESS HORMONES that cause blood vessels to constrict.

Dr. Airola suggests one week of eating nothing but WATERMELON to lower blood pressure. It is said that eating fruits and vegetables could decrease one's risk of having a STROKE by up to 40%. A RICE-FRUIT diet has also been shown to be effective for one or two weeks. As part of your own anti-hypertension campaign STEAM your vegetables. Boiling vegetables leaches away a good part of their potassium and magnesium.

✓ EXERCISE—Research has shown that regular aerobic exercise can lower your blood pressure by 4 or 5 points. Exercise forces the blood vessels to open up, and that makes the blood pressure come down. Regular exercise for 30 minutes a day 4 times a week can lower blood pressure by 5 to 20 points. It can lower it even if substantial weight loss is not achieved. Riding a bicycle for 1 hour 3 times a week for 10 weeks can drop 13 points off the blood pressure. Carrying a 1 to 3 pound weight in each hand while walking is good for weight loss and cardiovascular endurance, but it is bad for blood pressure, for it goes up. A group of people took a single brisk 40 minute walk and lowered their blood pressure significantly. This lowered blood pressure lasted a bit over two hours, which means that it must be kept up on a regular basis in order to have a more long-lasting effect. BRISK WALKING, which is 15 minutes per mile, can reduce the risk of stroke 80% as effectively as JOGGING.

The Harvard Alumni Study found that those people who did not exercise were 35% more likely to have HBP.

- ✓ GARLIC AND ONION—Many studies have indicated that garlic reduces blood pressure. It does so by dilating the blood vessels which has relieved HEADACHES, DIZZINESS, and ANGINA-LIKE PAIN and PAIN between the SHOULDER BLADES. Blood pressure is not reduced unless the salt intake is lowered to 1 or 2 gm per day. Garlic has been shown to decrease the systolic pressure by 20 to 30 points, and the diastolic pressure by 10 to 20 points. Onions have a similar lowering effect. Onions lower blood pressure because of the presence of PROSTAGLANDIN, a hormone-like substance that can lower blood pressure.

  The story is told of an electrical engineer who had a blood pressure of 375/220. He was told by his doctor to "Either bring down that sky-high blood pressure or get ready for a funeral…your own." He was told that such a reading could end his life at almost any moment. The problem was that he could not stand medication. Its side effects ranged from falling asleep at the wheel to painful spasms. He discussed the problem with a nutrition-minded physician who suggested that he should start snacking on GARLIC. He was to consume at least 4 garlic cloves daily, one at a time. He boosted his intake to 5 garlic clove "for good measure." In 3 days his reading dropped to 190/120. In 5 days he had a reading of 125/80. The garlic had saved his life.
- ✓ GRAINS—The best cereals are MILLET, OATS, RICE, and BUCKWHEAT which is rich in RUTIN.
- ✓ OLIVE OIL AND OTHER MONOUNSATURATED FATS—A Stanford University Study indicates that each tablespoon of MONOUNSATURATED FAT you eat per 1000 calories, will drop your systolic blood pressure 10 points. The best sources of monounsaturated fat is OLIVE OIL, CANOLA or RAPESEED OIL, and also PEANUT OIL.
- ✓ OMEGA-3 OIL—protects against strokes. Besides FISH it is contained also in SOYBEANS, WALNUTS, and WHEAT GERM. Vegetables such as SPINACH, BROCCOLI, and CAULIFLOWER contain small amounts of it.

  Dr. Singer of Berlin reduced his blood pressure from 140/90 to 100/70 after he started eating a small can of MACKEREL FILLET EVERY DAY. This was due to the OMEGA-3 FATTY ACIDS in the oil. They were as effective as the drug INDERAL, a commonly prescribed blood pressure medication.
- ✓ OTHER HELPFUL FACTORS— TRYPTOPHAN, an essential amino acid, is converted in the brain to SEROTONIN, which actually lowers your blood pressure. A HEARTY LAUGH causes a small but fleeting decrease in blood pressure. So be with people who make you laugh. Hence, the Bible says: "A merry heart doeth good like a medicine" (Pr. 17:22). Stroking a dog, rabbit, cat, or any other animal that is soft and cuddly can lower your blood pressure.

Herbs

- ✓ CAYENNE PEPPER—One patient from Florida wrote: "Several years ago I was on ALDOMET for high blood pressure. I went to a health lecture on folk cures and heard about CAYENNE RED PEPPER as a possible aid in controlling blood pressure problems. It worked wonders for me. For the first time in years my pressure became normal. It had been as high as 240/120, and was usually 190/110, even with the medicine. I was able to stop the medication I had been on for years."
- ✓ HAWTHORN BERRY—The leaves, berries, and the blossom of the HAWTHORN have blood pressure lowering effect due to their FLAVONOID compounds. They are effective also in reducing ANGINA attacks, as well as in lowering SERUM CHOLESTEROL LEVELS, and preventing the deposition of cholesterol in artery walls. Other beneficial teas for lowering blood pressure are ALFALFA, CATNIP, MINT, RED CLOVER, SAGE, SASSAFRAS, and WATERMELON SEED TEA.
- ✓ NORMALIZING BLOOD PRESSURE—The natural medicinals which aid in normalizing blood pressure include: GARLIC, CAPSICUM, SHEPHERDS PURSE, GOLDENSEAL, and PARSLEY.

Vitamins

- ✓ VITAMIN E—Vitamin E can help prevent a stroke because it prevents the clumping of platelets. The platelets become sticky when clumping takes place, and under those conditions a blood clot can form, and the blood clot can lead to a stroke.

- ✓ CHOLINE—Choline is a vitamin involved in the lowering of HBP. It is found in EGG YOLK, and as a constituent of LECITHIN in SOY BEANS. A deficiency of choline causes HBP. BREAST MILK contains a goodly amount of choline but COW'S MILK is lacking in it. It is also found largely in PEANUTS, LEGUMES, GREEN LEAFY VEGETABLES, SNAP BEANS, WHEAT GERM, and BREWER'S YEAST.

- ✓ VITAMIN C—Researchers have discovered that VITAMIN C might prevent healthy people from developing high blood pressure, and may even help in lowering slightly elevated blood pressure. It was found that the lower the blood levels of vitamin C, the higher the blood pressure. A new study has discovered that blood pressure readings taken at home are more accurate than readings taken at the doctors office.

Minerals

- ✓ CALCIUM (Ca)—Calcium is the natural medium and magic mineral which controls blood pressure. It stabilizes the arterial blood flow. The more calcium in your diet, the lower your blood pressure. 1000 mg per day is recommended. CALCIUM, MAGNESIUM, POTASSIUM, and LINOLEIC ACID can each individually lower blood pressure more safely than the most potent prescription drugs for HBP.

- ✓ MAGNESIUM (Mg)—Magnesium will reduce blood pressure, and fruits and vegetables are good sources of magnesium. Many magnesium depleted patients show high blood pressure, but their blood pressure returns to normal with magnesium supplementation.

- ✓ POTASSIUM (K)—Concentrating on foods high in potassium can be just as important as salt reduction. An imbalance with too little potassium causes the body to retain more sodium. Sodium and potassium must be in balance for proper body chemistry. Potassium is substantially lost when foods are canned or frozen. Good food sources of potassium are BLACKSTRAP MOLASSES, FRESH FRUITS SUCH AS BANANAS and WATERMELON, RAISINS, SUNFLOWER SEEDS, NUTS, WHEAT GERM, KELP, and fresh FRUIT and VEGETABLE JUICES. Also salt substitutes can be bought that have replaced the salt with potassium. Potatoes are also a potent source of potassium. They have almost twice as much potassium as bananas. In general we should take in about three times as much potassium as salt.

Increasing the POTASSIUM intake usually neutralizes some of the harmful effects of sodium. In a study of two normal groups, one went on a LOW SODIUM HIGH POTASSIUM DIET, and the other went on an AEROBIC EXERCISE program. After four weeks the blood pressure had dropped 10 points in both groups.

Things To Avoid

- ✓ ORAL CONTRASEPTIVES—In one test oral contraseptives increased blood pressure slightly in 95% of those who took them, and significantly in 5%.

- ✓ LOUD NOISE—A Japanese study determined that the higher the noise level to which you are exposed the higher your blood pressure.

- ✓ DRUGS—The drug RESERPINE used for HBP is causing CANCER in laboratory animals. It has been linked to MENTAL DEPRESSION, ANGINA, GLAUCOMA, and IMPOTENCE. CAFFEINE, DIET PILLS, and many prescription and over-the-counter drugs such as IBUPROFIN, ADVIL® or NUPRIN®, CIMETIDINE or TAGAMET®, ORAL CONTRACEPTIVES, and NOSE DROPS, can raise blood pressure significantly. Caffeine is found in most COLA drinks, COFFEE, TEA, CHOCOLATE, and COCOA.

- ✓ OVERWEIGHT—You can lose 1 point of systolic pressure for every two pounds of weight you shed.

HYPOGLYCEMIA—LOW BLOOD SUGAR

Nature Of The Disease

◆ *Excess Insulin Reduces Blood Sugar Level*

If DIABETES represents high blood sugar, then HYPOGLYCEMIA represents the opposite, namely low blood sugar. Hypoglycemia is defined as a blood GLUCOSE concentration of 50 mg/%. A normal blood sugar level is between 80 to 110 mg/%. The brain could not function more than 3 minutes without GLUCOSE. NATURAL SUGARS are surrounded by many other nutritional elements so that they don't enter the bloodstream in a flood of pure sugar as is true with pure SUCROSE. Hence, it places a great strain on the PANCREAS and on the LIVER, as well as on the ADRENAL GLANDS, which are involved in regulating the blood sugar levels. An excessive demand for INSULIN is brought about by the overuse of REFINED CARBOHYDRATES and it causes the pancreas to become oversensitive to INSULIN PRODUCTION in the body. In it the pancreas release more insulin than is needed. Hypoglycemia is often the forerunner of PARKINSON'S disease.

◆ *Refined Foods Overstimulate The Pancreas*

One sign of hypoglycemia is being constantly and ravenously hungry, particularly for starches and sugars. Other symptoms are MULTIPLE SCLEROSIS, a BAD MEMORY, and MIGRAINE HEADACHES. The answer to achieving a normal blood sugar level is to eliminate those foods which bring about a sudden, but short, rise in the blood sugar, which are generally refined sugars and simple starches, and replace them with plenty of FRESH FRUITS and VEGETABLES. This quick use of blood sugar is where the kick of coffee, the lift of cigarettes, and the euphoria of liquor come from. But such a lift is only temporary, for then the cycle starts over again There is no specific bodily need for refined sugar, for the body's need for glucose can be met by many carbohydrates. Dr. Jane Hungerford of California says that such sudden drops in blood sugar can TRIGGER VIOLENT IMPULSES such as WIFE-BEATING, CHILD ABUSE, DEPRESSION, and SUICIDE.

WHITE SUGAR throws the endocrine system out of balance. It depletes vitamins and minerals, especially CALCIUM. It should be classed as a drug, and not a food, because it causes sudden and dramatic changes in the body. WHITE FLOUR sticks to the bowel walls and slows elimination; FRYING disrupts the natural balance of fats, and it destroys LECITHIN, which is needed to balance cholesterol and other fats. When the body's natural defenses are weakened by poor living and eating habits, then any weak organ can break down. The weakest link always breaks first.

The Causes of Hypoglycemia

◆ *Caffeine And Theobromine*

Caffeine and theobromine which are found in chocolate, are often given as the cause of hypoglycemia, which is considered to be the forerunner of PARKINSON'S disease. Another symptom of hypoglycemia is considered to be MULTIPLE SCLEROSIS. Both of these diseases can be stopped with dietary measures, especially with vitamins and minerals which must be taken in megadoses.

◆ *High Sugar Consumption Causes Low Blood Sugar*

The main cause of functional hypoglycemia is the excessive consumption of concentrated REFINED STARCHES and SUGARS. Refined flour increases the load of the pancreas which is overstimulated thereby, and secretes an overabundance of INSULIN which reduces the blood sugar level to a below normal amount. It can be caused by JUNK FOODS or EMPTY CALORIES. Empty calories include foods such as SUGAR, WHITE FLOUR, WHITE RICE, SUGARED CEREALS, and ALCOHOL. Since empty calories have few or no nutrients, nor B-complex vitamins necessary for metabolization, the ISLANDS of LANGERHANS, which produce insulin, become overstimulated. Insulin takes glucose from the blood and places it inside the cells. This decreases the glucose in the blood, but the BRAIN is essentially cheated of this glucose supply on which it depends for energy. It does not itself store glucose, but other cells of the body can also get their energy from FAT.

◆ *Pure Sugar is Digested Too Quickly.*

Simple sugars are digested rapidly. The glucose is changed to PYRUVIC ACID, which is then broken down into HEAT ENERGY, WATER, AND CARBON DIOXIDE. THIAMINE (Vitamin B_1) is essential for pyruvic acid oxidation. If pyruvic acid does not get enough thiamine and other essentials, too much LACTIC ACID is then formed.

It can also be formed by insufficient secretion of adrenal hormones. Starch is changed to sugar by the body more quickly than WHOLE GRAINS, and therefore requires a quick need for insulin. Blood must have a proper level of sugar in order to function properly. It is the constant overconsumption of sweets which brings about a below normal level of blood sugar because of an oversupply of insulin. This sounds like a contradiction, but it is actually true.

MULTIPLE SCLEROSIS often represents a symptom of Hypoglycemia. Hypoglycemia is often the forerunner of PARKINSON'S disease, which can be helped if caught in the early stages. They can all be helped by following a nutritional program where vitamins and minerals are given in MEGADOSES.

The Effects of Hypoglycemia

✓ LEARNING DISABILITY—Dr. P.J. Dunn of Oak Park, Illinois, tested 144 children with learning disability and found that 78% had hypoglycemia.

Dr. Sydney Walker of La Jolla, California found that 44 of 48 children with LEARNING DISABILITY, POOR CONCENTRATION, and TEMPER TANTRUMS, had a blood sugar disorder. He put them on a sugar-free diet rich in fruits and vegetables. Almost all of them improved their behavior. The basic answer here may be that children naturally OVEREAT ON SWEETS.

✓ NEUROSIS—In a study of 700 mildly neurotic people, 600 had hypoglycemia.

✓ DIVORCE—Dr.R.J. Rogers of Florida says that America's high DIVORCE RATE, is caused in part, by hypoglycemia. Since insulin is dependent on ZINC, CHROMIUM, and MANGANESE for its normal functioning, he ameliorated many a situation by giving the parties these minerals as well as brewer's yeast.

✓ DEPRESSES BRAIN FUNCTION—Since the brain needs blood sugar to supply its energy needs, low blood sugar depresses all brain functions, which in turn depresses the whole array of metabolic processes in the body.

✓ COLDS—Those with low blood sugar tend to get more colds and flu, and thus take longer to recover from infections.

How To Heal Low Blood Sugar

✓ DIET—WHOLE GRAINS, SEEDS, and NUTS, should form the base of this diet. Nuts and seeds should be eaten raw. Grains should be cooked in the form of cereals. Cooked grain digests twice as slowly as raw grains. This is important for the nutrients are released more slowly into the blood stream.

✓ SALT—Avoid salt, for excessive salt consumption causes a loss of blood POTASSIUM which leads to a drop in blood sugar, while SODIUM is retained.

✓ EXERCISE—Exercise is an important part of the treatment for low blood sugar, because physical activity helps to control blood sugar fluctuations.

✓ HERBS—DANDELION ROOT exhibits hypoglycemic effects in experimental animals. It contains INULIN the precursor of INSULIN, which is a concentrated source of dietary fiber, whose carbohydrate substructure is FRUCTOSE. It buffers blood glucose levels, preventing sudden and severe fluctuations. LICORICE's role is to increase the effectiveness of the adrenal hormones, especially if low blood sugar is brought on by adrenal stress. It helps the body overcome adrenal failure which could lead to ADDISON'S DISEASE. It has the ability to maintain the proper electrolyte balance in the tissues. GINSENG's effect on blood sugar levels is an indirect result of its effect on the total organism. Any agent that improves general cellular health will have a positive effect on both low and high blood sugar levels. JUNIPER BERRIES and DANDELION ROOT TEA are very effective.

- ✓ VITAMINS and MINERALS—The B-VITAMINS are necessary for the assimilation of carbohydrates. VITAMIN B_1 is absolutely necessary for utilizing the energy in food. This is the reason why a person can eat enough to get fat, but never have any energy. CHROMIUM is needed to manufacture the GLUCOSE TOLERANCE factor which regulates blood sugar. Refined foods have also refined out many vitamins and minerals. These must be replaced.
- ✓ LECITHIN—It helps to burn body fat, and helps the body to utilize the oil-soluble vitamins A, D, E, and K. Lecithin is removed from commercial oil in the processing.
- ✓ JUICES—Fresh fruit and vegetable juices are helpful.

INFECTIONS

Nature Of The Disease

◆ *Defense Against Germs*

There are two types of germs in the human body, namely, those that are HELPFUL, and those that are HARMFUL. Human cells resent the presence of harmful germs, and the body's defense forces wage constant war against them. The apparently miraculous fact is that the body can distinguish between helpful and harmful germs. In many cases a natural substance, such as GARLIC, for example, will destroy harmful germs, but will leave the helpful germs untouched. Infectious diseases are becoming more rare. PNEUMONIA is the only infectious disease which is still in the top ten of diseases. On the other hand, DEGENERATIVE DISEASES are becoming more numerous due to the SUPPRESSION of infectious diseases with DRUGS.

◆ *A Weakened Resistance Causes Infections*

When our natural resistance to germs is weakened by STRESS or NUTRITIONAL DEFICIENCIES, or IMPURITIES in the system, germs, having less resistance to multiplying their numbers, and having fertile soil in which to do so, will multiply to such an extent that the resistance forces are overwhelmed. They will then cause diseases such as COLDS, FLU, KIDNEY or BLADDER PROBLEMS, SORE THROAT, TONSILLITIS, ETC., which may require healing assistance. CLEANLINESS, both internal as well as external, aids in both the acquiring and the spreading of germs. Germs will not settle where they cannot exist. Also the proper handling of food materials, both outside and inside the body, will limit the growth of germs, and avoid possible food poisoning.

◆ *Penicillin Destroys Both Helpful And Harmful Germs*

Many germs of different kinds, both helpful and harmful, are always in the body. The harmful ones are often not active because the resistance against them is too great, and the good bacteria overwhelm them so that they cannot multiply, because the army of antibodies is too large. ANTIBIOTICS, such as PENICILLIN, destroy many germs which in quantity cause many diseases. But they are really a mixed blessing, because they cannot distinguish between the helpful and the harmful bacteria, and hence, they destroy both the helpful as well as the harmful ones. They therefore cause harmful SIDE-EFFECTS and encourage the development of antibiotic-resistant germs. Some of the helpful bacteria in the intestines produce B-VITAMINS. Antibiotics destroy them too. TREATMENT: In order to restore the friendly bacteria in the digestive tract eat ACIDOPHILUS YOGURT daily, or take acidophilus capsules with each meal to counteract the possible damage done by antibiotics.

What To Avoid

- ✓ REFINED SUGAR—It should be avoided, but not honey, as it depresses the immune system, and impairs its ability to fight infections. Many authorities believe that high BLOOD-SUGAR levels encourage susceptibility to disease and infections.
- ✓ ANTIBIOTICS—When susceptible bacteria are suppressed by antibiotics, other YEAST-like organisms, such as CANDIDA ALBICANS, may appear and cause unpleasant side effects. VAGINAL and RECTAL infections are common effects. Dr. Eisenberg of New Hyde Park, N.Y., says that in the average hospital of the patients receive antibiotic injections three or four times a day. This means that bacteria that caused

no problems are now wiped clean of their enemies, and often themselves, by antibiotics. Dr. Reimann of Philadelphia says that relatively few infections can be cured by antibiotics, and cannot be prevented either. About 300 deaths annually are caused by penicillin, and less serious harm occurs in 15 to 30% of the recipients.

How To Heal Infections

✓ BLOOD POISONING—For infection around a wound, use hot and cold WATER to the infected part. Continue it until red streaks appear. Treatment: use PINE PITCH, CAYENNE PEPPER, GOLDEN SEAL, and CHARCOAL POULTICE.

✓ BOILS—infection with a single core. It is caused by too rich a diet whereby the body discharges poisons through the skin, Treatment: Apply hot and cold WATER.

✓ FUNGUS—The overuse of ANTIBIOTICS weaken the body's natural defenses, and thereby allows fungus disease to take hold because of the lack of the defending bacteria which have been destroyed. DRUGS and RADIATION upset the body's natural population of microbes also, and thus may give fungi a foothold ordinarily denied them. What most people don't realize is that they are all eating antibiotics without a doctors prescription. This is brought about through the penicillin which is put into the cows feed, and then gets into the milk we drink. They may be depleting our own native populations of bacteria, and are thereby opening the way to infestations by the fungus spore. For FUNGUS INFECTION apply a paste of BREWER'S YEAST and VITAMIN E OIL twice a day, which is often effective.

✓ GARLIC and ONIONS—Garlic is well known for its value in treating infections. A daily intake of 6 garlic cloves or the equivalent in pearls is suggested against infections. Onions have many of the same beneficial properties of garlic because of their high SULFUR content. A lady had a severe YEAST INFECTION problem, as well as a severe cholesterol problem of 350. She used OAT BRAN and CHARCOAL and got the cholesterol down to 305. But when she took the garlic preparation called KYOLIC, the cholesterol dropped to 220 after three months, and all other symptoms, including the yeast problem, were gone.

ONION TIP: To avoid the LACRIMATORY or tear-producing factor of onions, cut raw onions under water, for then the irritating factors dissolve in the water, and you won't notice them.

✓ HERB TEAS—Beneficial teas are SAW PALMETTO, COMFREY, ROSE HIPS, MULLEIN, GOLDENSEAL, HOPS, and RED CLOVER. One woman had a swollen PAROTID GLAND in her neck that was as hard and as large as a golf ball. She was given a tea made of two parts MULLEIN FLOWERS and one part LOBELIA. The tea was then reduced to of its original concentration to use as a compress over the affected area. Within two hours after she used this tea, the swelling had melted. In other cases the swelling will break, and the poison will drain externally.

✓ HYDROTHERAPY—The alternate applications of hot and cold water or packs, will improve the circulation in the affected area, and will help the body throw off the infection by increasing the number of friendly bacteria.

✓ IRON—It plays a major role in fighting infections. It helps make HEMOGLOBIN which carries oxygen to the cells. A healthy oxygen supply enables PHAGOCYTES to engulf and kill bacteria, and produces a sufficient level of T-cells.

✓ FRESH PINEAPPLE—It contains an enzyme called BROMELAIN, which is believed to destroy many kinds of infectious germs.

✓ TOMATOES—are a natural antiseptic, and therefore protect against infection.

✓ VEGETABLE JUICES—The important vegetable juices are CARROT, BEET, CUCUMBER, with small amounts of GARLIC and ONION juice added.

✓ VITAMINS—There is a great deal of evidence that vitamin C helps the body to repel the attack of COLD VIRUSES, SORE THROAT, and GERMS. VITAMINS A and E have similar good effects. Take 1000 mg of vitamin C per day. It will acidify the URINE enough to interfere with bacterial growth. VITAMIN B_6 acts as a natural antihistamine. For SINUS infection use vitamins B_6, C, and GARLIC. Vitamin A acts as a switch to turn on disease fighting T-cells. With a vitamin A deficiency, the switch doesn't get thrown on. BETA-CAROTENE stimulates the MACROPHAGES, the large cells that search out tumors, engulf them, and destroy them with a lethal chemical. It also increases the immunity against CANDIDA ALBICANS, a bacterium that causes YEAST INFECTION.

The WHITE BLOOD CELLS need vitamin B_6 to produce antibodies, and the THYMUS GLAND needs it to produce T-cells. A LOMA LINDA study showed that large doses of B_6 given to mice created stronger immune reactions in them than in those mice not given the vitamin. The T-cells are often destroyed by the AIDS virus. Vitamin C stimulates the production of INTERFERON which "interferes" with the production of the viruses. When 250 mg vitamin C was put in the drinking water of mice, the level of interferon in their blood increased, and their susceptibility to LEUKEMIA decreased. The interferon triggers the production of T-cells. Vitamin C also keeps the WHITE CELLS healthy, which produce antibodies needed to kill bacteria.

✓ YOGURT—One 8 oz. cup of plain acidophilus yogurt is reported to have an antibiotic value equal to 14 UNITS OF PENICILLIN.

✓ ZINC—Its deficiency causes a poor immune response to germs. It helps increase the antibodies which increase the resistance to infection. A FIT BODY IS THE BEST ANTIBODY.

KIDNEY AND BLADDER DISEASES

Nature Of The Disease

When the kidneys are in a healthy state, they PURIFY the BLOOD, and EXCRETE UREA, SALTS, and TOXINS. The presence in the urine of such nutritive substances as SUGAR, ALBUMEN, and MINERAL ELEMENTS, shows an abnormal condition of the organs, and is usually a precursor of destructive changes within the kidneys themselves. An excess ANIMAL PROTEIN diet often brings this about. Previous DRUG treatment for ailments such as FEVER, FLU, and other acute diseases, produce damage to the kidney structures as a result of suppressive treatments which drive the poisonous substances back into the system. The kidneys then have to work overtime in order to eliminate them.

Kidney Stones

Kidney stones are collections of systemic REFUSE and TOXIC matter around a nucleus, and brought there by the IMPURITIES in the blood to be discharged in the urine. The stones are composed of crystals of PHOSPHATE, or OXALATE of LIME, which are precipitated out of the urine into the KIDNEYS or the BLADDER. Kidney stones are composed of 75 to 85% CALCIUM SALTS, 5 to 8% URIC or OXALIC ACID, and 10 to 15% STRUVITE, the latter being crystals of MAGNESIUM AMMONIUM PHOSPHATE. Simply supplementing the diet with MAGNESIUM and VITAMIN B_6 in clinically controlled studies, has dissolved many kidney stones and prevented occurrence in 80 to 90% of patients. Normally, 60 to 70% of stones removed from the kidneys by surgery, tend to return, because the CAUSE of the problem has not been stoneremoved.

Men are 3 times as susceptible to kidney stones as women. They are now 10 times as prevalent as they were in 1900. Much of animal protein can form stones. The reason: eating animal protein can drive up the urine levels of the stones raw materials—CALCIUM, OXALATE, and URIC ACID. VEGETARIANS usually have only as many kidney stones as meat eaters. This is due to the fact that vegetarians eat twice as much FIBER which is recognized as an antidote to kidney stones, and they also excrete less calcium. Studies also show that when vegetarians are put on meat diets, they have increases of calcium in their urine.

The Causes Of Kidney Stone Formation

✓ IMPROPER ELIMINATION—Kidney trouble is the result of improper and insufficient elimination largely of the end-products of the excessive use of MEAT in the diet, which develops an excessive amount of URIC ACID.

✓ CARBONATED DRINKS—The consumption of large quantities of carbonated drinks produce a high incidence of kidney stones, because they contain excessive amounts of PHOSPHORUS which is known to drive CALCIUM from the bones and allows it to form stones. This contributes also to OSTEOPOROSIS, or the thinning of the bones. To get extra calcium through ESTROGEN THERAPY has recently been shown to produce UTERINE CANCER.

✓ DRUGS—Many drugs can cause kidney damage. These include the commonly used over-the-counter medications like ANTACIDS and ASPIRIN. The large amount of CALCIUM CARBONATE found in antacids is hard on the kidneys.

In one case a woman taking only the recommended dose of antacids came down with symptoms of NO APPETITE, NAUSEATED, DIZZY, CONFUSED, and CRANKY. Tests showed that her kidneys were in bad shape, and she was taken off antacids. A checkup a month later showed that her kidneys had healed.

In a study of patients with KIDNEY FAILURE, 20% of the cases were caused by ASPIRIN and other pain killers such as ACETOMINOPHEN and PHENACETIN. Some who were on a KIDNEY MACHINE were able to stop using the machine when they stopped taking the pain killers.

✓ LACK OF FIBER—21 patients who easily formed kidney stones had their low fiber intake of 6 gm per day raised to 18 gm per day, by the use of WHEAT BRAN and CORN BRAN biscuits. The result was that they sharply reduced the amount of CALCIUM in the urine. A high URINARY CALCIUM level is said to be a major risk factor for kidney stones which are largely composed of calcium oxalate.

✓ HIGH BLOOD PRESSURE—According to current belief, high blood pressure is a causative factor in practically all KIDNEY diseases.

✓ LACK of MAGNESIUM—Some have successfully taken MAGNESIUM, in the form of MAGNESIUM OXIDE, and VITAMIN B_6 to cure kidney infection. Recent ideas have indicated that stone formation is due to MAGNESIUM DEFICIENCY. In an experiment where rats were subjected to insufficient magnesium, increased amounts of calcium were deposited on the kidneys. One report indicates that kidney calcification increased when intakes of magnesium were low and intakes of phosphorus were high.

A man of 33 had been passing kidney stones every two weeks for years. Nothing he tried could stop it. Then his doctor recommended 420 mg of MAGNESIUM OXIDE tablets daily. He soon stopped passing stones and remained free of them.

✓ CHOLINE DEFICIENCY—Animal studies have shown that a deficiency of CHOLINE, one of the B-vitamins, can also destroy the kidneys. Adelle Davis has said that the kidneys are affected first when CHOLINE is lacking in the diet. Rapidly growing rats on a choline-deficient diet, develop NEPHRITIS, or inflammation of the kidneys within four to seven days, and most of them soon die. The choline deficient kidneys also cause a rise in blood pressure.

✓ MILK—The overconsumption of milk often results in the development of kidney stones. Also milk fortified with vitamin D results in lowered magnesium levels. Magnesium alone has been shown to be effective in preventing recurrences of kidney stones.

✓ LACK OF VITAMIN A—Experiments on ALBINO RATS indicated that diets deficient in vitamin A produced kidney stones, and that rich vitamin A feeding dissolved them. One patient with a stone completely filling one kidney got rid of it in 6 months with a diet consisting of high vitamin A foods.

✓ SALT—When one restricts SALT, it restricts the amount of calcium in the urine. Stone-formers usually overindulge in salt by eating 5 gm or more of salt a day. The average amount should be no greater than 2 gm per day.

✓ OXALATES—Stone-formers also have lots of OXALATE in their urine. While some vegetables have oxalates in them, the chances are that oxalates come from eating too much ANIMAL PROTEIN, for too much protein tends to enrich urine with oxalate. Limiting CALCIUM INTAKE is not the solution, for tests show that limiting calcium intake actually tends to increase oxalate, and increases kidney stones. Dr. Durham of Harvard thinks that calcium ties up food oxalate in the intestines and prevents it from entering the bloodstream and keeps it from going to the kidneys to form stones.

How to Heal Kidney Disease

✓ BRAN SUPPLEMENTATION—Eating more bran as well as changing from WHITE to WHOLE WHEAT BREAD has resulted in lowering urinary calcium.

✓ CRANBERRY JUICE—Cranberry juice is an old folk remedy which is also used by some doctors and clinics today. It contains QUINIC and BENZOIC ACIDS. It raises the acidity of the urine, thereby creating an unfavorable environment for pathogenic bacteria. One Chinese doctor suggested to his 85 year old patient with kidney infection that he drink a glass of cranberry juice every day. This did the trick. He had another patient, who started with a quart of cranberry juice a day, and then used 2 large glasses of the juice per day, to get rid of the kidney infection.

✓ GOAT'S MILK—A diet of raw goat's milk is very good. Drink nothing but goat's milk for a few days, and with it take 1000 IU of VITAMIN E, and 75,000 units of VITAMIN A.

✓ HONEY—Raw and unfiltered, has medicinal value in the treatment of kidney disorders.

✓ KIDNEY BEAN POD TEA—In Europe the kidney bean pod tea treatment is considered most effective for all forms of KIDNEY and BLADDER disorders such as EDEMA, due to kidney and heart conditions, KIDNEY INFLAMMATION, KIDNEY and BLADDER STONES, as well as in chronic GOUT, and DIABETES.

A woman, who had a case of DROPSY, drank a glass of KIDNEY BEAN POD TEA and thereupon began passing large amounts of crystal clear urine. After 3 weeks of this her dropsy was gone. This treatment also solved a case of KIDNEY BLOCKAGE. Stones and gravel were rapidly dissolved.

A lady with KIDNEY TROUBLE was kept on ANTIBIOTICS by her doctor, but the trouble didn't clear up. Another doctor found that she had a KIDNEY STONE as well as DIABETES. Her sugar count was 326. The doctor said that she would have to have an operation if the stone was not passed. When she got home she started drinking BEAN POD TEA, a quart a day. Two weeks later when she returned to the doctor, her sugar count was 128, and she no longer had a stone nor diabetes.

✓ MAGNESIUM—One modern strategy for preventing kidney stones is to fight mineral with mineral, that is, to fight unwanted calcium with magnesium. Magnesium supplements seem to inhibit new kidney stones from forming in people who are prone to them. Magnesium is one of the oldest cure for kidney stones, for it has been in use since 1697. Magnesium in the urine attaches itself to oxalate, and this union is less likely to form crystals. If magnesium is not present, then calcium will join with oxalate to more easily form crystals. High magnesium foods are NUTS and SEEDS.

Stones are more likely to form when the diet is low in FIBER, but high in FAT, ANIMAL PROTEIN, SALT, ALCOHOL, and refined CARBOHYDRATES such as SUGAR. Vitamins B_6, K, along with MAGNESIUM and POTASSIUM, are a few of the supplements that can lower the development of KIDNEY STONES. There is a current trend of prescribing ANTACIDS as a calcium source which may contribute to stone formation. In order to prevent OSTEOPOROSIS, doctors are now telling their patients that antacids are a cheap source of calcium. However, antacids also neutralize the stomach acid, thereby creating an ALKALINE situation which promotes stone formation.

✓ HERBS—PARSLEY acts as a solvent for URIC ACID when used as a tea or eaten after meals. It can be used with good effect for URINARY TROUBLES and PROSTATE pressures. It has also eliminated sugar from the urine in cases of DIABETES. It has also been found to be good medicine for strengthening the BRAIN.

PARSLEY PIERT is also called PARSLEY BREAKSTONE, is not related to common parsley, but its medicinal action is somewhat similar. It is classed as a DIURETIC and DEMULCENT. It acts on STONES and GRAVEL in the kidneys and bladder, and other urinary ailments. There has been developed a formula consisting of PARSLEY PIERT, MARSHMELLOW ROOT, GRAVEL ROOT, and PELLITARY, which is to be used as a tea on a daily basis. It is also helpful in CYSTITIS, or inflammation of the BLADDER, and DROPSY.

✓ SALT—Eliminate excess salt from the diet.

✓ FRESH VEGETABLES and FRUITS—CARROT, CELERY, CUCUMBER, GARLIC, PARSLEY, and WATERCRESS are excellent. Add to this their juices. Also drink plenty of vegetable BROTH. The best fruits are PAPAYA and BANANAS. Both have a healing effect on the kidneys. WATERMELON is excellent, but it should be eaten by itself, and not with any other food. Brown RICE is also good.

ASPARAGUS contains ASPARAGIN which is of great benefit in cases of KIDNEY DISFUNCTION. It can break up OXALIC ACID CRYSTALS in kidneys, and is good for RHEUMATISM and NEURITIS. One woman reports that asparagus cured her kidney disease. She had over 30 operations for KIDNEY STONES, and was receiving government disability payments for the inoperable kidney condition. She attributed her cure entirely to the ASPARAGUS THERAPY.

A lady had TOXIC POISONING as well as a case of PYELITIS or inflammation of the kidneys. She had seen a general practitioner for 2 years without much help. She had lost 50 lbs., and her pocketbook was merely a shadow of its former self. An acquaintance asked her to try PARSLEY TEA. The instructions he gave her were to take a fresh bunch of parsley, wash it in cold water, place it in a dish and cover it with scalding hot water, and replace cover. When cold, pour off the liquid and drink it during a 24 hour period. Repeat it daily until cured. This procedure has been recommended to many people, and it has never failed to bring a cure in about 3 weeks, regardless of whether it is a KIDNEY or BLADDER COMPLAINT.

✓ VITAMIN B_6—It lowers the amount of OXALATE in people who have a disposition toward kidney stones. WATER RETENTION and SWELLING can be relieved with B_6 where DIURETICS have failed. Use two 50 mg tablets of B_6 daily.

✓ VITAMIN C—in the Urine kills ESCHERICHIA COLI bacteria, the most common cause of urinary tract infection. CITRATE, or SALTS of CITRIC ACID supplementation have been shown to be quite successful in preventing recurring kidney stones.

✓ OTHER TEAS—CORN SILK tea is another proven remedy. Drink a glass of it several times a day, and continue this for several months. SARSAPARILLA is used for GENITOURINARY problems as it contains the hormones TESTOSTERONE, PROGESTERONE, and CORTIN. BUCHU is also an herb that has been recommended for the treatment of CYSTITIS, GRAVEL, URETHRITIS, PROSTATITIS, CATARRH, and IRRITATION of the BLADDER.

✓ WATER DRINKING—One cause of kidney stone development is that they are formed when there is too much calcium in the urine. The calcium joins with oxalates or phosphates to form crystals that precipitate out of solution when the solution is too concentrated. Hence, one way to keep the crystals from forming is to drink more water, at least 2 quarts daily.

✓ PINEAPPLE JUICE—One person with kidney stones found that upon drinking a can of pineapple juice when the kidney stone pain began, that he passed the stones the next day.

Bladder Problems

✓ CYSTITIS—INFLAMMATION of the BLADDER—represents difficulties or abnormalities in passing urine with respect to frequency, urgency, pain, or obstruction. The cure of cystitis with folk medicine includes CHERRY JUICE, CRANBERRY JUICE, CORN SILK TEA, and GARLIC. It is suggested that the patient drink a half cup of cranberry juice every two hours. Cherry juice works as well as cranberry juice. One lady said that after a week of eating 4 to 6 cloves of garlic a day her cystitis disappeared. VITAMIN C works well also. Take 2 gm of vitamin C by mouth every two hours to allow the vitamin C to accumulate in the urine where it heals the inflammation and neutralizes the poisons.

✓ CAUSES—Going too long without emptying

the bladder. It can be produced by drugs, or by eating too many acid foods and not enough green leaf foods, or by not drinking enough water

- ✓ TREATMENT—Use CORNSILK TEA in large quantities and often. Also SHAVE GRASS TEA works very well. A hot and cold SITZBATH with NETTLE TEA in it is helpful. Also drink diluted LEMON JUICE with a little HONEY in it.
- ✓ CRANBERRY JUICE—Cranberry juice can help eliminate the infection as well as prevent it. In 1985 a team of researchers from Ohio state University reported the discovery in cranberry juice of a substance that makes it difficult for the bacteria that cause urinary tract infection to cling to the walls of the bladder cells. The chemical kept the bacteria off the bladder cells for from 12 to 15 hours after the juice was drunk.
- ✓ CORNSILK TEA—Cornsilk tea has a soothing effect on KIDNEY, BLADDER, and URINARY problems, and it can clear up PUS, INFECTION, BURNING or SCALDING URINE. It seems to heal these diseased areas, and can flush out URIC ACID, TOXINS, and other POISONS.
- ✓ CHERRY JUICE—It has been shown to cure BLADDER TROUBLE. One person got a cherry concentrate from the health food store, and used one tablespoon in a glass of water every morning for complete relief.
- ✓ CRANBERRIES—One lady used fresh cranberries, chopped them up in a food chopper, mixed them with enough honey to make them palatable, and ate them for her BLADDER INFECTION. The symptoms were greatly relieved in 6 hours, and were completely gone in 12 hours.
- ✓ GARLIC—One lady chopped up 3 large cloves of GARLIC 3 times a day, put them on a teaspoon and into the mouth and washed it down with water. After 5 days of this procedure, the cystitis was gone.

LIVER TROUBLES

Nature Of The Disease

◆ *The Liver A Detoxifying Organ*

The liver is the detoxifying organ of the body which filters and stores poisons. It is involved in almost all conditions of ill health. It is the most important organ in metabolism. The health and vitality of an individual is to a large extent determined by the health and vitality of the liver. When there is serious liver damage, it will take a long time to get better. Patients should have the patience to stay on a special diet for from 3 months to a year if necessary. The SYMPTOMS of liver disease are FATIGUE, GENERAL MALAISE, DIGESTIVE DISTURBANCES, CHEMICAL SENSITIVITY, PREMENSTRUAL SYNDROME, and CONSTIPATION.

◆ *Animal Protein Is Harmful To The Liver*

The liver is the great barrier within the system to the inroads of foreign, harmful, and poisonous substances which could adversely affect the working of the organism. It also has a great deal to do with PROTEIN METABOLISM. The more of especially animal protein is included in the daily diet, the more excess protein there will be for the liver to break down into UREA, and get rid of it by way of the kidneys.

Liver Troubles And Their Causes

We are told that "All that is taken into the stomach above what the system can use to convert into good blood, clogs the machinery, for it cannot be made into either flesh or blood, and its presence burdens the liver" (CH160).

A few years ago the main two forms of hepatitis were form A and B. Now types C, D, and E have been added. Incidence of hepatitis E are rarely encountered in the U.S., since the virus is usually contracted from sewage-containing water. Hepatitis D is found only in the presence of B, but no one knows as yet why. Hepatitis C is the one that accounts for almost 40% of the estimated 800,000 cases of hepatitis in the U.S. each year, and it is implicated more and more in the rise of LIVER CANCER. The causes of liver troubles are:

- ✓ ALCOHOL—It is the most common cause of liver trouble. Alcohol ingestion causes fat to be deposited within the liver. This causes decreased liver function, and the risk of further damage to the liver. When one group was given foods high in FIBER and low in SUGAR, after 4 months on a no alcohol diet, they had less craving for a drink and less sugar consumption than those in the traditional group. Desire for ALCOHOL seems to be directly related to eating sugar. The craving for alcohol decreased from 80% to 17%. The researchers theorize that diets lacking in nutrients but high in sugar and caffeine may stimulate a thirst for alcohol. Diets lacking in the amino acid TRYPTOPHAN lower the body's supply of SEROTONIN, and low levels of serotonin are found in the brains of alcoholics.
- ✓ INFECTIOUS HEPATITIS—is an infection of the liver which is passed directly from person to person.
- ✓ SERUM HEPATITIS—is chiefly spread through contaminated blood transfusions.
- ✓ TOXIC HEPATITIS—is liver inflammation caused by chemicals or drugs.
- ✓ CIRRHOSIS—or hardening of the liver, may result from HEPATITIS. A recent study suggests that at least 20% of people with CHRONIC HEPATITIS will develop cirrhosis.
- ✓ MALNUTRITION—or an overabundance of SUGAR and SATURATED FATS in the diet, as well as too much ALCOHOL, results in nutritional deficiencies particularly of the B-VITAMINS.
- ✓ FATTY LIVERS—A diet low in CHOLINE and PROTEIN has produced fatty livers in animals.

How To Heal Liver Troubles

Adequate high quality PROTEIN is essential in liver diseases. The best complete proteins are obtained from BREWER'S YEAST, which is also high the the B-VITAMINS which are vital for liver health. Also RAW GOAT'S MILK, HOMEMADE COTTAGE CHEESE, SPROUTED SEEDS AND GRAINS, RAW NUTS, especially ALMONDS, SESAME SEED BUTTER called TAHINI, is especially beneficial because of its unusually high content of METHIONINE, an essential amino acid, UNSATURATED OILS, and CALCIUM.

- ✓ CHOLERETICS—Choleretics are substances that help to excrete bile from the liver, thereby lowering cholesterol levels, as well as decreasing the synthesis of cholesterol.
- ✓ DIET—The diet should be rich in FIBER and PLANT FOODS, low in refined sugar and fat, and as free from pesticides and pollutants as possible. Exclude all PROCESSED, CANNED, and REFINED FOODS. Avoid all CHEMICAL ADDITIVES in foods, POISONS in the air, WATER, and ENVIRONMENT if possible. Avoid SYNTHETIC VITAMINS, for they do not act exactly like natural vitamins in the system. No SALT, no SUGAR, no strong SPICES like MUSTARD, BLACK and WHITE PEPPER, no SUGAR, no ALCOHOL, for all of these will damage the liver. Use HONEY as sweetener. A diet high in saturated fat increases the risk of developing fatty infiltration, or bile slowdown. Heated fat should be avoided. The basic rule for liver patients is to eliminate all fried foods from the diet. A diet rich in water soluble FIBER will promote increased bile secretion.
- ✓ LECITHIN—Use one or two tablespoons of granules or the equivalent in capsules. Lecithin contains CHOLINE which helps prevent fatty degeneration, neutralizes some toxins, and is believed to improve liver function.
- ✓ VITAMIN A—Take 50,000 to 100,000 IU/day, then take 3 to 5 tablespoons of brewer's yeast daily.
- ✓ VITAMIN C—Use 3 to 10 grams/day. Many reports have been published regarding the effectiveness of 20 to 50 grams of vitamin C in clearing HEPATITIS in a matter of days It also acts as a preventative. It is nontoxic even in massive doses.
- ✓ VITAMIN E AND SELENIUM—Take 100–400 IU of vitamin E, and 100–200 micrograms (mcg) of selenium daily. Selenium increases the

effectiveness of vitamin E, and aids the liver's detoxification process.

✓ JUICES—RED BEETS and red beet JUICE are especially beneficial in liver disorders. Also ENDIVE, ARTICHOKE, CUCUMBER, GARLIC, and LEMON juices. For TOXIC LIVER engage in a special liver detoxifying JUICE FAST for 3 days as follows: Mix the fresh juice of 10 lemons in two quarts of water, sweeten it with honey, and drink one glass every two hours. Also twice daily, drink a GREEN VEGETABLE juice mixed with about 50% RED BEET juice.

✓ HERBS—Use DANDELION, PARSLEY, LIVER WORT, GOLDEN ROD, ST. JOHN'S WORT, and SARSAPARILLA TEA. Sarsaparilla is regarded as one of the finest liver remedies both as food and medicine. It enhances the flow of BILE, improves LIVER CONGESTION, BILE DUCT INFLAMMATION, HEPATITIS, GALLSTONES, and JAUNDICE. Dandelion causes contraction of the gallbladder, thereby promoting the flow of bile.

✓ EXERCISE—We are told that "Useful employment would bring into exercise the enfeebled muscles, enliven the stagnant blood in the system, and arouse the torpid liver to perform its work. The circulation of the blood would be equalized, and the entire system invigorated to overcome bad conditions." (HL593).

MULTIPLE SCLEROSIS

Nature Of The Disease

MULTIPLE SCLEROSIS is a disease of the central nervous system. More than 250,000 Americans are afflicted with it. It is a disease which usually strikes young adults without much warning. For some reason which is not clear, the protective covering of the nerves in the brain and spinal chord, called MYELIN, develops lesions so that nerve impulses are distorted, and the body cannot respond properly to them. The nerves are short-circuited, causing the STAGGERING WALK, DOUBLE OR BLURRED VISION, WEAKNESS OR NUMBNESS IN THE LIMBS, DIZZINESS, FAULTY EQUILIBRIUM, SHAKING, SLURRED SPEECH, as well as BOWEL and BLADDER trouble. It is said to be basically caused by MALNUTRITION, and is a degenerative disease, caused by nutritional deficiencies and metabolic disorders due to an unnatural, unbalanced diet of devitalized foods. Some believe that it is caused by too much LEAD in the diet, others by HYPERINSULINISM, and others from a lack of CALCIUM in the diet.

The Cause Of Multiple Sclerosis

◆ *Possible Lead Poisoning*

Scientists find that there seems to be a relationship between multiple sclerosis and LEAD POISONING. They discovered an unusually high incidence of the disease in a lead mining area. They theorize that lead may interfere with some essential mineral, vitamin, or enzyme reaction, and thereby precipitate the destruction of nerve sheaths. When 8 areas in Great Britain were investigated because of high MS incidence, they showed that in every instance rock, soil, and food samples contained from 2 to 10 times normal amounts of lead.

Some foods have a high lead content, which is suspected to be due to the spraying of LEAD ARSENATE INSECTICIDES. Among them were BAKING POWDER, SARDINES, DRIED GELATIN, PUFFED RICE, APPLE CIDER, and VINEGAR.

◆ *Lack Of Linolenic Acid*

Some believe that the lack of LINOLENIC ACID, an essential fatty acid, is a polyunsaturate which is important to the development of the brain and the spinal chord. Fresh FISH oils as well as SAFFLOWER, CORN, SUNFLOWER, COTTON SEED, and SOYBEAN oils, are particularly rich in linolenic acid, which the body itself cannot manufacture. Victims of MS do show a below normal amount of linolenic acid in their brains. In Japan, where people consume large amounts of fish, multiple sclerosis is almost nonexistent.

◆ *Fat Consumption*

Another theory relates MS to FAT CONSUMPTION. Studies seem to show that the disease increases as fat consumption increases. Other observations seem to indicate that the incidence was highest where farming and milk production were the chief industries, and where the diet consisted largely of milk and animal fat.

The Cure Of Multiple Sclerosis

- ✓ LINOLENIC ACID—It has been discovered that POLYUNSATURATED FATTY ACIDS are necessary to the development of the brain and of the spinal chord, the two vital areas affected by multiple sclerosis. Linolenic acid is particularly important.

- ✓ MOTHER'S MILK—is richer in UNSATURATED FATTY ACIDS than COW'S MILK. It has been shown that bottle-fed babies have a higher incidence of MS than breast-fed babies. Dr. Clausen of Denmark showed that rats fed a diet without unsaturated fats immediately developed symptoms of MS.

- ✓ USE ORGANICALLY GROWN FOODS—as well as whole unprocessed raw foods such as RAW FRUITS AND VEGETABLES, RAW MILK, PREFERABLY GOAT'S MILK, RAW SEEDS AND NUTS, RAW OATS, HOMEMADE COTTAGE CHEESE and SOURED MILK, WHEAT GERM OIL and other cereal germ oils as sources of ARACHIDONIC ACID, an unsaturated acid which is of specific value in the treatment of MS. SPROUTED SEEDS and GRAINS, especially sprouted WHEAT and RYE.

- ✓ LACTIC ACID FOODS—Daily use of FERMENTED LACTIC ACID FOODS such as SAUERKRAUT, SOUR PICKLES, AND LACTIC ACID VEGETABLES, ALL HOMEMADE. Sauerkraut can be made with seeds without the use of salt. Liquid WHEY, the liquid portion of soured milk, contains OROTIC ACID, which is of special value in MS. When raw cottage cheese is made at home, the liquid whey should not be thrown away but should be used for drinks.

- ✓ RAW UNFILTERED HONEY—is the only sweetener allowed.

- ✓ THE BEST VEGETABLES—are CARROTS, CABBAGE, RED BEETS, TOMATOES, and their juices.

- ✓ LINOLEIC ACID—Adding linoleic acid to one's diet reduces the incidence of MS severely, and can increase remissions. SAFFLOWER and SUNFLOWER SEED OILS are the richest in linoleic acid.

- ✓ COD-LIVER OIL—Dr. Swank believes that a low animal fat diet will arrest MS in a high proportion of cases, but he boosts unsaturated oil including one teaspoon full of cod-liver oil daily.

- ✓ SUNLIGHT—Dr. Paul Goldberg found that the more sunlight an area received, the lower was its rate of MS. This means that in the northern latitude the risk is greater than in a latitude closer to the equator. He also found less MS in the higher altitudes. The higher you live the more ultraviolet rays you receive, the more VITAMIN D your skin forms, the more CALCIUM your intestines absorb, and the lower your risk of MS. Hence, at the lower altitudes COD-LIVER OIL is the perfect supplement for MS.

- ✓ VITAMINS—Vitamin supplementation is a vital treatment for MS. Some doctors believe that it is caused by a lack of vitamin E in the diet, due to eating too many refined foods. Dr. Frederick Klenner uses megadoses of VITAMINS B_1, B_3, and B_6, as well as MINERALS, TRACE ELEMENTS, OILS, and AMINO ACIDS to heal people with MS. Both vitamins E, F, and essential fatty acids, are specifics for MS.

- ✓ MAGNESIUM—A lady had MS for over 20 years with relapses and remissions. She was taken to the Mayo clinic and told that nothing could be done about it, that it was incurable. She was numb over most of her body, especially in arms and legs. She discovered accidentally that MAGNESIUM in the form of DOLOMITE POWDER could control it, and all this happened in only one day.

- ✓ OTHER TREATMENTS—Herbalist Al. Wolfsen suggests—cleanse the BOWELS, take STEAM BATHS, eat 80% RAW FOODS, and also eat SEAWEED.

NERVE DISORDERS

Nature Of The Disease

NERVOUSNESS can be caused by OVERWORK, WORRY, CARE of CHILDREN, IMPROPER FOOD, and a LACK OF SLEEP. WASTE MATTER in the system gets into the blood and comes in contact with the nervous system, and especially affects the nerves in the brain, causing irritability, headaches etc. Food in the stomach affects the whole nervous system because what we eat and drink feeds and nourishes the nerves. We are told: "You should use the most simple food, prepared in the most simple manner, that the fine nerves of the brain be not weakened, benumbed, or paralyzed" (2T46).

The Causes Of Nerve Disorders

✓ TEA and COFFEE—We are told that tea has an influence to excite the nerves, and coffee benumbs the brain; both are highly injurious. "By the use of tea and coffee an appetite is formed for tobacco, and this encourages the appetite for liquors" (CD233).

✓ NEURALGIA—An eruption or pain along a nerve line, which happens in spurts. It is usually caused by TOXINS or POISONS in the system. It may be decayed teeth throwing poisons into the system, or it may be due to CLOGGED BOWELS. The treatment is cleansing the bowels by drinking a lot of water. HOT and COLD applications to the sore part, and going on a diet of RAW FOOD for one week.

✓ DAMPNESS—We are told that "Dampness gathers in the house, especially in wet seasons the sleeping rooms become damp, and those who sleep in the beds are troubled with RHEUMATISM, NEURALGIA, and LUNG COMPLAINTS, which generally end in CONSUMPTION" (HL615).

✓ DRUGS—A lady reports that one day she began to shake especially in the legs and elsewhere. The doctor said that it was "NERVES," and possibly the beginning of Parkinson's disease. A nurse told her that people on HIGH BLOOD PRESSURE MEDICATION will shake and tremble because the medication DESTROYS THE POTASSIUM in the system. The doctor finally gave her a prescription for potassium, and the improvement was noticeable within 3 days. She is free of the shaking now. Potassium tablets are available at the health food store.

✓ PARALYSIS—A 7 year old girl was hopelessly paralyzed by a virus that attacked her nervous system, and this condition is known as POLYNEURITIS. It keeps the white blood cells from doing their job of fighting viruses. Instead of doing this they attacked nerve tissue. In 3 weeks the girl was almost totally paralyzed, and doctors said that she would be paralyzed for life. They heard on TV of giving SUNFLOWER OIL to kidney transplant patients, to keep the white blood cells from rejecting the kidney. They decided to give the girl a teaspoonful of SUNFLOWER OIL 3 times a day. In 48 hours she began to move. Her father doubled the dosage and she continued to improve. Soon she could run and play like other girls, and she was back to complete normalcy.

How To Heal Nerve disorders

✓ THE BASIC NERVE TREATMENT—Cleanse the BOWELS, take STEAM BATHS, drink lots of WATER, EAT PROPERLY, go to BED at DARK, RELAX at your work, live in the open air by taking your sleeping bag and SLEEP ON THE GROUND, massage the BACK of the NECK. For NERVE RELAXING HERBS use CATNIP, HOPS, CAYENNE PEPPER, and LOBELIA teas. Also hot and cold FOMENTATIONS to the spine, stomach, liver, and spleen are very beneficial. A warm bath of an hour's duration is excellent. Gentle MASSAGES after the bath helps greatly. Use enemas and herbal laxatives for cleaning the system out. SKULLCAP is one of the best herbs for the nerves.

✓ CRAMPS—Muscles are controlled by electrical impulses from the nervous system which depend upon the B-VITAMINS for proper functioning. During periods of STRESS increased amounts of these vitamins are needed. Hence, any deficiency or imbalance of CALCIUM, MAGNESIUM, PHOSPHORUS, POTASSIUM

ETC. can cause MUSCLE SPASMS, TICS, or TREMORS. ALCOHOL, ALLERGIES, ANTACIDS, DIURETICS, TRANQUILIZERS, or other medication can upset the mineral balance. However, most of these muscular problems are believed to be the result of VITAMIN and MINERAL deficiencies.

A lack of CALCIUM generally, or also a deficiency of POTASSIUM and MAGNESIUM can bring on cramps. Excessive SUGAR in the diet can bring on a shortage of potassium, and with it cramps or other neuromuscular ailments. The richest sources of potassium are KELP, BREWER'S YEAST, SOYBEANS, WHEAT GERM, PARSLEY, SUNFLOWER SEEDS, ALMONDS, PEANUTS, VITAMIN B_6, VITAMIN C and E. Also the extra magnesium in these same foods can prevent CRAMPS, TREMORS, and TICS.

✓ LEG CRAMPS—or restless legs, can be relieved by supplements of CALCIUM and VITAMIN E, as well as with additional vitamins and minerals. LOW BLOOD SUGAR is at times also a factor. The leg cramps suffered by women during PREGNANCY, MENSTRUATION, or MENOPAUSE, can frequently be relieved by taking 1000 mg CALCIUM, 500 mg MAGNESIUM, 400 IU VITAMIN D, and 150 mg of VITAMIN B_6. TREMORS and FACIAL TICS have reportedly been corrected by the same supplementation plus several tablespoons of BREWER'S YEAST, or B-COMPLEX tablets. Exercising in heat and humidity can cause cramps from a DEPLETION of SODIUM. PAINFUL MUSCULAR CONTRACTIONS and STIFFNESS from unaccustomed exercise can be prevented by taking 500 mg VITAMIN C each hour during and after the activity. If a "charley horse" develops, it can be eased by pushing the foot against a resistance and MASSAGING the affected muscle, as well as by applying HEAT or ICE.

✓ One man reported that by wearing WARM CLOTHING in bed, and by not getting a cold, he could prevent leg cramps. A few months later he started taking daily 200 units of VITAMIN E, 500 mg of VITAMIN C, one DOLOMITE TABLET, some LIVER and YEAST. This therapy eliminated all cramps. As a side effect his hair is turning black, and he is 85 years of age.

✓ NEPHRITIS—or inflammation of the KIDNEYS. Use CORN SILK, SHAVE GRASS, and SLIPPERY ELM BARK teas.

✓ DIGESTION and INSOMNIA—CHAMOMILE tea has a well-established reputation as a remedy for SOOTHING the nerves, strengthening DIGESTION, and relieving certain forms of COLIC. The tea is a popular beverage in European countries where it is taken at bedtime for conditions of INSOMNIA. It is widely accepted as a domestic remedy for the treatment of NIGHTMARE and RESTLESS SLEEP, especially in children.

✓ HEADACHES—Some people have found relief from MIGRAINE HEADACHES with the use of ROSEHIPS VITAMIN C tablets, of from 250 to 300 mg. One woman who suffered from migraine headaches reports that she cured them by taking a tablespoon of HONEY as soon as she felt one coming on. If the headache returned she followed it with a second dose of honey and 3 glasses of water. Then it disappeared completely and didn't return.

A woman who was plagued by MIGRAINES for 6 years couldn't go anywhere without her bottle of the drug FIORINAL. Then she remembered an old man telling her that if he didn't take LECITHIN he couldn't control his temper. When she started taking lecithin she would still get headaches, but they were much milder. So instead of taking the drug she would take an extra dose of lecithin right when the headache started, and it worked. Another lady took 9 tablets of BREWERS YEAST per day and cured herself of the headache.

✓ FEVERFEW—Researchers in Britain are reporting success with feverfew especially in preventing and relieving MIGRAINE HEADACHE. WOOD BETONY is used for the relief of NERVOUS HEADACHES, MIGRAINE HEADACHE, and INSOMNIA, by placing two heaping teaspoons of the dried herb in a cup and adding boiling water.

✓ HOPS—Scientific research has shown that HOPS contains certain substances which act as a sedative in overcoming INSOMNIA. Hops pickers of yesteryear claimed that the strong ODOR of hops exerted a soothing influence on the nerves and produced drowsiness. Pillows stuffed with hops were used in place of ordinary pillows to insure a good nights sleep for sufferers of insomnia. A hop pillow is prepared by preparing a small muslin bag loosely with hops and attaching it to an ordinary pillow. To this day hop pillows have retained their popularity for allaying RESTLESSNESS and producing SLEEP in NERVOUS DISORDERS.

OSTEOPOROSIS

Nature Of The Disease

◆ *Calcium Absorption Slows With Age*

The PARATHYROID GLAND regulates CALCIUM and PHOSPHORUS metabolism. Its hormone, the PARATHYROID HORMONE, takes CALCIUM stored in the bones, and distributes it to the blood, nerves, muscles, and other cells. At age 40 the parathyroid slows down, and as a result calcium absorption slows down in both sexes. There is also a slowing down of ESTROGEN, a female hormone, which is needed to help the body absorb calcium and to build good bones. BONE BUILDING continues but lags behind BONE LOSS to the extent that over a 30 year period more than a third of the total calcium is lost. If the natural estrogen is replaced by a SYNTHETIC ESTROGEN, there develops the danger of its producing CANCER. VITAMIN D increases the absorption of CALCIUM, and EXERCISE not only halts bone loss, but actually stimulates the formation of new bone.

◆ *Estrogen Production Slows At Menopause*

Men are less likely to have osteoporosis because the MALE SEX HORMONE ANDROGEN is produced throughout life. On the other hand, the MENOPAUSE in women causes a diminishing supply of ESTROGEN in the female system. This leads to the demineralization of the bone structure, which is what osteoporosis is all about. As a result doctors attempt to give women the same life extension benefit that men have by replacing the lack of estrogen with more estrogen externally introduced. One problem in doing this is the development of CANCER. There then exists a 2 to 3 times greater risk of UTERINE cancer, a 4 to 8 times greater risk of OVARIAN cancer, and a 2 times greater risk of BREAST cancer among estrogen users.

At this time women who smoke will get PAIN in the bones because SMOKING starts an earlier menopause, and they are likely to get osteoporosis sooner. Aging significantly reduces the skin's capacity to produce vitamin D, which is needed for the assimilation of calcium. The skin of a 70 year old produces one half the vitamin D of the skin of a 20 year old.

The Causes Of Osteoporosis

✓ MAGNESIUM—It has been shown that individuals with osteoporosis have lower MAGNESIUM content, indicating a magnesium deficiency. An intake of dairy food results in decreased magnesium absorption. This seems to indicate that milk is not an appropriate food for preventing osteoporosis.

✓ NUTRITIONAL—Dr. Albanese said that osteoporosis may soon be regarded as a bone disease of nutritional origin, involving low CALCIUM intake, poor absorption of calcium, ALCOHOL abuse, a high PHOSPHATE diet emphasizing MEAT, CHEESE, COLA drinks involving PHOSPHORIC ACID, vitamin D deficiency, high CAFFEINE intake, and high PROTEIN intake, deficiencies of VITAMINS and MINERALS.

✓ CALCIUM IMBALANCE—If the body is in a negative calcium balance, it must pull some calcium out of the bones in order to maintain a balance. By the late 30's both men and women make fewer calcium deposits in the bone bank, partly because they are less able to absorb calcium from food. Then the bone bank is robbed and osteoporosis takes over. Bones may supply the rest of the body with adequate calcium, but they do so by sacrificing their own supply. One needs 1000 mg of calcium per day to maintain an adequate calcium balance according to Dr. B.L. Riggs of the Mayo Clinic. An 8 oz. glass of MILK has 300 mg of Calcium. An 8 oz. container of low fat YOGURT has from 350 to 450 mg. Vegetables have lots of calcium. One cup of BROCCOLI equals 150 mg.

Lifelong intake of calcium is the best hedge against osteoporosis. In one study women whose dietary calcium intake was 1000 gm per day had 60% to 75% fewer HIP FRACTURES than women consuming around 500 mg. If one doesn't consume enough calcium, the body will take calcium from the bones to make it available for life sustaining activities such as NERVE CONDUCTION, MUSCLE CONTRACTION, and BLOOD CLOTTING.

✓ ACID FOODS—Avoid more acid forming foods, for an oversupply of them causes the calcium to be pulled out of the bones. Concentrate on the alkaline fruits and vegetables, especially in their raw state.

✓ INSUFFICIENT ACTIVITY—It is diminished physical activity and loss of muscle strength that are contributing factors in senile osteoporosis.

✓ SALT—Too much salt helps destroy one's bones by robbing them of CALCIUM.

✓ COOKED FOODS—They cause osteoporosis because cooking deranges the mineral content of foods, so that the body cannot use the minerals that have been heated. For fruits and vegetables this means the loss of their alkaline properties and the development of acid tendencies.

How To Cure Osteoporosis

✓ NUTRITION—In order for you to obtain the 1000 mg of calcium daily, 5 glasses of milk would do it. Raw milk if possible, if not possible use GOAT'S MILK. Also 5 cups of yogurt on the same basis, or two pounds of COLLARD GREENS, or one pound of ALMONDS. Other high calcium foods are BROCCOLI, SOYBEANS, NUTS, SESAME and SUNFLOWER seeds. One can also make up the difference with calcium supplements of DOLOMITE, BONE MEAL, CALCIUM LACTATE, and CALCIUM GLUCONATE. EGG YOLKS contain a substantial amount of vitamin D. Generally, eat almost completely fruits and vegetables in their raw state.

✓ EXERCISE—In a test 13 men and 25 women over 70 walked for one hour every day for a year. They did not lose any bone mass during that year. Physical exercise of one hour three times a week has been shown to prevent bone loss. It will actually increase bone mass in menopausal women. Bones are like muscles. They will grow stronger as greater demands are placed on them. "Every faculty of the mind, every bone in the body, every muscle of the limbs, shows that God designed these faculties to be used, not to remain inactive" (4T411).

Plenty of regular physical exercise is necessary both for prevention and treatment of osteoporosis. When bones are subjected to pressure, an electric current is generated which draws calcium and other minerals out of the blood and into the bones, and allows the bones to become more dense. An increased density means stronger bones. Dr. Carlton Fredericks says that people with osteoporosis should SKIP ROPE, but WALKING can have the same effect.

✓ VITAMIN D—Vitamin D is essential for optimum absorption of calcium in the intestines, and one should get about 400 IU per day. 15 minutes to an hour per day outdoors where the sun is shining will give us a sufficient amount as a minimal basis.

What To Avoid

✓ CAFFEINE—It interferes with calcium absorption.

✓ MEAT EATING—Meat has a high phosphorous content. Avoid especially BEEF, which contains 25 times as much PHOSPHOROUS as CALCIUM. A high meat diet will lead invariably to calcium and magnesium deficiencies. Hence, meat eaters are more susceptible to osteoporosis.

✓ CORTICOSTEROIDS—Prolonged use of corticosteroids, frequently taken for arthritis, helps push calcium out of the body before it has a chance to settle in the bones. So does too much FAT, SALT, PROTEIN, and PHOSPHOROUS.

✓ COFFEE, ALCOHOL, and SMOKING—all induce a negative calcium balance, and are therefore associated with an increased risk of developing osteoporosis.

- ✓ ESTROGEN—Doctors used to prescribe estrogen for osteoporosis. It did stop the advance of osteoporosis, but it didn't make the bones stronger.

  Hence, estrogen should not be used because of side effects which give one a 10 times higher risk of inducing CANCER, such as cancer of the UTERUS and BREAST, a 6 times higher risk for developing BLOOD CLOTTING within the body which leads to THROMBOPHLEBITIS. It also leads to GALLBLADDER DISEASE, and an increase in HYPERTENSION. An excess of calcium with estrogen promotes KIDNEY STONES. For these reasons CALCIUM SUPPLEMENTATION is better than using estrogen.
- ✓ SOFT DRINKS—are damaging to the teeth. The PHOSPHATES in soft drinks speed up the depletion of calcium in the bones. For example, submerge a tooth in the bottle of a cola drink, and in 30 days it will be totally dissolved.
- ✓ VINEGAR—will dissolve calcium out of your bones.

PNEUMONIA

Nature Of The Disease

PNEUMONIA, called LUNG FEVER by Mrs. White, is an inflammation of the lungs that can be triggered by viruses and bacteria. The cilia in the lung tissue continuously propel mucus, in which the bacteria and viruses get stuck, continuously out of the lungs. This condition is much more common in winter with the entrance of cold air into the lungs. It is more often seen in individuals with a low immune function. Chronic lung diseases have increased due to the use of suppressive drugs and alcohol.

The Symptoms Of Pneumonia

It starts very much like a cold with a slight fever. The tiny air sacs in the lungs become inflamed and fill with mucus and pus. Thereupon follow fever, chills, cough, aching muscles, fatigue, sore throat, enlarged lymph glands, pains in the chest, and rapid and difficult breathing. sometimes small blood spots are noticed in the sputum.

The Causes Of Pneumonia

- ✓ VITAMIN A DEFICIENCY—Vitamin A is necessary for the health of the lining of the respiratory passages. A deficiency of the vitamin increases susceptibility to respiratory infections, which in turn can lead to pneumonia.
- ✓ VITAMIN C DEFICIENCY—at least 100 to 200 mg per day is needed as a minimum to maintain a good balance.
- ✓ DEVITALIZED FOODS—Refined SUGAR and refined and bleached FLOUR. Cold arms and legs. Swimming too long in cold water till the lips get blue.

How To Heal Pneumonia

- ✓ HIGH DOSES OF VITAMIN C—Dr. Fred Klenner has used massive doses of vitamin C against severe virus infections. One year he had a lady patient with VIRUS PNEUMONIA. She was unconscious, and had a fever of 106 degrees. He gave her 140 grams of VITAMIN C intravenously over a period of 72 hrs. By that time she was almost well, and she became completely well soon after. Pneumonia is a condition of extreme stress upon the body. Animals under stress manufacture many times more vitamin C than they do under normal conditions. Human beings cannot manufacture their own vitamin C. As a result the extra vitamin C given to humans from without, is of as much benefit to them as it is to animals producing their own vitamin C from within.

  Some suggest 500 mg of VITAMIN C every two hours. Of VITAMIN A 25,000 IU per day, ZINC lozenges, and 500 mg THYMUS EXTRACT twice a day. Vitamin C from ROSEHIPS being good for colds and flu, is also outstanding for pneumonia, and other respiratory problems.
- ✓ FLUIDS—Large amounts of fresh fruit juices as well as vegetable juices, but not at the same time. As well as vegetable BROTH. This will help nature to expel impurities.
- ✓ HERBS—DANDELION ROOT, besides being used for PNEUMONIA, has been used to treat liver disease as well as CANCER of the BREAST. In general it stimulates liver activity,

thereby encouraging the elimination of toxins in the blood. Other helpful herbs are ECHINACEA, GOLDENSEAL, and LICORICE. GARLIC has been highly recommended in France as a remedy for lung diseases. Although ANTIBIOTICS are effective in treating pneumonia, they will deplete the body of vitamins C and K, and the entire B-Complex.

✓ HOT BATHS—Take frequent hot baths. Drink some SEA WATER which is available in health food stores, and eat plenty of SEAWEEDS. Get at least four hours of sleep before midnight.

✓ MRS. WHITE'S EXPERIENCES—In (2SM304–6). Mrs. White relates how in 1864 her son WILLIE came down with LUNG FEVER. They had buried their oldest son with this disease, and decided this time not to send for a physician, but do the best they could by the use of WATER and PRAYER. His heart had an irregular beat and was in a constant agitated flutter. Water was used on his head, a compress was placed upon his lungs, and soon he became rational. His pain was subdued with cold water compresses. No drugs were used. In a dream she was shown that nature had done her work well to rid the system of impurities. He was given more air into the room. In a week he was better, the fever left him, and he recovered.

✓ JETHRO KLOSS'S EXPERIENCE—One time Jethro Kloss, herbalist, and author of the book *Back To Eden*, was called to see a young lady who had been given up to die by her doctors. She had PNEUMONIA with a high fever. He placed her between two cotton blankets and sponged her with tepid water. He gave her frequent sips of cold water, hot and cold applications to both chest and back. In two hours her lungs opened up. In 4 hours the body temperature had gone down two degrees. He placed a cold towel around her head and neck. He gave her a liquid diet and fruit juices. In four days her temperature was normal.

PREMATURE AGING

The Nature Of Aging

◆ *Lifespan Depends Upon Unchanging Laws*

When Adam was created he was given 20 times the vital power which men now possess. If he hadn't been given that much vitality, the human race would be extinct by now. As a result, "The patriarchs from Adam to Noah, with a few exceptions, lived nearly a thousand years" (CD112). During that time there was no record of an infant being born blind, deaf, crippled, or imbecile. People wore out rather than dying from some terrible disease. "Had men always been obedient to the law of the ten commandments, carrying out in their lives the principles of those precepts, the CURSE OF DISEASE now flooding the world would not exist" (CD118). "Intellectual power, physical strength, and longevity depend upon immutable laws" (CD29). Since disease is the result of violating God's laws. It may be that if we lived perfect lives, disease would not touch us, and we would wear out rather than die of disease. God would then place none of the terrible diseases upon us, for He is the Lord that heals us (Ex. 15:26). It was more than two thousand years before the violation of natural law was sensibly felt (CD117).

Isa 65:20 says: "There shall be no more thence an infant of days, nor an old man that hath not filled his days: for the child shall die an hundred years old; but the sinner being an hundred years old shall be accursed." Isaiah here describes the new heaven and earth that would have been brought about if Israel had heeded the message of the prophets following the restoration from captivity. A 100-year-old person would then still be a child, and longevity would then be the rule instead of the exception. Death at 100 would then be so premature as to resemble that of an infant.

The tendency for man has been downward, and disease has been increasing through successive generations. The animals have also decreased in size and length of years (2SM418). They have been made to suffer by the wrong habits of man. We are told that we can prolong our lives by the careful supervision of ourselves (CD162), and we can shorten it by the violation of the laws of life (3T140). Also by eating flesh food (CD373), by misuse of the body (CH41), by the misuse of our physical powers (COL346), by overtaxing our mental powers (3T34), by overtaxing the stomach (CD131), by keeping late hours, by gratifying appetite at the expense of health. When we do this we become guilty of ROBBERY toward God (CH41). As it is, the lifetime is too short to be squandered in harmful activities. It is too short to be trifled away. The principles of true religion should help us live a rich and full life here on earth. We are told that "Religion tends directly to PROMOTE HEALTH, to LENGTHEN LIFE, and to HEIGHTEN OUR ENJOYMENT of all its blessings" (PP600). Dr. Bernard Jensen said: "A long life may not be good enough, but a good life is always long enough." He also said that people who lived to a ripe old age in other countries, free of disease, emphasized the following factors:

☞ They ate more fruits and vegetables, nuts, and seeds, but little meat.

☞ They ate less than the average American, and

☞ They were more physically active.

Aging Due To Decreased Oxygenation Of The Cells

We are told that "vigor declines with age" (MH275). There is evidence that the AGING PROCESS is also largely a matter of DIMINISHED OXYGENATION of the cells of the body, resulting in energy loss. One of the biggest drops in efficiency during aging is the ability of the body to bring oxygen to the cells through the lungs. VITAMIN C has a great effect on improved cell breathing. Many doctors say that "you are as old as your arteries." Vitamin C is also the key factor in averting ATHEROSCLEROSIS, and thereby prevents heart disease which is our number one killer. Vitamin C has so many universal applications that it is almost impossible to find a disease condition vitamin C would not favorably influence.

◆ *Metabolism Slows Down*

There are many ways in which people can age. Each one seems to have a unique pattern of aging. The METABOLISM, the sum of all bodily reactions, slows with age at the rate of approximately 1% per year. CALORIE requirements decrease up to 8% for each decade of life past 20, but the QUALITY of the food in terms of vitamins and minerals should probably proportionately increase. The eating of the very best foods must be increased, and all others decreased. Aging impairs the body's ability to produce certain active forms of vitamin D, which in turn slows down the absorption of CALCIUM, resulting in an increased risk of faulty bone mineralization. Aging significantly slows down the skin's capacity to produce vitamin D. The skin of a 70 year old man can produce about the vitamin D_3 produced by a 20 year old man. Normal aging will cut the efficiency of the HEART as well as the RENAL or KIDNEY BLOOD FLOW in half by age 80. At this age the CEREBRAL or BRAIN BLOOD FLOW is reduced 20% from age 30.

◆ *Decrease of Functions*

Age decreases all metabolic functions. Among the early signs of old age are the partial loss of the SENSE OF BALANCE, partial loss of HEARING, partial loss of VISION or of ACCOMMODATION, decreased MUSCULAR STRENGTH, decreased JOINT FLEXIBILITY, loss of ENDURANCE, loss of PIGMENT in the HAIR, loss of HAIR, loss of a clear COMPLEXION, decreased sensitivity in the SKIN, decreased LIBIDO. Ecclesiastes says that with the process of aging a person's "desire shall fail" (Ecc. 12:9).

Other symptoms of aging such as BACKACHE, BONE PAIN, INSOMNIA, LOOSE TEETH, TREMORS of the fingers, can be associated with the lack of the assimilation of CALCIUM. In order to function properly calcium must be accompanied by the vitamins A, C, D, B_6, plus MAGNESIUM, PHOSPHORUS, and PROTEIN. Dr. Bortz studied the deleterious effects of bed rest, and concluded that at least a portion of the changes that are commonly attributed to aging are in reality caused by IMMOBILITY. Such lack of mobility may be caused by CALCAREOUS MINERAL MATTER that has been deposited in the tissues of the body, making them tough and rigid.

A study found that young adults between the ages of 21 and 31 years of age had 30 times more AMYLASE, a salivary enzyme that breaks down starch, than older adults between the ages of 69 and 100. This suggests that our enzyme reserve becomes depleted as we become older. In one study those women who appeared younger than their years were found to consume fewer CALORIES, and less total FAT.

Water—Nature's Life Extender

Most older people have to guard against drinking too little water. They do not get as thirsty as younger folks. They also try to control their loss of bladder control, or incontinence, by drinking less water, which action is almost always harmful. Water is the best and cheapest drink available. It makes you feel full with ZERO CALORIES. It holds down urinary tract infections by keeping the bladder well-flushed. It smooths out the skin and prevents tiny wrinkles from forming. In fact it is probably the best "ANTI-AGING VITAMIN" for the skin.

◆ *Water Cure Spas*

The water cure is an old tradition in Europe. Many towns and cities have been built around mineral springs. Here millions of people each year go to health spas or water resorts, take a water cure, and relieve themselves of ACHES and PAINS, of ARTHRITIS, HIGH BLOOD PRESSURE, DEPRESSION etc. Many people who go there are sent there by their doctor or by their company for REST, RELAXATION, and REJUVENATION. Those who have experienced the "baths" are enthusiastic in their praise of the many benefits they have received. Many are state-operated establishments that have been approved by the state medical association. Dr. Kellogg's Battle Creek Spa was one of the most famous ones here in the U.S. In the last part of the 19th century there were many spas in Florida, near Chicago, and on the West Coast. But with the advent of the chemical takeover of medicine, most of these spas have disappeared from the American scene.

BALNEOLOGY is the name for the science of baths and bathing. BALNEOTHERAPY is the use of baths in the treatment of disease. It is known that MINERAL WATERS do indeed have curative powers. This should be obvious since DISORDERED MINERAL METABOLISM and BIOCHEMICAL DERANGEMENT are at the root of many diseases. Doctors have demonstrated that mineral water is actually absorbed through the skin. With the spa treatments it is often possible for patients who have taken CORTICOSTEROIDS for years to do without them. They have beneficial effects on all types of diseases as well as on the IMMUNOLOGICAL and HEALING POWERS of the body.

◆ *Dr. Metchnikoff And Soured Milk Products*

Dr. Metchnikoff of Russia believed that AUTOTOXEMIA or SELF-POISONING through putrefaction of metabolic wastes in the large intestines was the main cause of PREMATURE AGING. He believed that if we could prevent the development of toxins in the colon, we could double the normal lifespan. He discovered that the bacteria of SOURED MILK products and WHEY prevent the development of harmful putrefactive bacteria. Whey is 77% LACTOSE, which is the natural food for the friendly ACIDOPHILUS and BIFIDUS bacteria in the intestines. He recommended the use of soured milk products, such as YOGURT, KEFIR, and ACIDOPHILUS MILK.

◆ *Dr. Johannes Kuhl and Lactic Acid Foods*

Dr. Johannes Kuhl of Germany is an expert on SOURED LACTIC ACID FOODS. He shows that the fermentation of grains makes many nutrients more easily available for assimilation in the intestinal tract. During the process of making sour dough bread, the PHYTIN is broken down, and valuable minerals and trace elements are released. During the fermentation valuable LACTIC ACID is produced.

◆ *Life Expectancy Can Be Improved*

Some say that LIFE EXPECTANCY for the ROMANS at the time of Christ was 22 years. It is 70 plus for Americans today, and a few years more than that for Adventists. 26 years of that increase was achieved during the last 100 years. Much of the credit must go to advances in SANITATION, control of INFECTIOUS DISEASES, and the reduction of INFANT MORTALITY. According to the Bible the average person's age is centered upon the principle of threescore and ten. The Psalmist says: "The days of our years are threescore years and ten; and if by reason of strength they be fourscore years, yet is their strength labor and sorrow; for it is soon cut off, and we fly away" (Ps. 90:10). The inheritance of a strong constitution can extend our life beyond eighty or more. Without a strong constitution one's life can be extended quite a few more years by the improvement of our lifestyle. Aging is susceptible to control the same as any other mental or physical process. We often emphasize emergency care for people who are ill, rather than providing preventive and supporting care for people who are still in good health. Everyone wants to die young late in life. In 1900 a baby was expected to live up to age 47. Now males can expect to live to age 71, and females to age 77. Being born FEMALE is still an advantage in the longevity stakes.

◆ *The Lifestyle Of Centenarians*

There are 25,000 men and women in RUSSIA that are over 100 years old. They have singled out HONEY for food and medicine more than any other substance for long life. It is used to treat patients with hard to heal SORES, NOSE—MOUTH—THROAT AILMENTS, EYE DISEASES, HEART, LIVER, STOMACH, KIDNEY, and INTESTINAL ULCERS.

There are more centenarians in BULGARIA than in any other country relative to the population. A study of 158 Bulgarian centenarians by Dr.E.M. Hoppe of Sweden regarding their lifestyle revealed the following facts:

- LACTO-VEGETARIANS—most of them were predominantly lacto-vegetarians whose diet consisted mainly of locally grown and stone ground whole grains, freshly ground; FRESH VEGETABLES and FRUITS from their own gardens; MILK and its products from sheep; only 5 of them ate meat regularly.
- YOGURT—All of them ate yogurt regularly, made mostly from sheep milk.
- HONEY—Almost all of them were beekeepers and used lots of honey in their diet.
- SUNFLOWER SEEDS—were eaten regularly by all of them.
- FERMENTED FOODS—were eaten by all, especially SAUERKRAUT
- WORKED HARD—all of their lives, mostly on farms. 13 lived in cities.
- EATING—110 were extremely poor and could not afford to overeat
- CONTENTED—They had no ambitions. They lived without a clock, and followed nature's rhythm. They went to bed with the sun and got up with the sun. All of the factor's which ruled their lives are scientifically proven as the most potent factors for preventing premature aging and prolonging life. Dr. Ray Walford of UCLA claims that UNDEREATING is the key to long life.

◆ *The Hunzakuts*

Happiness and long life are by-products of healthy nutrition, lifestyle, and other beneficial habits. Nutrition is PREVENTIVE MEDICINE, and food is the vehicle of its practice. Human beings are created from nature or natural substances. They were placed in a garden, and were involved with the processes of nature. Hence, they can only live and thrive within nature. We should therefore stay within nature in order to be perfectly healthy and satisfied. In Hunzaland almost everything is eaten raw, uncooked, just as nature intended. No meat, dairy products, or processed foods are eaten. The healthiest people seem to be those who have isolated themselves so that they could be completely within nature. Besides the people of Hunza, or the Hunzakuts, such healthy isolated societies are the VICABAMBA of Ecuador, people in the Caucasian region, and those of Pitcairn Island.

The HUNZA people attribute their exceptional health and longevity to the drinking of their naturally heavily mineralized water rich in SELENIUM. Besides this they eat lots of APRICOTS and CHILI PEPPERS. Scientific studies have shown that minerals in water help to prevent many killing diseases such as HEART DISEASE, DIABETES, and OSTEOPOROSIS. Dr. McGarrison said that the same grain when fertilized with manure was of higher nutritive value than when fertilized with artificial fertilizers. The source of all their health is also the quality of their soil. The guarantee against failing health lies in its wise management. In FINLAND the natives consider their hot SAUNAS to contribute to long life. Modern science has confirmed that periodic artificially induced FEVER, which a sauna bath creates, effect the general metabolic process, and helps to fight many diseases, including ARTHRITIS and CANCER.

◆ *Maintaining Fitness And Outlook On Life*

Recent scientific research has demonstrated that the aging process can be controlled and most senility prevented or reversed by natural means. ADEQUATE NUTRITION, a POSITIVE OUT-

LOOK on life, and MENTAL and PHYSICAL ACTIVITY, can impede degeneration. Anatomists have discovered that human brain tissue does not deteriorate until after age 80, if it has been CONSISTENTLY USED and PROPERLY NOURISHED. What we are accustomed to think of as normal old age is actually an abnormal premature phenomenon. Dr. Abram Hoffer has demonstrated that the mentally ill can be successfully treated with massive doses of NIACIN (B_3). He also believes that SENILITY is merely the result of prolonged chronic MALNUTRITION.

◆ *Macrobiotics*

MACROBIOTICS—is known as "the art of living longer in good health." The idea was developed by C.W. Hufeland of Berlin about 150 years ago. It has recently become very popular in the U.S. It is the study of fundamental factors essential for optimum health and longer life free from disease. Due to improved sanitation, and reduction in infant mortality, man's average life expectancy has increased. However, through technological and chemical advances, the harmony between man and his natural environment has been disturbed. This fact has brought upon man many so-called DEGENERATIVE DISEASES. Devitalized foods, a polluted environment, and physical and mental stresses of the competitive world, have resulted in a gradual deterioration of health. The basic causes of the diseases of civilization are to be found in our anti-biological way of living. These factors can be summarized as follows:

- ENVIRONMENTAL CHANGES—air, water, soil, and food pollution.
- CHANGES IN NUTRITION—health-destroying toxic food additives; foods grown in depleted soils; devitalized by processing; wrong selection of diet; overeating etc.
- DISTURBANCES IN LIFE RHYTHM—lack of exercise; haste and hurry; insufficient rest and exercise; use of health-destroying substances. With desire and effort all of these factors can be overcome.

The Causes Of Aging

◆ *Cell Production Reduced*

DR. ANA ASLAN—of Rumania discovered by accident that PROCAINE, a local anesthetic agent, has an age retarding property. She produced a formula from it which she called GEROVITAL, or KH-3. It is used extensively in Europe as a REJUVENATE and REVITALIZING substance. She claims that the aging process starts when the body's ability to produce new cells and replenish the old ones is diminished. Gerovital helps the body to regenerate new cell production.

◆ *Fat Diet*

Dr. Samuel Rosen of Mt. Sinai Hospital has linked hearing loss to a high fat diet. Fat apparently affects hearing by accumulating in the blood vessels of the ear

◆ *Denatured Foods*

will speed the process of aging.

◆ *Free Radicals—*

are chemicals which are unstable, and which develop by-products of metabolism as waste products. They form when high energy, such as ULTRA-VIOLET LIGHT or IONIZING RADIATION knocks an electron out of its orbit in an atom. This energy-charged electron seeks other atoms or molecules to latch onto, and when it does, it places the new molecule in an unstable condition as a free radical. These transfer their energy to nearby cells which they damage, and in which they damage the DNA (DEOXYRIBONUCLEIC ACID). They are dangerous by-products of oxidation, and they damage proteins and nucleic acids. Oxygen can have reactions which are beneficial as well as harmful to the body. The damage it causes to the DNA is now accepted as a major cause of aging.

A strong immune system can block free radical damage. However, uncontrolled free radicals can cause BRAIN DAMAGE, ARTHRITIS, PREMATURE AGING, and CANCER. The basic mechanism of cancer within the cell is the "cancer gene" or ONCOGENE, which however must be "switched on" by some carcinogenic factor.

Work with premature babies showed clearly that too much PURE OXYGEN can be toxic. With the extra oxygen they developed BLINDNESS caused by free radicals, and called RETROLENTAL FIBROPLASIA (RLF). Enzymes which defend the body against free radicals are CATALASE and GLUTATHIONE PEROXIDASE. In the external environment free radicals are chemicals like NITROGEN DIOXIDE, SOLVENTS, and PESTICIDES. They can make blood clot abnormally by destroying the body's anti-clot hormones. They are partially controlled by oxygen. Most brain damage is caused by insufficient oxygen due to free radicals.

Free radicals also cause AGE PIGMENT accumulation resulting in "AGE SPOTS" in the skin. They cause the loss of collagen support to the blood vessels, making them susceptible to injury. The tops of the hands are susceptible because they have already been damaged by sun exposure. Putting FRESH LEMON JUICE on them twice daily for 6 weeks will cause the spots to fade away. Also the enzyme BROMELAIN in fresh PINEAPPLE JUICE will cause them to fade. These age spots contain the pigment LIPOFUSCIN which is largely present in CARDIAC and SMOOTH MUSCLE CELLS. It damages our brain cells by clogging them so that vital nutrients cannot flow freely into the cells. Reducing calories in the diet reduces the production of free radicals. Increasing the number of antioxidants in the diet also reduces the number of free radicals.

If free radical injury could be lessened, the immune system would remain stronger, and would help to resist arthritic tendencies. When researchers fed subjects ANTOXIDANTS, there was seen a reduction of free radicals. Where there is a nutritional deficiency, the immune system is less able to recognize what belongs to the body, the self, and what doesn't belong to the body, the non-self. At times the body can even turn on itself and produce AUTOIMMUNE REACTIONS such as those which result in RHEUMATOID ARTHRITIS. Free radicals are often PEROXIDES. Their tendency is to oxidize any molecule they contact. THE NUTRITIONAL ANTIOXIDANTS, such as VITAMINS A, C, and E, and SELENIUM benefit the organism by endeavoring to prevent the free radical oxidation damage. SUPEROXIDE DISMUTASE (SOD) is an enzyme in our cells which helps to inactivate the PEROXIDE RADICALS. Peroxide radicals have an extra oxygen atom attached to them.

◆ *Free Radicals Harm Immune System—by*
- producing generic mutations
- damaging proteins
- destroying body cells
- producing inflammation
- damaging blood vessels
- decreasing the activity of the neurotransmitters
- damaging fats within the cells

◆ *Sources Of Excess Oxygen Radicals are:*
- air pollution
- cured meat
- fats used in frying
- inflammation
- pesticides
- tobacco smoke
- ultraviolet radiation
- X-rays

◆ *Oxygen Deficiency*

We can rationally come to the conclusion that the ultimate cause of all premature aging is a lack of oxygen in the cells.

◆ *Normal Aging*

will cut your heart's efficiency by 50% by age 80. As we age, our immune system protects us from BACTERIA, VIRUSES, CANCER, and ATHEROSCLEROTIC PLAQUES. Aging also reduces the neurotransmittors which are the chemicals with which nerves talk to each other. These chemicals are made by the brain cells. With the right nutrients we can improve the performance of our immune system. The IMMUNE SYSTEM, which consists of the THYMUS GLAND, THE WHITE BLOOD CELLS, THE BONE MARROW which makes some of the white blood cells, THE SPLEEN, LYMPH NODES and DUCTS, as well as ANTIBODIES, COMPLEMENT PROTEINS, and INTERFERON. As your body ages, you need FEWER CALORIES and MORE NUTRIENTS. The size of the thymus gland can be increased, as well as its functional capacity, with nutrients such as vitamins A, C, E, the amino acid CYSTEINE, the minerals ZINC and SELENIUM. Cysteine, found in EGGS, counteracts the aging process, by neutralizing poisons in the system. This is no doubt the reason why Mrs. White said that "eggs contain properties which are remedial agencies in counteracting poisons" (CD204). THEY ARE ALL IMMUNE SYSTEM STIMULANTS.

◆ *Overweight*

You are overweight if you are more than 10 lbs. heavier than you were at age 20. If you are more than 20 lbs. over your ideal weight you are OBESE. Being obese increases your blood pressure drastically, which in turn reduces your lifespan. CARBOHYDRATES in refined form produce weight gain, while in natural form they do just the opposite.

◆ *Heredity*

Dr. Clive McCay of Cornell University indicated that longevity has some relation to heredity. It appears that children and grandchildren may expect to live long if their ancestors did. Since there is nothing we can do about heredity, it would seem prudent for those who descended from short-lived parents to take special care with diet and other aspects of healthful living so that we may bequeath to our children a longer life expectancy.

Effects Of Aging

☛ BRAIN VOLUME—There is a 10% brain volume decrease after age 60.

☛ COORDINATION—A loss of coordination accompanies loss of muscular strength. This can be somewhat forestalled through exercise.

☛ ESTROGEN—The loss of estrogen predisposes women to an increased rate of bone loss, and the development of osteoporosis.

☛ GLUCOSE TOLERANCE—the ability to metabolize glucose diminishes with age, and hence diabetes and obesity increase. Doctors are suspecting that AEROBIC EXERCISE can improve glucose tolerance. JOGGING increases it. STRENGTH TRAINING improves it also because it increases muscles mass which takes up some of the excess glucose from the bloodstream.

☛ HEIGHT—up to the loss of 1 in. in height is noted by age 60 due to the degeneration of bones and joints.

☛ NEPHRONS—the structural and functional units of the kidneys, of which there are approximately 1 million in each kidney, are reduced in number as we age.

How To Lengthen The Lifespan

Ernst Wynder has said: "It should be the function of medicine to have people die young as late as possible," and many sages have equated good health with "living in harmony with NATURE." If you don't live right in later years, your life savings will be spent to pay the bills of illness.

✓ BEE POLLEN—Bee pollen is mentioned in some sacred writings such as the KORAN and the TALMUD as a source of perpetual youth and health. It has been found to contain nearly all of the nutrients which bring about internal revitalization. From 1000 TO 3000 mg in tablet or granule form is suggested for daily consumption.

✓ EXERCISE—One researcher found that older people who exercised regularly hardly ever fractured their bones when they fell, for their exercise program nourished their bones with minerals, and gave them both hardness and suppleness or resiliency. Those who had insomnia also slept better when they exercised at bedtime.

✓ GLUTAMINE—Is a nonessential AMINO ACID which is considered to be an ANTI-AGING, ANTI-WRINKLING factor. It is found in foods such as ASPARAGUS, BEETS, CABBAGE, CARROTS, CELERY, GREEN BEANS, PAPAYA, and PARSLEY. 500 to 1000 mg are recommended.

✓ KELP—is a seaweed which is eaten as a food in many parts of the world. It contains all the minerals that are found in the sea. In powdered form it is a healthful substitute for regular salt. It has a high vitamin and mineral content, and has long been believed to prolong health and vitality, which makes it a valuable supplement for the ELDERLY.

✓ LECITHIN—is a fatty substance of the group called PHOSPHOLIPIDS, which is found in blood, brain, egg yolk, and nerves. It can be split up into STEARIC ACID, GLYCEROL, PHOSPHORIC ACID and CHOLINE. It has been shown to prevent, slow, and even reverse the ravages of age. It can improve MEMORY by preventing nerve sheath destruction in the BRAIN, and since almost of the brain's substance is composed of lecithin, it can reverse the process of SENILITY. 3 or more of the 1200 mg capsules per day is suggested.

✓ MINERALS—CHROMIUM combats mental changes accompanying aging, regulates SUGAR LEVELS in the blood, assists in lowering HIGH BLOOD PRESSURE, and aids in reducing CHOLESTEROL and the HARDENING of the ARTERIES. 100 TO 300 MICROGRAMS (mcg) daily with meals is recommended. SELENIUM is an ANTIOXIDANT that works together with vitamin E to retard cellular aging. SOIL DEPLETION has made it almost impossible to acquire the 250 to 350 mcg needed each day without some supplementation.

✓ OXYGENATION AND BRAIN FUNCTION—Memory loss is not inevitable as we get older. As we get older the most common loss of memory is a selective one: We tend to have difficulty remembering the most recent things we learned, and may not be able to recall what happened in the past 24 hours, yet have no trouble remembering things that happened years ago. Also brain power does not necessarily decline as we get older. Eating well and exercising regularly helps to maintain brain function in healthy older people.

A group of 13 elderly male patients showing signs of senility were treated for 90 minutes, twice a day, for 15 days, in a PURE OXYGEN PRESSURE CHAMBER. Five others were put in the chamber with ordinary air. They were called the "control" group. The rationale was that SENILITY is often caused by a DEFICIENCY OF BLOOD FLOW to critical areas of the brain, with subsequent poor oxygenation of these tissues. To begin with the patients were given three standardized tests to evaluate efficiency of MEMORY, CONCEPT FORMATION, and PRESENCE of BRAIN DAMAGE. After the experiment they were tested again, and those breathing pure oxygen showed remarkable increases in their scores, while the control patients had no significant change in their scores. BLOOD SAMPLES showed a marked increase in the amount of oxygen in the blood of those breathing pure oxygen. The test seemed to indicate that increased oxygen in the blood can help the brain to function much more efficiently. Dr. Selye said that "one never dies of old age. We die because one vital part has worn out before the rest of the body." A Russian gerontologist said: "Brain and muscles age least if used most."

✓ ROSE HIPS TEA—is called the "Swedish Fountain of Youth."

✓ SIBERIAN GINSENG—In geriatric use, Ginseng has been proven beneficial in restoring mental abilities. It helps by directly affecting the ADRENAL and PITUITARY GLANDS, which effect is most often manifested as increased resistance to the effects of stress. It aids mental function by improving circulation, and memory, and it stimulates the central nervous system, thereby contributing to the prevention of senility.

✓ SYSTEMATIC UNDEREATING—is one of the secrets of LONG LIFE and YOUTHFUL VITALITY. It is the only method that has been scientifically proven to increase the maximum lifespan of warm-blooded animals, and has produced constant results for every species tested. It works by protecting the body's defense system, the immune system, from the wear and tear of normal aging. Extra weight ages you rapidly. Also PERIODIC JUICE FASTING can help you stay younger longer.

Clive McCay of Cornell University underfed rats by 40%, but added vitamin and mineral supplements, and he thereby extended their life by 33%. Rats and mice can live much longer lifespans, if their caloric intake is restricted early in life. They develop fewer CANCERS and other diseases. Being too well fed can lead to premature disease and death. Underfeeding reduces the free radical production rate. Lowering body temperature also reduces free radical production. If the PITUITARY GLAND of the SALMON is removed, thereby preventing it from spawning, instead of dying after spawning, it will live for many more years, whereas the spawning salmon dies within hours.

✓ VITAMINS—People with higher than normal intake of vitamin A, C, and NIACIN tended to live longer. A study by Dr. Michelson of 577 people over the age of 50 in the county of San Mateo, California, showed that people with higher than average intake of vitamin A, C, and

NIACIN tended to live longer than those with a lower intake. In this study, the vitamin A intake lowered the death rate by . It is generally acknowledged that VITAMIN A is the first line of defense against many diseases.

✓ VITAMIN B and BREWER'S YEAST—Brewers yeast is said to be the single most potent rejuvenative food with its rich source of NUCLEIC ACIDS, and all the anti-aging B-VITAMINS, ORGANIC ZINC, and 40% of HIGHEST QUALITY PROTEINS. A study at a Philadelphia hospital showed that there was a marked improvement in MEMORY and ability to THINK after all the B-VITAMINS were administered to elderly patients. In 1948 Dr. T.B. Gardner announced that while experimenting with FRUIT FLIES he had increased their lifespan by 45% by fortifying their diet with the B-vitamins PANTOTHENIC ACID, PYRIDOXINE, and YEAST NUCLEIC ACID. He commented on this experiment by stating that this clearly shows that we can also add years to our life and slow the process of aging.

✓ VITAMIN C—Vitamin C helps retard deterioration of DISKS, JOINTS, and other TISSUES, and delays old age because of its ANTIOXIDANT properties. Dr. Schlenker measured the average vitamin C and protein intake of 100 women over a period of 25 years. The women who had the higher intakes of vitamin C lived longer. Vitamin C has a profound stimulating effect on the ADRENAL glands which secrete over 20 steroid hormones. A decrease in the output of these hormones is responsible for the SYMPTOMS of AGING. A higher than normal intake appears to reduce the ACHES and PAINS to which older persons are prone. VITAMIN C has a great effect on improved CELL BREATHING, and thus prevents premature aging. According to Dr. Pauling, vitamin C in supplements of 10 gm/day, extended the lifespan of terminal cancer patients by an average of over 4 times, provided that they had not undergone immunosuppressive chemotherapy.

✓ VITAMIN E—Some research suggests that we should call vitamin E the "anti-aging" vitamin, because it was shown that vitamin E keeps the RED BLOOD CELLS from aging under stressful conditions. Dr. Harmon of the University of Nebraska discovered that vitamin E and other ANTIOXIDANTS can prolong the life of mice. They also help prevent the ACHES and PAINS common to old age. One study found that the lifespan of human cells was increased 100% when the cells were grown in a culture with vitamin E added, to a total of 100 doublings instead of the normal 50 doublings. From 100 to 1000 IU per day is recommended. Rats when given 100 mg of vitamin E per kilogram of food daily, increased their lifespan 2.3 times.

✓ WATER DRINKING—is the best anti-aging "vitamin" for the skin. It has been shown that older folks simply do not drink enough water. Several glasses of water each day is recommended, for water deficiency can cause senile behavior. When water intake is inadequate, the blood becomes thicker and reduces circulation to the brain.

✓ YOGURT—aids digestion and is thought to contribute to longevity. It was called "milk of eternal life," and is a staple food in Soviet Georgia, where many of the residents live well past the century mark. Other FERMENTED LACTIC ACID FOODS credited with revitalizing the digestive system and helping to rectify degenerative diseases are: KEFIR, SAUERKRAUT, SOUR MILK, and SOUR DOUGH BREADS.

✓ NUTRITION—the older you get the better your nutrition must be in order to maintain your efficiency.

✓ ALEXIS CARREL—kept the heart of a chicken alive for 25 years by feeding it nutrients and eliminating waste products.

✓ PANTOTHENIC ACID (B_5)—can greatly increase resistance to stress in both humans and animals. It increased the lifespan of mice by 20% when fed B_5 in the quantity of 12 mg/kg of body weight.

✓ EXERCISE—As we grow older, our circulation slows down, and most of the nourishment is directed toward our organs, while our muscles and connective tissue get less and less. For this reason, exercise seems to be the single best thing one can do to keep young.

✓ LIFTING WEIGHTS—A new study of the American Medical Association indicates that the secret to staying young is to lift weights. When 10 nursing home residents, ranging in age from 86 to 96, pumped iron with their legs for 8 weeks, the average STRENGTH GAIN was 174% in the right leg and 180% in the left leg. Also half of the volunteers were able to walk 1 times faster than before the leg-weight sessions. When these volunteers went back to their old ways of no exercise, they lost of their new found leg strength in 4 weeks. This indicates that EXERCISE needs to be continued indefinitely to maintain the benefits.

PROSTATE PROBLEMS

Nature Of The Problem

The PROSTATE is a gland which is the most common site of disorders in the male GENITO-URINARY SYSTEM. The most significant of these disorders are PROSTATITIS, which is an acute or chronic infection of the prostate, BENIGN PROSTATIC HYPERTROPHY (BPH), or enlargement of the prostate, and CANCER of the prostate. The symptoms are frequent and increased URINATION especially at night, LESSENING of the force of FLOW, and an accompanying BURNING SENSATION. The prostate encircles the urethra, so that the enlargement of the prostate reduces or entirely shuts down the flow of urine, resulting in URINE RETENTION. This causes frequent urination and pain connected with it. The retained urine under pressure backs up into the kidneys. This can damage the kidneys both by the pressure and by the contaminated urine.

BLADDER INFECTION or CYSTITIS can also develop. With the enlargement of the prostate, a pouch is formed at the base of the bladder in which fluid collects which cannot be entirely expelled. It can form CRYSTALS in the bladder which produce pain and infection which leads to a buildup of urinary wastes in the bloodstream. Cancer of the prostate is the third most common malignancy in men, following cancers of the lung and colon. It usually occurs in men over 60 years of age.

The Causes Of Prostate Problems

✓ ARTIFICIAL DIETS—Worldwide studies have shown that men who are still virile, in their 80's and 90's, and without prostate problems, are those who subsist on diets rich in natural foods, and whose diets are conspicuously lacking in refined sugar and refined flour.

✓ BACTERIAL INFECTION—Bacterial infection in other parts of the body may occasionally migrate to a man's prostate gland, resulting in an acute and painful inflammation, called PROSTATITIS.

✓ HORMONE INCREASE—Enlargement of the prostate is due to the increase of certain hormones with age, which are responsible for the overproduction of prostate cells which results in prostate enlargement.

✓ ZINC DEFICIENCY—Soil used for farming is often deficient in zinc, and unless one eats HUSKS of cereals, or BREWER'S YEAST, it is difficult to get much zinc in the diet. Zinc has been shown to reduce the size of the prostate by inhibiting the hormones which tend to enlarge it. VITAMIN B_6 is also needed in this process, for it enhances zinc absorption. PANCREATIC INSUFFICIENCY with age is also a factor, which may result in the decrease of zinc. ALCOHOL reduces zinc uptake and increases zinc excretion, leading to a zinc deficiency

✓ FATTY ACID DEFICIENCY—There seems to be an underlying essential fatty acid deficiency of LINOLEIC, LINOLENIC, and ARACHIDONIC ACIDS which lack can be supplied with LINSEED OIL, SUNFLOWER OIL, EVENING PRIMROSE OIL, SOY OIL, and OLIVE OIL. One teaspoon or 4 grams per day is usually sufficient. VITAMIN F represents the essential fatty acids.

✓ TOXIC CHEMICALS—It is possible that the tremendous increase in the occurrence of BPH in the last few decades is due to the effect that toxic chemicals have on our health.

✓ CHOLESTEROL—Dr. Mallouh, of the Metropolitan Hospital in New York found an 80% increase in cholesterol content of the prostate with BPH. Also there is a 4 times greater risk of PROSTATE CANCER among cases of BPH.

How To Heal Prostate Disorders

- ☛ WALKING—is the best possible exercise for keeping the prostate gland in good shape. One or two hours a day is not too much.
- ☛ PUMPKIN SEEDS—are very helpful because of their ZINC and essential FATTY ACID content. Among the gypsy tribes in Southern Europe, there is no identifiable prostate gland trouble among its men. This fact was traced to their habit of eating pumpkin seeds all day long.
- ☛ SITZ BATH—The hot sitz bath is the most common hydrotherapy technique used in the treatment of BPH. It can also be done with alternating hot and cold water which increases pelvic circulation and tones up the muscles in the region. Even better when CHAMOMILE TEA is added to the water.

HERBS:

- ☛ PARSLEY—is the foremost diuretic herb recommended when urination is painful and incomplete due to an enlarged prostate squeezing the urethra so tightly that urination is difficult. In one case a man suffered from PROSTATE ENLARGEMENT, and finally had complete stoppage of urine. He could not urinate without a tube. He was told that he needed surgery, but they could not operate because he had DIABETES. He was advised to try PARSLEY TEA. After drinking this tea he could urinate freely without a tube, for his sugar dropped to normal, and surgery was avoided. The SAW PALMETTO BERRY—acts directly on the enlarged prostate to reduce inflammation, pain, and throb. It also increases the bladder's ability to contract and expel its contents. ITS EXTRACT has been shown by scientific studies to be about 3 times more effective than the drug PROSCAR, for alleviating symptoms of prostatic enlargement, such as poor urinary stream, urinary retention, and nighttime urination. It has no toxicity whereas proscar causes IMPOTENCE, decreased LIBIDO, and could cause BIRTH DEFECTS in male children.
- ☛ CORNSILK—acts a lot like parsley. The gum-like substance is the active principle, but it also contains a lot of other helpful substances such as fatty acids, menthols, glycosides, thymol, saponins, steroids, vitamin C and K etc. It reduces painful symptoms and swellings due to infections.
- ☛ BUCHU LEAVES—are a urinary antiseptic, an important secondary consideration when treating prostate problems.
- ☛ KELP—ingestion on a daily basis gradually reduces the prostate in older men to the point that urination becomes painless. It may be achieved due to its general cleansing effect on the bloodstream, its antibiotic properties, and on the many essential elements that it supplies.
- ☛ TEAS made from GOLDENSEAL, JUNIPER BERRIES, SLIPPERY ELM, WILLOW HERB, and UVA URSI are also recommended.

- ✓ LOW FAT DIET—can lower the risk of prostatic cancer.
- ✓ RAW FRUITS and VEGETABLES, their JUICES, and SEEDS—Of the seeds use pumpkin, squash, sunflower, almonds, and sesame. They all contain high quality proteins, unsaturated fatty acids, and zinc. Tests have shown that all of these seeds do reduce an enlarged prostate. Folk remedies have suggested eating a handful of pumpkin seeds every day. Pumpkin juice is reported to be especially beneficial, as are also lemon and grape juices. A GARLIC DIET has been found helpful due to its mineral and chemical content. It contains compounds of SULFUR which have the power to fight germs and infection.
- ✓ BEE POLLEN—and pollen extract tablets worked like a miracle in the case of one man who took it three times a day. Use one to two teaspoons daily or three to nine tablets. Bee Pollen is believed to contain hormones beneficial to the prostate. It does not destroy bacteria, but it strengthens the prostate's ability to combat infection. It has been called the ELIXIR of perpetual youth for men.
- ✓ VITAMINS and MINERALS—recognized as helpful to prostate sufferers include the AMINO ACIDS, GLUTAMIC ACID, and GLYCINE, present to a great degree in soybeans. VITAMIN A is essential for the health of the

cells lining the prostate. Use 10,000 to 25,000 units per day, as well as 1 to 2 tablespoons of COD LIVER OIL. Also use the B-complex vitamins as well as brewer's yeast with added zinc.

✓ ZINC—is notably absent from the American diet, due to the refining processes which remove it. Numerous studies have shown that 15 to 50 mg of zinc per day is helpful. A zinc deficiency causes changes in the size, structure, and function of the prostate gland. 50 mg taken 3 times a day is generally the recommended dosage. When combined with BEE POLLEN and PUMPKIN SEED OIL, it has proven most effective. A man reports that he found relief from PROSTATE TROUBLE with ZINC GLUCONATE. This trouble had gotten him up several times nightly. He says that he is free from this problem as long as he takes this compound which is available in health food stores.

✓ GARLIC—Garlic detoxifies the system, and neutralizes and cleanses the poisons. In CHRONIC PROSTATITIS there is a deficiency in levels of ZINC. The GARLIC DIET, which includes other foods with the garlic, contains plenty of zinc from zinc-rich foods such as BREWERS YEAST, NUTS, MOLASSES, RICE BRAN, PEAS, BEANS, LENTILS, WHEAT BRAN, and WHEAT GERM. SUNFLOWER SEEDS and PUMPKIN SEEDS are the richest sources of zinc available in common foods. Sunflower seeds are of benefit also due to their UNSATURATED FATTY ACID content in combination with other factors. Dr. Devrient of Berlin has been curing patients of prostatic trouble by having them eat lots of pumpkin seeds. BEE POLLEN has been known to eliminate the symptoms of prostate problems. GARLIC has also been known to cure IMPOTENCE.

SKIN DISEASES

Nature Of The Disease

◆ *Impure Blood*

The skin is the largest of the body organs. It cools us down or conserves heat; it shields us from external and internal hazards; it houses our sense of touch; and it gives us signals about our state of health.

Skin diseases are caused by IMPURE BLOOD or INFECTION. When you have BOILS, CARBUNCLES, BLACKHEADS, PIMPLES, or a skin AFFECTION of any kind, go on a prolonged FRUIT, FRESH FRUIT JUICE, or FRESH VEGETABLE DIET. Take plenty of exercise in the fresh air where you will inhale plenty of oxygen to purify every part of the body. Drink a lot of RED CLOVER tea instead of water. Also use ROSE HIPS and ECHINACEA tea. Within a week or two the skin will become clear.

◆ *Purification Of Blood Underlies Healing*

The skin has many functions in the body. It is connected with the deeper tissues of the body by millions of capillaries and nerves from which it derives sustenance. The condition of the skin reflects the health of the underlying tissues. The skin also has functions which are strictly its own, such as BREATHING, PERSPIRING, SENSORY PROCESSING, and OIL PRODUCTION. Any skin ailments are best attacked from within rather than from without if it is to have lasting results. Attacking from within means concentrating on purifying the blood, and allowing the purified blood to eliminate skin conditions.

When you purify the blood, you are eliminating many other problems both on the skin and within the body. In the course of a day the skin will eliminate more than a pound of waste products in the form of SWEAT. Almost anything that the body tries to expel through the skin is a symptom of unwanted, impure, poisonous or waste products in the blood. Under these circumstances the skin is used as a greater WASTE ELIMINATION ORGAN, because of the fact that the normal channels of elimination are overloaded. On the other hand, if the pores of the skin are blocked an extra burden is placed upon the other eliminative organs (MH276).

The Causes Of Skin Diseases

✓ A FAULTY DIET—Researchers are discovering that even minor nutrition problems show up in the skin, often long before anyone is aware of their causes. For example, a VITAMIN C shortage may cause BLEEDING GUMS, SORE-

NESS in the MOUTH, and a SCALY RASH around the HAIR ROOTS. A VITAMIN B-COMPLEX deficiency can cause CRACKS and CANKER SORES in the corners of the MOUTH. Also deficiencies of COPPER, SELENIUM, VITAMINS A and E increase the risk of developing various kinds of SKIN CANCERS. Since doctors have not been strongly trained in nutrition and its effect upon health, they may not recognize the early signs of nutrition problems.

✓ ECZEMA—is a constitutional disease brought on by a WRONG DIET, and often by previous SUPPRESSIVE DRUG TREATMENT. The Spirit of Prophecy tells us "And the disease, which the drug was given to cure, may disappear, but only to reappear in a new form, such as SKIN DISEASES, ULCERS, painful DISEASED JOINTS, and sometimes in a more dangerous and deadly form" (2SM452). The skin is one of the main channels through which bodily impurities are eliminated from the system, and the ECZEMA of children is only another example of a natural healing crisis. It is the result of SYSTEMIC TOXEMIA, and chemical agents serve only to suppress the disease and make it chronic. By forcing it below the surface, they pave the way for some of the most dangerous diseases of childhood—diseases which may easily lead to INFANTILE PARALYSIS, TUBERCULOSIS and others. The real treatment for eczema lies in improving the elimination by cleansing and purifying the system, and for this purpose a PROPER DIET, SUN and AIR and WATER BATHING, ENEMAS and so on are necessary.

Small children should not be given EGGS up to one year of age. Studies showed that these children developed ECZEMA from eating eggs. The eczema cleared up quickly when eggs were withdrawn from their diet.

A young lady had been suffering from a severe case of ECZEMA since childhood. She was spending as much as $25 per week for drugstore preparations, which gave some relief, but did not cure the condition. An old lady told her about eating RAW POTATOES. She stopped taking the drugs, and after a few weeks on the raw potato diet, her face cleared up. She continues to eat one raw potato a day.

ECZEMA is based on immune system deficiencies. VITAMIN B_6 has brought improvement, as well as BETA CAROTENE which in tests gave great relief.

✓ BOILS—The cause of boils is a TOXIC BLOODSTREAM due to wrong dietetic habits and wrong living generally, especially the eating of excessive quantities of starchy and sugary foods. They usually make their appearance when the sufferer is in a run-down or devitalized condition. This results in BACTERIAL INFECTION through the sweat glands or hair follicles. It represents waste matter which the body has been unable to slough off through other eliminative channels, and calls upon the skin and pores for help. It is nature's emergency method of purging the organism when toxicity becomes too great. Then eruptions of the skin frequently appear (CD174). It was one of the ten plagues with which God afflicted the Egyptians (Ex. 9:10).

✓ PSORIASIS—is a chronic skin condition with lesions frequently appearing on the KNEES, ELBOWS, SCALP, CALVES, and HANDS. These conditions are considered to be almost incurable with modern medicines, which often resorts to STEROIDS and other medications that produce harmful side effects. Changes in DIET and the use of various herbs are often successful, and can produce significant improvement in 1 to 3 months. BURDOCK ROOT, DANDELION ROOT, and YELLOW DOCK ROOT are all traditionally used by herbalists in the treatment of chronic skin problems. Combine 1 tablespoon each of these herbs with tablespoon of LICORICE ROOT with 1 quart of water in a covered pot, and let it simmer for 20 minutes. Drink 3 cups daily. OINTMENTS made from COMFREY, CHICKWEED, GOLDENSEAL, or CALENDULA will soothe and heal skin lesions.

Healing Skin Diseases

✓ BLACKSTRAP MOLASSES—Cases of ECZEMA, DERMATITIS, and PSORIASIS have responded to the therapeutic power of blackstrap molasses.

- ✓ CASTOR OIL—Some people have shown that STIES and WARTS are effectively eliminated with applications of castor oil.

- ✓ FRUITS and JUICES—are especially beneficial in all skin diseases.

- ✓ LEMON JUICE—was found helpful in greatly reducing the irritation of the stings of a MAN-OF-WAR JELLYFISH. It also eliminated the sting of the STINGING NETTLE in a matter of seconds. Lemon juice also relieved the irritation of CHILBAINS, or the blistering of the skin due to cold exposure. It allays the irritation caused by BEE or HORNET STINGS, and the bite of GNATS or other similar insects. It sometimes alleviates SKIN BLEMISHES and DISCOLORATIONS.

- ✓ FASTING—Skin diseases have been successfully treated with fasting methods. Use the juices of BLACK CURRANTS, RED GRAPES, CARROTS, BEETS, and SPINACH. CUCUMBER juice used internally and externally is especially advised for the treatment of skin diseases. It possesses acknowledged cosmetic properties.

- ✓ HERB TEAS—The best teas are GOLDENSEAL, DANDELION, SASSAFRAS, RED and WHITE CLOVER, PENNYROYAL, PLANTAIN, and SPIKENARD. SARSAPARILLA was the wonder remedy of bygone days, and was considered a necessity for good health by many people. Successful use was made of it in the treatment of PSORIASIS. Its root contains the male hormones TESTOSTERONE, PROGESTERONE, and CORTIN. Testosterone is said to prolong youth and prevent premature aging. JEWELWEED has relieved ECZEMA, SKIN RASHES, POISON OAK, POISON IVY, and NETTLE STINGS. If the juice of this plant is put on the legs before going out into the woods, it will prevent the stings of poisonous plants. TINCTURE of MYRRH may be applied straight from the bottle to COLD SORES and SKIN IRRITATIONS. If diluted it produces a healing effect on MOUTH ULCERS, CANKER SORES, and IRRITATED GUMS. Drink the applicable teas freely in the place of water, and in a matter of a relatively short time the skin disease will disappear.

- ✓ LECITHIN—is valuable for treating PSORIASIS. Adelle Davis reported that psoriasis appears to result from the faulty utilization of FATS, and from excessive CHOLESTEROL in the skin and blood. Psoriasis usually clears up if the blood cholesterol is reduced to normal. It has also been helped by VITAMINS A and B_6.

- ✓ PROPOLIS—is the sticky resin present in the buds and barks of certain trees and plants. It is collected by bees for the purpose of repairing combs, filling cracks, and for making the entrance to the hive waterproof. It inhibits the reproduction of certain VIRUSES. PROPOLIS TINCTURE helps ACNE. When applied several times daily, it promotes rapid healing and forms an invisible coating which protects against renewed infection. Its tincture can be applied twice a day to eliminate WARTS. It eliminates SHINGLES if taken between meals twice daily.

  In a study of 21 cases of SHINGLES in Yugoslavia, Dr. Franz Feiks treated them with dressings of PROPOLIS TINCTURE. The PAIN disappeared in 48 hours in all 21 cases and did not return. In 19 cases the skin sores were completely healed.

  Doctors in Japan and Czechoslovakia showed that a PROPOLIS SUPPOSITORY PESSARY achieved curative result against CANDIDA ALBICANS.

  They concluded that propolis is remarkably effective for all fungal infections of the skin and body.

- ✓ SLIPPERY ELM—Poultices of slippery elm quickly disperses SURFACE INFLAMMATION and draws out IMPURITIES from the skin.

- ✓ VITAMINS—The Canadian Medical Association Journal told of 15 cases of skin diseases which were treated with injections of SYNTHETIC VITAMIN B. There was no improvement noted from these treatments until YEAST or LIVER EXTRACT was given. In another experiment with digestive disorders, patients treated with BREWERS YEAST EXTRACT had an excellent response in the loss of distressing symptoms. The patients were then taken off the yeast extract and given SYNTHETIC THIAMIN and RIBOFLAVIN, and as a result the symptoms returned.

- ✓ ZINC—The speed of healing eczema is enhanced by ZINC when combined with vitamins A, D, and E, plus ESSENTIAL FATTY ACIDS.
- ✓ SKIN AGING—A lack of elasticity of the skin is a readily observable sign of increasing age. Hold a fold of skin from the back of the hand for 5 seconds, and then see how long it takes for it to return to normal. Young skin snaps back right away. Old skin may take a minute or more to return to normal.

TUBERCULOSIS

Nature Of The Disease

Tuberculosis (TB) was in Mrs. White's day generally called CONSUMPTION or PULMONARY DISEASE. It was thought to be essentially wiped out in modern society, until the AIDS plague came along. In the 1960'S and 1970's TB was steadily decreasing, and experts were predicting its elimination by the turn of the century. In recent years it has been rising at the rate of 5% per year. Its revival is mainly linked to the AIDS epidemic, because people infected with the AIDS virus are unusually susceptible to TB. TB is a chronic WASTING DISEASE caused by the tuberculosis bacterium, which can be spread through the air by those who have active TB characterized by vigorous COUGHING, and large pockets of the germs in the lungs. TB is still endemic to many countries situated around the edges of the Pacific Ocean.

Causes Of Tuberculosis

◆ *A Faulty Diet*

- ✓ A MEAT DIET—We are told in the Spirit of Prophecy that "CANCERS, TUMORS, and all INFLAMMATORY DISEASES are largely caused by meat eating" (CD388). More specifically we are told that meat eating causes TUBERCULOSIS through meat that is filled with tubercular germs. If we eat meat of this type we should not assume that if we get sick from it, that it was a result of one of God's providential directions. God's direction was that we would possibly get sick if we ate that type of food of which we had been warned. We have been told for a long time that meat was never the best food for man, and that it is now doubly objectionable because of disease among animals which has developed proportionally with the sins among men.
- ✓ INADEQUATE DIET—predisposes one to TB. Such a diet inhibits the production of antibodies to fight the disease. In one sense TB is essentially a CALCIUM DEFICIENCY DISEASE, for it occurs only in a system depleted of organic lime, and one which is deficient in VITALITY. This means that MINERAL STARVATION of the tissues of the body is one of the main causes of the disease.
- ✓ EXCESSIVE MUCUS—in the system causes the propagation of the tubercular germ which is destructive to the tissues. Mucus is the natural breeding food for germs, and MILK is the most mucus forming food. Tuberculosis may result more from using pasteurized milk than from any other cause. However, if unpasteurized milk is drunk from infected cows, the disease can be transmitted in this manner also.
- ✓ DRUGS—Mrs. White tells of an infant whose arms and legs were exposed to cold air, and as a result the blood was driven to the lungs and head. He was given a poisonous drug and developed what she called DRUG-DISEASE, the most stubborn and incurable of all diseases. She said that if it recovered it must bear in its system the effects of that drug, which makes it liable to SPASMS, HEART DISEASE, DROPSY ON THE BRAIN, or CONSUMPTION. Some infants are not strong enough to withstand the drug poison and the infant often dies. (2SM 468).

TB has been checked because drug treatment has been largely abandoned and reliance has been placed on the healing value of NATURAL AGENTS such as FRESH AIR and SUNSHINE. The DEVITILIZATION of the SYSTEM and not the GERMS are the chief factor in the cause of the disease.

- ✓ LACK OF FRESH AIR and EXERCISE—We are told that "Many who are suffering from PULMONARY DISEASE might be cured if they would live in a climate where they could be out-of-doors most of the year. Many who have died of consumption might have lived if they had breathed more pure air. Fresh outdoor air is as healing as medicine, and leaves no injurious aftereffects" (2SM291).

✓ IMPROPER CLOTHING—The extremities should be kept as warm as the rest of the body with warm coverings. One cannot have health when the extremities are habitually cold. This means that there is less blood in them, while there is too much in other parts of the body. Perfect health requires perfect circulation. "Many women have become confirmed invalids when they might have enjoyed health, and many have died of CONSUMPTION and other diseases when they might have lived their allotted term of life, had they dressed in accordance with health principles, and exercised freely in the open air" (MH293).

✓ SLEEPING IN DAMP ROOMS—"In wet seasons the sleeping rooms become damp, and those who occupy them are troubled with RHEUMATISM, NEURALGIA, and LUNG complaints, which generally end in CONSUMPTION" (CH58). Also the decay of dead leaves poison the atmosphere around the house. Dwellings, if possible, should be built high and dry. If water settles around them for a time, FEVERS and LUNG DISEASES can be caused by it.

How To Heal Tuberculosis

☛ OUTDOOR EXERCISE—Plenty of exercise in the fresh air

☛ GOOD FOOD—such as SOYBEAN MILK, RIPE BANANAS, and POTASSIUM BROTH.

☛ TEAS—GOLDENSEAL, SLIPPERY ELM, and COMFREY TEA. Of these at least one quart per day.

☛ FRESH FRUIT—Go on a fresh fruit diet of three or four days.

☛ OLIVE OIL—We are told that OLIVE OIL "will be found beneficial to CONSUMPTIVES, and it is healing to an inflamed, irritated stomach" (MH298).

ULCERS

Nature Of The Disease

An ulcer in its simplest form is an inflammation or a sore in the STOMACH or the DUODENUM. Through continued irritation it turns into an ulcer. The term PEPTIC ULCER refers to both types. The term GASTRIC ulcer refers to the stomach. Duodenal ulcers are about 4 times as common as gastric ulcers. One cannot say that the HYDROCHLORIC ACID of the stomach is the primary cause of the ulcer, but it may be called a secondary cause. A normal stomach which constantly produces hydrochloric and other acids doesn't always suffer from ulcers. The natural view is that the hydrochloric acid could not eat into the stomach lining, if an inflammation did not already exist therein. The underlying cause must be placed upon the BILE from the gall bladder whose effect upon the stomach lining is disastrous. It produces the inflammation which is also entered into by the hydrochloric acid. Today there are approximately two men with ulcers for every woman who has them, because men in their business life are more subject to ANGER and TENSION. 75 to 90% of all ulcers recur.

The Causes Of Ulcer

◆ *Medications*

Some people produce 2 to 4 times as much digestive acid as others. Chronic conditions such as DIABETES, HYPOGLYCEMIA, or LUNG DISEASE may stimulate excess acid output. ASPIRIN, CORTISONE, and STEROID MEDICATIONS can adversely affect stomach lining cells. Some drugs used for stomach ulcers increase the risk of STOMACH CANCER. ASPIRIN as well as CORTICOSTEROID DRUGS can cause stomach ulcers. Aspirin is a gastric irritant that damages the lining of the stomach and predisposes individuals to ulcer development when taken regularly. It causes gastrointestinal BLEEDING even if it is injected under the skin rather than swallowed. One of the major side effect of CORTISONE is the "steroid ulcer."

Gastric ulcers are largely caused by ALCOHOL, ASPIRIN, DRUGS, TOBACCO, and COFFEE, both caffeinated and decaffeinated. Both types of coffee contain flavoring and aroma oils which irritate the lining of the stomach and intestinal tract. CAFFEINE PRODUCTS also cause an increased flow of digestive juices which are responsible for the irritation of the stomach lining. CHOCOLATE contains 68 mg of caffeine per cup, which is more than is contained in a cup of TEA.

◆ *Spicy Foods*

When you eat, the stomach secretes gastric juices which are the acids that digest the food. With SPICY food these acids are produced at a high rate. A slight sore in the stomach will be aggravated by these acids. The stomach reacts to the pain produced with violent SPASMS, which action may produce further damage. That is why stomach acids are so largely credited as the chief cause of ulcers.

When food is retained for an extended period in the stomach, it allows the acid more CONTACT TIME with the stomach lining, resulting in some part of the stomach being eroded to leave a raw sore. Experimental evidence points to FOOD ALLERGY as a prime causal factor. Milk seems not to be good for ulcers. To use MILK is using a highly allergic food which may contribute to the problem, because it promotes the secretion of GASTRIN, a hormone that triggers the release of more acid. On the other hand, milk, being somewhat alkaline, neutralizes some of the stomach acid. REFINED SUGAR tends to promote ulcers because it is acid forming. This is not true of NATURAL SUGARS. In general, foods that increase the acidity of the stomach should be avoided. These include COFFEE, REFINED SUGAR, and REFINED FLOUR.

◆ *Frequent Feedings*

There are no data to the assumption that frequent feedings are more beneficial in healing ulcers than are three meals a day. Frequent feedings are no more beneficial because the stomach releases digestive acids whenever it is fed. Food does buffer stomach acid somewhat, but it also causes the secretion of acid. When food is not THOROUGHLY CHEWED, it doesn't have a chance to mix thoroughly with a substance from the salivary glands called UROGASTRONE, a POLYPEPTIDE, which has an inhibitory effect on gastric secretions and protects the stomach lining from erosion. So thorough chewing may be the best safeguard against PEPTIC ULCERS.

◆ *Stress And Mineral Deficiencies*

In addition to the nutritional and metabolic causes, both gastric and duodenal ulcers can be caused by severe NERVOUS and MENTAL STRESS. Ulcers have been formed by stress alone, by the lack of essential nutrients, and by the combination of VITAMIN and MINERAL deficiencies. Ulcer patients as a group have been characterized as tending to repress emotions, possibly due to an excessive wish for dependency. This could be largely responsible for the ulcers. It is not the amount of stress, but the individual's response to it that is the significant factor.

◆ *Psychological Factors*

Before the nutritional and biological treatment can be successful, the psychological causes must be solved or eliminated. Persons with a predisposition for peptic ulcers should avoid all situations resulting in mental stress and prolonged nervous strain or irritability. Complete rest and relaxation from all pressing problems and worries is imperative.

◆ *Smoking*

Smoking is strongly linked to peptic ulcers because it decreases the PANCREATIC BICARBONATE secretion which is an important neutralizer of gastric acid. It increases the reflux of the bile salts into the stomach, and accelerates gastric emptying into the duodenum.

Substances And Methods Used To Control Ulcers

✓ ANTACIDS—ALKALIES in various antacids can irritate ulcers. The CALCIUM CARBONATE antacids such as TUMS and ALKA-2, may cause KIDNEY STONES. The SODIUM BICARBONATE antacids, such as ROLAIDS®, ALKA-SELTZER®, and BROMO-SELTZER, have a tendency to induce SYSTEMIC ALKALOSIS, and interfere with heart and kidney function. The ALUMINUM—MAGNESIUM compounds, such as MAALOX®, MYLANTA®, and DIGEL, may cause CALCIUM and

PHOSPHORUS DEPLETION, as well as possibly causing ALUMINUM TOXICITY, or the accumulation of aluminum in the BRAIN, and such accumulation has been linked to ALZHEIMER'S disease.

Studies indicate that commercial antacids provide only temporary relief, but they speed STOMACH-EMPTYING TIME to such a degree that ulcers are made worse by their longer contact with stomach acids. Antacids also interfere with VITAMIN C absorption. One test showed that antacids don't give any more relief than a PLACEBO.

✓ CIMETIDINE (TAGAMET®) NOT RECOMMENDED—Cimetidine, also called TAGAMET, is a drug which INHIBITS GASTRIC SECRETIONS, DISRUPTS NORMAL DIGESTIVE PROCESSES, and ALTERS the FUNCTION and STRUCTURE of the CELLS that line the digestive tract. While it is effective, there is a high relapse rate when the treatment is discontinued. A LICORICE ROOT EXTRACT has been discovered which works just as well as Tagamet, at a fraction of the cost, and with none of the risky side-effects.

✓ MEAL and BEDTIME—Ulcers can be irritated by not allowing enough time between supper and bedtime. While you are sleeping all of your body functions slow down. The stomach does not digest food quickly, and excessive acid is produced. To avoid irritating ulcers, doctors recommend that a person should not eat for 2 to 3 hours before going to sleep.

How To Heal Ulcers

◆ *Diet And Foods*

Some physicians feel that diet doesn't have very much influence on ulcers. Others advise a NATURAL diet with plenty of FIBER. Still others advise a BLAND diet. A British study showed that between a high fiber and a bland diet for patients with recently healed ulcers, the ulcers reappeared in 80% of the bland diet group, but in only 45% of the high fiber group. Fiber slows the passage of food, and there is no danger of natural roughage puncturing ulcer coverings, since only acids can penetrate the stomach's protective lining. A fiber diet is associated with a reduced rate of DUODENAL ulcers. Norwegian scientists have found that fiber can prevent and delay recurring ulcer attacks.

◆ *Vitamins:*

✓ VITAMIN A—retards ulcer formation by helping the epithelial cells to produce more mucus.

✓ VITAMIN C—was proved to be therapeutic in the treatment of PEPTIC ULCERS. Ulcer patients usually have very low levels of vitamin C. Absorption of vitamin C is improved in the presence of BIOFLAVONOIDS, which are in fruits and vegetables.

✓ VITAMIN E—has reduced ulcers and prevented them in rats.

✓ VITAMIN P or RUTIN—The appearance of an ulcer is usually preceded by inflammation of the stomach lining which in turn is the result of CAPILLARY WEAKNESS. Rutin is one of the 5 BIOFLAVONOIDS which are natural substances, largely contained in citrus fruits, which reduce the inflammation of the stomach lining and develop capillary strength. In all 36 cases treated by 3 doctors, the mucous membranes and duodenal contour returned to normal in about three weeks.

✓ VITAMIN U or CABBAGE JUICE—has been reported to cure ulcers. This was discovered by Dr. Garnett Cheney of the Stanford Medical School. Observation revealed a rapid healing of GASTRIC ULCERS in only the average time. DUODENAL ULCERS healed in about the average time. He healed 62 of 65 of his patients or 95%. Cabbage juice heals by strengthening the stomach lining's resistance to acid attack by generating increased mucous activity that regenerates ulcerated cells. Drink a quart of cabbage juice a day, and you will see results in 3 weeks. Vitamin U is contained in CABBAGE JUICE as well as in ALFALFA. Cabbage juice also contains METHIONINE, an amino acid, which plays an active role in the healing of ulcers.

Many ulcers have also been cured by RAW VEGETABLE JUICES other than cabbage juice, even though they do not contain significant amounts of methionine. Through the consumption of cup of cabbage juice several times a day for from 7 to 10 days, hundreds of patients have been totally cured of ulcers. But cooked cabbage has no effect. Some call ulcers a deficiency disease due to the lack of enough raw vegetables. Naturopath Tobe has said that there is no power on earth that can do what nature can do, and there is no healing power greater than a diet composed of RAW VEGETABLES, GRAINS, FRUITS, and NUTS. NATURE KNOWS NO INCURABLE DISEASES, and nature can easily defeat cancer, and the prevention of cancer is even easier.

◆ *Other Healing Substances And Methods*

✓ GOAT'S MILK—Drinking raw goat's milk is believed to help heal stomach ulcers.

✓ HEAT and COLD—One should avoid food or drink that is either too hot or too cold. Food should be, if possible, at ROOM or BODY TEMPERATURE.

✓ HONEY—Research has shown that a diet rich in honey decreases stomach acidity for those with gastric or duodenal ulcers. One man reported that he had been a sufferer from ULCERATED STOMACH for several years—part-time in the hospital and part-time in bed—and nearly all the time with much pain. He noticed that after eating HONEY he was much better, but he gave no thought to the reason but kept on eating honey because he relished it. He has had no attacks since. The great naturalist Father Kneipp stated: "Smaller ulcers of the stomach are quickly contracted, broken, and healed by honey."

✓ OLIVE OIL—Taking a spoonful of olive oil 3 times a day is a favorite folk remedy for easing ulcers.

✓ RAW POTATO JUICE—Mixed with a little cabbage juice is also excellent. It must be freshly made and drunk immediately, for even after one minute of waiting the medicinal value disappears because of rapid oxidation. CARROT JUICE is excellent also.

✓ RAW FRUITS and VEGETABLES—Some raw fruits and vegetables may have to be avoided for a while, since they may be irritating to the ulcers. The ones that will usually cause no problems are POTATOES, SQUASHES, YAMS, AVOCADOS, and BANANAS. PLANTAINS, a type of banana, tends to stimulate the growth of new stomach cells which help the ulcer heal. Heat will destroy the healing chemicals. Bananas stimulate the proliferation of cells and mucus to form a strong barrier between the stomach lining and the corrosive acid. Green plantains are a more potent medicine against ulcers than the ripe ones.

✓ ZINC—Zinc has been shown to have a protective effect in animals and humans, because of the fact that it increases the MUCIN FOUND IN MUCUS. Dr. Pfeiffer of Memorial University in St. Johns, Newfoundland, found that zinc supplements protected the stomach cells of rats, who had been given RESERPINE, a tranquilizer that can induce ulcers in humans and rats. An associate of Dr. Pfeiffer gave rats the drug METHACHOLINE, and as a result the stomach cells released HISTAMINE, which stimulated GASTRIC SECRETIONS, which caused ulcers. The zinc stopped the process. So there are many drugs which can induce ulcers. The stress which induces ulcers can often be prevented by the use of ANTIOXIDANTS.

✓ FASTING—It has proved to be an effective treatment for stomach ulcers, provided the patient is physically strong enough.

◆ *Herbs.*

✓ ALFALFA—Dr. Stanley Slinger of Canada suffered years of misery from Stomach ulcers until he tried ALFALFA TEA, and he has had no trouble since. The tea was able to accomplish what surgery and stomach freezing could not. From the very first dose he had almost immediate relief.

✓ CAPSICUM or RED PEPPER—stimulates the mucosa cells to release mucus to cover the walls of stomach and intestines with mucus. It represents the dog licking its wounds.

✓ COMFREY—has had a long history in the healing of ulcers. It has BONE-KNITTING and WOUND-HEALING properties. The leaves contain vitamins A, B, C, E, and also B_{12}, the ANTI-ANEMIA VITAMIN. It contains a valuable healing agent called ALLANTOIN, which is found in its leaves and roots. It can heal as well as prevent ulcers. A strong tea made from comfrey ROOTS and LEAVES, taken several times a day is an effective treatment. It has healed SUPPURATING ulcers, wounds which refused to heal, LEG ULCERS, BED SORES, and SPRAINED ANKLES. A poultice applied to the wound works well. Mix comfrey powder or leaves in water to make a paste. Also use an infusion to bathe swollen joints in RHEUMATISM and BRUISES.

A 16 year old girl suffered from a BLEEDING STOMACH ULCER. The doctor gave her the usual DIET with MEDICATION. In a matter of days she was completely healed. She later confessed that she never took a drop of the doctor's medicine. All she did was to sip strong COMFREY TEA until she felt healed.

✓ LICORICE—and its constituent GLYCIRRHIZINIC ACID, was the first compound proven to promote the healing of gastric and duodenal ulcers. It stimulates the normal defense mechanisms that prevent ulcer formation by increasing the mucus secreting cells, improving the quality of the mucus, and increasing the lifespan of the surface intestinal cells. Scandinavian scientists found that licorice compounds REDUCED ACID, STIMULATED MUCUS SECRETION, and helped stomach wall CELLS REPAIR THEMSELVES.

VARIOUS AFFLICTIONS

Alcoholism

A recovery rate of 71% has been achieved in a 2 year study of 507 alcoholics on massive doses of VITAMIN B_3, NIACIN, according to Dr. Smith, the alcoholism expert of Brighton Hospital, Detroit, Michigan. Some of the benefits of the B_3 treatment are the marked ability of B_3 to reduce the MOOD SWINGS and INSOMNIA common to alcoholics. It reduces alcohol tolerance and the severity of the withdrawal symptoms. It also stabilizes behavior in such a way that traditional treatments function more efficiently.

In an experiment rats given a JUNK FOOD diet, and being given a choice of drinking water or alcohol, chose alcohol above water. A 16 week rat experiment at Loma Linda University brought out the fact that a carbohydrate junk food diet encourages the tendency to drink more alcohol. It is also known that animals who are made deficient in the B-VITAMINS will prefer alcohol to water. This definitely seems to apply to the human tendency also. A good diet seems to reduce or eliminate a craving for alcohol. The vitamins A, C, and E as well as the minerals MAGNESIUM, SELENIUM, and ZINC, will protect the liver from damage by alcohol.

Another experiment involving laboratory mice on a DEFICIENT DIET showed that NIACIN DEFICIENCY caused both male and female mice to turn to ALCOHOL rather than WATER. When the diet was made nutritionally adequate with plenty of B_3 available, the consumption of alcohol dropped.

According to a University of California study, rats which inhaled only polluted air during a 2 month experimental period, chose to drink ALCOHOL RATHER THAN WATER. For the first three weeks all the rats chose water rather than alcohol, but then the group exposed to AIR POLLUTION switched over to drinking alcohol. It is an indication that STRESS tends to a desire for a deficient diet. We should remember that cigarette smoke contains carbon dioxide and carbon monoxide just as traffic air does, and this polluted air has no doubt had a part in leading many into the drinking habit.

Bruises, Burns, Cuts, Sores, Wounds, And Stings

◆ *Spirit Of Prophecy Statements*

"God has provided a balm for every wound. There is a balm in Gilead, there is a physician there. In every trial plead with Jesus to show you a way out of your troubles, then your eyes will be opened to behold the remedy and to apply to your case the healing promises that have been recorded in His Word" (2SM273). "God's healing power runs through all nature. If a tree is cut, if a human being is wounded or breaks a bone, nature begins at once to repair the injury. Even before the need exists the healing agencies are in readiness; and as soon as a part is wounded, every energy is bent to the work of restoration" (ED113). "Always study and teach the use of the simplest remedies, and the SPECIAL

BLESSING OF GOD may be expected to follow the use of these means which are within the reach of the COMMON PEOPLE" (Herbs, EGW p. 25).

◆ *Various Methods Of Healing*

✓ ALOE VERA—The aloe liquid is a folk remedy that seems to work, although no one knows exactly why. Dozens of laboratory tests have proven that the GEL will soothe small injuries, scrapes, cuts and burns.

Aloe is used for SUNBURN, RADIATION BURNS, and BURNS of all kinds. It has a remarkable power of REGENERATING the SKIN and damaged tissues. It relieves PAIN quickly, REDUCES INFLAMMATION, and PREVENTS BLISTERING. It has been successfully used to treat WOUNDS, BEDSORES, ULCERS, ERYSIPELAS, SHINGLES, POISON OAK, POISON IVY, PSORIASIS, and HEMORRHOIDS.

✓ ICE WATER—In the case of burns ICE WATER will prevent BLISTERS. Keep on ice pack or cold water until pain is gone. In case of SHOCK, use CAYENNE PEPPER TEA. A smashed ONION POULTICE will also relieve the pain, as well as a mashed RAW POTATO POULTICE.

✓ CAYENNE PEPPER—is very effective for internal or external BLEEDING. Mixed with water it will stop bleeding and relieve SHOCK. For BLACK SPIDER bites suck out as much poison as possible, and then drink cayenne pepper mixed with water.

✓ CHARCOAL—We are told that "one of the most beneficial remedies is pulverized charcoal in a bag and used in fomentations. This is a most successful remedy. If wet in SMARTWEED, it is still better. I have ordered this in cases where the sick were suffering great pain, and when it has been confided to me by the physician that he thought it was the last before the close of life. Then I suggested charcoal, and the patient has slept, the turning point came, and recovery was the result" (2SM294)

"To students, when injured with BRUISED HANDS, and suffering with INFLAMMATION, I have prescribed this simple remedy with perfect success. The POISON of inflammation is overcome, the PAIN removed, and the HEALING goes on rapidly. The more severe INFLAMMATION of the EYES will be relieved by a poultice of charcoal, put in a bag and dipped in hot or cold water will best suit the case. This works like a charm.... For some forms of INDIGESTION, it is more efficacious than drugs. A little OLIVE OIL into which some of this powder has been stirred tends to CLEANSE and HEAL. SNAKE BITES and the sting of REPTILES and POISONOUS INSECTS could often be rendered harmless by the use of charcoal poultices.

"I write these things that you may know that the Lord has not left us without the use of simple remedies which when used will not leave the system in the weakened condition in which the use of DRUGS so often leave it." (Herbs, EGW p. 24–27).

✓ COMFREY—A lady said that her granddaughter caught her heel in the spokes of her bicycle. She applied COMFREY OINTMENT to the wound, and now her heel is better, and the proud flesh has almost disappeared. COMFREY BURN PASTE is made with equal parts of COMFREY LEAF POWDER, WHEAT GERM OIL, and HONEY. A person accidentally scalded his hand with hot oil during a kitchen fire and acquired 3rd degree burns. The emergency doctor cleaned the burn and told him that he would need SKIN GRAFTING. He used the comfrey paste instead. After a few weeks he was able to move his hand, and has now total use of his hand.

Two boys were playing with gasoline and matches, and their hands were burned up to their wrists with THIRD-DEGREE BURNS. One boy was taken to the hospital and treated for nearly a year with SURGERY and SKIN GRAFTING. When he went home his hands looked "mummified." The other boy's parents applied the comfrey burn paste, and in a few months his hands were completely healed, looking as perfect as before.

✓ HONEY—was used by the Egyptians for ULCERS, BURNS, and SKIN DISEASES. Dr. Robert Bloomfield of England states that he has used HONEY in the accident and emergency departments where he works with a dry dressing, and found it to promote the healing of ULCERS and BURNS better than any other local application. One lady had a severe BURN on her wrist. Her husband applied honey to the affected area and covered it with a bandage. Within 10 minutes the pain was gone. After 20 hours the bandage was removed, and she had no sign of blistering or damage to the skin. Another lady put honey on an ABSCESS plus a dressing, and it shriveled down to a small lump in two weeks, and soon after that disappeared. Antibacterial factors in raw honey sterilize the wound. A honey dressing lifts off the burned area effortlessly because honey converts slowly to HYDROGEN PEROXIDE and WATER.

A man was scalded all over his head, hands, and feet. Large pieces of linen were daubed with HONEY and put on his head, neck, hands, and feet. Instantly the pain ceased, and from then on the healing made steady progress.

A woman was admitted to the hospital with GANGRENE of the foot. After examining her the doctors decided that she could not survive an amputation. It was decided to try HONEY. The foot was tied into a large bag of honey. To everyone's amazement the foot soon healed, and she walked out of the hospital under her own power.

- ✓ HORSETAIL or SHAVEGRASS—has been shown to possess HEMOLYTIC or blood clotting and antibiotic activities which contribute to the healing process. A poultice can be formed to apply to external wounds. This remedy was practiced by the American Indians and by the Chinese. Horsetail also supplies CALCIUM, the primary mineral required for the healing of bones. It is also rich in several other minerals that the body uses to rebuild injured tissue.

- ✓ MARIGOLD—a well-known garden plant, was used during World War I and had a remarkable healing effect on the wounds of injured soldiers. It is considered to be one of the best antiseptics. This quality is said to be due to its content of NATURAL IODINE. It is used as TINCTURES, OINTMENTS, or CREAMS which are effective for CUTS, SPRAINS, BRUISES, ULCERATIONS, and SEVERE BURNS.

- ✓ PINE PITCH or BALM—Use on OPEN WOUNDS. BALSAM, or the clear pitch of the pine or fir trees, is the best to put on CUTS, WOUNDS, or NAIL PUNCTURES. It is a most powerful healer both inside and out. As second best TURPENTINE is very good.

- ✓ PLANTAIN—The plantain leaf has been used on people who have contracted POISON IVY. The itching subsided immediately and did not return. It is also effective on RINGWORM. Early American Physicians used plantain for almost any SKIN infection or inflammation. For SNAKEBITE mix plantain with ECHINACEA TINCTURE into a paste and apply it on the wound.

- ✓ SEA WATER—For burns over of the body use a SEA WATER BATH. Leave the patient in it night and day. This method was discovered at Dunkirk for wounds from flame throwers.

- ✓ SLIPPERY ELM—became a popular herb in this country as a poultice for wounds and as a remedy for BROKEN BONES after the settlers noticed its use by the Indians. Since then it has been used for about any condition involving injured or infected tissue or bone.

- ✓ Vitamins A & E—BURNS can be relieved with capsules of 25,000 units of VITAMIN A and 400 IU of VITAMIN E. They should be mixed and then applied. Repeat application every 4 hours, so that blisters do not form, and so that healing can proceed promptly.

- ✓ LEMON JUICE—A young man accidentally sat in some POISON IVY, and his entire body broke out in one massive inflammation, with itching that could be relieved only by soaking in a tub. Then he remembered that LEMON JUICE is valuable in many SKIN CONDITIONS such as ACNE, ECZEMA, ERYSIPELAS, BOILS, CARBUNCLES, BLACKHEADS, DANDRUFF, SORE HANDS ETC. He also remembered that it would relieve the ITCH of INSECT BITES, as well as the irritation caused by POISON OAK or IVY. Thereupon he rubbed lemon juice all over his body. In less that 5 minutes his skin looked completely normal, and he felt complete relief.

- ✓ RAW ONION—The juice of a sliced RAW ONION is alkaline, and it will relieve the acid VENOM from a WASP or a BEE, if applied immediately. So does HONEY and WHEAT GERM OIL.

Leprosy

◆ *Produced By The Eating Of Pork*

In Hawaii there exist both cancer and the leprosy. There it is said that those who live in the warmer climate below the FROST LINE and eat PORK get the LEPROSY, and that those who live above the frost line and eat a lot of pork get CANCER. There is a contagious phase and a noncontagious phase to leprosy. There are two kinds of leprosy or HANSON'S DISEASE. One causes large nodules under the skin which often become ulcers. The second kind of leprosy affects the nerves causing large white patches and a loss of feeling. Parts shrivel up and fall off. A nurse from North Africa said that people who don't eat MEAT don't get the leprosy, but people who eat CROCODILES would generally get the leprosy, because crocodiles eat mainly rotten flesh.

Leprosy was called by the Jews "the stroke," and "the finger of God" (DA262). It was said to be contagious and incurable, and to the Jews it was regarded as a judgment of God on account of sin. By the ritual law the leper was pronounced unclean as though he were already dead. As a result he was shut out from society. Whatever he touched was unclean, and even the air was polluted by his breath. He bore the heaviest burden, the burden of sin.

◆ *Eating Pork Was Forbidden By The Law Of Moses*

We are told that "pork, although one of the most common articles of diet, is one of the most injurious. God did not prohibit the Hebrews from eating swine's flesh merely to show his authority, but because it was not a proper article of food for man. It would fill the system with SCROFULA, and especially in that warm climate produced LEPROSY, and diseases of various kinds. Its influence upon the system in that climate was far more injurious than in a colder climate. But God never designed the swine to be eaten under any circumstances.... It is impossible for the flesh of any living creature to be healthy when filth is their natural element, and when they will feed upon every detestable thing" (2SM417). Eating the flesh of pigs was forbidden to the Jews by the law of Moses (Lev. 11:7). A strict Jew would not even mention swine by name. He would always use the term "the abomination." Israelites considered themselves polluted if they were even touched by a swine's bristle. So the lepers whom Christ healed had undoubtedly been eating swine's flesh in contradiction to all of the principles of the Jewish economy.

◆ *Remedy*

Drinking a lot of CHAPARRAL TEA, and eating only RAW FOODS for a whole year. An angel gave this instruction to a lady in a dream, and she followed the advice and recovered.

Headaches

◆ *Lifestyle And Headaches*

A headache is a symptom of a total body response. It is not a disease in itself, but a symptom of a total body irregularity. For some headaches are an occasional painful nuisance, while for others they represent a "crown of thorns" they bear constantly, wondering what terrible sin they have committed which makes them endure such suffering. Headaches should help us examine our lifestyles to determine what changes in our life have brought them on. We should ask ourselves if we are exposed to new environmental chemicals at home or in our place of work; if we have been eating and drinking food that does not agree with us, or to which we are allergic; if we have been getting too much sun; if we are not getting enough sleep; if we are subject to withdrawal symptoms of some kind; if we are not exercising enough; or if we are not breathing enough fresh air.

◆ *Causes Of Headaches*

Headaches can also be caused by many abnormal conditions within the body. To avoid them with respect to children we are told that "regularity should be the rule in all the habits of children" (CD242). The matter of EATING BETWEEN MEALS is one of the important factors in causing headaches, because such a bad habit causes the stomach to become deranged and the foundation is laid for present and future suffering because of such errors in diet. What disturbs the stomach will cause pain in the head. What the young need most of all is self control, and for parents to teach them self-denial.

✓ THE PILL—One lady tells her experience of how after a year or two of headaches she read that the Pill can cause a VITAMIN B DEFICIENCY, which sometimes causes MIGRAINES. She took vitamin B_6 for a while and then quit. As soon as she quit she got more headaches. She did this several times with the same results. She never quit taking B_6 again. A while later she decided to take the whole B-COMPLEX, and she hasn't had a headache since. Another lady took two heaping tablespoons of BREWER'S YEAST for migraine each morning in her juice, and within two weeks all signs of pain in the head had disappeared.

✓ COFFEE and TEA—cause headaches (4SG128). "The money expended for tea and coffee is worse than wasted. They do the user only harm, and that continually." (CD422). "Tea is intoxicating; though less in degree, its effect is the same in character as that of spirituous liquors. Coffee has a greater tendency to becloud the intellect and benumb the energies. It is not so powerful as tobacco, but is similar in it effects. The arguments brought against tobacco may also be urged against the use of tea and coffee" (CD426). "Tea and coffee drinking is a SIN" (CD425).

✓ OVEREATING—Often this intemperance is felt at once in the form of HEADACHE, INDIGESTION, and COLIC. A load has been placed upon the stomach that it cannot care for, and a feeling of oppression comes. The head is confused, and the stomach is in rebellion. It may become paralyzed and the digestive organs may lose their vital force, and undermine the foundation of the human machinery. (CD101).

✓ COLD EXTREMITIES—"When the extremities…. are not properly clad, the blood is driven to the head, causing HEADACHE or NOSEBLEED; or there is a sense of fulness about the chest, producing cough or palpitation of the heart, on account of too much blood in that locality; or the stomach has too much blood, causing indigestion" (2T531).

✓ IMPROPER CIRCULATION—"Whatever hinders the circulation forces the blood back into the vital organs, producing congestion. HEADACHE, COUGH, PALPITATION of the heart, or INDIGESTION, is often the result" (MH272). Headaches are caused by INTESTINAL DISTURBANCES. Putrefactive processes develop gases which enter the liver through the portal vein, and then find their way into the bloodstream, and the headaches result from the POISONS circulating in the bloodstream. They are also caused by an insufficient blood supply to the brain. This can be relieved by the use of GINKGO TEA.

✓ MENSTRUAL CYCLE—One young lady was bedridden with migraines on the 3th and and 15th day of her menstrual cycle from age 13 to 23, for from 1 to 5 days a month. She had taken drugs and alcohol. At age 23 she went into treatment as an alcoholic. The first thing her new doctor did was to put her on VITAMIN B_6, 100 mg per day. She also took VITAMIN B_3 or NIACIN on the recommendation of her fellow recovering alcoholics. She followed both recommendations and hasn't had a MIGRAINE since.

✓ ICECREAM—may cause a headache by a response of the warm tissues of the mouth to a cold substance. Two nerves there carry the impulse to the head causing the pain.

✓ SINUS—One lady had suffered for years from sinus headaches and received no relief from any medication except pain killers. Then she began to take 100 mg of NIACIN three times a day, and her sinus headaches disappeared.

✓ HYPOGLYCEMIA—When the sugar content of the blood drops, blood vessels swell, causing vascular headaches. Migraine headaches may be caused by the ingestion of a great amount of MONOSODIUM GLUTAMATE (MSG).

✓ CHINESE RESTAURANT SYNDROME—MSG, which is put into Chinese soups, will cause headaches. They are most pronounced if you eat the soup on an empty stomach.

✓ SALT HEADACHE—When SALT hits the stomach lining, says Dr. John Brainard, it stimulates the VAGUS NERVE, which carries the impulse to the brain causing the headache.

◆ *Factors That Alleviate Headaches*

✓ LECITHIN—One individual had been bothered with migraines for six years. He wouldn't go anywhere without a painkilling drug. Then he remembered that an old man had told him that if he himself didn't take lecithin, he couldn't control his temper. Then the young man said to himself that he was an extremely nervous person, and if lecithin helped the old man's TEMPER it might also help my NERVES. He took the lecithin and instead of taking the drug also, he would take an extra dosage of lecithin right when the headache started. This did the trick for him and the migraine soon disappeared.

✓ GINGER—Ginger affects PROSTAGLANDINS that help control inflammatory responses, involving HISTAMINE and PAIN. It blocks prostaglandin synthesis leading to reduction in inflammation and pain. For MIGRAINE HEADACHES take teaspoon of powered GINGER 4 times a day.

✓ FEVERFEW—According to a report in Science News, feverfew is an herb that can cut the number and severity of migraine headaches. Taking daily capsules of ground FEVERFEW LEAVES will reduce migraine headache discomfort and also relieve the NAUSEA that sometimes accompanies migraine headaches.

✓ MOIST HEAT—Moist heat will help improve the circulation which will speed up the cleansing of the blood. A warm BATH or SHOWER will do wonders in this regard. HOT TOWELS, HEATING PADS, or a HEAT LAMP will produce similar results. Some headaches are due to the DILATION of the ARTERIES that surround the brain. In such cases COLD PACKS or ICE PACKS can become soothing healers. Also IMMERSING the FEET in cold water causes the relaxation of the blood vessels around the brain, which draws away congestion and redistributes the circulation of the blood which will eliminate the causes of the headache.

✓ INHALING HERBAL VAPORS—Inhaling VIOLET VAPOR is said to ease the distress of a headache. Inhaling the vapor of a mixture of 2 oz. each of LAVENDER, MARJORAM, BETANY, ROSE LEAF, and ROSE PETALS, plus oz. of CLOVES placed in a small pillow is said to relieve a headache.

In a vial place 12 drops of OIL OF LAVENDER, 8 drops of OIL OF MARJORAM, 8 drops of OIL of CLOVER, 10 drops of OIL OF MINT, and 8 drops of OIL OF ROSE. Upon the onset of a headache inhale the vapor for relief.

✓ MORNING HEADACHE—For a morning headache drink one glass of ORANGE JUICE with 1 or 2 tablespoons of HONEY stirred in. The natural fruit sugar in the orange juice with the vitamins and minerals in the honey will stimulate a sluggish GLANDULAR SYSTEM to secrete a flow of enlivening hormones.

◆ *Various Facts Regarding Headaches*

✓ WOMEN vs. MEN—It is known that women are more likely than men to suffer from MIGRAINE HEADACHES in the ratio of about 10:1 On the other hand, men are more likely to suffer from CLUSTER HEADACHES, the severe and devastating headaches that come in bunches, such as four or five a day, and then disappear for weeks and months.

✓ PERFECTIONISTS—There is plenty of circumstantial evidence that migraine headaches are more common among people with perfectionist personalities who want to be in total control of their lives as well as their surroundings.

✓ AIR PRESSURE—It has been established that when the BAROMETER goes down, then incidence of migraines goes up. And when the air pressure goes up, the incidence of migraines goes down.

✓ BRUSHING THE SKIN—Brushing the skin will relieve chronic headaches far more efficiently than do painkillers.

The Natural Elimination Of Pain

◆ *Pain—A Result Of Disobedience*

Pain is one of the afflictions that sin brought into the world. Along with sin and sickness Satan brought pain into the world. Sickness and pain are always closely associated. They are to be a reminder to man and all created beings of the cost of sin. Pain is always unpleasant. It is the opposite of happiness and joy which was to reign in God's perfect creation.

But we are to realize that "it was SIN which marred God's perfect work; that thorns and thistles, sorrow and pain and death, are all the result of DISOBEDIENCE TO GOD" (6T358); that it is the fruit of transgression(3T492); that God does not cause pain and suffering, but "man through his own ignorance has brought this condition upon himself" (6T280); that God does not desire His creatures to suffer pain (DA207). Jesus made it clear to His disciples that "not a sigh is breathed, not a pain felt, not a grief pierces the soul, but the throb vibrates to the Father's heart" (DA356).

◆ *The Origin Of Pain In The System*

✓ ARTIFICIAL FOODS—It is artificial foods, foods that have been processed, that are liable to cause aches and pains. As far as possible they should be eliminated from the diet to reduce the possibility of future aches and pains. Reduce SALT as far as possible, as well as REFINED SUGAR. Eat all natural foods, fruits, and vegetables, dates, and figs. DAIRY PRODUCTS in limited quantities, are good calcium foods as well as containing other minerals needed to coat the body's nervous system and guard against aches and pains. Fruits are good sources of vitamins, minerals, and enzymes which can give help in developing better digestive health.

✓ PROSTAGLANDINS—Pain starts with an injury—a cut finger for example. PROSTAGLANDINS and other chemicals at the injured point stimulate nerve endings that send the pain message through the spinal chord to the brain. ASPIRIN is believed to work at the site of the injury, diminishing the pain by blocking prostaglandin production. At the THALAMUS in the brain, the message is consciously recognized as pain, and in the CORTEX, the location and severity of the pain are perceived. The signal then descends down to the SPINAL CHORD where the pain's intensity is thought to be modulated by ENDORPHINS, released from the brain to block pain signals. This explains also why some athletes who are injured during a contest can continue playing without pain. SEVERITY of PAIN depends upon how many nerve endings are involved. Your thoughts often influence endorphin release, as is true in the case of giving the patient PLACEBOS. Endorphins may also explain why ACUPUNCTURE sometimes relieves pain. Through complex nerve pathways, messages of stimulation from acupuncture needles trigger production of endorphins which relieve the pain.

✓ CONDIMENTS AND SPICES—such as KETCHUP, MUSTARD, and PEPPER should be eliminated from your diet. Instead, use natural HERBS. The condiments will inflame the lining of the stomach, and possibly cause excessive HEART BEAT, HEART PAIN, and HEART TROUBLE in general. We are told that "CONDIMENTS are injurious in their nature. MUSTARD, PEPPER, SPICES, and PICKLES, and other things of a like character, irritate the stomach and make the blood feverish and impure…. They would irritate and inflame the delicate coating of the stomach…. SODA causes INFLAMMATION of the stomach, and often poisons the entire system" (CD339, 340, 342).

✓ ENDORPHINS—Electrodes may also stimulate peripheral nerves and then stimulate the pain centers of the brain which then produce endorphin secretions. It appears that endorphins are able to relieve pain whether induced by thought or nutrition.

✓ FAT AND CHOLESTEROL—Reduce the intake of fat and cholesterol foods, and you will eliminate the possible pain of arthritis.

✓ LACTIC ACID—WASTE MATTERS may be piling up in the blood due to WORRY, LACK of SLEEP, OVERWORK, TENSION, and NERVOUS EXHAUSTION. There may be an accumulation of LACTIC ACID in the muscles or other waste products which cause a harsh reaction in the muscles. This creates INFLAMMATION and SPASMS.

◆ *God's Pain Relief Methods And Remedies In Nature*

Pain is indirectly beneficial. It is supposed to act as a benefit t to the body. It is to tell us that we should slow down, rest, or stop. If we take a drug, pill, or shot to eliminate the pain, great damage may be done to the organs of our body because of inattention, and due to the lack of investigation of the cause of the pain. The pain is a God-given mechanism that is trying to tell us that there is something wrong in the system that should be looked after to see if a process of healing is to be initiated. A pain killer will cover up the trauma that might exist as though it weren't there. It represents an act of ignoring and not listening to the body to that which may be harmful to the whole system.

Pain is subjective. We can never really experience someone else's pain. Nobody can grasp the pain you feel. Pain is a great MOTIVATOR. So is pleasure. Pleasure moves people to do things that are PRO-SURVIVAL. Pain moves people to avoid things that are ANTI-SURVIVAL.

"There are simple remedies provided by God to alleviate pain and to aid nature in her work. This is not a denial of faith, but rather is in strict harmony with the plans of God (CH381). Hours of pain should be made hours of prayer (2SM240). Pain may be relieved on the sabbath (DA207). Invalids should rise above their pain through useful employment (MH246).

We are told that "many are living in violation of the laws of health and are ignorant of the relation their habits of eating, drinking, and working sustain to their health. They will not arouse to their true condition until nature protests against the abuses she has suffered, by ACHES and PAINS in the system" (CD304) The persons who suffer PAIN become impatient. They are not willing to use SELF-DENIAL, and suffer a little from HUNGER. They are determined to get relief at once, and then take powerful drugs prescribed by a physician, and sometimes drug themselves to death (2SM450–1).

Natural pain relievers or ANALGESICS, created by God in nature, besides alleviating pain also at the same time help to promote the healing process of the body, and alert the body's self-healing powers. When they heal, they apply their healing powers to the whole body. This drugs cannot do, for they are not healing substances. They relieve the SYMPTOMS of disease, but not the CAUSES of disease. Because of the fact that they are used to suppress symptoms, DRUGS often contribute to the development of more serious physical, mental, and emotional disorders.

◆ *Eliminating Harmful Substances Reduces Pain*

✓ EXCESSIVE USE OF SALT—Too much salt constricts the arteries and can cause HARDENING of the ARTERIES or ARTERIOSCLEROSIS. Instead, use natural HERBS which contain healthful nutrients.

✓ ELIMINATE REFINED SUGAR PRODUCTS AS FAR AS POSSIBLE—Instead, use HONEY, but in moderation, and satisfy your sweet tooth with DATES, FIGS, RAISINS, GRAPES, and BERRIES.

✓ ELIMINATE WHITE FLOUR PRODUCTS—Replace them with WHOLE GRAIN FLOUR FOODS. Whole grains are prime sources of vitamins and minerals which are needed to soothe the nervous system, and protect against HEADACHES and chemical bleaches that produce NERVE-CAUSED PAIN.

✓ GIVE UP CAFFEINE - CONTAINING FOODS AND BEVERAGES—They irritate the nerve cells and cause nervous symptoms ranging from EMOTIONAL UPHEAVAL to HEADACHES and INSOMNIA. Drink HERB TEAS instead.

✓ GIVE UP ALCOHOL IN ANY FORM—It depletes the body's store of nerve-healing B-complex vitamins and creates emotional distress and headaches.

✓ GIVE UP CONDIMENTS—such as KETCHUP, MUSTARD, and PEPPER. They inflame the lining of the stomach and cause excessive HEARTBEAT, and may predispose to HEART TROUBLE. Use HERBS instead and your food will taste much better also.

✓ ACID FOODS—Reduce acid foods to a normal recommended diet of no more than 20%, and you will eliminate the possible PAIN of ARTHRITIS.

◆ *Substances And Procedures That Help Reduce Pain*

✓ BEE STINGS—There are many followers of the folk therapy that indicates that bee stings relieve arthritis pain, sometimes for good. Analysis shows that BEE VENOM contains two proteins—MELITTIN and APAMINE—that cause the pituitary and adrenal glands to produce more CORTISONE. It is an effective anti-nflammatory substance that is often prescribed by doctors to reduce pain and swelling. It is important to note, however, that cortisone produced naturally in your body does not create the devastating effects of artificial cortisone, or cortisone taken from animals.

✓ CALCIUM—Calcium produces a coating action upon the MYELIN SHEATH covering the network of nerves. This represents a natural insulation against STRESSES and STRAINS which deplete the myelin sheath. It is a mineral that can relieve headaches.

For a MINERAL PAIN RELIEVER, in a glass of skim milk stir a teaspoon of BREWERS YEAST and a tablespoon of HONEY. The calcium of the milk is taken up by the B-complex vitamins of the brewers yeast and then energized by the natural sugars of the honey for speedy assimilation into the bloodstream. The calcium is then used to soothe the nervous system, and will promote relief from general body pains.

✓ CAPSAICIN—CHILI PEPPERS possess a traditional reputation for curing ARTHRITIS. Scientists no longer scoff at the use of chili peppers since it was found that the active ingredient is capsaicin. It also suppresses PAIN by inducing a reduction in the nerve cells of a neurotransmitter called SUBSTANCE P which delays pain sensations to the central nervous system, so that capsaicin actually "short-circuits" the perception of pain. Merely rubbing an ointment of capsaicin on the skin numbs the pain.

✓ CHARCOAL—"One of the most beneficial remedies is PULVERIZED CHARCOAL, placed in a bag and used in fomentations. This is a most successful remedy. If wet in smartweed boiled, it is still better. I have ordered this in cases where the sick were suffering great pain, and when it has been confided to me by the physician that he thought it was the last before the close of life. Then I suggested the charcoal and the patient slept, the turning point came, and recovery was the result" (2SM294). In a case in Australia a woman with a fever was not expected to live, but Mrs. White suggested that they get pulverized charcoal, make a poultice of it, and lay it over her stomach and sides. Relief was said to have come in less than half an hour after the application of the poultices. She also said that she had ordered the same treatment for others who were suffering great pain, and it brought relief and has been the means of saving life. Her mother had told her that SNAKE BITES, THE STING OF REPTILES, and POISONOUS INSECTS could often be rendered harmless by the use of charcoal poultices (2SM295).

In another case a man was taken sick with INFLAMMATION OF THE BOWELS and BLOODY DYSENTERY. The thought came to Mrs. White like a communication from the Lord to take PULVERIZED CHARCOAL, put water upon it, and give this water to the sick man to drink, putting bandages of the charcoal over the bowels and stomach. The result was that in half an hour there was a change for the better (2SM299). A little 18 months old boy had a painful swelling on the knee from possibly some poisonous insect. Pulverized charcoal, mixed with FLAXSEED, was placed upon the swelling, and the poultice gave relief at once. The child had screamed with pain all night, but when the poultice was applied, he slept. She says that we should thank the Lord to become intelligent in using the simple things within our reach to alleviate pain, and successfully remove its cause. (2SM300). It is presumption to ask the Lord to relieve pain when we are too indolent to make use of these remedies within our power, it is simply presumption (2SM297). Charcoal absorbs intestinal gas when taken after a meal.

✓ ENDORPHINS—are morphine-like substances that block pain signals. They are the body's own PAIN KILLERS. They help ARTHRITIS pain. They are contained in OATS, NONFAT WHEAT, CORN, and LIMA BEANS. MAGNESIUM boosts the protective endorphins to inhibit the dispersion of the pain. Eating spicy foods seasoned with CAPSAICIN, the substance that makes chili peppers hot, renders the skin insensitive to pain by depleting substance "P," the chemical in peripheral nerves, that sends the pain message to the brain. It actually increases the endorphins.

✓ EXERCISE—is a natural PAIN RELIEVER. With exercise the body develops its own CORTISONE which prevents the pain of CALCIUM SEDIMENTS. It loosens tight muscles and improves the circulation which protects against

LEG ACHES.

- ✓ FIBER—Fiber will soften the STOOL, cut the amount of time that food takes to work its way through the digestive system, and reduces the pressures inside the GUT that cause PAIN. The fiber soaks up fluids like a sponge, so that drinking the proper amount of fluids is very important.
- ✓ HEAT—The application of heat with a heating pad or hot fomentation will often give pain relief.
- ✓ HOP POULTICES—over the stomach will relieve pain (2SM297).
- ✓ MASSAGE—is a technique that can relieve muscle tightness and soreness. It would be good for every household to have at least one member who is skilled in the art of giving a pain-relieving massage.

A MINERAL PAIN RELIEVER—In a glass of skim milk, stir one teaspoon of BREWER'S YEAST, and one teaspoon of HONEY. Drink slowly. The calcium of the milk is taken up by the B-complex vitamins of the brewer's yeast and is then energized by the natural sugars of the honey for speedy assimilation into the bloodstream. The calcium is then used to soothe the nervous system and promote relief of head and general body pains.

- ✓ NATURAL ANALGESICS—Because of the fact that drugs suppress symptoms, they often contribute to the development of more serious PHYSICAL and EMOTIONAL DISORDERS. ACHES and PAINS are NATURE'S SIGNALS that something has gone wrong with the body. Drugs interfere with the body's natural way of healing aches and pains. Natural pain relievers treat the body toward health at the same time that they are relieving pain. All body systems are interdependent, and a disturbance in one may cause a disturbance in another. By treating the whole body, the parts are being treated also. Medications often become CRUTCHES. The habitual use of ASPIRIN, a TRANQUILIZER, a PEP PILL, a SLEEPING PILL, a MUSCLE RELAXANT, an ARTHRITIC PILL, may create many other medicine-caused reactions and diseases, so that the ailment produces other ailments, and makes the conditions worse than before.

In Japan GARLIC is used as a pain killer. Sulfur compounds from garlic inhibit CARCINOGENS, and inhibit the enzymes that allow cancer to spread.

- ✓ OXYGEN—DEEP BREATHING helps to get more oxygen into the tissues, and it then combines with poisonous substances, neutralizes them, and keeps them from causing painful situations.
- ✓ PHENYLALANINE—is one of the essential AMINO ACIDS which the body does not produce, but which must be obtained from food sources. It strengthens the immune system to reduce painful symptoms. It has been found effective against the chronic pain of OSTEOARTHRITIS, RHEUMATOID ARTHRITIS, LOW BACK PAIN, JOINT PAINS, MENSTRUAL PAIN, WHIPLASH, MIGRAINE HEADACHE, and BONE PAIN. It has no side-effects, is nonaddictive, and nontoxic. It works by stimulating the body's hormones to block the pain signals from the brain. It is called "nutritional aspirin." It is found in dried NONFAT MILK, PEANUTS, PEANUT BUTTER, WALNUTS, WHEAT GERM, OAT FLAKES, GRANOLA, and COTTAGE CHEESE. For an amino acid pain stopper in 8 oz. of COTTAGE CHEESE or YOGURT, mix one teaspoon of WHEAT GERM, and 1 teaspoon of OAT FLAKES, and eat it slowly with a spoon. It should gradually stop arthritic pain. It is not fast acting, so allow from 3 to 6 weeks for it to really take effect.
- ✓ TRYPTOPHAN—Tryptophan, an essential amino acid, is also an effective PAIN RELIEVER. It seems to increase the body's production of substances in the brain which act on the brain's pain center to lower pain signals coming from the body. It has the ability to initiate the release of SEROTONIN, a neurotransmitter, which helps to block the pathway of pain. It is most effective against chronic BACKACHE and LEG PAIN. It coats the neurotransmitters, controls their intensity, keeps them in check, and protects them against runaway impulses.

The immune system needs to be nourished with foods containing tryptophan. At the same time VITAMIN B$_6$ and FOLATE, another B-complex member, are needed to stimulate the activity of tryptophan to manufacture the soothing serotonin to ease and minimize the pain of ARTHRITIS. The immune system of the arthritic often shows a deficiency in tryptophan. Such a person is advised to take 1 gm of tryptophan per day to be obtained from the health food store. Good food sources of tryptophan are ALMONDS, EGGS, MILK, BREWERS YEAST, and YOGURT. For a tryptophan TONIC blenderize in a glass of milk, 1 teaspoon of brewers yeast, and some almonds.

✓ VITAMIN B$_1$—It promotes a soothing relaxation of the nervous system. It especially nourishes the MYELIN SHEATH around nerves, so that they are naturally insulated against corrosive acids. It is found in WHEAT GERM, BREWERS YEAST, and most WHOLE GRAIN FOODS.

✓ VITAMIN B$_{12}$—Nutritional deficiencies cause ACHES, predispose to problems of SORENESS, WEAKNESS of the LIMBS, DIMINISHED REFLEXES, SENSORY PERCEPTION, changes in TEMPERATURE of parts of the body, and difficulties in WALKING.

A woman who suffered from painfully weak legs was given large amounts of vitamin B$_{12}$. She had LATERAL SCLEROSIS, which is a degeneration of the nerves controlling motion in the spinal chord. With the vitamin she soon walked normally. When cooking soybeans, the water in which you cook contains vitamin B also, so one should make use of it for sauce or dressing.

✓ VITAMIN C—In burns it alleviates pain, hastens healing, combats the accumulation of toxic poisons, and reduces the time needed for skin grafting.

✓ VITAMIN E—In an Israeli study vitamin E gave relief of pain to some people with OSTEOARTHRITIS. Of 29 people divided in two groups, the vitamin E group and the inert pill or placebo group. 15 of the vitamin E group experienced a marked relief of pain, while only one of the placebo group did so.

✓ WATER—Water can be used in many ways to relieve suffering. Drafts of clear, hot water taken before eating, half a quart more or less, will never do any harm, but will rather be productive of good. For LUNG FEVER or PNEUMONIA, Mrs. White used water freely upon her son Willie's head and a compress upon his lungs, and he soon became as rational as ever. His pain on the right side was subdued with cold water compresses (2SM304).

Water helps in washing away TOXIC ACIDS and debris. This helps the kidneys and liver in their work, and eases the distress symptoms of COLITIS and CONSTIPATION, for water is a natural laxative. A hot as well as a cold shower will speed up the circulation of the blood, purify it, and take away aches and pains.

✓ WILLOW BARK—The Willow Bark contains a substance called SALICIN, which the body converts into SALICYLIC ACID to alleviate pain. This is no doubt the NATURAL WAY in which God wanted us to use this pain reliever. The synthetic derivative of salicylic acid is called ASPIRIN. It is one of the most widely used ANALGESICS and ANTIPYRETICS against fever. It is often misused, and is one of the most frequent causes of accidental poisoning in children. In case of a cold it makes much more sense to swallow a couple of vitamin C tablets. They truly have the power to help heal a cold, not just relieve the symptoms, and there is no danger involved with them. Experiments have shown the overwhelming superiority of the natural pain reliever salicin over aspirin.

Aspirin reduces SWELLING the same way it reduces PAIN: by inhibiting the production of PROSTAGLANDINS, which send pain messages, but allow the white blood cells to cover the area where you hurt, thereby causing a swelling. It LOWERS BODY TEMPERATURE by influencing the internal thermostat, the HYPOTHALAMUS.

✓ WALKING—Walking helps loosen up the tight muscles and improves the CIRCULATION. This oxygenates the blood and thereby eliminates poisonous substances. A better blood flow sends nutrients to the capillaries and protects against LEG ACHES.

✓ WORMWOOD—A tincture of this herb applied externally has been used as a pain reliever for women during labor and against TUMORS and CANCERS. It also relieves the soreness of

ACHING MUSCLES, ARTHRITIC JOINTS, SPRAINS, DISLOCATED SHOULDERS, and FRACTURED BONES.

◆ *Backpain*

In general a lower backpain can be traced to INADEQUATE EXERCISE, EXCESSIVE STRAIN on the SPINE, DETERIORATION, and PRESSURE on the SPINAL CHORD. Here a spinal manipulation can loosen up pockets of CONGESTION along the spinal column, and help promote greater flexibility, thereby relieving discomfort. The primary cause for backpain is MUSCLE TENSION, brought on by PSYCHOLOGICAL or EMOTIONAL STRESS. Lifting a heavy object or other physical strain can bring on the condition, but many authorities claim that muscle tension was present long before the pain came about. Most back pain is caused by the compression on nerves and spinal disks. Once a disk goes out of alignment, it can press against the SCIATIC NERVE that runs along the spinal column and down the leg. So the best treatment is to relieve the tension and the pressure. A contributing cause of back pain is WEAK STOMACH MUSCLES, which place a greater burden on the spine to support the upper body. To alleviate this we must do exercises which strengthen the stomach muscles. It is said that a WATER BED is an excellent reliever of BACK PAIN.

◆ *Arthritis Pain*

Arthritis is often traced to the accumulation of toxins within the system that create a corrosive action, which manifests itself in the form of joint pain. The use of drugs known as SALICYLATES as well as other preparations tend to mask the cause of arthritis by suppressing the symptoms. Dr. Bingham has helped many arthritics by restoring better metabolism through better nutrition. He says: "No person who is in good nutritional health develops RHEUMATOID- or OSTEOARTHRITIS." DR. Bingham recommends 2000 mg of VITAMIN C, 3 glasses of RAW MILK, which contains protein and calcium, and which has an ANTI-STIFFNESS FACTOR which is destroyed by pasteurization, and which will gradually ease arthritic pain and promote healing.

✓ HEAT—Use an approved infrared HEATING LAMP, an ELECTRIC LIGHT BULB, an ELECTRIC HEATING PAD, or a HOT WATER BOTTLE. Use for up to 20 minutes. This will loosen up and expand constricted muscles that may be causing the pain.

✓ COMFREY—Comfrey is a natural pain reliever. Make a poultice with it or a hot compress and apply to the aching part. Let it remain until cool, then heat again and make repeated applications. The warmth of the comfrey poultices opens the pores, and sends natural healing medications to the tissues, cells, and muscles.

✓ EARACHE—A folk healer calls for placing a small slice of garlic loosely in the ear. Let it remain there for 30 minutes. This works wonders in syphoning off toxins and promoting a natural healing. For another method try a HOT PAD applied to the ear. For EAR DROPS try warm OLIVE OIL. Lie on the side and let the olive oil go into the ear. Keep ear warm with a hot pad.

✓ HELIOTHERAPY—Expose your aching back to sunlight for 30 to 60 minutes at a time. The sunshine activates small glands beneath the surface of the skin to manufacture vitamin D which strengthens weak or porous bones, and builds resistance against arthritic infection. It also facilitates better CALCIUM ABSORPTION, and calcium is also a natural pain reliever.

✓ HOT BATH—Fill a tub with comfortably hot water and soak yourself for 30 to 45 minutes at a time. The warm water will soothe the hurting nerves that cause the ache.

✓ HOT TOWEL—Fold a towel into 6 layers thick. Dip it in hot water, put on the back and cover with a dry towel to help hold the heat in. Apply until it cools off. Then repeat. This also will relieve the backache.

✓ ICE MASSAGE—Rub the back with an ICE PACK, a plastic container filled with ice. Put some ice in a towel. Lie face down. Let a friend rub the ice over your back. After 3 minutes your back grows numb. Continue for 15 to 20 minutes until the pain is gone. This procedure should give relief for an extended period of time. The ice will cool down the inflamed nerves and arteries that abound around the spinal column. This causes a natural cooling of the inflammation of the region, and thereby eases the pain.

✓ MUSCLE PAIN—MUSCLE SPASMS—are helped by a sunshine exposure of 20 minutes the first day, 45 minutes the 2nd day, 90 minutes the third day, 2 hours the fourth day, and 3 to 5 hours the fifth day. The rays of the sun stimulate the oil glands to manufacture vitamin D. It mobilizes CALCIUM and PHOSPHORUS transport from body glands into the bloodstream. These minerals nourish the tissues and cells of the muscles to eliminate the spasms.

✓ HYDROTHERAPY—produces the benefit of opening up the body pores, to permit a form of self-cleansing and the casting out of TOXIC WASTES that might be the cause of aching muscles. Take a bath with a handful of HEALING HERBS that have been soaked in the warm water. The medicines from the herbs will enter the body through the pores.

Indians troubled with NEURALGIA or MUSCULAR SORENESS, would make a tea of ROSE PETALS, PEPPERMINT, LINDEN LEAVES and LEMON PEEL, sweetened with honey and lemon juice.

WHIRLPOOL BATH—offers an additional natural healer in the massage action of the water, without using up energy in massaging. It alerts sluggish cells, boosts circulation, and limbers up arms and legs. Natural analgesics work to help the body create CHOLINESTERASE, a substance that destroys ACETYLCHOLINE, which is produced by the nerve endings and produces pain.

✓ NOISE POLLUTION—Noise is unhealthy for the entire body. It upsets BALANCE and EQUILIBRIUM that creates good hearing and overall health. It causes the heart to beat faster, the muscles to tense, and the blood pressure to shoot up. It doesn't matter what the source of the loud noise is as to whether it comes from a HORN, a SCREAM, or an EXPLOSION. Persistent noise upsets

☛ the output of glandular hormones.

☛ boosts the secretion of stomach acid.

☛ adversely affects the heart and the blood vessels, and

☛ interferes with the correct functioning of the ears and eyes.

✓ OIL MASSAGE—Blend 1 part of OIL of LAVENDER and 3 parts of OLIVE OIL. Massage into the muscles of your lower back. The oil will seep into the body through the pores. Do this before going to bed, and by morning the muscles should feel a lot better.

✓ PAPAYA—The papaya contains the valuable enzyme group known as PAPAIN. It also has additional enzymes such as AMYLASE, LIPASE, and PECTASE. These enzymes alert the digestive system to break down fatty tissues. It also contains PROTEOLYTIC or protein digesting enzymes such as ALPHA and BETA PAPAIN and CHYMOPAPAIN. They all aid in the better digestion of food.

✓ SCIATICA, BURSITIS, AND NEURALGIA PAINS—SCIATICA—generally refers to many pains in the HIPS and LEGS, which are the consequence of muscular imbalance.

✓ BURSITIS PAIN—usually involves the SHOULDER, ELBOW, or KNEE. In these areas tendons and muscles glide across each other and rub against bony prominences. The body tends to ease the abrasive friction by forming smooth-lined pockets of tissue. These become sore and painful.

✓ NEURALGIA—is an ailment affecting the PERIPHERAL NERVES and also involves nerve inflammation. A natural analgesic program will re-establish nerve equilibrium.

✓ STOMACH GAS AND CHEST PAINS—Stomach pains cannot be balanced with ANTACIDS which cause worse distress with long-term health risk. Most antacids are extremely ALKALINE. They neutralize gastric acid, the cause of stomach ache, but the loss of such gastric acid creates what is called an ACID REBOUND. This means that as a result of neutralizing the stomach acid, the digestive system produces more acid, and this creates a dangerous cycle. It hinders digestion, for the system needs this acid for metabolism and absorption, and it can cause serious injury to the lining of the stomach, leading to ulcers and cancers.

These pains may occur from eating fatty rich foods. Gas accumulates in the higher portions of the stomach. It is often felt as a CHEST

PAIN, and then as a distressful eruption. It is recommended that you DO NOT SWALLOW AIR WHILE YOU EAT, and chew only small portions of food. DO NOT EAT HURRIEDLY. DO NOT BOLT DOWN YOUR FOOD. Also avoid foods into which a lot of air has been beaten.

MASSAGE OILS—that can be used for chest pain as self-massage oils are YERBA SANTA and WINTERGREEN in OLIVE OIL. An HERBAL BALM is one made with equal parts of BALM of GILEAD, VERVAIN, and MARJORAM in OLIVE OIL. It is believed that the NATURAL MEDICINES IN THESE HERBS seep through the pores of the chest to help relieve congestion.

CHEST CONGESTION—may be relieved with the following HERB TEAS: HYSSOP, CAMOMILE, COMFREY ROOT, WINTER GREEN. Sweeten them with lemon juice and honey. SWEET MARJORAM—is a healing herb that has also healed chest congestion. It is made with honey and applied to the chest as a natural ointment.

CHEST COUGHS—Mix equal amounts of LICORICE, HOREHOUND, and PENNY ROYAL herbs and use 1 heaping tablespoon in a cup of boiled water. Let it steep for 15 minutes. Strain and add honey and lemon juice. Drink throughout the day. The ingredients in the herbs are said to be soothing to the bronchial tubes and they will clear up tight chest feeling.

✓ VITAMIN C—Vitamin C helps create a healing relationship between the building of the BONE, BLOOD VESSELS, CARTILAGE, and COLLAGEN in the spinal column. A deficiency of vitamin C produces a fragility of these tissues due to the breakdown of COLLAGEN, the intercellular cement, resulting in easy breakage of any or all of these connective tissues. Dr. Syed suggests that muscle stiffness can be prevented by taking massive doses of vitamin C, such as 500 mg every few hours. This may mean that a BACKACHE represents a vitamin C deficiency.

✓ WATER—HYDROTHERAPY—Water represents another natural pain reliever. Take a warm shower for 10 minutes the first thing in the morning, and follow it with a 30 second comfortably cold shower. Invigorate the painful area with a good brushing with a stiff bristled brush. Finnish with a towel rubbing. By this time you should feel warm all over. This indicates that your sluggish metabolism has been alerted and that your circulation has been speeded up. Your endocrine glands have been stimulated to reactivate their hormone-producing function, so that especially the adrenal gland can produce its natural supply of CORTISONE.

◆ *The Survival Value Of Pain*

✓ IMMEDIATE REACTION—If a person steps on a nail, the pain causes the individual to immediately withdraw the foot in order to prevent further damage.

✓ LEARNING EXPERIENCE—The pain avoidance that prevents further injury serves as a basis for learning, so as to avoid injurious objects or situations which may occur in the future.

✓ LIMIT ACTIVITIES—Pains due to damaged joints, infections, diseases, or serious injuries set LIMITS on activities, and enforce inactivity and rest which are often essential for the body's insurance of recovery and survival.

PSYCHOGENESIS — THE MENTAL CAUSE OF DISEASE

The Interrelations Of Mind And Emotions

It can be safely stated that one of the greatest causes of disease has to do with the interrelatonship between the MIND and the EMOTIONS. We are told that of the diseases from which men suffer have their foundation in the mind (CH324). Mental and emotional stress can tear your health down faster than inadequate nutrition can. It can cause, TOXIC GOITER, ULCERS, MIGRAINE HEADACHES, ANGINA, GLANDULAR DISTURBANCES, ARTHRITIS, APOPLEXY, ASTHMA, STROKES, DIABETES, HIGH and LOW BLOOD PRESSURE, HEART TROUBLE, and CANCER. Emotional DEPRIVATION may cause stunted and RETARDED GROWTH, and IMMATURITY.

Studies show that when children from a broken home are placed in a foster home or an orphanage, they will continue to flourish. But when such children are returned to their old homes, they stopped growing and lost weight. We must believe that a positive outlook on life, a contented spirit, a cheerful disposition, and a faith that natural processes, which God has established, will do their part in helping to maintain and restore our health, if we do our part.

A positive emotion can be a double negative emotion. For example, hate is emotionally harmful, but not if it is applied to HATING SIN. Positive emotions like love, acceptance, and forgiveness will stimulate the immune system positively. The feeling that you, with God's help, can control what is happening seems to enhance the immune system.

◆ *What Causes Mental Disease*

We are told that "Thousands who might have lived, have prematurely passed into their graves, physical, mental, and moral wrecks. They had good powers, but they sacrificed all to the indulgence of APPETITE, which led them to lay the reins upon the neck of lust" (3T562). Many more suffer from mental disease than we imagine (3T184). "The mind becomes depressed because it sympathizes with the weariness of the body" (1T306). "Disease of the soul, such as bigotry and unbelief, are worse than leprosy and palsy" (DA271). We are also told that mental disease is caused by FAMILY TROUBLES; ERRONEOUS DOCTRINES, REMORSE FOR SIN (5T444); and by SELFISHNESS, which causes sickness of soul which no earthly balm can heal (COL 418), and that under those circumstances one cannot distinguish between right and wrong (Te37).

In a strong emotional reaction HORMONES are secreted, and your BODY CHEMISTRY is altered. This can affect your ENDOCRINE BALANCE, your BLOOD SUPPLY, INHIBIT your DIGESTION, CHANGE your BREATHING, and change the TEMPERATURE of your SKIN. A sustained emotional state may cause changes that lead to disease. CRYING provides an emotional outlet. TEARS carry away toxins that are produced during emotional shock. They are one of nature's safety valves. Stress may also be caused by external changes to which we have not adjusted ourselves. Even CANCER has been linked to the emotions of those who feel HOPELESS.

The Mind-Body Unity

We are viewed as a mind-body unity. The mind will affect the body, and the body will affect the mind. There is a mutual influence of one upon the other. They react upon each other. If one is hurt, the other sympathizes. A very close relationship exists between the two. The emotional state can play a direct role in the production of bodily illnesses. The human organism is so arranged that the mind is to have control over the body, and the body's organs are made to be servants of the mind (FE26). As far as possible it is to control bodily functions. Whenever the mind becomes unable to rule, then the mind follows the body to the destruction of both. It is also a fact that the body cannot be cured without the POSITIVE INFLUENCE of the mind. When the mind is suppressed, so is the body, and when the body is ill, it affects the state of the mind.

The results of a Yale University Study showed that if you believe that you are healthy, you will live a longer healthier life.

Emotions Suppress Or Enhance The Immune System

◆ *Emotions Affect Lymphocites*

Our responses to the ups and downs of every day life are translated by the brain into chemicals which have the ability to either SUPPRESS or ENHANCE the IMMUNE SYSTEM. Negative emotions suppress the immune system, while positive emotions enhance it. If you are TRUSTING, CARING, and OPTIMISTIC, you are more likely to stay well. The immune function drops immediately after SEPARATION or DIVORCE, and women with poor marriages have poor immune function. A study of 15 WIDOWERS showed that they had a significant drop in the ability of their LYMPHOCITES to fight invading GERMS. A 20 year Chicago study of 2000 electric company workers showed that depressed employees were almost twice as likely to die of a deadly disease than those who had a more positive emotional outlook.

Many studies have shown that positive feelings such as LOVE, SECURITY and FAITH, help to strengthen the immune response, thereby giving the body a better chance of fighting disease. At the same time negative feelings such as TENSION, WORRY, and DEPRESSION seem to undermine the immune system. Many of such negative emotional states have been linked to diseases such as CANCER, CORONARY HEART DISEASE, KIDNEY MALFUNCTIONS, LUNG AILMENTS, DIABETES, MIGRAINE HEADACHES, and many other ailments.

A study of 1500 people revealed that those who practiced their faith regularly had better health as compared to those who were not actively involved in religious activities.

◆ *Depression*

"Many of the diseases from which men suffer are the result of MENTAL DEPRESSION. GRIEF, ANXIETY, DISCONTENT, REMORSE, GUILT, DISTRUST, all tend to break down the life forces and to invite decay and death" (MH247).

DEPRESSION is usually one of the early signs of NUTRITIONAL DEPLETION, such as a DEFICIENCY OF CALORIES, STARVATION, or a CRASH DIET. DRUGS can cause depression by neutralizing many nutritional elements in the body. For example, the PILL increases the need for FOLIC ACID, VITAMIN B and ZINC.

◆ *Mental Attitudes In Disease*

☛ RESIGNATION—An individual can have a negative psychological attitude or disposition which may slow or be harmful to his discovery.

☛ WORRY AND ANXIETY—Such people were found to have a deficiency of RED BLOOD CELLS, but no alteration in the WHITE CELLS was discovered.

☛ FIGHTER—Such a person had the desire to overcome the illness through direct and purposeful action. They showed a higher than normal WHITE BLOOD CELL count.

Emotional Factors That Lead To Disease

The emotional factors that lead to disease are WORRY, FEAR, HATE, ANXIETY, ENVY, and JEALOUSY. Also DEPRESSION, UNHAPPINESS, DEPRIVATION of LOVE, and LONELINESS. Our inability to look into the future, and perceive the outcome of a present train of events, processes, or procedures, places the Christian in a position where he must substitute FAITH in GOD for a lack of discernment of future events. This gives him something to get hold of to control and steady his emotions, which factor non-Christians lack.

So-called TYPE A BEHAVIOR is marked by impatience, aggressiveness, and hostility which may hurt the heart enough to kill you. It also suppresses the immune system. Paul said: "I have learned in whatsoever state I am, therewith to be content" (Phil. 4:11). "And having food and raiment let us be therewith content" (1 Tim. 6;8). And "Be content with such things as ye have" (Hebr. 13:5). These attitudes have the ability to eliminate type A behavior.

◆ *Worry*

✓ WORRY IS BLIND—Worry represents a concern for the negative outcome of future events which we cannot control. Most worries are anticipatory worries. We are afraid of what might happen. But all negative emotions affect the health of the individual in the negative direction toward the incidence of disease. The Christian has an escape hatch under these circumstances. When we are worried we are told to "flee to Christ" (2T81). If we do not do this then we are worrying ourselves out of the arms of Christ. WORRY IS BLIND and cannot discern the FUTURE. But when we flee to Christ, we are fleeing to one who can see the end from the beginning, (MH481), one who sees the future, and who has made provision for our future welfare. We are told that "the health is ill-affected by worry about self" (5T315), and that "the life forces are worn out by continual worry" (DA330). We are therefore admonished to lay aside this yoke of bondage.

"When we really believe that God loves us and means to do us good, we shall cease to worry about the future. Christ said: 'My grace is sufficient for thee'" (MB101; 2 Cor. 12:9). "Those who accept the one principle of making the service and honor of God supreme, will find perplexities vanish, and a plain path before their feet" (DA339). And "those who take Christ at his word, and surrender their souls to His keeping, their lives to His ordering, will find peace and quietude…. In perfect acquiescence there is perfect rest" (DA331).

✓ LET WORRY BE GOD'S PROBLEM—God continually thinks thoughts of peace toward us (Jer. 29:11). "A plant is not in continual worry about its growth" (ML103), and neither should we be. "God is not pleased by a life of worry" (2SM242). It grieves the Holy Spirit (2SM253). In quietness and confidence should be our strength (Isa 30:15). The assumption of a NEGATIVE outcome causes worry. Hence, THINKING POSITIVELY, as many preachers have indicated, is the proper attitude. If we have done all we can in a situation, we should cease worrying and go calmly about other pressing duties. It is then no longer our problem but God's (5T347). Then for the Christian to leave things in God's hands is the most beneficial mental attitude. (TM201).

✓ WE TRY TOO HARD—God is our helper in any condition of life, but many times we feel that we have to do these things all by ourselves. We are often trying to do things which we should allow God to do. "We try too hard to take care of ourselves. We are uneasy and greatly lack a firm trust in God. Many worry and work, contrive and plan, fearing they may suffer need. They cannot afford time to pray or to attend religious meetings, and in their care for themselves leave no chance for God to care for them. And the Lord does not do much for them, for they give Him no opportunity. They do too much for themselves and BELIEVE and TRUST in God too little." (2T196).

✓ WE SHOULD LET GOD PLAN OUR FUTURE—We are told that it is not for us to shape our future, because we do not have enough wisdom to plan our own lives. "Christ, in His life on earth, made no plans for Himself. He accepted God's plan for Him, and day by day the Father unfolded His plans. So should we depend upon God, that our lives may be the simple outworking of His will. As we commit our ways to Him, He will direct our steps…. God never leads His children otherwise than they would choose to be led, if they could see the end from the beginning, and discern the glory of the purpose which they are fulfilling as coworkers with Him" (MH478–9). So we are admonished, "Do not worry. By looking at appearances and complaining when difficulty and pressure come, you reveal a sickly, enfeebled faith" (7T212). By our words and works we are to show that our faith is invincible.

"God is our refuge in sickness and in health. But many do not leave their cases with Him; they encourage weakness and disease by worrying about themselves. If they would cease repining and rise above depression and gloom, their recovery would be more certain" (5T315)

◆ *What Science Has Discovered About Worry*

✓ UNCERTAINTY—is the No. 1 stressor regarding those future "what ifs." and past "if only's." It is those things that we don't know and can't do anything about that can really hurt us. Here is where the Christian again has a great advantage over the worldling. If our life is in the hand of God, He will see us through the difficulties of life as well as through the pleasant experiences, and we can safely trust our future in His hands without worrying about it.

Rats given electric shocks WITHOUT WARNINGS developed gastric complications at a greater rate than when they were given WARNINGS. This means that we also perform best when we are given some idea of what to expect. With God the future is an open book. That is why God has given us PROPHECIES regarding the future so we know what to expect so that we can make adjustments beforehand.

✓ PEPTIC ULCERS—increased by 50% among people living in the center of London during World War I

Extended periods of FEELING HELPLESS can depress the immune system and increase disease possibilities. Men internalize their feelings more, hold their anger, and cover up their worries more than do women. They also get more ulcers than women.

✓ PROBLEMS WITHIN AND OUTSIDE OUR CONTROL—The ones outside our control are not worth worrying about. To remain in mental health, we must act on problems that are within our power to resolve. ULCERS are the rewards earned by worries.

✓ EXERCISE and TALKING TO FRIENDS— are two remedies for allaying worries.

◆ *Fear*

✓ THERE IS NO FEAR IN LOVE—1 John 4:18 tells us, "There is no fear in LOVE, but perfect love casteth out fear: because fear hath torment. He that feareth is not made perfect in love." Also we should not fear what other people might do to us (Isa 8:12), we should let God be our fear (Isa 8:13). There is also no fear with Christ, "The Lord is my helper and I will not fear what man shall do unto me" (Hebr. 13:6). God says: "Fear not for I am with thee" (Isa 43:15), and He wants us to know that He has redeemed us (Isa 43:1). As David once said, "I will fear no evil for thou art with me" (Ps. 23:4), and God admonishes us to abide with Him and fear not (1 Sam. 22:23). "God has not given us the spirit of fear; but of power, and of love, and of a sound mind" (2 Tim. 1:7). "The fear (or respect) of the Lord is the beginning of wisdom" (Prov. 9:10).

ABSENCE OF FAITH BRINGS FEAR— It is the absence of faith and trust that brings distressing fear (2T140). Those who have little faith are always fearing and borrowing trouble (GW261). Those who continue to fear create greater fears (4T558). A lack of fear comes from DEPENDENCE UPON DIVINE POWER. It gives us a peaceful attitude if we do not overemphasize our feelings and emotions (TM518). Mahatma Ghandi once said, "There is nothing to fear, but fear itself," and President Franklin D. Roosevelt echoed the same sentiments. To achieve peace of mind, we have to give ourselves to God and others, and thereby achieve the removal of fear. Health is inner peace, therefore healing is letting go of fear.

✓ A GUILTY CONSCIENCE BRINGS FEAR— There develops an attitude of fear if we have a guilty conscience due to doing what we shouldn't have done. Guilt creates fear (PP330). If we will confess our sins we will quiet our fears and will have peace with God (2T301), We should not fear because God is with us (Isa 43:5), but if God is not with us, then Satan can use fear to rule our conscience (GC591), but the sense of God's presence will banish all fear (Ed. 255). If we lack faith, then our perplexities will increase. If we fear that FOOD will hurt us, then it certainly will (2T530). Someone has said that since fear in the form of hell fire and brimstone is no longer preached from the pulpit, people are living longer. A morality which is kept in bounds by fear is health-destroying. Man was taught to fear God and to love Him at the same time, but wherever fear is real, there is no love. To respect God is wisdom (Pr. 1:7).

✓ TRUSTING IN RICHES WILL INCREASE OUR FEAR OF LOSING THEM—If in the world we put our trust in money, it will increase our fear of losing it (CO51). We are told not to trust in uncertain riches (1 Tim. 6:17). Where our treasure is there will our heart be also (Luke 12:34). We have nothing to fear of the future, except as we forget how God has led us in the past (TM31).

✓ FEAR OF MAN—We should say, "The Lord is my helper, and I will not fear what man shall do unto me" (Hebr. 13:6). We are told not to fear them "which kill the body, but are not able to kill the soul: but rather fear him which is able to destroy both soul and body in hell" (Matt. 10:28). Witherspoon said, "It is only the fear of God that can deliver us from the fear of man."

The story is told of a man by the name of Jim Vaus, who had been a wiretapper for an infamous underworld gang of Mickey Cohen in Los Angeles. He was converted during one of Billy Graham's crusades there. The newspaper gave him a big write-up. He read the write-up and thought about what action the gangsters might take about this matter. After all he knew a host of secrets that might send some of the gang members to the penitentiary or to the gas chamber. From the gang's viewpoint he had become a traitor to them. He didn't have long to wait, for as he looked out of the window, a big limousine stopped in front of his house. Jim recognized the men who emerged as some of the most heartless killers of the underworld. Looking carefully up and down the street, they approached his front door. Did he become panicky and make for the back door? He had reason to flee but he didn't. In his earlier life he would have run or fled for his life. That morning when he opened his Bible he had read from Proverbs 16:7: "When a man's ways please the Lord, he maketh even his enemies to be at peace with him." He opened the door and they told him that a wiretapping job had been assigned to him in St. Louis. Jim told him that he couldn't do it because the Lord had changed his heart. When he described his conversion his visitors looked bewildered and left. Jim knew that the Lord had protected him from fear and had preserved his life and his health — Love casteth out fear.

✓ SCIENCE AND FEAR—Fear produces conditions that makes a person less healthy. It is a degenerative and decaying influence.

- ☛ Fear grows with indulgence.
  In a study students who felt that they didn't "fit in" had a lower number of natural killer cells than students who felt comfortable with themselves and their environment.
  When a 6 month old monkey is separated from its mother, its ability to fight off an infection is reduced 10 fold. Even if mother and baby are reunited on the same day, the immune function may stay depressed for weeks and months. This means that bad experiences may leave us open to infection and disease for a long time after the experience.
- ☛ Fear inhibits action. It takes courage to let the unexpected happen. Fear of death immobilizes us.
- ☛ Fear of all kinds inhibits learning, such as the fear of failure.
- ☛ Fear depletes the body of nutrients, and prevents healing.
- ☛ Fear in both children and adults, is the greatest of all causes of ENERVATION
- ☛ Fear can cause the BLOOD to DRAIN from the FACE, the HEART TO POUND, the PALMS to SWEAT, the MUSCLES to TREMBLE. Emotional distress can lead to HYPERTENSION, ALLERGIES, SKIN ERUPTIONS, COLITIS, as well as MENTAL and NERVOUS BREAKDOWNS.

✓ OVERCOMING FEAR—The only meaningful choice is between LOVE and FEAR. FORGIVENESS is the way to true health and happiness. By not judging others we release the past and let go of our fear of the future. One solution to fear is to limit our thoughts largely to the present. COURAGE, HOPE, FAITH, SYMPATHY, and LOVE, promote health and prolong life. A contented mind, a cheerful spirit, is health to the body and strength to the soul. "A merry heart doeth good like a medicine" (Prov. 17:22). The most powerful force is the force of a warm, loving, caring relationship, marked by openness, honesty, and sharing.

✓ PHOBIAS—are IRRATIONAL FEARS. There is no logical reason for them. Knowing that fears are unfounded doesn't lessen the panic, The body cannot sustain this aroused level of anxiety indefinitely. It is involuntary and inappropriate to the situation. TRANQUILIZERS are not effective. The typical diet of a PHOBIC include 8 cups of coffee a day, and a lot of sweets. In some cases a change in DIET has worked. Irrational fears obstruct our goals, blocking us from taking action.

When a woman stopped drinking coffee her fear level dropped by half. Phobics are often linked with HYPOGLYCEMIA or low blood sugar. It is suggested that phobics eat NUTS, RAISINS, and SEEDS to bring up their blood sugar levels. They are often addicted to SWEETS, to HYDROGENATED FATS, WHITE BREAD and OVERPROCESSED CEREALS, which produce MALNUTRITION.

PUBLIC SPEAKING is the premier fear of Americans, followed by fear of HEIGHTS, BUGS, MONEY PROBLEMS, DEEP WATER, SICKNESS, DEATH, FLYING. and LONELINESS.

◆ *Hate*

✓ TRUE CHRISTIANS CANNOT HATE—The Bible tells us to LOVE our ENEMIES, to BLESS them that CURSE us, to do GOOD to them that HATE us, and to PRAY for them that despitefully use us and PERSECUTE us (Matt. 5:44). A heart of love cannot hate anyone. Everyone for whom Christ died is our brother, whom we therefore cannot hate (Lev. 19:17). We should not respond in the same hateful manner in which others may treat us. God's love subdues enmity in converted hearts (4T223), and changes enmity into love (MB77). We should remember that we have enemies only because others make themselves our enemies, but we should never make ourselves their enemies.

✓ RESPOND TO HATE WITH LOVE—Matt. 5:44 tells us to do good to them that hate us. This means that we should respond to those who hate us with an attitude opposite to that which they show toward us. "Be not overcome of evil, but overcome evil with good" (Rom. 12:21). First of all we may say that hate breeds hate, but also that love breeds love. When we respond with love, we are responding with good emotions which safeguard our own well-being. Secondly, we are responding in such a manner as to possibly create a better attitude, that of love, in the other person. We should remember that "a soft answer turneth away wrath" (Pr. 15:1). We are also told that it is our privilege to help change the world for the better. Furthermore, we are admonished to not let there be any "shadow of hate, or ill will, no bitterness or sourness of expression. Nothing but kindness and gentleness can flow from a heart of love" (2T52). The Holy Spirit alone gives love for hatred (MB75). This means that we should pray to have the Holy Spirit live in our hearts, so that only love will reign therein. Hatred cannot exist in a heart that is at peace with God and fellow men (MB28). Love is a brain tonic and a healer.

✓ THE ONLY THING THAT WE SHOULD HATE IS EVIL—If we have love in the heart for the Lord, we will hate evil (Ps. 97:10). If we have fear or respect for the Lord, we will also hate evil (Pr. 8;13). We will not only refrain from engaging in a wrong emotion, which is destructive to us and others, but we will take a positive attitude of doing good to them that hate us. The WORDS OF HATE are registered in the books of heaven (AH362), and they are listed under the general heading of JEALOUSY (4T385).

✓ SATAN PROMPTS MEN TO HATE—It is Satan who influences men to hate one another. (PP337). The spirit of hate originated with him (MB56). It represents his principle (7T126). In the final analysis hatred leads to murder, and Satan was a murderer from the beginning (Jo. 8:44). That is his nature, and when we are living out his principles, then we are on his side, helping the cause which he espouses, and are doing our part to advance it. The TEN COMMANDMENTS, which are a decalogue of love, forbid the spirit of hatred (PP308). It is contrary to God's nature, and as children of God, it should be contrary to ours. Sinners are Satan's helpers, and like Satan they are at enmity with God and with one another (DA305).

✓ SCIENCE AND HATE—People who are hostile, who act as though the whole world is against them, are the ones who die early.

You can tell that you are hostile if you find that you are imputing evil motives to other people.
One way to get rid of hostility is to be more religious. Every one of the world's religions tells us to treat others the same way we want to be treated. If you do this then there is no room in your heart for hostility.
Feelings of hostility are responsible for increasing the death rate 5 to 7 times among otherwise healthy people.
A study revealed that OPTIMISTS healed faster, went home sooner, had fewer complications' and were significantly less likely to experience a heart attack after surgery than pessimists.
Physical problems which originate in emotional problems require that the emotional problem

be released first. No doctor can help a patient with arthritis who refuses to give up hate and resentment.

No case of ulcers can be really healed until the marriage or job problem is taken care of.

The asthma and allergies cannot be cured until mother and father give the child the love it needs.

Excessive excitement can break down the CEREBELLUM. The breaking down of the cerebellum can produce HEADACHES, LOSS of AMBITION, FEAR of SOCIETY, and an INCLINATION to SOLITUDE.

The EXECUTIVE DILEMMA is that there is a high price to pay, brain-wise, for coping with high responsibilities, stress, important decisions, and critical thinking.

HOSTILITY is the key trait that puts the "Type A' personality at risk of an early HEART ATTACK.

◆ *Anxiety*

✓ TAKE NO THOUGHT FOR TOMORROW—"Take no thought for your life, what ye shall eat, or what ye shall drink; nor yet for your body, what ye shall put on. Is not the life more than meat, and the body more than raiment? Behold the fowls of the air: for they sow not, neither do they reap, nor gather into barns; yet your heavenly father feedeth them. Are ye not much better than they? Which of you by taking thought can add one cubit to his stature? And why take ye thought for raiment? Consider the lilies of the field, how they grow; they toil not neither do they spin: and yet I say unto you, that even Solomon in all his glory was not arrayed like one of these. Wherefore if God so clothe the grass of the field, which today is, and tomorrow is cast into the oven, shall he not much more clothe you, O ye of little faith?" (Matt. 6:25–30)

✓ ANXIETY CANNOT REMEDY A SINGLE EVIL—"When we take into our hands the management of things with which we have to do, and depend upon our own wisdom for success, we are taking a burden which God has not given us, and are trying to bear it without his aid. We are taking upon ourselves responsibility which belongs to God, and are really putting ourselves in his place. We may well have anxiety, and anticipate danger and loss; for it is certain to befall us. But when we really believe that God loves us, and means to do us good, we shall cease to worry about the future. We shall trust God as a child trusts a loving parent. Then our troubles and torments will disappear, for our will is swallowed up in the will of God. Faith lightens the burden of anxiety" (PP600). Anxiety cannot remedy one evil (AH431). ANXIETY, DISTRUST, GRIEF, GUILT and REMORSE all tend to break down the life forces and to invite decay and death.

✓ GOD'S GRACE IS SUFFICIENT FOR US—Christ has given us no promise of help in bearing today the burdens of tomorrow. God has said, "My grace is sufficient for you" (2 Cor. 12:9). This grace is bestowed daily, for the day's need. "If you have given yourself to God to do his work, you have no need to be anxious for tomorrow. He whose servant you are, knows the end from the beginning. The events of tomorrow, which are hidden from your view, are open to the eyes of him who is omnipotent. Like the hosts of Israel in their pilgrim life, we may find morning by morning the bread of heaven for the day's supply. One day alone is ours, and during this day we are to live for God. For this one day we are to place in the hand of Christ, in solemn service, all our purposes and plans, casting all our care upon Him, for He careth for us" (SD119).

✓ ANXIETY AND DISEASE—"Because God's love is so great, and so unfailing, the sick should be encouraged to trust in Him. To be anxious about themselves tends to cause weakness and disease. If they will rise above depression and gloom, their prospect of recovery will be better; for the eye of the Lord is upon them that hope in His mercy" (MH22). Anxiety breaks down health (MH241); It is generally harmful (AH431); It means borrowing trouble (2T72); It cannot remedy a single evil (AH431); The life forces are crushed by it. It is usually about worldly things which should not be made supreme (CS159); and we are told that we should have no anxiety regarding whether we are saved or not (SC72).

✓ SCIENCE AND ANXIETY—It has been scientifically established that emotional stresses and disturbances can cause practically any disease in the medical dictionary, including ARTHRITIS, ULCERS, CONSTIPATION, ASTHMA, STROKES, DIABETES, HIGH and LOW BLOOD PRESSURE, ANGINA, GLANDULAR DISTURBANCES, ETC. Happy people rarely get these diseases.

Disclosing feelings of mental pain and distress suffered in the past by the hands of relatives or loved ones hurts, and is emotionally upsetting, but getting them off one's chest is a liberating feeling, and mentally beneficial in the long run. Such people have few health complaints, and fewer doctor visits. Confession is good for the soul as well as for the body. In the mind a covered-over negative event, composed of negative thoughts and feelings is never finished. That is why CONFESSION, SELF-DISCLOSURE, and CONFIDING IN OTHERS is so rewarding mentally and physically. Confiding in God is best of all.

According to president Carter's Commission on Mental Health 15% of all Americans (32 million) require some form of mental health services. 25% of the population suffers severe emotional stress. That means that 40% require some mental health treatment. Is it any wonder that tranquilizers sell so well?

Repression can fool only the mind, not the body. The body responds to unconscious processes.

Anxiety is a nameless dread. When one concentrates on ones pain, it becomes more acute.

PLACEBOS help the patient get better 35% of the time.

Anxiety can be converted into bodily symptoms. It is harmful when it interferes with our effectiveness, achievement of goals, or emotional comfort.

HOW TO OVERCOME ANXIETY—We should not allow the perplexities of every day life to cloud our vision. Life is what we make it, and we will make it much better with Christ, with laying all our burdens upon Him. Anxiety shows upon our faces, and as Christians, it gives the wrong impression to others. We must cultivate the attitude of cheerfulness instead of being anxious about the solutions to problems that come our way. If we succumb to them, we are sacrificing health and happiness to a morbid imagination (AH430). Such expressions of emotions are a great injury to us health-wise.

They interfere with our nutrition by hindering the process of digestion (AH431). We are told that Mrs. White was never fearful in adversity. She said that she had a faith which forbad her being anxious. It is a lack of genuine religion that produces gloom, despondency, and sadness. We are to bring cheer to others and make the world a better place through our having lived here. But this we cannot do when we can't even cheer ourselves up.

GOD'S ATTITUDE TOWARD ANXIETY—Anxiety displeases God (CS159), and grieves the Holy Spirit (PP294). Christ rebukes our anxiety (CS227), and asks us to lay off such a heavy yoke which He does not want us to bear (PP294), for it does not help us in our spiritual growth. Anxiety can be lightened by faith (PP600). God watches everything that happens to us. There are no tears shed that God does not notice. If we could fully believe this, then we would not regard anxiety as a necessary part of life. If we regard Him in faith, our life would not be so filled with disappointments, for then everything would be left in the hand of God. He wants us to present all our anxieties to Him, and leave them with Him for Him to take care of.

◆ *Envy*

✓ BE CONTENT WITH WHAT YOU HAVE—ENVY is a resentful awareness of an advantage enjoyed by another, and a desire to enjoy the same advantage. It is implied that we are unhappy about the advantage possessed by someone else. It is caused by a lack of HOLINESS (2T445). Phil. 4:11 tells us that in whatever state we are in, we are to be content therewith. And Hebr. 13:5 tells us "Be content with such things as ye have." We should be content with what we have, for that is the amount that God believes we can handle at the moment. In this connection we should remember the parable of the talents. It teaches us that God has distributed various diverse talents to people, and that we should be satisfied with what has been given us, provided that we are making the best use of them. God has distributed them as he sees fit, and we should accept that fact. For this reason we are told that we should not envy one another (Gal. 5:26).

✓ ENVY IS THE OFFSPRING OF PRIDE—To envy a person is to believe him to be superior, and pride will not permit any concessions (5T56). "Envy is the offspring of pride, and if it is entertained in the heart, it will lead to hatred, and eventually to revenge and murder" (PP651). It is a sinful emotion (1SM217). It was envy that made Saul miserable and put David in danger of his life.

✓ LOVE ENVIES NOT—If we have a loving attitude toward our brethren and fellowmen, we will not envy what they have either in personal talents or in other possessions. 1 Cor. 13:4 tells us that LOVE does not envy. And especially should we not envy those who are not living up to all of the light which the Lord has shed upon their pathway, nor should we envy evil men. We are admonished to lay aside all envies (1 Pet. 2:1)

✓ ENVY IS SATAN'S WORK—Envy began with Satan in heaven (5T56), which means that it began with sin (CG79). It is an attribute of Satan, a part of his character (FE278), the fruit of pride and ambition (5T242). Since it is part of his character, he seeks to incite envy among the brethren of God's people (PP403). In heaven envy caused discord and strife (PP385). It changed the good into that which is evil. Jam. 3:16 says, "Where envy is there is confusion and every evil work." It is engendered by those individuals who are accusers of the brethren (3BC1162). The Holy Spirit must uproot it from the heart (AH196).

✓ THE RESULTS OF ENVYING—We are told that the envious shuts his eyes to the good qualities and noble deeds of others, and that envy disorders all of man's faculties (5T56). Pr. 14:30 says: "A sound heart is the life of the flesh: but envy the rottenness of the bones." In the case of its development in children, it is caused by parental neglect (FE67). Every cherished envy leads to evil deeds which include HATRED, REVENGE, and MURDER. (PP651). The heart cannot harbor envy and still be at peace with God or men (MB28). God's law condemns the emotion of envy (SD61), and it will finally exclude a man from heaven (4T453).

◆ *Jealousy*

✓ JEALOUSY—A HOSTILE ATTITUDE—Jealousy is a hostile attitude toward a person who is believed to enjoy an advantage. Envy and jealousy are attitudes of comparison between people. Since people are created unequal in many ways, it is not good to compare ourselves with others, for God has given different people different talents, and it is therefore not good for them to size themselves up to others with more or others with fewer talents. Paul tells us that they who measure themselves by themselves and compare themselves among themselves are not wise (2 Cor. 10:12). We are told that emulation and rivalry foster selfishness the root of all evil (Ed. 226). Jealousy is a poisonous plant sown by Satan (AH196). When it comes to comparing ourselves with anybody, the only person that we should compare ourselves with is Christ. Here we are told that "He who possesses love compares only the loveliness of Christ and his own imperfect character" (COL402).

✓ JEALOUSY—A SINFUL EMOTION—Jealousy is a negative, destructive, and sinful emotion which God's law condemns. It represents a hostile attitude toward others for whom Christ has died also, and whom we should therefore also love as our friends. Regardless of what advantage someone else may enjoy, we should rejoice with him for such an advantage, which he may be able to use for better service in God's cause. For this we should be glad. Continued jealousy causes mental unhappiness (1T708), and has a destructive influence upon the whole being. God does not want us to destroy our body temple. It is the fruit of selfishness, a sin which we should put away. Other negative attitudes that follow from Jealousy are ENVY and MALICE, which is a wish to cause someone else harm.

✓ SATAN—THE INSTIGATOR OF JEALOUSY — Jealousy began with sin, which means that it began with Satan (CG79), the originator of this sin, when he desired to occupy a place in heaven which was the prerogative of Christ alone. Christ had a higher position than Satan in heaven, and Satan coveted that higher position. Jealousy is one of Satan's attributes, and if we partake of Jealousy it blinds us to the reality of what actually exists (PP383). With such an attitude we become one of Satan's instruments for creating more evil in this world. Jealousy represents a demonic attitude, for in the case of Saul, we are told that the demon of jealousy entered him (PP650). Saul was jealous of David because the people praised David more highly than Saul. They said that Saul had slain thousands, but that David had slain ten thousands. The brother of the prodigal son harbored jealousy, because after the prodigal son had made a big mistake in his life, he was treated more royally than his brother who had not made any big mistakes. Eve was jealous of God because He withheld the forbidden fruit from her.

✓ THE RESULTS OF JEALOUSY—Jealousy interprets to us things to the injury of others (5T95). We should therefore not allow jealousy to come into our hearts (TM505). It closes our door to the Holy Spirit (AA271). Children learn jealousy from their parents (4T196). We are told that DOUBT is caused by jealousy (1T708). ENVY usually follows jealousy, and REBELLION follows after that (3T346). Jealousy manifests itself in the countenance (CSW113), which is a result of the mental unhappiness it causes (1T708). It further leads to unrest and dissatisfaction. (2T572).

✓ GODLY JEALOUSY—Jealousy can be something good if it is applied to something good. For example, Paul says to the Corinthian believers, "I am jealous over you with godly jealousy" (2 Cor. 11:2). God says that He will be jealous "for my holy name" (Eze. 39:25). In Joshua He tells us that He is a jealous God (Joshua 24:19). Throughout history God has been jealous for His people, His commandments, His principles. This means that He has such a high regard for them all, that He is going to protect them at all times.

◆ *Anger And Wrath*

✓ RIGHTEOUS INDIGNATION—ANGER represents a strong feeling of displeasure. WRATH is a vengeful anger. There is such a thing as RIGHTEOUS ANGER or INDIGNATION, when that which is good is made of none effect, or when that which is holy is desecrated. This is no doubt of what Christ felt when He cleansed the temple twice. Generally, however, we should not readily give in to anger or wrath. It is said of God that He is slow to anger (Ps. 145:8), and we should be such likewise. It is said that "He that is slow to wrath is of great understanding" (Pr. 14:29) When we are facing a wrathful person we are also admonished that "A SOFT ANSWER turneth away wrath" (Pr. 15:1), and sometimes it is best to say nothing at all in the face of anger, for we are admonished that "anger quickly dies away when met with SILENCE" (MH486).

✓ IT IS BEST TO AVOID ANGER AND WRATH—In most cases anger and wrath are such upsetting emotions that it is better to avoid them if at all possible. They have a ruinous effect on health (Ed. 197). We are therefore to "cease from anger and forsake wrath" (Ps. 37:8). We are told to "give place unto wrath" (Rom. 12:19), and that what is done in anger is not excusable (4T243), for anger has an effect on the mind, so that under such circumstances we cannot think straight, for anger dethrones reason (4T431) Anger and wrath are commonly engaged in as forms of revenge, but God has told us, "Vengeance is mine; I will repay, saith the Lord" (Rom. 12:19).

✓ PARENTS SHOULD NOT PUNISH CHILDREN IN ANGER—Eph. 6:4 tells us, "And, ye fathers, provoke not your children to wrath; but bring them up in the nurture and admonition of the Lord." When children need correction, the parents should ask the Lord to give them wisdom in dealing with them. The child to be punished should never be given the feeling that they have been punished in anger, for in doing so a greater evil will be worked.... "Be firm with them, but do not let Satan control them. Discipline them only when you are under the discipline of God" (CG245). What is done in anger is not excusable (4T243) If you are OUT OF CONTROL, you cannot develop SELF-CONTROL in the child. Anger opens the heart to Satan. (DA310). An uncontrolled anger is a demonic anger. Those who practice the casting out of demons have found that a demonic anger allows Satan to move from the mother into the child to possess it, so that the indulgence of anger makes us servants of sin and of evil (2T52).

To Trust In God Means To Eliminate Our Bad Habits

◆ *Our Faith Must Be Made Perfect By Works*

We are told that "It is labor lost to teach people to go to God as a healer of their infirmities, unless they are educated also to lay aside every wrong practice" (HL1015). "Many have expected that God would keep them from sickness merely because they have asked Him to do so. But God did not regard their prayers because their faith was not made perfect by works. But God will not work a miracle to keep those from sickness who have no care for themselves, but are continually violating the laws of health, and make no effort to PREVENT DISEASE. When we do all we can on our part to have health, then we may expect that the blessed results will follow" (HL1016). You will suffer for every sin which you commit against yourself. Not one such sin is forgiven, meaning that the consequences of such sins will remain, and will exercise an effect upon the system. Every act or practice has either a good or a bad effect. "Whatsoever a man soweth that shall he also reap" (Gal. 6:7).

◆ *The Prayer Of Faith Shall Save The Sick*

"Is any sick among you? let him call for the elders of the church; and let them pray over him with oil in the name of the Lord: And the prayer of faith shall save the sick, and the Lord shall raise him up; and if he have committed sins, they shall be forgiven him" (Jam. 5:14–5). But "If we regard iniquity in our hearts, the Lord will not hear us" (Ps. 66:18). God is always willing to restore the sick to health, but He expects them to do what they can to have health. They must change the natural causes of their disease which they can control. In one test 86% of the people said that prayer helped relieve their tension.

◆ *Every Precious Promise Will Be Fulfilled*

"Christ is the same compassionate physician now that he was during his earthly ministry. In Him there is healing balm for every disease, restoring power for every infirmity. His disciples in this time are to pray for the sick as verily as the disciples of old did. And recoveries will follow; for 'The PRAYER OF FAITH shall save the sick'. We have the Holy Spirit's power, the calm assurance of faith, that can claim God's promises" (MH225–7). "If we live according to his word, every precious promise He has given will be fulfilled to us" (MH227).

Take your troubles to God in prayer. Jesus will forgive your sins if you ask Him. For He has promised, "If we confess our sins, He is faithful and just to forgive us our sins, and to cleanse us from all unrighteousness" (1 Jo. 1:9). If we lack wisdom to do what we ought to do, we should ask God, and He will give it to us (Jam. 1:5).

Sinful Desires

◆ *Our Desires Must Conform To God's Moral Standard*

Everyone has desires to do this and that, to have this and that, and to be this or that. Many desires are beneficial to the individual if accomplished, and some may be harmful to him if he realized them. From God's standpoint our desires must conform to God's moral standard; they must come from a conscience illuminated by divine grace (FE118).

◆ *Sinful Desires Strengthen The Soul's Aversion To God*

There may be desires which are not in harmony with God's moral standard, and such desires will turn out to be harmful to the individual and possibly to others also. They may be called SINFUL DESIRES which oppose the teachings of the standards which God has set up for our conduct, and which are conducive to harm and self-destruction. We are told that "Sinful desire strengthens the soul's aversion to God, and will eventually neutralize all the power of the gospel" (SC34). If we look at the 10th commandment of the Decalogue, this commandment regarding coveting is a commandment which forbids sinful or selfish desires (SD65). It demands purity in such desires. Sinful desires allows Satan to get a foothold in our heart, and induces us to compromise our integrity and to contaminate the soul (DA125).

◆ *Children Should Not Be Allowed To Indulge In Selfish Desires*

We are also admonished not to allow children to indulge in selfish desires (CT113), for sinful acts spring from selfish desires. We are told that unholy desires are created by the reading of immoral books such as novels (MYP277). Such bad habits must be changed. But alone we cannot change them. "God alone can give victory over evil desires, man cannot conquer them" (MB 142). With the help of God we must exercise severe discipline so as to hold our desires in subjection to reason and conscience (5T177).

All Negative Emotions Represent Stress

◆ *Accepting Bible Principles*

We are told that "they that are Christ's have crucified the flesh with the affections and lusts" (Gal. 5:24). One doctor has said that the sincere acceptance of the principles of Christ with respect to the life of mental peace and joy, the life of unselfish thought and clean living, would at once wipe out more than half the difficulties, diseases, and sorrows of the human race, and that it would pay any man or woman to live the Christlike life just for the mental and moral rewards here in this present world. A clear conscience is a great step toward barricading the mind against NEUROTICISM. Henry C. Link, the author of *The Return To Religion,* said: "The emphasis on SIN has largely disappeared from the teachings of religion at the very time when psychology has discovered its importance and extended meanings."

What a person eats is not as important as the bitter spirit of hate and the feelings of guilt that eat him. We must eliminate the acids that destroy body, mind, and soul. The medicine is given in Col. 3:13–14 — "Forbearing one another, and forgiving one another, if any man have a quarrel against any: even as Christ forgave you, so also do ye. And above all these things put on CHARITY, which is the bond of perfectness." Love is the antidote that can save man from the many diseases produced by the emotions of our evil nature.

◆ *Stress Can Cause Disease*

Stress tends to shut down the immune system, and the possibility to disease is increased. Good health depends LESS ON MEDICINE than on ADAPTATION TO THE ENVIRONMENT. Stress can cause increased PLATELET CLUMPING, VASOCONSTRICTION, or the narrowing of blood vessels, a SUPPRESSION of the IMMUNE SYSTEM which can cause a HEART ATTACK, a STROKE, or other diseases. We know that such stressful situations as ASTHMA and PEPTIC ULCER are more common in urban centers than in rural areas. We probably need to give modern civilization the credit for allowing us to achieve heightened enjoyments but at certain stressful costs to the human system. When too many adjustments have to be made by the human organism in an environment that is changing too fast for us to adjust ourselves to, there develop conditions of maladjustment which conditions represent great stresses upon the system. It doesn't matter that much whether or not the events are good or bad.

◆ *Mental Stress Brings On Physical Stress*

Excitement in almost any form is a stress upon the organism, and a stress being a depriver of organic energy, can, if repeated too often, bring about a disease condition. For example, the death of a spouse can very likely bring about a disease condition. A woman with cancer had a remission for 3 years, but when her son went into the army she had a relapse. Even a small infant whose mother is not too interested in him can develop a peptic ulcer. We are told that "depressing emotions do great injury to health by hindering digestion, and interfering with nutrition."(AH431). We are even told that ROBBING GOD brings sickness (2T199). Researchers Holmes and Rahe studied 5000 individuals with reference to their reactions to events in their life, ranging from Christmas to the death of a spouse. They found that the higher your total stress score, the more likely you were to become ILL. On a scale of a hundred the most stressful event is the DEATH OF A SPOUSE (100), the next stressful event is DIVORCE (73), and the next is the death of a MEMBER OF THE FAMILY (63). Marriage has a 50 point stress rating.

How To Overcome Mental Disease

◆ *Overcoming Sin*

Sin is no doubt the greatest problem in mental disease. Doing wrong is detrimental to both mind and body. Doing right and keeping our thoughts in the right channels is beneficial mental discipline (MYP149), and strict compliance with God's requirements is beneficial to mental health. Remorse for sin undermines the constitution and unbalances the mind. The physician must first gain the confidence of the individual and then point him to the Great Healer (MH244). Sometimes sympathy and tact is of more benefit than treatment. We should give more expression to our faith, rejoice more in the blessings that result from appreciating the goodness and love of God. (MH253). We should not talk of our lack of faith and of our sorrows and sufferings. Also we should not dwell on the great power of Satan to overcome us. Often we give ourselves into his hands by talking of his power.

◆ *Center Your Mind Upon Others*

One of the surest hindrances to the recovery of the sick is the centering of attention upon oneself (MH256). We should forget self and place our INTEREST IN OTHERS—those who are more needy than ourselves, then we would realize the promise "then shall thy health spring forth speedily" (Isa 58:8). "The CONSCIOUSNESS OF RIGHT DOING is one of the best medicines for diseased bodies and minds. GOOD DEEDS are TWICE A BLESSING, benefiting both the giver and the receiver of the kindness" (MH257).

◆ *A Good Lifestyle*

If you have built for yourself a strong foundation by eating a good kind of diet, and by maintaining sufficient physical activity, you will be able to stand more stress. We must distinguish between an unhealthy stress and a healthy stress. A healthy stress is a challenge of some type, while an unhealthy stress is an enervating unpleasant experience. An unhealthy stress, as well as some healthy stresses that are overdone, produce ADRENALINE which causes blood flow restriction and can trigger a heart attack. Modifying one's activity to avoid stress is as important as any other lifestyle recommendation. COMPULSIVE EATING is in general not a good way to relieve stress. Such a habit will contribute to excess weight, and it will stress your gastrointestinal system. The drug stress relievers of TOBACCO, ALCOHOL, and CAFFEINE are not recommended as stress relievers. They tend to change stress to disease in their effect upon the human constitution. Caffeine can cause HEADACHES, RESTLESSNESS, DIGESTIVE PROBLEMS, HEART ARRHYTHMIAS, AND HYPERTENSION. The one activity that is really beneficial in relieving stress is AEROBIC EXERCISE. It will immediately and directly provide tangible benefits in reducing stress and promoting relaxation by releasing ENDORPHINS in the body which reduce pain and thereby contribute to bodily comfort. REST and SLEEP are also excellent eliminators of stress. Dealing with stress effectively is a matter of dealing with life effectively. Talking about one's true feelings, fears, worries, and hopes with a friend without having to worry about being embarrassed is very helpful. And the best friend we have is Jesus Himself. We are admonished to speak to Him as to a friend.

APPLYING THE THREE A'S OF ACCEPT, APPROVE, AND ADORE

Accept—Appreciation

✓ Accept things as they are. You cannot readily change them. You will be happier if you adjust yourself to them.

✓ Practice the art of accepting. In so doing we come to see that everyone is our teacher, and that every circumstance is an opportunity for growth in happiness, peace, and love. Wrong emotions disappear when the mind is focused on loving peace.

✓ Our inner peace will be transferred to others once we accept it for ourselves.

✓ Healing proceeds faster when people accept each other's feelings, and when they are expressed to others. Share your experiences. The only condition is not to be judgmental but forgiving.

✓ "Every 'Thou shalt not' implies a promise. If we obey it blessing will attend our steps" (MH114)

✓ "Come unto me,...and I will give you rest" is a prescription for the healing of physical, mental, and spiritual ills" (MH115).

✓ "Faith in God's power to heal infirmities is dead unless the one diseased improves the light God has given him by bringing his habits into line with right principles" (MM262).

Approve—Praise

✓ Try to be agreeable if at all possible. It will make you feel good.

- ✓ "The assurance of God's approval will promote physical health. It fortifies the soul against doubt, perplexity, and excessive grief, that so often sap the vital forces and induce nervous diseases of a most debilitating and distressing character" (LS270)
- ✓ Positive thinking is beneficial.

Adore—Love

- ✓ To receive affection show affection. Lose yourself in others. It will block out depression, make us less aware of our inadequacies, and help surmount our personal problems.
- ✓ Resolve that we look for signs of love in another person. Put others before yourself.
- ✓ Giving is receiving. Thereby fear is removed, and we accept healing for ourselves.
- ✓ When alone spend time creatively. Loneliness may be affection deprivation.
- ✓ Pets can satisfy the need for affection, and they can help improve one's rapport with people.
- ✓ The heart must be filled with hope, love, joy, in order to have health (CH587).
- ✓ Psychiatrist Alfred Adler wrote: "The most important task imposed by religion has always been 'Love Thy Neighbor'. It is the individual who is not interested in his fellow man who has the greatest difficulties in life and who provides the greatest injury to others. It is from such individuals that human failures spring." He observed that the "lack of love" was indicated in all human failures after analyzing thousands of patients. Evil emotions must be overcome by good emotions, and the greatest good emotion is LOVE (1 COR. 13:13)

THE WORK OF OUR SANITARIUMS

PURPOSE OF OUR SANITARIUMS

To Reform The Medical Practices of Physicians

Mrs. White says that "The light was first given to me why institutions should be established, that is, sanitariums were to reform the medical practices of physicians.... In His mercy God has made the sanitarium such a power in the relief of physical suffering that thousands are drawn to it to be cured of their maladies, and very often they are not only cured physically, but from the Saviour they receive the forgiveness of their sins, and they identify themselves completely with Christ, with His interests, His honor" (MM27).

"The purpose of our health institutions is not first and foremost to be that of HOSPITALS" (MM27). "If a sanitarium connected with the closing message fails to lift up Christ and the principles of the gospel as developed in the third angel's message, it fails in its most important feature, and contradicts the very object of its existence" (MM27–8). "Let us present the gospel to the sick, connecting Jesus, the Great Healer, with the simple remedies used; and our living faith will be answered. But those who come to the Great Healer must be willing to do His will, to humble their souls, and confess their sins. As we lay hold of divine power with faith that will not be denied, we shall see the salvation of God" (MM29).

There is need of reform because of the fact that 6 patients out of a hundred admitted to hospitals will contract some kind of infection, one they didn't have upon admission, and that over a 100,000 patients in the U.S. will die from them. Those infections acquired in hospitals costs over $2 billion each year in prolonged hospital stays.

Established To Use Hygienic Methods

"The treatment we gave when the sanitarium was first established required earnest labor to combat disease. We did not use drug concoctions; we followed hygienic methods. This work was blessed of God. It was a work in which the human instrumentality could cooperate with God in saving life" (2SM293).

Since the Spirit of Prophecy condemns the use of drugs as a matter of principle, it does also logically deny their use and application in our sanitariums. Whatever is bad in principle should not be called good in practice. Patients in our sanitariums should be treated with God's chosen methods, his hygienic methods, nature's own provisions which are God-given. We are told that "Our sanitariums are to be conducted on hygienic methods.... Habits of cleanliness with regard to that which is INTRODUCED INTO THE MOUTH, should be observed" (MM227). In such a sanitarium maladies are to be "cured by NATURE'S OWN PROVISIONS, and where the people may be taught how to TREAT THEMSELVES WHEN SICK" (Te88), without drugs (Te87). The restorative agencies that the Lord has provided should be made use of (Ms19, 1911). "There is a work to be done in treating the sick with water and teaching them to make the most of the sunshine and physical exercise. Thus in simple language, we may teach the people how to preserve health, and how to avoid sickness. This is the work our sanitariums are called upon to do."

The Emphasis Is To Be On Sanitariums Rather Than Hospitals

Elder F.D. Nichols wrote in the Review of Sept. 5, 1974 the following: "Did God set us in the world to compete with hospitals? No! To have hospitals we must be close to cities. Private physicians would claim that their patients should be admitted. We were to offer what the world doesn't offer. Sanitariums have three therapeutic procedures, 1. MENTAL HYGIENE, 2. PHYSICAL MEDICINE, and 3. DIET THERAPY. Educationally and spiritually they exist in an atmosphere of faith and prayer where men will be taught to live aright. They should be specialized institutions — there should be many small sanitariums — away from the cities — among nature — to use THERAPIES WHICH THE PATIENT HIMSELF CAN USE when he returns home. It will not only relieve the immediate malady, but help the patient permanently. INSTRUCTION should be in COOKING, LIFE-STYLE, and PHYSICAL THERAPY. This will not only cure the malady but prevent its return. " Such instruction is to be blended.

Mrs. White said that we should "operate MANY SMALL SANITARIUMS outside of large cities" (8T223), that we should "practice HYGIENIC TREATMENTS" there (MM27), which is "one of God's means for healing the sick" (MM233). We are to supply the sick with good food, WITHOUT DRINKS OR DRUGS, and follow rational methods, and our instruction should be blended with the study of the Bible. However, what we are actually doing is 1. using DRUG THERAPY and we are operating HOSPITALS, 2. We are following SECULAR PRACTICES, hygienic practices are discouraged, and 3. We are giving patients TEA, COFFEE, MEAT, DRUGS, and allow them to SMOKE. The great final test is to come to the churches "in connection with TRUE MEDICAL MISSIONARY WORK, a work that has the Great Physician to dictate and preside in all it comprehends" (Loma Linda Messages, p. 62). This may mean that there will come a division in the church between NATURAL HEALING and ALLOPATHIC HEALING, between God's method and the worldly method. Sanitariums are to break down prejudice against the truth.

The Functions Of Sanitariums

The functions of sanitariums is to deal largely with helping people to regain their health and strength under quiet surroundings, and be treated with the provisions of nature which are positively restorative. With these functions sanitariums would have mostly those patients who have overworked themselves indiscreetly, who need REST and SUPPORT in order to allow nature's restorative powers to assert themselves toward the patient's condition of normal health. They are to be conducted on different lines from those of worldly institutions. "They were to be founded and conducted upon Bible principles as the Lord's instrumentality" (CH205). The Spirit of Prophecy implies that in general people come to the sanitarium not with the most serious diseases, who were not at the point of death, and who were not in the condition just before breathing their last, and had no other place to turn to.

"There is a work to be done in treating the sick with WATER and teaching them to make the most of the SUNSHINE and PHYSICAL EXERCISE. Thus in simple language, we may teach the people how to preserve health, how to avoid sickness. This is the work our sanitariums are called upon to do, This is TRUE SCIENCE" (MS 105, 1898).

If God's people applied strictly the health principles and directions given to them to their own lives, such serious conditions would not arise, unless they had already lived a full life. That is why the directions given are simple directions which everyone can apply to himself, and need not call a doctor any sooner than they would call a lawyer. This does not mean that God's medicines cannot cure SERIOUS DISEASES. They can cure any and all diseases including the ones medicine finds INCURABLE. With God there are no incurable diseases. There may be incurable people, however. It simply means that if God's people live according to health reform, they will not find themselves in the condition, where the methods of the sanitarium would not be sufficient for their medical needs.

Drugs Were To Be Left Out Of Our Sanitariums

The application of God's methods of healing in our sanitariums would have no use for any DRUGS, or any substance of a poisonous nature to be introduced into the system of any patient. Drugs as poisonous substances would defile the body temple, which is the temple of God. Paul says: "If any man defile the temple of God, him shall God destroy; for the temple of God is holy, which temple ye are" (1 Cor. 2:17)

In our sanitariums special instruction was to be given in the art of treating the sick without the use of poisonous drugs, and in harmony with the light that God had given. Students were to come forth from the school without having sacrificed the principles of health reform. If instruction was given against the use of drugs, then certainly drugs would not and could not be used within the sanitarium itself (SOHM378). In CH394 we are told that "It is the Lord's purpose that his method of healing without drugs shall be brought into prominence in every large city through out medical institutions."

According to MS115, 1903, we are told that "It would have been better if from the first all drugs had been kept out of our sanitariums, and use had been made of such simple remedies as are found in PURE WATER, PURE AIR, SUNLIGHT, and some of the SIMPLE HERBS growing in the field. These would be just as efficacious as the drugs used under mysterious names, and concocted by human science, and they would leave no injurious effects in the system." HEALTH REFORM was to take a leading part in the work of our sanitariums (Te247).

Sanitariums Were to Teach Self-treatment And Self-denial

We are told that in the "early history of our work many were healed through prayer, but were not educated in healthful living, and so they repeated their bad habits. Hence, sanitariums were to be established to educate these in respect to healthful living. (CH469). In such an institution people were to be taught how to DRESS, BREATHE, and EAT PROPERLY, how to PREVENT SICKNESS by proper habits of living" (CD444). They were to be taught the principles of healthful living, and the values of self-denial and self-restraint (CH212), and to be taught how to cooperate with God in seeking health (CD303), so that the people may be able to TREAT THEMSELVES when sick (CD281). To treat oneself would not mean that a large number of technical apparatus would be needed to maintain health.

God's doctors of REST, EXERCISE, SUNLIGHT, DIET, WATER, TEMPERANCE, FRESH AIR, and TRUST IN DIVINE POWER are available to every person. God's medicines, the HERBS, are available and usable without the need for a doctor. And the knowledge of how to use them properly can be self-acquired largely without the need for a professional teacher. If we all made use of them, we would to a great extent reduce the need for doctors, and their numbers would be greatly reduced. The study of healthful living is a lifelong study in which everyone should be engaged every day, in which learning never ends, in which improvement should continue daily, and in which new procedures give us more joyful and evermore beneficial experiences.

Sanitariums Were To Advance Present Truth

We are told that "our sanitariums are to be established for one object—the advancement of present truth" (CH272). "The truth is to come to the attention of thousands who are influenced by the work of the sanitarium" (CH510). In order for our sanitarium to influence people in the truth, it must itself practice and live the truth. It cannot do this if in its general practice it is dispensing drugs which action is contrary to the light of present truth. They should pray for the sick, ministering to their necessities, not with drugs, but with nature's remedies, and teaching them how to regain health and avoid disease (CH397).

Counsel was given us that the peculiar principles of our faith were not to be hidden in our institutions in order to obtain a large patronage (SOHM295). There is to be no covering up of any phase of our message. The truth for this time is to be given to the souls who are ready to perish. Those who hide the truth dishonor God, and upon their garments will be the blood of souls (8T153–6).

The Sanitarium Diet

If we are to uphold the principles of present truth in our sanitariums, then those things that are against those principles should not be used and applied in them. The principle here is that "It is right that no TEA and COFFEE or FLESH MEAT be served in our sanitariums. Their place should be taken by wholesome palatable food (CD283). To serve flesh food is not pleasing to God (CD414). A diet without flesh food would be more effectual in healing the sick (CD304). There is one exception made. Those patients who demand flesh food should eat it in their own rooms (CD290). It is easily seen that the principles of our health reform message would not be served, if meat were served in the dining hall where everyone could see that we are not really practicing what we preach in regard to health principles.

Healing Of Soul More Important Than Healing Of Body

Since a large number of illnesses are illnesses of the mind, it is important to pay attention to correcting the mental attitudes of patients while at the same time paying attention to the body. Before Christ healed the man with the palsy, and while this man was still at home, the Savior had brought conviction to his conscience. When he repented of his sins and believed in the power of Christ to make him whole, the burden of sin rolled off his shoulders. His sins were pardoned and his soul healed (DA268). Similarly, we are told that "the principle involved here is that the healing of the soul of a patient is far more important than the healing of the body" (7T96). We are told that "the paralytic found in Christ healing of both soul and body. The spiritual healing was followed by physical restoration. This lesson should not be overlooked" (DA270). Christ does not heal just to heal. If sin is involved, repentance must precede the physical healing, before true physical healing can occur. If repentance of wrongdoing does not occur, then the patient will in time commit the same sins which caused his illness in the first place. This principle of "Go and sin no more" is missing in the procedures of television healers. That is why such healing cannot be very effective.

Loma Linda

Regarding Loma Linda Mrs. White tells of her experience. She says, "One night I was awakened and instructed to write a straight testimony regarding the work of our school at Loma Linda. By that school a solemn and sacred work was to be done. The teachings of health reform were to stand out clearly and brightly, that all the youth in attendance might learn to practice them. All our educators should be strict health reformers" (MM63). "Facilities should be provided at Loma Linda that the necessary instruction in medical lines may be given by instructors who fear the Lord and who are in harmony with His plans for the treatment of the sick" (MM62). Loma Linda was designated as a center for the training of MEDICAL MISSIONARY EVANGELISTS (SOHM369). It was to be conducted on the principles of the ancient SCHOOLS OF THE PROPHETS where the Word of God will be regarded as essential, and where obedience to its teachings was to be taught (SOHM374)

The students that would come to Loma Linda were to obtain a medical education that would enable them to pass the examinations required by law of all those who practice as regularly qualified physicians. In order to pass those examinations they would no doubt know something about the nature of drugs, in theory and in their interrelationships. However, since the Spirit of Prophecy condemned the use of drugs, such knowledge did not have to be personally applied to the patients, but needed to be known and understood. This would be especially true for patients who came from other outside institutions where drugs were administered to them. It would be similar to students in biology knowing about evolution without believing in and applying its principles.

Loma Linda was NOT TO COMPETE WITH WORLDLY MEDICAL SCHOOLS, nor with the WORLD'S METHOD of medical practice by exacting large fees for physicians' medical services. The less dependent it was upon worldly methods of education the better it would be for the students, for they were to come forth from the school without having sacrificed the principles of HEALTH REFORM. (SOHM378). On June 17, 1971 Kenneth H. Wood, editor of the ADVENTIST REVIEW wrote the following in the editorial: "The Church has failed to live by the principles and counsel given to it through INSPIRATION. It has been a mere imitator. It has conformed to the influences from FALSE SCIENCE and SECULAR MEDICINE. Its schools have too often merely met the standards of accrediting associations; its medical institutions, instead of being unique. They have no special identity. The Church has muffled its marvelous HEALTH MESSAGE. It has largely substituted DRUG THERAPY for NATURAL REMEDIES."

Pastor Thomas M. Kopko indicates the deterioration of our HEALTH REFORM PRINCIPLES in a statement of his December 1984 publication of his paper "God's Physicians" under the heading "What We Are Doing" as follows:

✓ Operating ALLOPATHIC (drug therapy) hospitals, usually one to a conference.

✓ Giving DRUGS freely—The definition of allopathy, "the method of treating disease by the use of agents producing effects different from the disease treated."

- ✓ SECULAR PRACTICES are followed, and HYGIENIC, RATIONAL THERAPIES discouraged.
- ✓ HYDROTHERAPY (water treatment) departments in our hospitals disbanded, or seldom used.
- ✓ The sick are treated with DRUGS, SURGERY, and RADIATION. For all practical purposes our hospitals are treating the sick completely opposite to E.G. White's counsel. Recent studies have shown hospital food, if continually eaten, causes MALNUTRITION.
- ✓ TEA and COFFEE are served. Patients are allowed all types of DRUGS; they are not discarded, and ALCOHOL is winked at too often.
- ✓ FLESH FOOD is allowed and served.
- ✓ SMOKING is permitted in patients rooms.

More and more liberties are taken in doing BUSINESS on the SABBATH.

Most employees are not SDA's, and therefore there is little SPIRITUAL ADVENTIST INFLUENCE.

☞ Most hospitals give ABORTION on demand.

Medical Missionary Work

We are told that every Christian born into this world is born to be a missionary. It means that we endeavor to help every individual that we come in contact with to understand the principles of healthful living and how to apply them to their own lives. We are told that "We have come to the time when every member of the church should take hold of medical missionary work. The world is a lazar house filled with victims of of both physical and spiritual diseases. Everywhere people are perishing for lack of the knowledge of the truths that have been committed to us" (CH425). Medical missionary work is THE GOSPEL IN PRACTICE, the gospel practically carried out. Soon there will be no work done in ministerial lines but medical missionary work. It will give us access to people. Their hearts will be touched as we minister to their necessities (SOHM308). "It will give us the privilege of participating in Christian help work in our homes with neighbors and friends (SOHM436). In every place the sick may be found, and those who go forth as workers for Christ should be true health reformers, prepared to give to those who are sick the simple treatments that will relieve them, and then pray with them. This will open the door for the entrance of truth" (MM320). "Every gospel worker should feel that the giving of instruction in the principles of healthful living is part of his appointed work" (CH40).

THE WORK OF THE DOCTOR

The Physician's Work Is To Cooperate With God

◆ *The Work Of Healing Is The Lord's*

The doctor, in his work of assisting the patient to overcome his disease, must cooperate with God, and he must give this same attitude of cooperation to the patient. He must indicate to the patient that in every step taken in harmony with the laws of God he may expect the help of divine power (MH118). He must give the patient to understand that God alone is the one who can heal. Hence, he must encourage the patient to lay hold of divine strength through obedience to the commandments of God. "The Lord will be the helper of every physician who will work together with Him in the effort to restore suffering humanity to health, not with drugs, but with nature's remedies…. He gives success to those who work in partnership with Him" (Letter 142, 1902). "The physician ministers to the body in healing, yet all the work is the Lord's" (MM119). That is why the praise given to the physician for saving the patient's life belongs to God. Physicians are too often given honor for health that God restores (CH456). HIPPOCRATES said: "Nature heals, the physician is only nature's assistant."

"To educate the human family that the doctor alone knows all the ills of infants and persons of every age is false teaching, and the sooner we as a people stand on the PRINCIPLES of HEALTH REFORM, the greater will be the blessing that will come to those who would do true medical missionary work" (MS. 105, 1898).

◆ *It Is Proper For Physicians To Help Heal On The Sabbath*

Physicians are acting in Christ's stead. They are used by God to heal the sick (MM55), not only PHYSICALLY, but SPIRITUALLY also. That is why all physicians in our sanitarium should be CHRISTIANS (6T229), so that he can point them to Christ the GREAT PHYSICIAN. Presenting Christ the Restorer to patients is the REAL SCIENCE OF HEALING for body and soul (MH244). "While the physician uses nature's remedies for physical disease, he should point his patients to Him who can relieve the maladies of both soul and body" (MH111). Since it is proper to do good on the Sabbath day, and since Christ therefore also healed on the Sabbath, it is also proper for the physician to relieve suffering on the Sabbath (MM50).

The physician needs more than human wisdom and power that he may know how to minister to the perplexing cases of disease of the mind and heart with which he is called to deal. If he is ignorant of the power of divine grace, he cannot help the afflicted one, but will aggravate the difficulty; but if he has a firm hold upon God, he will be able to help the diseased, distracted mind (5T444).

The Physician Should Be A Health Reformer

◆ *There Is Danger In Departing From God's Instruction*

In order for the physician to help in healing the patient, he himself must be a health reformer. In fact all of our educators should be HEALTH REFORMERS, as well as OUR MINISTERS (Ev. 546). "The reason why many of our ministers complain of sickness is, they fail to take sufficient EXERCISE and indulge in OVEREATING" (CH595) Angels are at the side of godly physicians to give them wisdom and skill (6T229). "There is danger in departing in the least from the Lord's instruction. When we deviate from the plain path of duty, a train of circumstances will arise that seems irresistibly to draw us farther and farther from the right" (CH458).

◆ *Drugs Mask The Real Causes*

"Physicians and ministers are to unite in an effort to lead men and women to obey God's commandments. Physicians are in greater danger of falling under TEMPTATION than are ministers (CH584). They need to study the intimate relationship existing between OBEDIENCE and HEALTH" (CH321). "If a doctor himself uses drugs, he cannot condemn them in others, for he then would be condemning himself" (CH322). What drugs accomplish is 1. to MASK the difficulty, 2. they do NOT ELIMINATE it, 3. they CONTAMINATE the internal environment, 4. they create a DEPENDENCY on the part of the patient, 5. they ERASE VALUABLE CLUES as to the real source of the trouble. You do not have a HEADACHE because your system lacks ASPIRIN. Aspirin is a non-biological weapon. It covers up trouble which needs more fundamental attention. It disguises symptoms which may interfere with the task of finding the real cause behind the symptom.

Doctors Are Not Well Trained In Nutrition

The most basic weapons in the fight against disease are the numerous NUTRIENTS that the cells of our bodies need. CLINICAL NUTRITION is not taught very much in medical schools. Doctors are not well trained to identify MALNUTRITION. We should not depend upon any INORGANIC MATERIAL or MODIFIED ORGANIC MATERIAL as a solution to the health problem. Even the chemical "purification" of an organic substance, such as the SALICYLATES whose natural source is the WILLOW BARK, is more harmful when refined, or if made artificially in the chemical laboratory. Salicylates are irritating to both skin and mucous membrane, and represent a poison to the system.

It is therefore easy to see that a MEDICINE must be a part of the composition of the food or herb that is COMPATIBLE WITH THE ORGANISM. We can develop new chemicals in the test tube, but we cannot improve the organism therewith. INORGANIC SUBSTANCES as MEDICINES can only develop a disease in the organism. Some years ago Family Weekly carried an article of a girl who had LEUKEMIA. She was given up to die. Her parents grew desperate and sought out a "nature curist" who discontinued her medicines and put her on a strict diet of natural foods. On this diet she improved and became free of leukemia. The doctors could not explain her recovery and called it a miracle. It had become obvious that the poisonous medicines were killing her.

Physicians Should Teach Patients How To Prevent Disease

◆ *It Is Better To Keep Well Than To Know How To Cure Disease*

We are told that physicians do not pay enough attention to PREVENTION, and that they should instruct patients in prevention. Their first work is to educate the sick and suffering to prevent disease (Te86) "Physicians dwell too much upon the WORKING OF DISEASE, but do not as a general rule arouse the attention of the patient to the laws which must be sacredly and intelligently obeyed to prevent disease" (MM223). One author says: "We are still a profession thinking more about CURING than PREVENTING by attacking the basic causes of disease" They generally avoid the teaching of the principles of PREVENTIVE MEDICINE. "The distinction between PREVENTION and CURE has not been made sufficiently important. Teach people that it is better to KNOW HOW TO KEEP WELL than how to cure disease" (MM221).

The physician should educate the sick and suffering how they can best prevent disease. But this they are for the most part reluctant to do because from their standpoint, doing this seems to work against their best financial advantage. Since drugs do not heal, the patient will come to the physician over and over again, and such actions will give the physician more and more monetary rewards. To teach prevention is not a paying proposition because there is no money in it. But the Christian physician should look at the matter from the standpoint of how he can best help the patient, and not from the standpoint of monetary reward. One doctor said to his apprentice student: "If you want to be a good doctor, you have to do more than diagnose and treat. You must educate the patient by telling him how he got the disease, and what he can do to prevent it from recurring."

◆ *Healing Honor To Be Given To God Instead Of To Physician*

The intelligent physician will have an increasing knowledge of the connection between SIN and DISEASE and is in the best position to teach the patient to eliminate sinful practices from his life in order to remain in health, and avoid sickness. We are told that when sickness is the result of transgression of natural law, they do not seek to correct the error, but resort to physicians. "If they recover they give to DRUGS and DOCTORS all the HONOR." (CH456).

Physician Should Not Follow Practices Condemned By God

◆ *Our Institutions Should Not Employ Physicians Prescribing Meat*

We are told that "Our physicians should be wise educators warning all against self-indulgence, showing that abstinence from the things that God has prohibited is the only way to prevent ruin of body and mind" (MM221). "He should follow God's way with suffering humanity" (MM188) The "believing physician must follow no CUSTOM, TRADITION, or PRACTICE condemned by God" (MM122). This would include the use of drugs, and even the matter of eating meat. First of all we are told that SDA institutions should not employ physicians who use flesh food and prescribe it to their patients, because in doing so they are prescribing that which makes them sick. Herein he is not reasoning from cause to effect, and is leading the patient to indulge perverted appetite (CD290). "The physicians employed in our institutions should be reformers in this respect and in every other" (CD291). It is stated that the SUPERINTENDENTS of our health institutions are DISQUALIFIED if they recommend a diet of FLESH (CD294). And we are also told that the physician who encourages MEAT EATING makes a necessity for DRUGS (MM222).

◆ *Doctors Must Be Interested In Health Instead Of Only Disease*

Dr. Stuart Berger said: "Doctors learn how to use SCALPEL, DRUGS, RADIATION BEAMS TO DESTROY CANCER, but not how the right food and lifestyle could help PREVENT cancer. The medical system is one of REACTION to ILLNESS, instead of one of PREVENTION and HEALTH. Our medical MYOPIA sentences millions of Americans to ANGUISH, POOR HEALTH, PREMATURE AGING, and DEATH." Sir George Newman said: "The IDEAL MEDICINE is the prevention of disease, and the necessity for curative treatment is a tacit admission of its failure. To do this the attitude of physicians must turn around. He must be INTERESTED in HEALTH, and not only in disease. When doctors think entirely in terms of disease, they are then ignoring opportunities to make people healthier."

Physicians Should Teach By Means Of Cause And Effect

◆ *Cooperation with God*

"The physician should teach his patients that they should cooperate with God in the work of RESTORATION. The physician has a continually increasing realization of the fact that disease is the result of sin. He knows that the LAWS OF NATURE as truly as the DECALOGUE, are divine, and that only in obedience to them can health be recovered or preserved. He sees many suffering as a result of hurtful practices who might be restored to health if they would do what they might for their own restoration. They need to be taught that every practice which destroys the physical, mental, or spiritual energies is SIN, and that HEALTH is to be secured through obedience to the laws that God has established for the good of all mankind" (MH113).

◆ *Trace Disease To Its Cause*

When a physician has identified a disease, he should try to determine what possibly brought the disease about. And if he is intelligent regarding this matter, he will be able to trace disease to its cause (5T440). Once he has discovered the cause of the disease he should not keep silent about it, but tell the patient exactly what habits of life might have contributed to it (MM49). He is doing the patient an injury, if he does not point out that the patient's ailment was caused by improper eating and drinking (CH353).

◆ *The Whole Truth Cannot Always Be Told To The Patient.*

At times it may be unwise to conceal the nature and cause of the disease to the patient. This may give him a false hope of recovery. It may not always be best to explain to the patient the full extent of his danger. This might alarm him and retard and even prevent recovery. Nor can the whole truth always be told to those whose ailments are largely imaginary. Christ said to His disciples "I have yet many things to say unto you, but ye cannot bear them now" (Jo. 16:12). If all of the truth may not be presented, it is never justifiable or necessary to deceive, or stoop to prevarication. He who does this places himself where God cannot cooperate with him (MH246).

◆ *Health Cannot Be Restored Without Removal Of Cause*

On the other hand, Mrs. White also says that the physician who tells the TRUTH about disease will have an UPHILL BUSINESS (Te86). But as a physician he should be an example in healthful living, so that the patient will respect his authority along this line (MM264). The enlightened physician will talk plainly of the ruinous effect of SELF-INDULGENCE in EATING, DRINKING, and DRESSING; of the OVERTAXATION of the vital forces that have brought his patients where they are. If the physician never makes a genuine search for causes, he is not in the position to give the patient any sound advice. Without the REMOVAL OF CAUSE, health cannot be restored. He will not increase the evil by administering drugs till exhausted nature gives up the struggle, but will teach the patients how to form CORRECT HABITS and to aid nature in her work of restoration by a wise use of her own simple remedies (CH451–2). We are told that "our workers should use their knowledge of the laws of life and health. They should study from cause and effect. Read the BEST AUTHORS on these subjects, and obey religiously that which your REASON tells you is TRUTH" (CH566).

◆ *Doctors Must Treat Causes, Not merely Symptoms Or Effects*

Whenever a doctor prescribes a PAIN RELIEVER, he doesn't assume that he is removing the cause of the ailment. Whenever he removes an affected organ, he also does not pretend that he is removing the cause of the affection. When a URINE TEST shows sugar in the urine, this fact does not reveal the cause of the GLYCOSURIA. He who treats disease with PALLIATIVES, treats EFFECTS and ignores CAUSES. An ANTACID does not remove the cause of the gastric distress. When a drug is taken to silence pain, we defy the warnings of nature, and pretend that no warning has been given. We set aside the LAWS of BIOLOGY and resort to the LAWS of CHEMISTRY to solve health problems. To excise a kidney stone does not remove the cause of the stone. Hence, another stone may form a little later.

◆ *Doctors Can Eliminate Infectious Diseases*

Doctors generally can eliminate INFECTIOUS DISEASES caused by germs, because DRUGS are designed to DESTROY GERMS, but they do this not entirely without harm to the patient. The diseases which are not largely caused by germs, namely the DEGENERATIVE DISEASES which are largely caused by CHEMICAL IMBALANCES, are generally considered to be INCURABLE by the medical profession. These include ARTHRITIS, DIABETES and CANCER. However, NATUROPATHIC PHYSICIANS do not find them entirely incurable. One arthritis patient was cured of his arthritis by drinking nothing but lots of water for 5 to 6 weeks. Bernard Baruch said: "There is no such thing as incurables. There are only things for which man has not found a cure."

◆ *Doctors' Strikes Improve Health Of Communities*

The poisonous nature of drugs is indicated by the fact that about 4 million people each year are poisoned so seriously by their physicians, that they require hospitalization. This is about 10% of all those who are hospitalized. Of these over 40,000 die. The story is told of some towns in North Dakota which were looking for a doctor because they had none. A survey of the health departments of those towns, however, revealed that their health norm was far above the national average.

When doctors go on strike, it seems that the health conditions of the people improve. In 1973 there was a doctors strike in Israel. The statistics of the Jerusalem Burial Society showed that the death rate went down 50%, for there were 50% fewer funerals. The New York Times noted that this was a predictable statistic, for in a similar situation in Israel 20 years before, the death rate had decreased by about the same ratio. The physicians in Israel were saving the lives of their patients by remaining away from their bedsides. The statement was also made that the sick would be better off to pay the doctors $10 to stay away, than to pay them $5 to come to their bedsides. However, the people of Israel had apparently not learned the lesson of the previous strike. Similar results were obtained from doctors strikes in both Canada and the Netherlands. All their rates went up again when the strikes ended.

◆ *Life Without Drugs Lengthens Life*

In 1929 Dr. Herbert Shelton, a Hygienist, suggested that if we abolished medicine in all its forms, human life would increase the lifespan by an average of 10 years in a decade. After he had published an article on the dangers of medicine Dr. Shelton was arrested in New York City, and the above statement was read, to his surprise, in court as evidence that he was practicing medicine without a license. In answer the judge said that many thousands of people held that same view. The Spirit of Prophecy holds a similar view when it says: "If people would reason from cause to effect, and would follow the light which shines upon them, they would pursue a course which would insure health, and MORTALITY would be far less"(2SM443). And on page 450 of 2SM it states: "More deaths have been caused by drug taking than from all other causes combined. If there was in the land one physician in place of thousands, a vast amount of PREMATURE MORTALITY would be prevented." Dr. Kugler says that the average lifespan of men who do everything wrong is about 60 years.

How The Doctor Treats Disease

The forces of the patient's own system must be employed in fighting disease, else all of the physician's medicines will be useless. The act of the physician is grounded on cooperation with NATURE. His present role has tended to de-emphasize the human element in the disease fighting equation, which is the patient's contribution. It has made the doctor think almost exclusively in terms of combating the manifestations of illness, rather than the health of the body as a whole. Deficiencies in the body environment constitute a major cause of disease. Medicine has become addicted to the administration of vast quantities of non-biological medications which have no known connection with the disease. The Spirit of Prophecy tells us that "there are many ways of practicing the healing art, but there is only ONE WAY THAT HEAVEN APPROVES. God's remedies are the SIMPLE AGENCIES OF NATURE, that will not tax or debilitate the system through their powerful properties. PURE AIR and WATER, CLEANLINESS, a PROPER DIET, PURITY of LIFE, and a firm TRUST IN GOD, are remedies for the want of which thousands are dying, yet these remedies are going out of date because their skillful use requires work that the people do not appreciate. Fresh air, exercise, pure water, and clean, sweet premises are within the reach of all with but little expense; but DRUGS are EXPENSIVE, both in the outlay of means and the effect produced upon the system" (CH323).

Doctors And Nutrition

Of 127 medical schools in the U.S., only 24 require courses in nutrition. Only one school, the University of Rochester, requires a full-fledged course in PREVENTIVE MEDICINE. HEW director Califano estimated that 67% of all diseases could have been prevented. Dr. Stare of Harvard said that most physicians know almost nothing about determining the nutritional status of patients. Some nutrients taken in inappropriate amounts can be toxic, but are constructive when taken in reasonable amounts. Drugs are toxic in any amount, for they are usually substances which are foreign to our bodies and not adaptable to them. For this reason non-biological drugs are not needed by the cells of the body. It is NATURAL NUTRIENTS that are needed.

How The Doctor Treats The Patient

◆ *Drugs Hinder Nature's Effort*

"When persons are in distress they send for the doctor, and trust their bodies in his hands, with the expectation that he will make them well. He deals out to them drugs, the nature of which they know nothing, and in their blind confidence, they swallow anything that the doctor may choose to give. Thus POWERFUL POISONS are often administered which fetter nature in all her friendly efforts to recover the abuse the system has suffered, and the patient is hurried out of this life.

The mother who has been but slightly indisposed, and who might have recovered by ABSTI-

NENCE FROM FOOD for a short period, has instead of doing this sent for a physician. But the physician who should give a few simple directions and RESTRICTIONS IN DIET administers POISONS, which, if he were sick, he would not venture to take himself. The patient grows worse, and poisonous drugs are more freely administered. The mother dies as a result. She was drugged to death. Her system was poisoned beyond remedy. She was murdered.... Her untimely death dishonored God. Heaven wanted her to live. With some there is sufficient life force to expel the poison from the system. No credit should be given to the drugs for they HINDERED NATURE in her effort. All credit should be given to nature's restorative powers. If the patient recovers, the effort that nature had to make, injured the constitution and shortened the life of the patient. Physicians, by administering drug poisons, have done very much to increase the DEPRECIATION of the RACE PHYSICALLY, MENTALLY, and MORALLY.(2SM441–2).

◆ *Poisonous Medicines Destroy*

A poison by any other name, such as MEDICINE, is still a poison. Is there a person who would deliberately poison his body, or let anyone else do it? But where they are called MEDICINES people readily assent. From DEATH-DEALING substances they have now become LIFE-ENHANCING substances. A change in name has now "changed" the character of the substance. If the honest physician would say: "I am going to give you a dose of this poison three times a day, and if that doesn't work, I will switch to a more powerful poison," then who would continue to patronize such a physician? Poisons add problems instead of solving them.

Drugs furnish no nutrients. They have no intelligence to create new cells, and repair damaged tissue. Instead they form chemical unions that PARALYZE NERVES, DESTROY CELLS, and SUSPEND VITAL ACTION, thereby causing symptoms to disappear. The person so treated is sicker than before, even though he may feel better. Drugs and treatments rise to glory on the back of the SELF-HEALING POWERS of the body.

The "Cures" Of Medicine

✓ MEDICAL "CURES" ARE SHORT-LIVED—The "cures" of medicine are peculiar in that they do not long remain cures. New "cures" have to be found to supplant the old ones, until they also lose their effectiveness. Each year the drug companies put on the market about 4000 new drugs. Of the discovery of new "cures" there seems to be no end. This fact is a direct indication that the "old cures" really didn't work as they were supposed to work. They were "cures" that did not cure. This is to be assumed since the Spirit of Prophecy tells us that "drugs never cure." An old French physician once said to a patient, "Take this while it is still a remedy." People are "cured" repeatedly, for the "cures" don't stick, because the "cures" are not cures. Furthermore, a disease really cannot be cured, if the cause of the disease is not removed, which in many cases demands a LIFESTYLE CHANGE. A few years ago a weekly magazine estimated that there were 130,000 remedies for 407 diseases. With so many remedies, why should anybody be sick or die of disease?

✓ "CURES" GIVE ONLY TEMPORARY RELIEF—Cures are what people want, and cures are what physicians pretend to give. However, at most only temporary relief is given, a postponement of the inevitable. Nature returns to normal only when enervating habits are given up. Modern "cures" are based upon the principle of thinking from EFFECT (disease) to cause, which is mostly unknown, rather than from cause to effect. When the effect is discovered, the cure is to "cut it out." This is accomplished with the surgeon's knife. This usually implies that the reason for the effect has not been discovered. This shows that such action is a non-intelligent or non-rational way of dealing with the effect. The rational way to deal with it is to discover why an organ has failed to function properly.

✓ TO PREVENT DISEASE CAUSE MUST BE KNOWN—If the cause is not known, how is PREVENTION possible? The idea that a disease can be made to cure itself by means of VACCINES which are made from the products of disease, is an end product of pathological thinking. If "cure" means producing the disease itself, then such a "cure" is exactly what is not wanted. It is not the disease itself but rather the cause that we need to know in order to prevent the disease. One doctor said that he was mistaken in his DIAGNOSES about 50% of the time, and that he had proved it by his POSTMORTEMS. Diagnoses may mean discovering of effects or SYMPTOMS which as such give little or no information regarding what the cause might have been.

✓ STUDY HEALTH IN ORDER TO PREVENT DISEASE—The proper way to study disease is to STUDY HEALTH, and every influence favorable or unfavorable to its progress, for every influence that lowers NERVE ENERGY becomes disease producing.

Dealing With Symptoms

◆ *Symptoms Are The Superficial Indications Of Abnormal Conditions*

DISEASE SYMPTOMS are evidences that the body is trying to purify and heal itself. They may be evidences of a disease in the body, but they are not the disease. To analyze a woman's tears does not tell us the cause of why she is crying. The CAUSES of disease are not found in its symptoms. If the cause is not known, then PALLIATION OF SYMPTOMS is all that can be hoped for. A symptom may be an external response to an inner condition.

◆ *Treating Symptoms Only Masks The Disease*

By overemphasizing and overtreating the symptoms of disease, doctors do not get at the causes of disease which are largely due to FAULTY HABITS of eating and drinking "(MH295; CH90). Without knowing the cause of a disease, a true remedy of the disease cannot be effected. Taking away symptoms is not taking away disease. It is said of PAIN as a symptom of disease, that it is a RED FLAG of DANGER, indicating that something is out of balance within the system. Alleviating merely the symptom of pain tears down the red flag of warning and makes the patient feel that the ailment has been removed, when this is not at all the case. The disease itself is an even bigger red flag which should make the individual consider that there is within his system a threat to life itself.

◆ *The Main Cause Of Disease Is TOXEMIA*

Drugs are quick relievers of symptoms. They are favored because they quickly give the patient a sense of WELL-BEING and SECURITY. Such security is often false because it is superficial, for it does not get at the real cause of the ailment. Natural methods of healing are rather slow and gradual, but they do get at the basic cause of the impure conditions within the system. Dr. Arbuthnot Lane said: "There is but one cause of disease — POISON, TOXEMIA, most of which is created within the body by faulty living habits and faulty elimination." Henry Lindlahr said: "Every acute disease is a result of a cleansing and healing effort of nature." Hippocrates said: "Leave thy drugs in the chemist's pot if thou canst heal the patient with food." This is the reason why doctors should use herbs and other natural substances because they cleanse the system, for housecleaning is needed more often than the destruction of germs, and cleansing the system is what herbs, which are Christ's remedies, do (2SM289).

◆ *Drugs Are Anti-vital Substances*

If we place toxic MUSTARD OIL on the skin of a healthy child, it will occasion a blister. Here the blister is a sign of a healthy internal condition. The body is responding to that which is annoying. If, on the other hand, the mustard oil is placed on the skin of a person with a WEAK VITALITY, it will not produce a blister. This is due to the fact that the vitality is so low that the body does not have the strength to resist the toxic mustard oil. Here the body indicates that it does not have enough power to protect itself from an irritating ANTI-VITAL substance. No reaction also means that the body has a greater toleration for a poisonous substance, and that it will take a greater load of the poisonous substance before reacting at a greater crisis point. The response to only a greater toxic load means that the crisis, when it happens, will be of a more serious nature, and that the patient is nearer death than he would otherwise be. This indicates that a poisonous substance can only move a patient nearer to death, rather than in the direction of recovery. A double dose of such a substance, or an added dose of another poisonous substance would continue the movement of the condition in the wrong direction. The body's reaction shows the strength of its vitality. Hence, people with strong vitalities live longer because their bodies find it easier to eliminate poisonous substances from the system.

Surgery

There will arise EMERGENCY CIRCUMSTANCES when there is a need for surgery. Doctors like to think of every case as being a case of life and death. With such an attitude high fees can be charged, for a person will give almost everything to save his life, if that is indeed the case. Many surgery conditions could indeed be of this type. We are told that "If there is need of a surgical operation, and the physician is willing to undertake the case, it is NOT A DENIAL OF FAITH to have the operation performed." (2SM284) We are told that under those circumstances the physician should ask Christ's aid before the operation (MH118), that angels will then be by the side of the surgeon during the operation (2SM285). "The Lord is to be the efficiency of every physician. If in the operating room the physician feels that he is working only as the Lord's visible helping hand, the Great Physician is present to hold with His invisible hand the hand of the human agent and to guide in the movements made" (MM34–5). When the patient sees the physician on his knees, it inspires him with hope and confidence which is a means of making the operation a success. Such a prayer, even if made before an unbeliever, sweeps away the shadow by which Satan has darkened the mind, and when it is over, TRUTH takes the place of doubt and unbelief (MM35). Many times it is also mentioned that physicians should not charge exorbitant fees for operations.

Operations Are Not Without Danger

In spite of the fact that some operations may be necessary, operations as such are not without danger. Every year a great many people put their lives at unnecessary risk because their IMMUNE SYSTEMS are not up to the stress of battle they will be forced to fight. ANESTHESIA, STRESS, LACK OF SLEEP, and POOR NUTRITION before surgery increase the risk of complications by suppressing the immune system. Major surgery has been shown to reduce immune function by 50%. PAINKILLERS like MORPHINE can reduce the function of individual immune system cells by up to 80%. Malnourished patients going into surgery with low lymphocyte count are 20 times more likely to die than patients without this risk factor. The risk of blood infection doubles if patients immune system does not respond positively to a SKIN-TEST. It was shown that people who are under a lot of stress before an operation will have more complications, need 3 times more pain killers, and will need to spend an extra 5 or 6 days in the hospital. People who had a ROOMMATE in the hospital were less anxious before surgery, got out of bed faster after surgery, and went home sooner. OPTIMISTS healed faster, had fewer complications, went home sooner, and were less likely to experience a heart attack after surgery than pessimists.

Treating Oneself — Self-Healing — Being Your Own Doctor

◆ *With God's Remedies We Can Be Our Own Doctor*

Treating oneself cannot be done very well with the medicines prescribed by a doctor, because they are in control of those medicines, for only doctors can prescribe poisonous substances. The beauty of God's medicines is that they are nonpoisonous substances which anyone can use for himself, and as Mrs. White repeatedly mentions, with their use one need not call a doctor any sooner than one would engage a lawyer. The only way in which we can profitably use God's remedies is 1. if we trust in God supremely; 2. if we believe in the efficacy of God's remedies; and 3. if we are willing to leave off all bad habits in eating and drinking in order to obtain the greatest possible benefit from them. We cannot allow the good that we are endeavoring to do for ourselves to be overcome by habits which counteract the good effects, and might possibly neutralize them. With God's remedies we can be our own doctor.

◆ *We Should Know How To Treat Ourselves*

We are told that "the sick should have confidence in nature's great blessings which God has provided; and the most effective remedies for disease are PURE SOFT WATER, the blessed God-given SUNSHINE coming into the rooms of the invalids, LIVING OUTDOORS as much as possible, having HEALTHFUL EXERCISE, and eating and drinking foods that are prepared in the most HEALTH-

FUL MANNER" (MM225). "You can do the very best HOME MISSIONARY WORK by taking care of GOD'S TEMPLE.... Do not presume to OVERTAX this wonderful machinery, lest some part give way and bring your work to a standstill. I am pained as I have presented to me students who are being educated to work for the salvation of the souls and bodies of those perishing around them, but who will themselves perish before they can accomplish that for which they are striving so earnestly. Will all teachers and students learn before they go any further how to TREAT THEMSELVES, that they may intelligently cooperate with God, to bear His message, to do his work, and not to be cut off, at the very time when they are most needed" (MM80–1)?

If we practice medicine on our own with herbs, under the first amendment of the constitution the law of the land will allow us to do so, for then we are simply practicing and applying our religious beliefs with reference to the Bible and the Spirit of Prophecy. Then no one can come and tell us that we are practicing medicine without a license. We can also build structures in which to give treatments, and if they are built as temporary structures, then no taxes need to be paid on them.

◆ *Most Diseases Represent Nutritional Deficiencies*

One author says that the responsibility of the health care professions should be to help us HEAL OURSELVES. The principle of healing ourselves can be accomplished rather easily if we remember that most health problems result from nutritional deficiencies, hence, the vital need is NOURISHMENT. When one is ill we are told that "Nature will want some ASSISTANCE to bring things to their proper condition, which may be found in the simplest remedies, especially in the use of nature's own furnished remedies — PURE AIR.... PURE WATER.... plenty of SUNLIGHT.... All of these are powerful in their efficiency.... If the sick and suffering will do only as well as they know in regard to living out the PRINCIPLES of HEALTH REFORM perseveringly, then they will in NINE CASES OUT OF TEN recover from their ailments" (MM223–4).

◆ *Our Complaints Are Caused By Our Own Actions*

We are told that "thousands who are afflicted might recover their health if, instead of depending upon the drugstore for their life, they would discard all drugs and live simply, without using TEA, COFFEE, LIQUOR, or SPICES, which irritate the stomach and leave it weak, unable to digest even simple food without stimulation"(MM229). "Thousands need to be educated patiently, tenderly, but decidedly, that of their complaints are created by their own course of action. There is intemperance in eating and in the many varieties of food taken at one meal.... Those who ignore these things, who take no precautions in regard to getting PURE AIR to breathe and PURE WATER to drink, cannot be free from disease" (MM225, 226). God will not do for us what he has left for us to do (MM226).

HEALTH REFORM

THE PRINCIPLES OF HEALTH REFORM

It Is Part Of The Third Angel's Message

◆ *The Principles Are Contained In The Word Of God*

The Health reform is a message that we should present to our people as a part of the THIRD ANGEL'S MESSAGE. (CD32). It is as closely allied to the third angel's message as the ARM is to the BODY. (CD38). It is a part of the truth for the last days as verily as are other features of the gospel work. The gospel includes it in all of it phases. All of the principles of Health Reform are found in the WORD OF GOD (CD75). In the time of the end, God's peculiar people will exercise temperance in all things. (CH116). "Our natural inclinations and appetites.... were divinely appointed.... It was God's design that REASON SHOULD RULE the appetites, and that they should minister to our happiness. And when they are regulated and controlled by sanctified reason, they are holiness unto the Lord." (Te12)

◆ *Purpose is To Lessen Suffering And to Purify The Church*

We are told that "The work of Health reform is the Lord's means for LESSENING SUFFERING in our world and for PURIFYING THE CHURCH" (CD20). It is one branch of the great work which is to fit a people for the COMING OF THE LORD (CD69). "True conversion to the message of present truth embraces conversion to the principles of health reform." The object of health reform "is to teach the people HOW TO LIVE so as to give NATURE a chance to REMOVE and RESIST DISEASE" (1T643). Other purposes are: to give physical and spiritual health (1T546); to keep many from physical, mental, and moral degeneracy (6T378); to prepare minds for the reception of truth (CH22); and to aid in the preparation for Christ's coming (CH20).

Another object is the highest development of MIND, SOUL, and BODY (CD23). Health Reform was also given in order for us to guard against the evils of a DEBASED DIET. Some have been taught that we should never learn to treat ourselves, or to hire a minister to tell us what to believe. Mrs. White tells us that "To educate the human family THAT THE DOCTOR KNOWS ALL THE ILLS IS FALSE TEACHING, and the sooner we as a people stand on the principles of health reform, the greater will be the blessing to those who would do true medical missionary work. It says nurses should learn to use HERBS, and every family should learn how to use them 'intelligently'. That puts no premium on ignorance, but requires us to learn how to use these natural remedies for ourselves and in medical missionary work."

It Increases Spirituality

◆ *Lack Of Health Reform Caused By Lack Of Spirituality*

In the process of hygienic reform, "the spiritual truths were to be developed first before the health reform." (SOHM34) "If Seventh-day Adventists practiced what they profess to believe, if they were sincere health reformers, they would indeed be a SPECTACLE to the WORLD, to ANGELS, and to MEN. And they would show a far greater zeal for the salvation of those who are ignorant of the truth. Greater reforms should be seen among the people who claim to be looking for the soon appearing of Christ. Health reform is to do among our people a work which it has not yet done" (CH575).

"As a people we have been given the work of making known the principles of health reform. There are some who think that the question of DIET is not of sufficient importance to be included in their evangelistic work. But such make a great mistake." (9T112). "We need to learn that IN-

DULGED APPETITE is the greatest hindrance to MENTAL IMPROVEMENT and SOUL SANCTIFICATION" (9T156). "A diseased body and a disordered intellect.... make sanctification of the body and spirit impossible" (CD44). "It is impossible for those who give reins to appetite to attain to CHRISTIAN PERFECTION" (2T400). On the other hand "If man will cherish the light that God in mercy gives him upon health reform, he may be sanctified through the truth and fitted for IMMORTALITY" (Te19).

◆ *Eliminate All Health-Destroying Substances*

Elder Robinson tells us, "The cause of HEALTH REFORM might well be begun by discarding the use of DRUGS, adapting a RATIONAL DIET, and using WATER and other NATURAL AGENCIES as REMEDIES for disease" (SOHM203). Also TOBACCO, TEA, and COFFEE were involved in the first steps of reform. "We should not give the sick that which will keep them sick" (CD415). "Health reform was to be carried forward as described in Isa 61:1–4 and in Christ's commission to his disciples, 'and gave them power to heal all manner of sickness, and all manner of disease'

"(SOHM307). "People must be educated to understand that it is a SIN to destroy their PHYSICAL, MENTAL, and SPIRITUAL ENERGIES, and they must understand how to cooperate with God in their own restoration" (Te89).

"All are personally exposed to the temptations that Christ overcame, but strength is provided for them in the all-powerful name of the great Conqueror. And all must, for themselves, individually overcome" (Te21). If an individual maintains impure conditions in his system, then his system is more likely to crave unhealthful and stimulating food. It was proven with rats that when they were given a deficient diet, and they had the drink-choice between water and alcohol, they chose the alcohol. This was not so when they were given an all-around complete diet.

◆ *Ignoring Health Reform Causes Harm*

"The light which God has given upon health reform cannot be trifled with without injury to those who attempt it" (CD38). "The greatest objection to health reform is that this people do not live it out" (2T486). "Guilt rests upon us who as a people have had much light, because we have not appreciated or improved the light given upon health reform" (HL35). "Health destroying indulgences counteract the influence of health reform" (CD455).

◆ *Teaching Health Reform*

"There is great need of instruction in regard to dietetic reform. Wrong habits of eating and the use of unhealthful foods are in no small degree responsible for the intemperance and crime and wretchedness that curse the world. In teaching health principles, keep before the mind the great OBJECT of REFORM—that its purpose is to secure the HIGHEST DEVELOPMENT of body, mind, and soul. Show that the laws of nature, being the laws of God, are designed for our good; that obedience to them promotes happiness in this life, and aids in the preparation for the life to come. Every gospel worker should feel that to teach the principles of healthful living is a part of his appointed work. Of this work there is great need and the world is open for it" (CH 389–90). "The Saviour's commission to the disciples included all the believers in Christ to the end of time" (DA822). "Where there is no active labor for others, love wanes, and faith grows dim" (DA825).

"Of all people in the world, REFORMERS should be the most UNSELFISH, the most KIND, and the most COURTEOUS....Let words fall gently when seeking to win men from ERROR" (MH157). "Health reformers, above all others, should be careful to AVOID EXTREMES" (CD91). "Those who advocate an unpopular truth should above all others, seek to be consistent in their own life. They should not try to see how different they can be from others, but how near they can come to those whom they wish to influence, that they may help them to the positions they themselves so highly prize" (CH153). And especially should ministers and their families live up to health reform (CD399), for they are setting the example for the whole congregation. They are the ones who are being looked up to and imitated. However, many times ministers manifest little interest in health reform because instruction in TEMPERANCE in all things is opposed to their PRACTICE of SELF-INDULGENCE.(CD453).

It should be said to all HYGIENIC REFORMERS that they live up strictly to the convictions of their own enlightened minds. That they not be led into indulgence by the entreaties of friends. That they live reform at home; and when they go abroad, that they carry the principles of health reform with them. That they should live it, and at proper times, in proper places, and in a proper manner, talk of and defend its principles. (CH447). "Special instruction should be given in the art of treating the sick, without the use of poisonous drugs, and in harmony with the light that God has given. Students should come forth from the school without having sacrificed the principles of health reform" (Letter 90, 1908).

The Need For Temperance

◆ *The Law Of Temperance*

1 Cor. 9:25 tells us, "Every man that striveth for the mastery is temperate in all things." We are also told that intemperance lies at the foundation of all the evil in our world (Te165). It is the basis of all suffering.(2SM411). Intemperance is the hurtful indulgence of any appetite or passion (Te137), and strict temperance is the total abstinence from every injurious or debasing indulgence (CD29). The law of temperance must control the life of every Christian, and in every respect it should control what we EAT, DRINK, how we DRESS, and EVERY PHASE OF LIFE (CD406). In the extreme "victims of intemperance are under the power of a DEMON and are not SANE MEN" (MH172).

◆ *The Appetite Has Controlled Reason*

From the standpoint of human nature, unless we have been strictly trained, appetite is not a safe guide (CD126). From birth the appetite and inclinations of the mother have been transmitted to the children (Te292).

"Appetite and passions should be under the control of reason" (CH112). "If our appetites are not under the control of a sanctified mind, we are not temperate in all our eating and drinking" (Te15). Daniel's parents had trained him in his childhood to habits of strict temperance.(Te190). On the other hand, Eve was intemperate in her desires, in that she wanted to eat the fruit of the tree of the knowledge of good and evil which God had forbidden her to eat of. For the sake of gratifying taste, Eve transgressed the command of God. Since the fall intemperance of every form has existed. The appetite has controlled reason to an alarming degree. Man has run to excess in about everything, and disease has steadily increased. (4SpG120).

◆ *One Of Satan's Strongest Temptations*

The first great temptation of Satan was upon the point of APPETITE; the second was upon the point of PRESUMPTION; and the third was upon the LOVE OF THE WORLD. "One of the stronger temptations that man has to meet is upon the point of appetite" (CH108). "Satan is constantly on the alert to bring the race fully under his control. His strongest hold on man is through appetite, and this he seeks to stimulate in every possible way" (Te13). "Through the temptation to indulge appetite, Adam and Eve first fell from their high, holy, and happy state, and it is through the same temptation that the race have become enfeebled" (Te15). "It will prove the ruin of thousands, when if they had conquered on this point they would have moral power to gain victory over every other temptation of Satan" (Te16). We are told that if Israel had been willing to deny appetite, FEEBLENESS and DISEASE would have been unknown among them. (CD378).

◆ *Slaves to Appetite Cannot Perfect Christian Character*

"It is impossible for those who indulge in appetite to attain to Christian Perfection" (CD22). "Youth in general are governed by impulse, and are slaves of appetite" (CD231). The appetite can be depraved to the extent that it desires not what is good for the body. Under these circumstances good food will not taste good to the person, it will taste flat or insipid. If people are willing to gratify their appetites at any cost, then "God will not miraculously save them from the consequences of their indulgence" (CD25). "The Spirit of God cannot come to our help and assist us in perfecting Christian characters, while we are indulging our appetites to the injury of health and while the pride of life controls" (CD57). "We need to learn that indulged appetite is the greatest hindrance to MENTAL IMPROVEMENT and SOUL SANCTIFICATION" (CD127).

◆ *Overeating*

For every pound of excess weight you gain after 30, you shorten your life by 6 months. With every excess pound after 50, you shorten your life by 1 year. 31% of men and 38% of women in the U.S. weigh more than they should. A 1% reduction in body weight produces a 2 point reduction in blood pressure. Weight loss specialists say that no one is meant to be fat. Solid fats enhance weight gain more than liquid vegetable oils. In the U.S. weight gain peaks at 50 for men and 64 for women. Dr. Kelly Browell gives us some suggestions for breaking the links of the chain that leads to overeating. He says:

- Don't go shopping when you are hungry.
- Don't buy food you shouldn't eat.
- Don't leave tempting food on the kitchen counter.
- Don't put yourself in overeating situations, such as meeting your friends in a restaurant.

Those who watched TV more than 3 hours per day were more than twice as likely to be obese than those who watched it less than that. Water will help to cut down on water retention because it acts like a diuretic. It also dulls the appetite when you drink it a while before meals. The John Hopkins Health, Weight, and Stress Clinic observed that when slow relaxing tunes were played at dinner, people took fewer bites per minute, chewed more, and swallowed before taking another bite. They ate less even though the meals were 15 minutes longer.

◆ *Anorexia—Loss Of Appetite*

30 female patients who were hospitalized for ANOREXIA were unable to taste the BITTER and SOUR tastes. When they were given 30 mg of zinc, they increased their ability to taste, and their APPETITE increased also. What can bring it on also is eating too little to supply the nutrients which generate hunger. Also the inability to experience the full range of tastes. DRUGS will also generate a loss of appetite.

✓ DIGITALIS—When digitalis is used in large quantities to treat heart disease, it can bring on anorexia.

✓ ALCOHOLICS—can develop a sharp decrease in appetite due to the depletion of VITAMIN B_1, PROTEIN, and ZINC. CIRRHOSIS of the LIVER as well as MILK INTOLERANCE can also do so.

✓ ANOREXIA NERVOSA—This is an intense fear of becoming OBESE. Such fear does not diminish as weight loss progresses. The patient claims to feel fat even when emaciated. No known physical ailment accounts for the weight loss. He may lose as much as 25% of his original weight. Young girls can be helped by giving them 30 mg of ZINC, and a 50 mg capsule of the B-COMPLEX vitamins. This will increase their ability to taste food as well as improve their appetite.

✓ CELIAC DISEASE—Celiac disease represents an intestinal MALABSORPTION of FATS and CALCIUM which leads to DIARRHEA, MALNUTRITION, and HYPOCALCEMIA. This disease also responds to eliminating WHEAT and RYE from the diet because they contain the GLUTEN protein which seems to trigger it. Celiac disease is often treated with APPLES, BANANAS, and the B-COMPLEX vitamins. Researchers have restored the appetite of children with celiac disease with 2 or 3 bananas daily. Foods rich in vitamin B_1 are BREWERS YEAST, WHEAT GERM, SUNFLOWER SEEDS, and SOY BEANS.

The Results Of Intemperance

◆ *Physical Intemperance*

"Those who consider the matter of eating and drinking of too little consequence will find that what seemed to them unimportant was not so regarded by God. 'Thus said the Lord' is to be our rule in all things.—Daniel did not vacillate between principle and inclination.—A strict compliance with the requirements of God is beneficial to health of body and mind." (RH1-25-81). "The SIN of intemperate eating, eating TOO FREQUENTLY, TOO MUCH, and of rich UNWHOLESOME FOOD, destroys the healthy action of the DIGESTIVE ORGANS, AFFECTS THE BRAIN, PERVERTS JUDGMENT, PREVENTING RATIONAL CALM, HEALTHY THINKING AND ACTING" (CD50).

◆ *Intemperate In Quantity And Quality Of Food Eaten*

Intemperance is often the cause of SICKNESS. We can get sick on good food as well as bad food. Good food can also be used injudiciously. For example we are told that "It is a sin to be intemperate in the quantity of food eaten, even if the quality is unobjectionable" (CD102). "We are constantly tempted to excess. There is danger in abundance" CD29). "Abstemious in diet is rewarded with mental and moral vigor" (CD126). "Often the intemperance is felt at once in the form of HEADACHE, INDIGESTION, and COLIC" (CD101). "DEGRADATION, CRUELTY, WRETCHEDNESS, and STRIFE follow as the natural results of intemperance" (Te54).

◆ *Food Must Be Good And Not Only Taste Good*

All too often people consult their taste first without reference to health. The question we should ask first is, "Is it good food?" If good food is not at first tasty to us, one can get used to it in time. Today, processed food is made tasty by adding a lot of SALT and SUGAR to it. Such action bypasses the real NATURAL flavor of food by superimposing an artificial flavoring device. The addition of salt and sugar to food has increased steadily in the last two or three decades. But natural food will taste good to the person who has not perverted his taste buds by the use of condiments and stimulants. "We cannot be safely guided by the CUSTOMS OF SOCIETY. The disease and suffering that everywhere prevail are largely due to ERRORS IN DIET" (CD127).

◆ *Mental And Spiritual Intemperance*

"The HEALTH REFORM is one branch of the great work which is to fit a people for the COMING of the LORD. It is as closely connected with the THIRD ANGEL'S MESSAGE as the hand is with the body" (CH20–1) "Whether therefore ye EAT, DRINK, OR WHATSOEVER YE DO, do all to the glory of God" (1 Cor. 10:31). "The grace of Christ must be the abiding principle for temperance" (CD35). "Temperance in all things is necessary. Intemperance weakens PHYSICAL and MORAL POWER" (CD18). It is impossible for the intemperate to value the ATONEMENT, and to be susceptible to the TRUTH. (CD83; 451). It will also blunt the HOLIER EMOTIONS. (CD55). In order for us to reach the highest standard in moral and intellectual achievements, we must observe strict temperance in all the habits of life "Intemperance dethrones REASON; SENSUAL INDULGENCE, STRIFE, and BLOODSHED follow" (CH460). "It is impossible for an intemperate man to be a Christian, for his higher powers are brought into slavery to the passions" (CH36). The reason for this is that intemperance of any kind BENUMBS the PERCEPTIVE ORGANS and so weakens the BRAIN NERVE POWER that ETERNAL THINGS are not appreciated, but placed upon a level with the COMMON. (Te12).

Temperance Begins In The Home

◆ *Self-Control Must Be Taught Early*

We are told that "temperance and self-control should be taught from the cradle up" (CD246). "Regularity should be the rule in all the habits of children. Mother's make a great mistake in permitting them to eat between meals Even young children should be educated to deny their appetites and restrict their desires. If this is not done, then they become SELFISH, EXACTING, DISOBEDIENT, UNTHANKFUL, and UNHOLY" (CD238), and then they are not "doing all things to the glory of God." We are also told that there is little need for temperance crusades if RIGHT PRINCIPLES in regard to temperance are implanted in the Youth. (CD237). Often intemperance begins in the home. By the use of rich unhealthful food, the appetite is educated to crave continually something stronger, the system becomes more or less filled with poison, and it creates a thirst for strong drink (CD123). Even our eternal destiny depends upon strictly temperate habits of eating and drinking (CD234).

◆ *Wine, Strong Drink, And Cider*

"The Lord has given special directions in His Word in reference to the use of WINE and STRONG DRINK. He has forbidden their use and enforced His prohibition with strong warnings and threatenings, so that they may escape from the evil results of indulgence in wine and strong drink" (Te53). He says, "Wine is a mocker, strong drink is raging: and whosoever is deceived thereby is not wise" (Prov. 20:1).

The apple is the king of the fruits, and the juice made from it is equally beneficial. However, if fresh apple juice stands around for a week or two it begins to ferment, which means that ALCOHOL starts to develop in it. Alcohol is a harmful drug.... "LICENTIOUSNESS, ADULTERY, and VICES of almost every description are committed as the result of indulging the appetite for wine and cider. A professor of religion who loves these stimulants, and accustoms himself to their use, never grows in GRACE. He becomes gross and sensual; the animal passions control the higher powers of the mind, and virtue is not cherished. MODERATE DRINKING is the school in which men are receiving an education for the drunkard's career" (CD433). We are told that "Cider drinking leads to the use of stronger drinks. The stomach loses its natural vigor, and something stronger is needed to arouse it to action" (CD434).

◆ *Licensing Liquor Is Licensing Crime*

"After the 1906 San Francisco earthquake all liquor stores were closed, and there was a remarkable freedom from violence and crime.... By legalizing the sale of liquor.... they are virtually licensing the commission of crime. It buys WRETCHEDNESS, POVERTY, DISEASE, DEGRADATION, LUST, CRIME, and DEATH" (Te26). "He who is thoroughly converted will abandon every injurious habit and appetite. By total abstinence he will overcome his desire for HEALTH-DESTROYING INDULGENCES.... ABSTINENCE from all hurtful food and drink is the FRUIT of TRUE RELIGION" (CD29).

The Development Of Self-Control

◆ *Two Meals Are Better Than Three*

When it comes to eating, it is important to develop REGULARITY. This means that there should be a specific time for eating, and that nothing should be eaten between those times. Most people regularly eat three meals a day. Between those three meals there should at least be two 5 hours of rest before the next meal is eaten. However, if it can be established for the family, it is better to eat two meals than three a day, especially if large portions are served at each of two meals. "Most people enjoy better health while eating two meals a day than three;.... Let no one think himself a criterion for all—that everyone must do exactly as he does" (CH156). If anything the evening meal should be very light so that all the food will have been digested before bedtime comes along. This will give also the stomach a rest during the night.

◆ *Eat Less And Less Food With Age*

We should realize that as we get older the organs of digestion become less efficient. This means that we need to eat fewer and fewer calories per day, without losing weight, to maintain the organs in health. Eating more than that would have to be considered excessive. At a certain age it may be even best to change from two meals to one meal a day. This may be all that is necessary for an individual at a more advanced age to keep up his weight. Many individuals found that that is what they had to do in order not to gain excessive weight. We are told that "Excessive indulgence in eating, drinking, sleeping or seeing, is SIN" (CD141).

◆ *Food Needs To Be Eaten Slowly*

We are told that those who are upset or excited do not produce the necessary digestive juices in order to digest their food properly. Under these circumstances it is better for one not to eat, and to wait until one is calmed down and more rested. Food needs to be EATEN SLOWLY so that the saliva is properly mixed with it and the digestive juices are called into action. (CD107). It is also best that at each meal only two or three kinds of simple foods are served, and that no more is eaten than what is required to SATISFY HUNGER (CD138). Mrs. White says of her own habits, "I eat enough to satisfy the wants of nature, but when I get up from the table, my appetite is just as good as when I sat down" (CD485). We should never present the idea that it is of little importance what we eat.

◆ *What We Should Not Use*

✓ ALCOHOL AND TOBACCO—"are poisons, and their use is a violation of God's law." (Te87). "There is no natural appetite for tobacco in nature unless inherited" (Te56). They pollute the blood of men, and thousands of lives are yearly sacrificed to these poisons (Te57)

✓ BAKING POWDER—"The use of baking powder in breadmaking is harmful and unnecessary. Soda causes inflammation of the stomach, and often poisons the entire system.... Hot biscuits raised with soda or baking powder should never appear upon our tables. Such compounds are unfit to enter the stomach. Hot raised bread of any kind is difficult of digestion (CD342-3).

✓ CONDIMENTS—Condiments are FLAVOR ENHANCERS and are usually injurious in their nature. MUSTARD, PEPPER, SPICES, PICKLES, and other things of like character, irritate the stomach and make the blood feverish and impure.... Soon ordinary food does not satisfy the appetite. The system feels a want, a craving, for something more stimulating (MH325). "Food prepared with condiments and SPICES inflames the stomach, corrupts the blood, and paves the way to stronger stimulants. It induces nervous debility, impatience, lack of self-control. Tobacco and the wine cup follow" (Te57). The false feeling of strength which stimulants impart is an ILLUSION. FOOD also acts as a stimulant, giving us a feeling of strength when a meal is eaten. It is probably because of this fact that many people feel "weak" when food is withheld. "Do not eat largely of salt, avoid the use of pickles and spiced foods, eat an abundance of fruit, and the irritation that calls for so much drink at meal time will largely disappear." (MH305).

According to Dr. Rosenvoldt "Certainly the stronger spices such as PEPPER, GINGER, MUSTARD, NUTMEG, CURRY, VINEGAR, and other commonly used condiments deserve no place at all in a healthful dietary. We are amazed how many SDA Christians will have CATSUP on their tables. Why should we dishonor God with these health-destroying practices. Condiments destroy the natural taste for food by masking or overpowering the NATURAL FLAVORS" (Modern Manna, p. 156). He also says that CURRY will readily produce STOMACH ULCERS. After the stimulating effects of condiments have worn off, the individual lapses into an emotional condition as much below par as he was raised above par by these stimulants.

"Some who have powerful constitutions can recover from abuses to which they may subject the system. While others, whose hold on life is not as strong, who possess enfeebled constitutions, have never recovered from receiving into the system even one dose, and many die from no other cause than the effects of one portion of this poison. Its effects are always tending to death" (2SM449).

"When the appetite for SPIRITUOUS LIQUOR is indulged, the man voluntarily places to his lips the draft which debases below the level of the brute him who was made in the image of God. Reason is paralyzed, intellect is benumbed, the animal passions are excited, and then follow crimes of the most debasing character. When they are under the influence of the liquid poison, they are in SATAN'S CONTROL. He rules them, and they cooperate with him" (Te23-4). Then there is no crime which he will not commit; for he has put into his mouth that which has intoxicated him, and made him, while under its influence, a DEMON (Te36). The Lord makes the liquor dealer responsible for every penny that comes to him from the earnings of the drunkard (Te40). We are told that HOLIDAYS increase the evils of intemperance. They are no help to morality or to religion. On them men spend in drink the money that should be used to supply the necessities of their families; and the liquor sellers reap their harvest.

In this manner thousands of families are deprived of the comforts of life, acts of violence and crime are multiplied, and disease and death hurry myriads of victims to a drunkard's grave (Te30-1). The houses of liquor dealers are built with the wages of unrighteousness, and upheld by violence and oppression (Te27). For the money they receive no useful equivalent is returned. Every dollar they add to their gains has brought a curse to the spender (Te28). The millions of dollars invested in drink that will make a man like a brute, and destroy his reason, could accomplish untold good if it were used in the support of missions. God is being robbed of that which is rightfully His (Te29).

✓ STIMULANTS—Through stimulants the system becomes filled with poison, and the more debilitated it becomes, the greater is the desire for these things. One step in the wrong direction leads to another. (MH334). "Every organ, every fiber of our being is to be sacredly guarded from harmful practices" (CD19), because our body is the temple of God. "The use of unnatural stimulants always tends to excess, and it is an active agent in promoting PHYSICAL DEGENERATION and DECAY" (MH325).

✓ THE EFFECTS OF CAFFEINE—The average American consumes from 150 to 225 mg of caffeine per day, 75% of which comes from coffee. Caffeine consumption raises the BLOOD PRESSURE; stimulates INSULIN OUTPUT which then lowers the BLOOD SUGAR; causes high urinary loss of CALCIUM, MAGNESIUM, SODIUM, and CHLORIDE, which loss may cause "fuzzy thinking" upon awakening; accelerates BONE LOSS. Regular coffee is 95% caffeine free, decaffeinated coffee is 97% caffeine free; a 12 oz. cola contains 35 mg caffeine. The intake of caffeine has been positively related to MENTAL ILLNESS in PSYCHIATRIC patients.

Caffeine is a close cousin to NICOTINE. One cup of coffee or tea will excite a demand for a cigarette. The chemical used to decaffeinate coffee is CAFFEOL which gives coffee its aroma and flavor. It is a CARCINOGEN, and it also irritates the STOMACH, LIVER, KIDNEYS, and BLADDER, and in some cases causes cancer of the bladder. Caffeine prevents the blood cells from carrying OXYGEN to the cells by restricting the capillaries. Under these circumstances the sugar which the cells burn is turned into alcohol. The cell becomes a wild cell which can produce one kind of CANCER.

Caffeine causes the blood sugar level to rise rapidly and then fall just as rapidly. When this happens the individual feels tired, uncomfortable or hungry, and eats something else that is sugary, or gets a LIFT from a cup of coffee. Caffeine stimulates the ADRENAL CORTEX to produce more of its hormones, which in turn induce the liver to break down GLYCOGEN into GLUCOSE which flows into the bloodstream to give the body a lift. If not enough INSULIN is produced DIABETES results. If too much insulin is produced HYPOGLYCEMIA occurs. Essentially hypoglycemia is SUGAR STARVATION. Since the nourishment of the brain is exclusively glucose, many hypoglycemia victims suffer from frequent HEADACHES, because their brains as well as their bodies cry out for nourishment.

Coffee and cola beverages are highly addictive due to their "quick fix" caffeine content. Some teenagers drink 2 to 3 quarts of cola a day. A TOXIC DOSE of caffeine is 500 mg; a 10 oz. bottle of coke contains 100 mg caffeine. Research shows that the entire ENDOCRINE SYSTEM is disoriented completely by excessive amounts of caffeine in the circulating blood plasma. It turns the body immunity into a teeter-totter immune function.

✓ TEA AND COFFEE—Tea and coffee are neither wholesome nor necessary. They are of no use as far as the health of the body is concerned, but practice in their use becomes a habit (Te78). The money expended for tea and coffee is worse than wasted. They do the user only harm, and that continually. (Te79). The drunkard sells his reason for a cup of poison. Satan takes control of his REASON, AFFECTIONS, CONSCIENCE. Such a man is destroying the temple of God.

Tea drinking helps to do this same work "Tea acts as a stimulant, and, to a certain extent, produces intoxication. The action of coffee and many other popular drinks is similar. They stimulate the nervous system, and decrease the ability of the LYMPHOCITES TO FUNCTION. They also decrease GAMMA GLOBULIN, which is a protein formed in the blood, which has the ability to resist infection. Smokers also have decreased amounts of gamma globulin. There have been reports that coffee drinking is related to some types of CANCER. More than 2 cups of coffee a day produce higher CHOLESTEROL levels. The first effect is exhilarating. The nerves of the stomach are excited; these convey irritation to the brain, and this in turn is aroused to impart increased action to the heart, and short-lived energy to the entire system. Fatigue is forgotten; the strength seems to be increased. The intellect is aroused, the imagination becomes more vivid."(MH326). Yet how many there are who place these destroying agencies on their tables, thereby quenching the divine attributes. "OPIUM, TEA, COFFEE, TOBACCO, and LIQUOR are rapidly extinguishing the spark of vitality still left in the race" (CD423). The only safe course is to TOUCH NOT, TASTE NOT, and HANDLE NOT any of these substances (CD428). Every penny expended for them is worse than wasted. CAFFEINE causes a high urinary loss of CALCIUM, MAGNESIUM, SODIUM and CHLORIDE. In a Norwegian study of 15,000 adults, coffee intake of 9 cups daily for men, and 6 cups daily for women was associated with higher CHOLESTEROL LEVELS.

Tea and coffee drinking is a SIN, an injurious indulgence, which like other evils, injures the soul. These darling idols create an excitement, a morbid action of the nervous system. By the use of tea and coffee an appetite is formed for TOBACCO and the use of tobacco encourages an appetite for LIQUOR. (Te79–80). An acute HEART ATTACK has been found to correlate with coffee consumption. There is strong evidence supporting an association of caffeine consumption and FIBROCYSTIC BREAST DISEASE, which is a precancerous condition.

A waitress in a Chicago restaurant told an herbalist that she kicked the coffee habit for good by the use of the herb VALERIAN. To 3 cups of boiling water, she would add a level teaspoon of the dried chopped root and let the mixture simmer on low heat for 10 minutes, and then steeped it for an additional 30 minutes.

An animal experiment found that INSTANT coffee blocks the opiate receptors in rat brains. If that can apply to man, then the body's natural opiates, the ENDORPHINS, which are part of the body's mechanism for controlling PAIN, would cause them to be blocked, and would make the body more sensitive to pain.

✓ WINE—"The Bible nowhere sanctions the use of intoxicating wine. The wine that Christ made from water at the marriage feast of Cana was the PURE JUICE OF THE GRAPE…. It was Christ who, in the Old Testament, gave the warning to Israel, 'Wine is a mocker, strong drink is raging; and whosoever is deceived thereby is not wise' (Prov. 20:1). He Himself provided no such beverage. His whole life was an example of self-denial…. Christ did not contradict His own teaching. The unfermented wine that He provided for the wedding guests was a wholesome and refreshing drink." (MH333).

Reasoning From Cause To Effect

◆ *Some Foods Will Not Agree With All People*

We should investigate our habits of diet, and study the effect of food on our system from cause to effect. Some foods will not agree with all people. We must search out what benefits us and what doesn't. Most peoples' chief anxiety is how to get rid of the pain and inconvenience. This means that they are impatient to get well, and they resort to those things that quickly change the way they feel at the moment. Many will not take the trouble to find out the cause of their illness. But we should look for the cause in all of our sicknesses. Unhealthful conditions should be changed, and wrong habits corrected (CH89).

◆ *We Can Often Do More For Ourselves Than The Doctor*

"When the abuse of health is carried so far that sickness results, the sufferer can often do for himself what no one else can do for him. The first thing to be done is to ascertain the TRUE CHARACTER of the sickness, and then go to work intelligently to remove the cause. If the harmonious working of the system has become unbalanced by OVERWORK, OVEREATING, or other IRREGULARITIES, do not endeavor to adjust the difficulties by adding a burden of poisonous medicines" (MH235). People need to "wake up and reason from cause to effect. They themselves need to realize that they are disease producers because of their ignorance upon the subject of proper eating, drinking, and dressing"(Te196).

◆ *We Can Be Our Own Doctors*

"The PHILOSOPHY OF HEALTH should compose one of the important studies for our children. It is all-important that the human organism be understood, and then intelligent men and women CAN BE THEIR OWN PHYSICIANS. If people would reason from cause to effect and follow the light which shines upon them, they would pursue a course which would insure health, and mortality would be far less. But the people are too willing to remain in inexcusable ignorance, and trust their bodies to the doctors, instead of having any SPECIAL RESPONSIBILITY in the matter THEMSELVES" (2SM443).

◆ *The Intelligent Physician Studies The Sin-Disease Connection*

The intelligent physician has an increasing knowledge of the connection between SIN and DISEASE. He is constantly striving to perfect his knowledge of the relation between cause and effect, and is constantly trying to educate medical workers and patients to be strictly temperate in all things, because a failure to care for the living machinery is an insult to the Creator. There are divinely appointed rules which will keep human beings from disease and PREMATURE DEATH (MM49).

The Use Of Fiber

◆ *Fiber Is Necessary To Maintain Health*

Modern food processing methods remove much of the fiber from our food, which leads to CONSTIPATION and HIGH BLOOD PRESSURE as well as other health problems. Most Americans eat very little fiber. They eat WHITE BREAD, WHITE RICE, and everything that is soft. Such low fiber diets have been linked to HEART and ARTERY DISEASE, APPENDICITIS, COLON CANCER, DIVERTICULOSIS, CANCER, HEMORRHOIDS, DIABETES, and OBESITY.

✓ DIETARY FIBER—is found only in plant foods — WHOLE GRAINS, FRUITS, and VEGETABLES. Fiber ABSORBS WATER as it moves through the digestive system. The result is an INCREASE IN STOOL BULK and a FASTER TRANSIT TIME, which makes such fiber a natural protector against constipation and intestinal cancer. There are two types of fiber, INSOLUBLE and SOLUBLE.

✓ INSOLUBLE FIBER—The insoluble fiber is not digested. It is found in the STALKS, STEMS, PEELS, and SKINS of fruits and vegetables, and in the BRAN or SEED COAT of whole grains. Bran is 85% dry material, but it has the property of absorbing large amounts of WATER, up to 8 or 9 times its own volume.

✓ SOLUBLE FIBER—is found in PECTIN, GUMS, and MUCILAGE. Soluble fiber is virtually all digested. It doesn't have the bulk of insoluble fiber, but it forms a kind of GEL as it absorbs water. It lowers the LDL or low density lipoprotein cholesterol levels. PECTIN is found in most vegetables, especially in ONIONS, LEEKS, and ASPARAGUS, as well as in the flesh of fruits such as APPLES, or in the stringy membranes of CITROUS SECTIONS. GUM is found in OAT BRAN, and every LEGUME contains its own gum-like soluble fiber. Mucilage is a substance that keeps the plant from drying out, and is found primarily in SEEDS. 30 gm of fiber a day such as wheat bran, oat bran, fruits, vegetables, whole grain breads, and cereals will lower BLOOD PRESSURE.

✓ EAT FIBER FOODS SLOWLY—If you eat fiber foods slowly, you may end up eating less, because you will reach a feeling of fullness before your meal is finished. Also, food fiber HINDERS ENERGY or CALORIE intake. It also requires more vigorous CHEWING, which slows intake, and limits the amount of food which can be consumed. Fiber inhibits CARCINOGENIC substances as well as NEUTRALIZING all kinds of POISONS in the intestines.

Fiber And Disease

✓ INTESTINAL DISEASE AND REFINED FOODS—It used to be rare, but it is now running rampant. We are starting to find out that it is our own fault; a consequence of tampering with our food by refining it. REFINING is partially destroying good food and with it our DIGESTIVE SYSTEM. Refining removes a vital component from food, which is necessary for maintaining intestinal health. Enriching and fortifying doesn't put the fiber back. The scarcity of fiber is the key factor behind the soaring rates of BOWEL DISEASE in the civilized world. Refined foods do not fully distend the stomach, and hence, the stomach does not contract as much to push the contents into the bowels. Food remains in the stomach longer. When wheat is processed, a substantial amount of PROTEIN is lost. Protein acts as a buffer against the HYDROCHLORIC ACID (HCL) protecting the stomach walls from acid attacks that lead to ULCERS. CORONARY THROMBOSIS is caused by a lack of fiber.

✓ CHOLESTEROL—A deficiency of fiber and an excess of sugar interfere with BILE FUNCTION and CHOLESTEROL FUNCTION, and allows cholesterol to build up in the bloodstream. People on high fiber diets EXCRETE more cholesterol.

✓ DIABETES—is not found among people who rely on unrefined foods for their carbohydrates.

- ✓ WHEAT BRAN—is the most readily available fiber. It is the outer coat of the wheat kernel which is removed when it is milled into white flour. Its absence can cause the variety of diseases mentioned above. It is a DRUGLESS NATURAL REMEDY that really works. It is easy to use, readily available, and it is cheap. BULGAR WHEAT, BROWN RICE, OATMEAL, and BUCKWHEAT are fine sources of ROUGHAGE. Bran as a normalizer of bowel function can relieve DIARRHEA as easily as CONSTIPATION.

- ✓ A CIVILIZED DIET IS HARMFUL TO CIVILIZATION—To be civilized and modern, when it comes to diet, is harmful to civilization. Many of our most familiar diseases are seen among PRIMITIVE PEOPLE only to the extent that they become civilized. To become civilized is to die from civilized diseases. These diseases used to be believed to be a consequence of growing old. Many of these ailments existed only in rare instances before the 20th century. Most of them can be prevented by a few dietary modifications.

- ✓ REFINED FOODS CAUSE OVERWEIGHT—The Africans eat twice the CARBOHYDRATES of the Englishmen, but they do not grow fat, while the Englishmen do. OBESITY is not so much the result of overeating, but of having more carbohydrates absorbed by FIBERLESS FOODS, which do not tell us soon enough when to stop eating, because they do not allow water to increase their bulk sufficiently enough. Hence, the refined carbohydrate foods supply us with too much energy in relation to our needs. This implies that unrefined carbohydrates should not be fattening, and this is exactly what the statistics show. NATURAL FOODS DO NOT FATTEN A PERSON.

- ✓ DR. D.P. BURKITT'S DISCOVERY—Dr. D.P. Burkitt of Great Britain, discovered the link between diet and intestinal disorders, when he was for ten years a missionary in Uganda. He discovered that BOWEL DISEASE is almost unknown among rural Africans. In civilized nations, COLON CANCERS account for 12 to 14% of all cancers. The African eats food high in fiber which is not refined. He eats largely of fruits, vegetables, seeds, and roots. What we need are foods that provide BULK in the lower intestines, those high in cellulose. In the civilized world, WHITE BREAD has practically all of the fiber removed. Sugar is completely digested, but it has no fiber at all. Animal fats and dairy products have no fiber. As a result, it takes Westerners 3 days transit time for food to pass through the system, while it takes only 1 days for rural Africans. FIBERLESS FOOD can't absorb enough water to move easily through the colon.

Applying Self-Discipline

◆ *We Are To Set An Example In Christian Temperance*

In order for an individual to maintain himself in health, he cannot allow his feelings, his inclinations, and the desires based on them to rule and control him. They must all be under the control of a well educated mind. Such a mind must help him to become the ruler of his lower nature. He must become the ruler of his own INCLINATIONS with the help of the power of God (Te110, 112). In order to accomplish this everything depends upon the right action of the WILL. We must yield the will to God; we must choose to serve Him (Te 112). The will is the governing power in the nature of man. It is not the inclination but the CHOICE (Te113). We are all to set an example of CHRISTIAN TEMPERANCE. We are to do all in our power by SELF-DENIAL and SELF-SACRIFICE, to control our APPETITES (Te 119). "Everyone should exercise reason and self-control and should act from principle" (CD138).

◆ *Children To Be Trained In Self-denial From Babyhood*

"The time of trouble will require God's people to deny self, and to eat merely enough to sustain life" (CD202). We are also told that self-denial should be taught to children, and enforced upon them, so far as consistent, from babyhood (CD234), for the greatest danger of the young is from lack of self-control. They must be educated not to follow inclination. The habit which we form in this life affect our eternal interests. Eternal destiny depends upon strictly temperate habits of eating and drinking. Hence, we should be admonished by Paul's statement that "Whether ye therefore eat or drink, or whatsoever ye do, do all to the glory of God" (1 Cor. 10:31).

Acting From Principle

◆ *We Must Control The Mind To Act From Principle*

We are told that "Education in HEALTH PRINCIPLES was never more needed than now" (Te247). "What seems unimportant is not so regarded by God" (CD30). "The strange absence of PRINCIPLE which characterizes this generation is astonishing, and it is shown in their disregard of the laws of life and health, which is a PERSONAL DUTY. They indulge the depraved appetite in the use of slow poisons, which corrupt the blood, and undermine the nervous force, and in consequence bring sickness and death" (CD119). It is from the standpoint of principle that we should discard the use of those things which irritate the stomach and destroy health (CD196).

◆ *What It Means To Act From Principle*

TO ACT FROM PRINCIPLE means to act on an idea on the basis of trust and faith, which we believe will give us long-range beneficial results, although we do not always see immediate beneficial results. Our own actions should be an example to others. We should therefore "Teach by example. Let your self-denial and your victory over appetite be an illustration of obedience to right principles. We should always act from principle and not from IMPULSE (CD484).

◆ *The Principle We should Follow*

The principle we should follow is the following: "In regard to that which we can do for ourselves: There is a point that requires careful, thoughtful consideration. I must become acquainted with MYSELF. I must be a LEARNER always as to how to take care of this building, the BODY God has given me, that I may preserve it in the very best condition of health. I must EAT those things which will be for my very BEST GOOD physically, and I must take special care to have my CLOTHING such as will conduce to a healthful circulation of the blood. I must not deprive myself of EXERCISE and AIR, I must get all the SUNLIGHT that it is possible for me to obtain. I must have WISDOM to be a faithful guardian of my body.

"I should do a very unwise thing to enter a cool room when in a PERSPIRATION; I should show myself an unwise steward to allow myself to sit in a draft and so expose myself so as to take cold. I should be unwise to sit with cold feet and limbs and thus drive back the BLOOD from the EXTREMITIES TO THE BRAIN OR INTERNAL ORGANS. I should always protect my FEET in damp weather. I should EAT REGULARLY of the most HEALTHFUL FOOD which will make the best quality of BLOOD, and I should not WORK intemperately if it is in my power to avoid doing so. And when I violate the LAWS God has established in my being, I am to REPENT and REFORM, and place myself in the most favorable condition under the doctors God has provided—PURE AIR, PURE WATER, and the healing, precious SUNLIGHT" (MM230).

◆ *The Body Should Be Servant To The Mind*

We are told that the appetite should ever be in subjection to the MORAL and INTELLECTUAL powers. The BODY should be servant to the MIND, and not the mind to the body (Te138). We should cultivate the higher powers of the mind and there will then be less strength of growth of the animal (CD63). Those who are governed by principle will SHUN EXTREMES both of INDULGENCE and of RESTRICTIONS. But no one should consider himself a criterion for all. Some cannot use MILK while others thrive on it (CD198). This is due to the fact that in some people the production of LACTASE which breaks down the LACTOSE in milk before it reaches the colon, decreases as they grow older, until at times there is none left to digest the lactose. This can cause frequent DIARRHEA. "One person cannot lay down an exact rule for another. Everyone should exercise reason and should act from principle" (MH310). "Every violation of principle in eating and drinking BLUNTS the PERCEPTIVE FACULTIES, making it impossible for them to appreciate or place the right value upon ETERNAL THINGS" (CH38).

BIBLIOGRAPHY

ADAMS, Rex, *Miracle Medicine Foods*, Parker Publishing Company, Inc., West Nyack, New York, 1977.

ADAMS, Ruth, *The Big Family Guide To All The Vitamins*, Keats Publishing, Inc., New Canaan, Connecticut, 1992.

——————, & MURRAY, Frank, *Vitamin C*, Larchmont Press, New York, 1972.

AIROLA, Paavo O., *Are You Confused?*, Health Plus Publishers, Phoenix, Arizona, 1971.

——————, *Health Secrets From Europe*, Parker Publishing Company, West Nyack, New York. 1970.

——————, *How To Get Well*, Health Plus, Publishers, Phoenix, Arizona, 1974.

——————, *Hypoglycemia: A Better Approach*, Health Plus, Publishers, Phoenix, Arizona, 1977.

——————, *Rejuvenation Secrets From Around The World*, Health Plus Publishers, Phoenix, Arizona, 1974.

ARONOFF, Michael S., *Sleep And Its Secrets*, Plenum Press, New York, 1991.

ATKINS, Robert C., *Dr. Atkins Nutrition Breakthrough*, William Morrow and Company, Inc., New York, 1981.

BALBOA, David and Deena, *Walk For Life*, The Putnam Publishing Group, New York, 1990.

BALCH, James F., and BALCH, Phyllis A., *Prescription For Nutritional Healing*, Avery Publishing Group, Garden City Park, New York, 1990.

BENJAMIN, Harry, *Everybody's Guide To Nature Cure*, Health For All Publishing Co., Surrey, Great Britain, 1967.

BERGER, Stuart M., *What Your Doctor Didn't Learn In Medical School*, William Morrow and Company, Inc., New York, 1988.

BEVERLY, Cal, *Proven Home Remedies And Natural Healing Secrets*, FC&A Publishing, Peachtree City, Georgia, 1993.

——————, *1001 Home Health Remedies*, FC&A Publishing, Peachtree City, Georgia, 1993.

BRAGG, Paul C., *The Shocking Truth About Water*, Health Science, Burbank, California, 1970.

BRICKLIN, Mark, *Medical Healing Yearbook 1991*, Rodale Press, Emmaus, Pennsylvania, 1991.

——————, *The Natural Healing Annual 1984*, Rodale Press, Emmaus, Pennsylvania, 1984.

——————, *The Natural Healing Annual 1985*, Rodale Press, Emmaus, Pennsylvania, 1985.

——————, *The Natural Healing And Nutrition Annual 1990*, Rodale Press, Emmaus, Pennsylvania, 1990.

——————, *The Natural Healing And Nutrition Annual 1991*, Rodale Press, Emmaus, Pennsylvania, 1991.

——————, *The Natural Healing And Nutrition Annual 1993*, Rodale Press, Emmaus, Pennsylvania, 1993.

——————, and HOFFMAN, Matthew, *The Natural Healing And Nutrition Annual 1994*, Rodale Press, Emmaus, Pennsylvania, 1994.

——————, *Natural Healing*, Rodale Press, Emmaus, Pennsylvania, 1983.

——————, *The Natural Healing and Nutrition Annual 1992*, Rodale Press, Emmaus, Pennsylvania, 1992.

——————, *Natural Home Remedies*, Rodale Press, Emmaus, Pennsylvania, 1982.

BUCHMAN, Dian D., *Herbal Medicine*, Wings Books, New York, 1979.

——————, *The Food Pharmacy*, Bantam Books, New York, 1988.

BUTLER, Kurt, and RAYNER, Lynn, *The Best Medicine*, Harper & Row, San Francisco, California, 1985.

CALBOM, Cherie, *Nutrition and Cancer*, The Center for Alternative Cancer Research, 1990.

CAMERON, Myra, *Lifetime Encyclopedia of Natural Remedies*, Parker Publishing Company, West Nyack, New York, 1993.

CANNON, Walter B. *The Wisdom Of The Body*, W.W. Norton & Company Inc., New York, 1967.

CARPER, Jean, *Food Your Miracle Medicine*, HarperCollins Publishers, New York, 1993.

CARROLL, David, *The Complete Book Of Natural Medicines*, Summit Books, New York, 1980.

CARTWRIGHT, Frederick F., *Disease And History*, Dorset Press, New York, 1972.

CASTLEMAN, Michael, *The Healing Herbs*, Rodale Press, Emmaus, Pennsylvania, 1991.

CHEN, Philip S., *Soybeans For Health Longevity And Economy*, The Chemical Elements, South Lancaster, Massachusetts, 1962.

——————, *Mineral Balance In Eating For Health*, Rodale Books, Emmaus, Pennsylvania, 1969.

CHERASKIN, E. and RINGSDORF, W. M., *Predictive Medicine*, Pacific Press Publishing Association, Mountain View, California, 1973.

COLBIN, Annemarie, *Food And Healing*, Random House, Inc., New York, 1986.

COON, Nelson, *Using Plants For Healing*, Hearthside Press Inc., New York, 1963.

CLASSIC, Carl, *Secret To Hunza Superior Health,* Center For Human Natural Nutrition, Sherman Oaks, California, 1989.

COWARD, Rosalind, *The Whole Truth,* Faber & Faber, London, 1989.

CROOK, William G., *The Yeast Connection,* Professional Books, Jackson, Tennessee, 1984.

DAVIS, Adelle, *Let's Eat Right To Keep Fit,* Harcourt, Brace And Company, New York, 1954.

DAVIS, Ben, *Rapid Healing Foods,* Parker Publishing Company, Inc., West Nyack, New York, 1980.

DREHER, Henry, *Your Defense Against Cancer,* Harper & Row Publishers, New York, 1988.

DRURY, Neville & Susan, *The Illustrated Dictionary Of Natural Health,* Sterling Publishing Co., Inc., New York, 1989.

EHRET, Arnold, *Mucusless-Diet Healing System,* Ehret Literature Publishing Co. Los Angeles, California, 1924.

————, *Rational Fasting,* Ehret Literature Publishing Co., Dobbs Ferry, New York, 1965.

ELLIS, John M., & PRESLEY, James, *Vitamin B_6 The Doctor's Report,* Harper & Row, New York, 1973.

EVANS, William, and ROSENBERG, Irwin H., *Biomarkers,* Simon & Schuster, New York, 1991.

FAELTON, Sharon, *The Allergy Self-Help Book,* Rodale Press, Emmaus, Pennsylvania, 1983.

FEINSTEIN, Alice, *Training The Body To Cure Itself,* Rodale Press, Emmaus, Pennsylvania., 1992.

FELTMAN, John, *Food And Nutrition,* Rodale Press, Emmaus, Pennsylvania, 1989.

FERRELL, Vance, *The Water Therapy Manual,* Pilgrim's Books, Altamont, Tennessee, 1986.

FINKEL, Maurice, *Fresh Hope With New Cancer Treatments,* Prentice-Hall, Inc., Englewood Cliffs, New Jersey, 1984.

FISCHER, William L., *Miracle Healing Power Through Nature's Pharmacy,* Fischer Publishing Corporation, Canfield, Ohio, 1986.

————, *Breakthroughs In Arthritis,* Fischer Publishing Corporation, Canfield, Ohio, 1992.

FISHER, Jeffrey A., *Rx 2000,* Simon & Schuster, New York, 1992.

FREDERICKS, Carlton, *Nutrition: Your Key To Good Health,* London Press, North Hollywood, California, 1964.

GARTEN, M.O. *The Health Secrets Of A Naturopathic Doctor,* Parker Publishing Company, Inc., West Nyack, New York, 1967.

GERSON, Max, *A Cancer Therapy,* The Gerson Institute, Bonita, California, 1986.

GRIFFIN, Edward G., *World Without Cancer,* American Media, Westlake Village, California, 1974.

HARBERT, Virgil, *Sensible Living,* William Morrow and Company, Inc., New York, 1988.

HARRIS, Coleman M., and SHURE, Norman, *All About Allergy,* Prentice-Hall, Inc., Englewood Cliffs, New Jersey, 1969.

HARRIS, Lloyd J., *The Book Of Garlic,* Holt, Rinehart and Winston, New York, 1975.

HAUGHT, S. J., *Has Dr. Max Gerson A True Cancer Cure,* London Press, North Hollywood, California, 1962.

HAUSMAN, Patricia, *Foods That Fight Cancer,* Rawson Associates, New York, 1983.

HEALTH RESEARCH, *Is Cancer Curable?,* Health Research, Mokelumne Hill, Ca., 1954, 1962.

HUNTER, Beatrice Trum, *Consumer Beware,* Simon and Schuster, New York, 1971.

HURLEY, J.B., *The Healing Foods,* Rodale Press, Emmaus, Pennsylvania., 1989.

HEINERMAN, John, *Double The Power Of Your Immune System,* Parker Publishing Company, West Nyack, New York, 1991.

————, *Heinerman's Encyclopedia Of Fruits, Vegetables, And Herbs,* Parker Publishing Company, West Nyack, New York, 1988.

HENDLER, Sheldon S., *Anti-aging Nutrients,* Simon & Schuster, New York, 1985.

HILL, Ann, *Unconventional Medicine,* Crown Publishers Inc., New York, 1979.

HOFFMAN, Jay M., *The Missing Link,* Professional Press Publishing Company, Valley Center, California, 1982.

HOFFMAN Matthew, and LEGRO, William, *Disease Free,* Rodale Press, Emmaus, Pennsylvania, 1993.

HUNT, Teresa, *Growing Older, Living Longer,* The Bodley Head, London, 1988.

HURDLE, Frank J., *A Country Doctor's Common Sense Health Manual,* Parker Publishing Company, Inc., West Nyack, New York, 1975.

ISRAEL, Richard, T*he Natural Pharmacy Product Guide,* Instant Improvement, Inc., New York, 1991.

JAIN, K. K. *Health Care In New China,* Rodale Press, Emmaus, Pennsylvania, 1973.

JENSEN, Bernard, *Beyond Basic Health,* Avery Publishing Group, Inc., Garden City Park, New York, 1988.

————, *You Can Master Disease,* Bernard Jensen Enterprises, Los Angeles, California, 1952.

JOCHEMS, Ruth, *Dr. Moerman's Anti-Cancer Diet,* Avery Publishing Group, Inc., Garden City Park, New York, 1990.

KADANS, Joseph M., *Encyclopedia of Fruits, Vegetables, Nuts and Seeds For Healthful Living,* Parker Publishing Company, West Nyack, New York, 1973.

————, *Modern Encyclopedia Of Herbs,* Parker Publishing Company, Inc., West Nyack, New York, 1970.

KELLER, Jeanne, *Healing With Water,* Parker Publishing Company, Inc., Wesy Nyack, New York, 1968.

KEOUGH, Carol, *Water Fit To Drink,* Rodale Press, Emmaus, Pennsylvania, 1980.

KIME, Zane R. *Sunlight,* World Health Publications, Penryn, California, 1980.

KINDERLEHRER, Jane, *How To Feel Younger Longer*, Rodale Press, Emmaus, Pennsylvania, 1974.

KIRSCHNER, H. E., *Nature's Healing Grasses*, H. C. White Publications, Riverside, California, 1960.

KIRSCHHEIMER, Sid, *The Doctor's Book Of Home Remedies*, Rodale Press, Emmaus, Pennsylvania, 1993.

KITTLER, Glenn D., *Control For Cancer*, Warner Books, New York, 1963.

KLOSS, Jethro, *Back To Eden*, Longview Publishing House, Coalmont, Tennessee, 1939.

KNEIPP, Sebastian, *My Water Cure*, Health Research, Mokelumne Hill, California, 1956.

KORDEL, Lelord, *Health Through Nutrition*, The World Publishing Company, New York, 1950.

KOWALCHIK, Claire, and HYLTON, William H., *Rodale's Illustrated Encyclopedia Of Herbs*, Rodale Press, Emmaus, Pennsylvania, 1987.

KUGLER, Hans J., *Doctor Kugler's Seven Keys To A Longer Life*, Fawcett Crest, New York, 1978.

LEE, William H., *Run-Away Healers*, Instant Improvement, Inc. New York, New York, 1991.

————, *The Complete Home Encyclopedia of Food Miracles*, Instant Improvement, Inc., New York, 1991.

LEVENSON, Frederick B., *The Causes And Prevention Of Cancer*, Stein and Day Publishers, New York, 1984.

LEY, Beth M., *Health Talks*, 1989.

LIBERMAN, Jacob, *Light—Medicine Of The Future*, Bear And Company Publishing, Santa Fe, New Mexico, 1991.

LINDEMANN, Alan R. *Modern Medicine: What You're Dying To Know*, Personal Best Press, Fargo, North Dakota, 1992.

LOWE, Carl, and NECHAS, James W., *Whole Body Healing*, Rodale Press, Emmaus, Pennsylvania, 1983.

LYNES, Barry, *The Healing Of Cancer*, Marcus Books, Queensville, Ontario, Canada, 1989.

MALKIN, Mort, *Walking—The Pleasure Exercise*, Rodale Press, Emmaus, Pennsylvania, 1986.

LUST, John B. *Raw Juice Therapy*, Benedict Lust Publications, New York, 1967.

MARGEN, Shelden, *The Wellness Encyclopedia Of Food And Nutrition*, The University of California at Berkeley, 1992.

MENDELSOHN, Robert S., *Confessions of a Medical Heretic*, Contemporary Books, Inc., Chicago, Illinois, 1979.

MERVYN, Leonard, *Vitamins And Minerals*, Thorsons Publishers, Inc., Rochester, Vermont, 1987.

MICHAUD, Ellen, FEINSTEIN, Alice, *Fighting Disease*, Rodale Press, Emmaus, Pennsylvania, 1989.

————, ANASTAS, Lila L., *Listen to Your Body*, Rodale Press, Emmaus, Pennsylvania, 1988.

MINDELL, Earl, *Earl Mindell's Food As Medicine*, Simon & Schuster, New York, 1994.

MONTE, Tom, *The Way Of Hope*, Warner Books Inc., New York, 1989.

MORGAN, Brian and Roberta, *Brainfood*, The Body Press, Tucson, Arizona, 1987.

MOSKOWITZ, Reed C., *Your Healing Mind*, William Morrow and Company, Inc., New York, 1992.

MOWREY, Daniel B., *The Scientific Validation Of Herbal Medicine*, Keats Publishing, Inc., New Canaan, Connecticut, 1986.

MOYER, Anne, *The Fiber Factor*, Rodale Press, Emmaus, Pennsylvania, 1976.

MURRAY, Michael, and PIZZORNO, Joseph, *Encyclopedia of Natural Medicine*, Prima Publishing, Rocklin, California, 1990.

NEWBOLD, H.L., *Mega-Nutrients The Body Press*, Los Angeles, California, 1987.

NOLFI, Kristine, *Raw Food Treatment of Cancer*, TEACH Services, Inc., Fort Oglethorpe, Georgia, 1995.

OLSEN, Kristin G., *The Encyclopedia of Alternate Health Care*, Simon & Schuster, New York, New York, 1989.

OPPENHEIM, Michael, *The Best Medical Care*, Rodale Press, Inc., Emmaus, Pennsylvania, 1992.

————, *The Complete Book of Better Digestion*, Rodale Press, Inc. Emmaus, Pennsylvania, 1990.

PADUS, Emrika, *Your Emotions And Your Health*, Rodale Press, Emmaus, Pennsylvania, 1986.

PASSWATER, Richard A. *Cancer And Its Nutritional Therapies*, Keats Publishing Inc., New Canaan, Connecticut, 1978.

PAULING, Linus, *Vitamin C And The Common Cold*, W. H. Freeman and Company, San Francisco, California, 1970.

————, and CAMERON, Ewan, *Cancer and Vitamin C*, Warner Books, New York, 1979.

PEARSON, Durk, and SHAW, Sandy, *Life Extension*, Warner Books, Inc., New York, 1982.

————, *The Life Extension Companion*, Warner Books, Inc., New York, 1984.

PETRIE, Sidney, *Fat Destroyer Foods*, Parker Publishing Company, West Nyack, New York, 1974.

PFEIFFER, Carl C., *Mental and Elemental Nutrients*, Keats Publishing, Inc., New Canaan, Connecticut, 1975.

PINCKNEY, Edward R. and Cathey, *The Cholesterol Controversy*, Sherbourne Press, Los Angeles, California, 1973.

PREVENTION MAGAZINE EDITORS, *The Complete Book of Vitamins*, Rodale Press, Emmaus, Pennsylvania, 1984.

————, *Cancer Prevention*, Rodale Press, Emmaus, Pennsylvania, 1988.

————, *The Complete Book of Vitamins And Minerals For Health*, Rodale Press, Emmaus, Pennsylvania, 1988.

————, *Everyday Health Tips*, Rodale Press, Emmaus, Pennsylvania, 1988.

————, *Giant Book of Health Facts*, Rodale Press, Emmaus, Pennsylvania, 1991.

————, *Intensive Healing Diets*, Rodale Press, Emmaus, Pennsylvania, 1988.

———, *LifeSpan-Plus,* Rodale Press, Emmaus, Pennsylvania, 1990.

———, *New Encyclopedia of Common Diseases,* Rodale Press, Emmaus, Pennsylvania, 1984.

———, *Healing Remedies and Techniques,* Rodale Press, Emmaus, Pennsylvania, 1992.

———, *Pain-Relief System,* Rodale Press, Emmaus, Pennsylvania, 1992.

———, *Positive Living and Health,* Rodale Press, Emmaus, Pennsylvania, 1990.

———, *Surgery And Its Alternatives*, Rodale Press, Emmaus, Pennsylvania, 1980.

———, *Symptoms Their Causes & Cures,* Rodale Press, Emmaus, Pennsylvania, 1994.

———, *Visual Encyclopedia of Natural Healing*, Rodale Press, Emmaus, Pennsylvania, 1991.

PRITIKIN, Nathan, *The Pritikin Program For Diet & Exercise,* Grosset & Dunlap, New York, 1979.

QUILLIN. Patrick, *Healing Nutrients*, Contemporary Books, New York, 1987.

READER'S DIGEST ASSOCIATION, INC., *Family Guide To Natural Medicine,* Pleasantville, New York, 1993.

READER'S DIGEST ASSOCIATION, INC., *Magic And Medicine of Plants*, Pleasantville, New York, 1986.

REAMS, Carey A. *Choose Life or Death,* Holistic Laboratories, Tampa, Florida, 1978.

REUBEN, David, *The Save-Your-Life Diet,* Random House, New York, 1975.

REVIEW AND HERALD PUBLISHING ASSOCIATION, *Youth's Instructor,* Washington, D.C., 1986.

RICHARDSON, John A., & GRIFFIN, Patricia, *Laetrile Case Histories*, American Media, Westlake Village, California, 1977.

RICHTER, John T., *Nature The Healer,* The Provoker Press, St. Catherines, Ontario, 1972.

RINZLER, Carol Ann, *Feed A Cold, Starve A Fever*, Facts On File, New York, 1991.

ROBINSON, D.E., *The Story of our Health Message*, Southern Publishing Association, Nashville, Tennessee, 1965.

RODALE, J., *Arthritis, Rheumatism, and Your Aching Back,* Rodale Press, Emmaus, Pennsylvania, 1970.

———, *Best Articles From Prevention*, Rodale Press, Emmaus, Pennsylvania, 1967.

———, *Cancer, Facts and Fallacies,* Rodale Press, Emmaus, Pennsylvania, 1969.

———, *The Complete Book Of Food And Nutrition,* Rodale Press, Inc., Emmaus, Pennsylvania, 1961.

———, *The Health Builder*, Rodale Press, Pennsylvania, 1957.

———, *Your Diet And Your Heart,* Rodale Press, Emmaus, Pennsylvania, 1969.

ROE, Daphne A., *Drug-Induced Nutritional Deficiencies*, The Avi Publishing Company, Westport, Connecticut, 1976.

ROLFE, Lionel, and LENNON, Nigey, *Nature's 12 Magic Healers,* Parker Publishing Company, West Nyack, New York, 1978.

ROSENFELD, Isadore, *The Best Treatment,* Simon & Schuster, New York, 1991.

———, *Modern Prevention: The New Medicine,* Simon and Schuster, New York, 1986.

———, *Symptoms,* Simon & Schuster, New York, 1989.

SALAMAN, Maureen, *Foods That Heal,* MKS, Inc., 1989.

SAMUELS, Mike, and SAMUELS, Nancy, *The Well Adult*, Summit Books, New York, 1988.

SANFORD, David, *Hot War on the Consumer,* Pitman Publishing Company, New York, 1969.

SANTILLO, Humbart, *Natural Healing With Herbs,* Hohm Press, Chino Valley, Arizona, 1984.

SCALA, James, *Prescription for Longevity*, Dutton Books, New York, 1992.

SCHNEIDER, L. L., *Old—Fashioned Health Remedies That Work Best,* Parker Publishing Company, West Nyack, New York, 1977.

SEHNERT, Keith W., *How To Be Your Own Doctor*, Grosset & Dunlap, New York, 1981.

SHELTON, Herbert M., *Exercise*, Natural Hygiene Press, Chicago, Illinois, 1971.

———, *Fasting Can Save Your Life*, Natural Hygiene Press, Chicago, Illinois, 1964.

SHIMER, Porter, *Fitness Through Pleasure,* Rodale Press, Emmaus, Pennsylvania, 1982.

SIMONE, Charles B., *Cancer and Nutrition,* Avery Publishing Group Inc., Garden City Park, New York, 1992.

SHUTE, Wilfrid E., *Health Preserver,* Rodale Press, Emmaus, Pa., 1977.

SHUTE, Wifrid E., and TAUB, Herald J., *Vitamin E For Ailing And Healthy Hearts,* Pyramid Publications, New York, 1969.

SOLTANOFF, Jack, *Natural Healing*, Warner Books, New York, 1988.

STITT, Paul A., *Why George Should Eat Broccoli,* The Dougherty Company, Milwaukee, 1990.

SUSSMAN, Aaron, and GOODE, Ruth, *The Magic Of Walking,* Simon and Schuster, New York, 1967.

SUSSMAN, Vic, *The Vegetarian Alternative*, Rodale Press, Emmaus, Pennsylvania, 1977.

TAPLEY, Donald F., *Complete Home Medical Guide,* Crown Publishers, Inc., New York, 1985.

TAYLOR, Renee, *Hunza Health Secrets for Long Life and Happiness*, Prentice Hall, Englewood Cliffs, New Jersey, 1964.

TENNEY, Louise, *Today's Herbal Health*, Woodland Books, Provo, Utah, 1992.

THOMAS, Clayton, L., *Taber's Cyclopedic Medical Dictionary* (16th Edition), F. A. Davis Company, Philadelphia, Pennsylvania, 1989.

TKAC, Debora, *The Doctor's Book of Home Remedies*, Rodale Press, Emmaus, Pennsylvania, 1990.

TOBE, John H., *How To Prevent and Gain Remission, From Cancer*, Provoker Press, St. Catherines, Ontario, 1975.

——————, *Cataract, Glaucoma, and Other Eye Disorders*, Provoker Press, St. Catherines, Ontario, 1973.

——————, *Proven Herbal Remedies*, Pyramid Publications, New York, 1969.

VOGEL, H.C.A., *The Nature Doctor*, Keats Publishing, Inc., New Canaan, Connecticut, 1991.

WADE, Carlson, *Eat Away Illness*, Parker Publishing Co., West Nyack, New York, 1992.

——————, *Helping Your Health With Enzymes*, Parker Publishing Company, West Nyack, New York, 1966.

——————, *The Miracle of Organic Vitamins For Better Health*, Parker Publishing Company, West Nyack, New York, 1974.

——————, *The Natural Way To Health Through Controlled Fasting*, Parker Publishing Company, West Nyack, New York, 1968.

——————, *Nature's Cures*, Award Books, 1972.

——————, *Nutritional Healers*, Parker Publishing Company, West Nyack, N.Y. 1987.

WAGNER, Edward M., *How To Stay Out of the Doctor's Office*, Instant Improvement, Inc., New York, 1992.

WARMBRAND, Max, *The Encyclopedia of Natural Health*, Groton Press, Brooklyn, New York, 1962.

WEIL, Andrew, *Natural Health, Natural Medicine*, Houghton Mifflin Co., Boston, Massachusetts, 1990.

WERBACH, Melvyn, *Healing Through Nutrition*, Harper Collins Publishers, New York, 1993.

WEINER, Michael A., *Earth Medicine-Earth Foods*, The MacMillan Company, New York, 1972.

WEISS, Gaea and Shandor, *Growing and Using The Healing Herbs*, Rodale Press, Emmaus, Pennsylvania, 1985.

WHITE, Ellen G., *The Acts of The Apostles*, Pacific Press Publishing Association, Mountain View, California, 1911.

——————, *The Adventist Home*, Review and Herald Publishing Association, Takoma Park, Washington, D.C. 1980.

——————, *Child Guidance*, Review and Herald Publishing Association, Takoma Park, Washinton, D.C., 1954.

——————, *Christ's Object Lessons*, Review and Herald Publishing Association, Takoma Park, Washington, D.C., 1941.

——————, *Colporteur Ministry*, Pacific Press Publishing Association, Mountain View, California, 1953.

——————, *Counsels on Diet And Food*, Review And Herald Publishing Association, Takoma Park, Washington, D.C., 1938.

——————, *Counsels on Health*, Pacific Press Publishing Association, Mountain View, California, 1951.

——————, *Counsels to Parents, Teachers, and Students*, Pacific Press Publishing Association, Mountain View, California, 1943.

——————, *The Desires of Age*, Pacific Press Publishing Association, Mountain View, California, 1940.

——————, *Early Writings of Ellen G. White*, Review and Herald Publishing Association, Takoma Park, Washington, D.C., 1945.

——————, *Education*, Pacific Press Publishing Association, Mountain View, California, 1952.

——————, *Fundamental of Christian Education*, Southern Publishing Association, Nashville, Tennessee, 1923.

——————, *Gospel Workers*, Review and Herald Publishing Association, Battle Creeek, Michigan, 1901.

——————, *Healthful Living*, TEACH Services, Inc., Fort Oglethorpe, Georgia, 1997.

——————, *Life Sketches of Ellen G. White*, Seventh-day Adventist Publishing Association, Battle Creek, Michigan, 1888.

——————, *Medical Ministry*, Pacific Press Publishing Association, Mountain View, California, 1963.

——————, *Ministry Of Healing*, Pacific Press Publishing Association, Mountain View, California, 1909.

——————, *Selected Messages, Books 1-3*, Pacific Press Publishing Association, Mountain View, California, 1958, 1980.

——————, *Sons and Daughters of God*, Review and Herald Publishing Association, Washington, D.C., 1955.

——————, *Spitual Gifts*, Seventh-day Adventist Publishing Association, Battle Creek, Michigan, 1945.

——————, *Temperance*, Pacific Press Publishing Association, Mountain View, California, 1949.

——————, *Testimonies For The Church, Volumes 1 9*, Pacific Press Publishing Association, 1948.

——————, *The Medical Missionary Manual*, Harvestime Books, Altamont, Tennessee, 1992.

——————, *Welfare Ministry*, Review and Herald Publishing Association, Washington, D.C., 1952.

WIGMORE, Ann, *Be Your Own Doctor*, Avery Publishing Group, Wayne, New Jersey, 1982.

——————, *The Hippocrates Diet*, Avery Publishing Group, Wayne, New Jersey. 1984.

——————, *Why Suffer*, Hippocrates Health Institute, Boston, Massachusetts, 1964.

WILLIAMS, Roger J., *Nutrition Against Disease*, Pitman Publishing Corporation, New York, 1971.

WINICK, Myron, *The Columbia Encyclopedia of Nutrition*, G. P. Putnam's Sons, New York, 1988.

WOLFSEN, Al, *Healing By God's Natural Methods*, TEACH Services, Inc., Fort Oglethorpe, Georgia, 1997.

YABKER, Gary & BURTON, Kathy, *Walking Medicine*, McGraw-Hill Publishing Company, New York, 1990.

YIAMOUYIANNIS, John, *Fluoride—The Aging Factor*, Health Action Press, Delaware, Ohio, 1983.

YOUNG, DOBOZIN, MINER, & EDITORS OF CONSUMER REPORTS BOOKS, Consumers Union of the United States, Inc., New York, 1991.

YUDKIN, John, *Sweet And Dangerous*, Peter H. Wyden, Inc., New York, 1972.

ZERDEN, Sheldon, *The Best Of Health*, Four Walls Eight Windows, New York, 1889.

GLOSSARY OF TERMS

ADULTERANT—to make impure by mixing
ALKALOID—an organic nitrogenous compound
ALLERGEN—producing a specific susceptibility
ALTERATIVE—producing a healthful change
ANODYNE—relieves pain
ANTHELMINTIC—an agent that expels worms
ANTIPYRETIC—an agent that will reduce fever
ANTISCORBUTIC—will prevent scurvy
ANTISEPTIC—an agent that will inhibit microorganisms
ANTISPASMATIC—relieves or prevents spasms
APERIENT—a gentle laxative
APERITIVE—will stimulate the appetite
ASTRINGENT—a substance that shrinks the tissues
AROMATIC—a medicinal substance with a strong fragrance
CARMITIVE—an agent that aids in expelling gas
CATHARTIC—a strong laxative
CHOLAGOGUE—increases the flow of bile
CONDIMENT—a flavor enhancer
DEMULCENT—usually an oily substance that relieves inflammation
DIAPHORETIC—increases perspiration
DIURETIC—increases the flow of urine

EMETIC—produces vomiting
EMMENAGOGUE—promotes menstruation
EMOLLIENT— soothing to inflamed parts
EXPECTORANT—promotes the discharge of mucus
FEBRIFUGE—an agent that expels worms
FLATULENCE—distention of the intestines by gas
HEMOSTATIC—promotes blood clotting
HEPATIC—a remedy for diseases of the liver
INFUSION—steeping an herb for its medicinal properties
MUCILAGINOUS—soothes inflamed parts
NARCOTIC—a agent that promotes insensibility
NERVINE—allays nervous excitement
POULTICE—a medicinal mass spread on cloth and applied to sores
PULMONARY—pertaining to the lungs
PURGATIVE—a powerful laxative
RENAL—pertaining to the kidneys
RUBEFACIENT—an agent that reddens the skin
SEDATIVE—a tonic for the nerves
SUDORIFIC—produces perspiration
TINCTURE—an alcoholic solution of herbs
VASODILATION—the dilating of blood vessels
VERMIFUGE—an agent that expels worms

INDEX

Abortion, 249, 305, 317, 324, 461
Abscess, 111, 143, 147, 167, 348, 431
Abstemious, 13, 15, 33, 79, 113–114, 475
Abstinence, 15, 20, 98, 109–110, 113–114, 119, 221, 370, 464, 473, 476
Acerola, 238, 296
Acetaminophen, 288, 366, 398
Acetate, 224, 251, 296
Acetic, 47, 130, 132, 153, 185, 289
Acetonemia, 187
Acetylcholine, 251, 287, 441
Acetylsalicilic, 154
Acid balance, 197
Acid-alkaline, 129, 255, 260–262
Acidophilus, 131, 162, 193, 196, 198–200, 215, 278, 339, 345, 363–364, 369, 395, 397, 412
Acidosis, 129–131, 160, 164, 166, 173, 260, 295, 309–310, 360
Acne, 142, 183, 194, 230, 234, 278–281, 348, 423, 431
Acrolein, 127
Activated charcoal, 156, 278; *see also* Charcoal
Acupuncture, 435
Addiction, 187
Adenoid, 61, 188, 202, 293
Adolescence, 218, 278–279
Adrenal glands, 22, 70, 81, 99, 146, 149–150, 153, 191, 206, 215, 227, 237, 246, 256, 273, 295, 298–299, 357, 388, 393–394, 417–418, 436, 442, 478
Adrenaline, 22, 54, 105, 269, 301, 455
Adrenocortical, 206
Adriamycin, 247
Advil®, 392
Aerosol, 219, 310
Aesculapius, 137
Aflatoxin, 164, 174, 339
Albumen, 306, 397
Albumin, 70, 284
Alcohol, 36, 76, 127–128, 132, 146, 161, 191, 197, 203, 221, 228, 235, 255, 259, 266, 288, 291, 302, 317, 359, 387, 393, 399, 402, 406–409, 419, 425, 429, 433, 436, 455, 461, 472, 476, 478
Aldehydes, 309
Aldosterone, 261
Algae, 102, 148, 282
Algin, 93, 268
Alginate, 148, 268
Alkali, 129–133, 221, 255, 272, 293–294, 327, 426

Alkaline, 64, 108, 129–133, 142, 148, 160–161, 165–167, 172–173, 177–178, 180–182, 184, 188–190, 204, 221, 231, 260, 262–263, 267, 271, 283, 290, 293–295, 302, 309, 338–339, 343, 360, 375, 399, 408, 426, 431, 441
Alkaloid, 138–139, 142, 149, 153, 182, 280, 345, 489
Allantoin, 139, 141–142, 278, 294–295, 428
Allergen, 90, 283–286, 300, 318, 375, 489
Allergy, 48, 99–100, 168, 183, 186, 193, 195, 199, 204, 218, 237, 260, 279, 283–285, 292, 300–301, 356, 363, 370, 406, 426, 447, 449, 484
Allicin, 169–170, 364
Alliin, 168, 170
Alliinase, 170
Almond, 117, 130, 174, 183, 220, 232, 257–258, 260, 328, 339, 342, 355, 365–366, 402, 406, 408, 420, 439
Aloe vera, 92, 134, 139–140, 219, 278, 430
Alphaoxide, 105
Alphatocopherol, 245–246, 248, 250
Alum, 267, 287
Aluminum, 69, 89, 100, 225, 257, 267, 286–287, 289–290, 302, 310, 359, 426–427
Alzheimers, 145, 286–289, 427
Amaranth, 366
Amenorrhea, 365
Amino acids, 67, 100, 107, 113, 117, 123, 127, 131, 140, 163, 170, 174, 179, 184–185, 192–193, 197, 215, 220, 222, 229, 231, 234, 264, 273, 282, 287, 289, 294, 296, 298, 315, 342, 346, 358, 372, 386, 391, 402, 404, 415–416, 420, 427, 438
Ammonium, 128, 166, 214, 221, 261, 305–306, 310, 397
Amygdalin, 174, 327
Amylase, 131, 133, 144, 195, 411, 441
Amyloid, 223
Anaerobic, 47, 210, 306, 310–311, 323, 341
Analgesic, 140, 151, 257, 259, 436, 438–439, 441
Analytical, 226
Anaphylactic, 194, 201, 283–284, 356
Androgen, 407
Anemia, 93, 111, 129, 142–143, 149, 160–161, 165–169, 180, 184–185, 193, 201, 231, 233–236, 246, 250, 252–254, 265–267, 282, 289–290, 314, 324, 328, 366, 428
Anesthesia, 469
Anesthetic, 140–141, 150, 251, 414
Aneurysms, 265
Angina, 62, 93, 147, 154, 171, 206, 247, 249, 267, 378, 380–381, 383–384, 386, 391–392, 443, 450
Animalism, 134, 213–214
Anise, 295, 370, 376

Ankle, 84, 232, 261, 296, 350, 383, 429
Anorexia, 474
Antacid, 69, 142, 231, 257, 286–287, 289, 324, 355, 374, 398–399, 406, 426–427, 441, 465
Anti-inflammatory, 140, 143–144, 149, 170, 175, 277, 280, 295–296, 301
Anti-perspirants, 286–287
Antibacterial, 140, 149, 170, 186, 278, 280, 317, 330, 345, 431
Antibiotic, 48–49, 57, 70–71, 75, 89, 94, 138–139, 141–143, 145–146, 164, 168, 170, 185–186, 194, 199, 228, 237, 240, 260, 268, 277–282, 297, 317, 344–345, 363, 367, 369, 380, 395–397, 399, 410, 420, 431
Antibody, 47, 49, 173, 193–194, 199, 201, 212, 234, 237, 248, 277, 281, 292, 299, 351, 356, 395, 397, 415, 424
Anticandidiasis, 345
Anticoagulant, 139, 171, 245, 258
Anticonvulsant, 139, 153
Antidepressants, 81
Antidiabetic, 317
Antifungal, 143, 170, 345
Antihistamine, 59, 106, 285, 301, 317, 351, 370, 397
Antimicrobial, 146, 170
Antioxidant, 105, 142, 145, 152, 170, 176–177, 229, 237, 246, 248–249, 265–266, 269, 282, 288, 297–298, 305, 316, 333–334, 346–347, 352, 383, 389, 415, 417–418, 428
Antiprotozoan, 170
Antipyretic, 59, 154, 439, 489
Antiseptic, 136, 141, 153–154, 170, 172, 185, 280, 297, 353, 376, 396, 420, 431, 489
Antispasmodic, 147, 366, 374, 383, 489
Antithrombin, 245–246, 248
Antitoxin, 93, 285, 348
Anxiety, 2, 17, 19, 23, 66, 87, 140, 146–147, 153–154, 320, 363, 444, 447, 449–450, 479
Apamin, 298
Apoplexy, 4, 214, 443
Appendicitis, 216–217, 222, 332, 374, 480
Apple juice, 159–161, 178, 360–361, 372–373, 376, 476
Applesauce, 118, 146, 364
Apricot, 21, 161, 228, 238, 262, 266, 290, 328, 333, 366, 413
Arachidonic acid, 179, 291, 295, 382, 404, 419
Aromatherapy, 353
Arrhythmias, 68, 455
Arsenic, 100, 160, 225, 241, 342
Arteriosclerosis, 162, 180, 189, 191, 211, 222, 234, 263, 293, 314, 324, 378–381, 383, 387, 436
Arthritis, 30, 70, 84, 97, 100, 102, 112, 127, 135, 140–141, 143–144, 147, 151, 154, 160, 165–169, 172–173, 179–180, 188–189, 194, 197, 210, 212, 216, 218, 222, 227, 237, 239, 252, 257, 260, 262, 264–265, 274, 288–300, 315, 327, 332, 340–341, 379, 408, 412–415, 435–440, 443, 449–450, 465, 484, 486
Artichoke, 132, 335, 360–361, 372, 376, 403
Ascorbic acid, 69, 208, 237–241, 288, 330
Asparagus, 263, 333, 400, 416, 480
Aspartame, 192
Aspilia, 138

Aspirin, 61, 68–70, 94, 135, 139, 145, 154, 239, 247, 268, 277, 286, 288, 291, 295–298, 300, 317, 324, 353, 365–366, 368–370, 385, 398, 425, 435, 438–439, 463
Asthma, 16, 60, 89, 91, 99, 109, 142, 146, 150, 161–162, 164–165, 168, 183, 185, 188, 191, 193, 200, 237, 263, 266, 284–285, 295, 299–301, 443, 449–450, 454
Astringent, 136, 149, 154, 489
Atherosclerosis, 96, 99–100, 106, 148, 170, 172, 174, 195, 210, 222, 236, 240, 249, 258, 263, 288, 306, 357, 359, 378–383, 385–387, 411, 415
Atkins, Dr. Robert, 325, 483
Autistic, 231, 233
Autoimmune, 269, 292, 415
Autointoxication, 83, 160, 292
Autotoxemia, 222, 412
Avocado, 124, 208, 211, 234, 262, 279, 428

Bacillus, 48, 57, 128, 150, 168–169, 198–199, 215, 369
Backache, 171, 233, 365, 375, 411, 438, 440, 442
Bad breath, 48, 113, 376; *see also Halitosis*
Baking powder, 204, 267, 286, 358–359, 403, 476–477
Baking soda, 133, 204, 236, 238, 278
Baldness, 237, 274
Balm of Gilead, 135, 442
Balneology, 96, 412
Balsam, 13, 92, 154, 431
Banana, 142, 161–162, 428
Barberry, 345
Barbiturate, 237, 367
Barium, 148
Barley, 117, 135, 162, 166, 208, 221–222, 296–297, 322, 339
Basal, 102, 104
Basil, 94
Bayberry, 366, 370
Beano®, 163
Bedsores, 136, 180, 277, 430
Beef, 202, 213, 215–217, 294, 306, 408
Beets, 187, 230, 259, 266, 270, 283, 290, 333, 346, 348, 355, 366, 372, 376–377, 380, 390, 396, 403–404, 416, 423
Benjamin, Harry, 13
Bentonite, 287
Benzaldehyde, 167, 174
Benzine, 219
Benzoic acid, 131, 229, 231, 399
Benzopyrene, 94, 309, 312, 328
Beriberi, 188, 225, 232, 382
Bernard, Claude, 57
Beta carotene, 105, 161, 180, 228, 288, 329, 333, 383, 422
Bicarbonate, 129, 204, 262, 358, 426
Bilberry, 347
Bile, 48, 97, 113, 142, 146, 150, 175–176, 206, 208, 210, 255, 306, 312, 322–323, 332, 334, 336, 344, 370–373, 376, 382, 402–403, 425–426, 480, 489
Bioflavonoid, 94, 238, 269, 277, 285, 296, 342, 345, 367, 427
Biotin, 231, 236, 356
Black plague, 50
Blackhead, 112, 279, 421, 431

Blackstrap molasses, 193, 375, 392, 422
Bladder, 97, 100, 128, 131, 140, 147–150, 153–154, 160–161, 164–166, 171–172, 178–179, 181, 189, 191–192, 214, 216, 222, 230, 240, 242, 263, 308–309, 314, 317, 321, 328, 334, 371–372, 376, 382, 395, 397, 399–401, 403, 412, 419–420, 425, 478
Blindness, 93, 165, 225, 269, 345, 359, 376–377, 389, 414
Blister, 91, 141–142, 227, 278, 280, 350, 369–370, 423, 430–431, 468
Bloating, 69, 195, 376
Blood pressure, 20, 56, 70, 77, 84, 86–87, 92, 94, 97, 104, 106, 109, 128–129, 141, 145, 147, 149, 151, 153, 160–162, 165–166, 168–171, 176, 178, 180, 182, 198, 211–212, 218, 236–237, 253, 258, 260–261, 263–264, 271, 273–274, 284, 288, 291, 293, 328, 335, 349, 358–359, 377–378, 380–381, 383–384, 386–392, 398, 405, 412, 416–417, 441, 443, 450, 474, 478, 480
Blueberry, 170, 266, 290, 362, 364
Boric acid, 233
Boron, 184
Botulism, 170, 315
Brazil nuts, 130, 332, 334, 346
Breadmaking, 477
Breakfast, 97, 103, 120, 122, 132, 143, 182, 208, 235, 372–373, 375
Breast cancer, 84, 105, 147, 162–163, 171, 179, 193, 210, 212, 249, 304–305, 309, 312, 314, 316–318, 321–324, 326, 331, 334, 336, 361, 407
Breastfed, 193, 201
Breathlessness, 384
Brewer's yeast, 93, 123, 170, 179, 198, 222, 231–237, 264–267, 269–270, 299, 329–330, 343, 346, 372, 385, 392, 394, 396, 402, 406, 418–419, 421, 433, 438
Broccoli, 163, 289–290, 331–332, 337, 346, 366, 388, 391, 408, 486
Bromelain, 295–296, 298, 380, 396, 415
Bronchial tubes, 299–301, 351, 442
Bronchitis, 14, 58, 60, 91, 109, 136, 146, 150, 152–153, 161, 167–168, 180, 240, 301
Bruising, 237, 239, 250, 330
Brussels sprouts, 163–164, 264, 266, 331–332, 337
Buchinger, Dr. Otto, 112
Buchu leaves, 420
Buckwheat, 117, 130, 184, 220, 238, 339, 360, 366, 391, 481
Bulgar, 481
Burroughs, John, 88
Bursitis, 297–298, 441
Buttermilk, 192, 196, 198, 237, 339
Butyric acid, 130
Cabbage, 127, 139, 163–164, 187, 227, 238, 256, 262–264, 266, 286, 289–290, 323, 331, 337, 345, 365, 374–375, 404, 416, 428
Cabbage juice, 164, 427–428
Cactus, 362
Cadmium, 148, 178, 267–268, 389
Caffeic acid, 143, 164, 172

Caffeine, 130, 147, 182–183, 255, 273, 284, 299, 317, 364, 366, 374, 377, 382, 392–393, 402, 407–408, 426, 436, 455, 478–479
Calamus, 134, 373
Calciferol, 103, 243, 258
Calcium oxalate, 131, 180, 256, 293, 398
Calendula, 280, 422
Calomel, 75
Calorie, 22, 82, 86, 102, 120, 122, 147–148, 161, 163, 166, 176–177, 182, 187, 189, 198, 209–211, 217, 220–221, 224, 249, 318, 323, 336, 360–361, 368, 385–386, 391, 393, 411–412, 415, 444, 476, 480
Calotropin, 140
Camomile, 442
Camphor, 152–153, 351
Cancer, 302–344
Precancer, 167, 306, 321, 324, 329–330, 479
Skin cancer, 103–106, 141, 229, 240, 248, 256, 296, 316–318, 321, 324–325, 329–330, 422
Cancerous, 62, 105, 149–150, 152, 215, 229, 233, 237, 258, 306, 310–312, 316, 318, 321, 323–324, 326, 329, 333, 337–338, 382
Candida albicans, 63, 140–141, 143, 146, 280, 282, 344–345, 395, 397, 423
Canker sore, 20, 140, 233, 422–423
Canola oil, 192, 209, 211–212, 382, 391
Cantaloupes, 228, 262
Capsaicin, 151–152, 360, 437
Capsicum, 144, 151, 360, 366, 391, 428
Caraway, 275
Carbon dioxide, 88, 91, 94–95, 103, 132, 225, 237, 260, 263, 266, 293, 316, 394, 429
Carbon monoxide, 93, 219, 225, 241, 267, 318, 384, 429
Carbuncles, 143, 186, 348, 421, 431
Carcinogen, 105, 128, 139, 143, 159, 163, 165, 172, 174, 177, 180, 209–210, 214, 221, 241, 248–249, 258, 303–309, 311–318, 322–323, 328, 330–333, 336, 338–339, 342–343, 346, 382, 414, 438, 478, 480
Carcinoma, 102, 317
Cardiovascular disease, 176, 210, 261, 264–265, 267, 359, 379, 382, 385
Carnitine, 358
Carob, 34, 182–183, 363–364
Carotene, 102–103, 105, 139, 164–165, 224, 228–230, 285, 288, 324, 329, 337, 346, 353, 371, 383, 397
Carotenoids, 163, 180, 228, 238, 333
Carpal tunnel syndrome, 161, 235, 299
Carrageen, 148
Carrot, 21, 132, 149–150, 164–165, 172, 180, 187, 208, 224–225, 228, 234, 262, 265, 270, 273, 280, 283, 285, 290, 295, 328–329, 332–333, 335, 337, 346, 348, 355, 359, 363–364, 377–378, 380, 389–390, 396, 400, 404, 416, 423, 428
Cartilage, 147, 172, 190, 255, 290–291, 293, 442
Casein, 201
Castor oil, 175, 423
Cataract, 187, 196, 232, 240–241, 244, 249, 288, 317, 338, 345–347, 359, 487

Catarrh, 56, 160, 164, 190, 300, 400
Catnip, 150, 155, 157, 355, 368, 370, 374, 391, 405
Cauliflower, 132, 163, 180, 238, 331, 337, 375, 391
Cavity, 102, 166, 189, 221, 234, 239, 257, 335, 344, 351
Cayenne pepper, 151–152, 350, 352–353, 355, 367, 370, 374, 380, 391, 396, 405, 430
Cedar, White, 173
Celandine, 250, 373
Celery, 166, 246, 262–264, 270, 273, 295, 300, 360, 380, 390, 400, 416
Celiac disease, 161, 363, 474
Cellulose, 175, 323, 327, 332, 481
Cerebellum, 449
Cervix, 314, 324, 328
Chamomile, 94, 140–141, 144, 297, 345, 347, 353, 370, 373, 376, 406, 420
Chaparral, 141, 150, 278, 297, 334–335, 347–348, 432
Charcoal, 136, 156, 175, 278, 364, 370, 376, 396, 430, 437
Chard, 180, 230, 262–263, 265, 290, 372
Cheese, 129, 131, 133, 192, 194, 196–198, 200, 204, 206, 286, 300, 304, 306, 322, 341, 344, 348, 367, 371, 407
Chelation, 268, 287
Chemotherapy, 60, 247, 281, 290, 304, 308, 325–326, 334, 418
Cherry juice, 165, 264, 291, 294–295, 400–401
Chickenpox, 142
Chickweed, 422
Chilbains, 153, 423
Childbirth, 70, 153, 251
Chili peppers, 360, 413, 437
Chiropractors, 269, 321
Chlorine, 61, 95, 100, 166, 181, 203, 225, 249, 254, 262–263, 269–271, 284, 309, 363, 384
Chloromycetin, 146, 225
Chlorophyll, 139, 149–150, 163–164, 228, 240, 258, 282, 326
Cholecalciferol, 242
Cholera, 50, 146, 168–169, 201, 214
Cholesterol, 48, 82, 102–105, 111, 119, 139, 144, 146–147, 151, 160–163, 166, 170, 172–177, 179–180, 182, 193, 196, 198–200, 206–212, 215–216, 222, 233–234, 237, 240–241, 247–248, 255, 260–261, 264, 274, 288, 306, 312, 314–316, 324, 332, 335–336, 339, 357, 361, 371–373, 378–386, 388–391, 393, 396, 402, 417, 419, 423, 435, 478–480, 485
Cholestyramine, 172, 208
Choline, 141, 164, 180, 215, 231, 236, 251, 287, 311, 392, 398, 402, 416
Cholinesterase, 286, 441
Chromium, 184, 242, 264–265, 280, 357, 360–362, 379, 381–382, 394–395, 417
Chronic disease, 14, 30, 45, 56, 60, 284, 308, 328
Cigarette, 91, 203, 230, 242, 287, 310, 312, 330, 386, 393, 429, 478
Cimetidine, 139, 392, 427
Cinnamon, 134, 141, 152, 336
Cirrhosis, 128, 142, 236, 265, 341, 402, 474
Citric acid, 131, 172–173, 181, 185, 400
Clabbered milk, 196, 339, 355, 366
Clofibrate, 170

Clove, 169–170, 178, 208, 282, 288, 352–353, 391, 396, 400–401, 434
Clover, 155, 423, 434
Cobalamin, 235
Cobalt, 161, 164, 169, 235, 254, 265
Coconut oil, 207, 209
Cod liver oil, 164, 186, 227, 229, 252, 265, 353, 355, 421
Codeine, 288, 374
Coenzyme Q, 288
Colic, 150, 364, 374, 406, 433, 475
Colitis, 96, 99, 140, 144, 161, 167, 188, 217, 261, 263, 310, 363, 375, 439, 447
Collagen, 100, 147, 237, 277, 285, 296, 320, 330, 377, 415, 442
Collard greens, 163, 180, 323, 331, 346, 408
Colon, 47–48, 54, 64, 84, 103, 112, 126, 128, 160, 162–164, 198, 209–210, 215–216, 284, 289, 297, 300, 305–306, 308–309, 311–312, 317, 323, 328, 331, 333–334, 336–337, 361, 375, 412, 419, 480–482
Color therapy, 20
Colorectal cancer, 302, 336
Colostrum, 193, 236, 322
Coma, 259, 261, 360
Comfrey, 139, 141–142, 235, 278, 280, 290, 295, 297, 300–301, 355, 370, 373, 380, 390, 396, 422, 425, 428–430, 440, 442
Complexion, 160, 164–165, 168, 173, 183, 185, 228, 411
Conception, 246, 251, 329, 340
Coneflower, 143
Congestion, 21, 84, 87, 135, 144–145, 147, 149–150, 155, 157, 193, 249, 273, 351, 353, 367, 370, 403, 433–434, 440, 442
Congestive heart failure, 147, 386–387
Conjunctivitis, 168
Constipation, 83, 125, 128, 142, 160, 162, 168, 172–173, 175, 188, 195–196, 198–199, 204, 216, 223, 237, 261, 279, 306, 325, 327, 352, 361, 374–375, 401, 439, 450, 480–481
Contraceptives, 230, 241, 302, 314, 387, 392
Contraction, 147, 256, 354, 369, 373–374, 403, 406, 408
Convulsions, 113, 165, 195, 214, 255
Corn oil, 103, 106, 166, 176, 209–210
Cornea, 377
Cornmeal, 348
Cornsilk, 400–401, 420
Cortex, 286, 295, 435, 478
Corticosteroid, 69, 106, 293, 377, 408, 412, 425
Cortin, 153, 400, 423
Cortisol, 92, 104, 149, 320, 340
Cortisone, 54, 70, 97, 99, 149, 207, 227, 260–261, 277, 295–298, 344, 374, 425, 436–437, 442
Cottage cheese, 117, 131, 198, 200–201, 339, 360, 366, 402, 404, 438
Cottonseed oil, 209
Couscous, 221
Cow's milk, 192–194, 199–202, 223, 233, 236, 240, 257, 274, 284, 290, 322, 339, 356, 374, 392, 404
Cowpox, 319
Cramp, 48, 68, 140, 150, 153, 195, 214, 245, 247, 255, 284, 354–355, 365–367, 374, 376, 378, 380, 405–406
Cramping, 83, 255, 348, 363

Cranberries, 166, 204, 301, 328, 390, 399–401
Creatinine, 388
Credence, 153, 175
Creosote, 141, 297, 334
Crib death, 194, 201, 355–356; *see also SIDS*
Crotonaldehyde, 168
Cruciferous, 163, 324, 331, 346
Cucumber, 168, 263, 278, 286, 355, 360, 372, 396, 400, 403, 423
Cyanide, 328
Cyanocobalamin, 235
Cysteine, 220, 346, 415
Cystic breast disease, 364
Cystine, 264
Cystitis, 400–401, 419

Dandelion, 142–143, 230, 290, 348, 355, 366, 372, 375, 403, 423
Dandelion root, 142, 280, 373, 394, 409, 422
Dandruff, 231, 236, 431
Daylight, 145, 195
DDT, 93, 100, 194, 268, 308; *see also Insecticide*
Deafness, 70, 112, 179, 272
Decomposition, 121, 132, 165, 180, 184, 197, 305–306
Degenerative disease, 30, 57, 67, 114, 120, 124, 189, 198, 203, 234, 315–316, 332, 380, 395, 403, 414, 418, 465
Dementia, 233, 286–287, 363
Denatured foods, 119, 123, 302–303, 339, 358, 414
Dentures, 239, 318
Deodorants, 286–287
Depression, 17, 19, 84, 97, 105, 118, 138, 145, 147, 153, 191, 232–234, 236, 269, 273, 320, 365–366, 392–393, 412, 444–445, 449, 456
Dermatitis, 233, 236, 363, 422
Dermatologist, 272, 279
Dextrins, 184
Dextrose, 133, 183–184, 186, 226
Diabetes, 14, 21, 58, 60, 75, 84, 97, 99, 106, 108, 112, 128–129, 140, 142–143, 145, 148–149, 152, 160, 162, 164–165, 170, 174–176, 178–179, 183, 186–187, 189, 191, 195, 214, 216, 229, 234, 239, 244, 246, 248–250, 252–253, 259–261, 265–266, 269, 274, 277–279, 294, 300, 314–315, 324, 332, 344–347, 356–363, 371, 383–384, 389, 393, 399, 413, 416, 420, 425, 443–444, 450, 465, 478, 480
Diallyl sulfide, 333
Dialysis, 178, 287
Diarrhea, 14, 47, 60, 70, 113, 139, 146, 150–151, 160–162, 169–170, 178–179, 182, 185, 195, 199–200, 226, 233, 257, 281–282, 284, 286, 319, 363–364, 474, 481–482
Diastase, 184, 195
Diastolic pressure, 162, 171, 176, 211, 387, 390–391
Digitalis, 68, 70, 137–138, 147, 385, 474
Dill, 388
Diphtheria, 168, 356
Disaccharide, 133, 183–184, 189
Disinfectant, 146, 151, 185
Distilled water, 95–96, 283, 285
Diuretic, 106, 142, 147, 149, 152–153, 163, 168, 170, 259, 261, 271, 317, 324, 355, 366, 374, 399–400, 406, 420, 474, 489

Diverticular disease, 336, 376
Diverticulitis, 175
Diverticulosis, 144, 374–375, 480
Dizziness, 91–92, 144–145, 171, 192, 315, 378, 387, 391, 398, 403
Dogwood, 370
Dolomite, 252, 255–257, 259–260, 365, 404, 406, 408
Dopamine, 84
Doughnut, 189, 191, 312
Dramamine®, 144
Dropsy, 140–141, 273, 399–400, 424
Drowsiness, 144, 226, 348, 357, 366, 407
Dubois, Dr. Rene, 57
Duodenal ulcers, 161, 164, 173, 425–429
Duodenum, 370, 425–426
Dysentery, 47, 50, 57, 136, 156, 168–170, 182, 185, 198–199, 222, 363–364, 437
Dyspepsia, 85, 124, 132, 142–143, 150, 160, 177, 180, 199, 221, 375–376
Dysplasia, 329

Earache, 144, 169, 440
Echinacea, 143, 278, 280, 335, 348, 353, 410, 421, 431
Eczema, 97, 103, 140, 142–143, 146, 152, 175, 178, 193, 200, 204, 234, 236–237, 284, 295, 422–424, 431
Edema, 234, 249, 273, 307, 366–367, 399
EDTA, 289
Eggplant, 208, 292, 335, 379
Eggs, 75, 104, 119, 129–131, 133, 155, 157, 176, 179, 184, 188, 195, 206–209, 215–216, 220, 222, 224–225, 228, 231, 234–236, 240, 242, 246, 258, 264, 267, 279, 284, 304, 306, 317, 339, 360, 371, 376, 387, 392, 408, 415–416, 422, 439
Egg yolk, 179, 184, 206–208, 215–216, 222, 225, 228, 231, 234–236, 242, 246, 264, 279, 339, 360, 392, 408, 416
Elderberry, 143, 297
Embolism, 247, 380
Embryo, 238, 249, 251, 317, 342, 355
Emetic, 272, 489
Emphysema, 89, 91, 93, 109, 221, 252, 267, 301
Enamel (tooth), 100, 259, 267–268
Endive, 295, 376, 403
Endocrine, 146, 354, 380, 393, 442–443, 478
Endorphins, 22, 82, 86, 321, 338, 435, 437, 455, 479
Enema, 149, 341, 343, 368, 375, 405, 422
Ephedra, 301, 366
Epilepsy, 113, 136, 153, 191, 234, 259–260, 274, 386
Epinephrine, 357
Epsom salt, 97, 260, 268, 280, 301
Epstein-Barr virus, 63
Erysipelas, 168, 430–431
Escherichia coli (E-coli), 141, 363, 400
Esophagus, 161, 165, 310, 333, 374
Estradiol, 323, 331–332
Estriols, 323
Estrogen, 48, 105, 128, 149, 234, 250, 279, 314, 322–324, 331, 333, 340, 342, 344, 364–365, 372, 389, 398, 407, 409, 416
Estrone, 128, 323, 332

Ether, 140, 168
Eucalyptus, 94, 156–157, 186–187, 266, 351, 353, 370
Expectorant, 170, 489
Eyesight, 178–179, 359, 378

Febrifuge, 144–145, 489
Fennel, 373–374, 376
Fenugreek, 143–144, 208, 290, 341, 362, 364, 370, 375
Fenulin, 144, 375
Fermentation, 118, 121, 125, 132, 161, 171, 188, 190, 197, 199, 222, 235, 262, 267, 291–293, 298, 309–310, 329, 339, 342, 348, 371, 412
Fetus, 251, 317, 321, 340
Feverfew, 138–139, 272, 370, 406, 434
Feverish, 114, 119, 151, 173, 347–348, 369, 435, 477
Fibrin, 169
Fibrocystic disease, 248–249, 252, 364–365, 479
Fibroid tumor, 314
Filberts, 204, 339
Fish liver oil, 103, 123, 225, 227–228, 230, 242–243, 245, 258, 385
Flatulence, 136, 141, 144, 163, 168, 199, 364, 375–376, 489
Flavone, 140, 238
Flavonoid, 139–140, 147, 164, 288, 391
Flaxseed, 156, 192, 295, 313, 322, 339, 382, 386, 437
Flu, 89, 144, 146, 149, 152, 160, 168, 170, 172, 240, 301, 350, 352–353, 394–395, 397, 409
Fluoride, 69, 95–96, 100, 219, 225, 242, 259–260, 287, 302, 308–309, 318, 488
Folic acid, 69, 231, 268, 290, 292, 324, 329, 365, 375, 444
Fomentation, 142, 157, 353, 405, 430, 437–438
Footbath, 144, 149, 176
Formaldehyde, 168, 219
Foxglove, 138
Fractures, 62, 83, 141–142, 244, 255–256, 296, 365, 408, 416, 440
Frankincense, 134–135, 288
Fructose, 183–185, 187, 189, 360, 362–363, 394
Fungicide, 152, 280, 293
Fungus, 140–141, 143, 146, 164, 170, 173, 280, 292, 335, 339, 344–345, 396

Galactose, 196, 241, 345
Gallbladder, 48, 60, 176, 179, 370–373, 403, 409
Gallstone, 140, 142, 160, 173, 176, 206, 236, 256, 361, 371–373, 403
Gangrene, 136, 143, 164, 169, 246, 355, 359, 431
Garlic, 87, 117, 139, 145, 148, 162–163, 168–171, 178, 208, 232, 241, 265, 271, 280, 282–283, 285, 295, 297, 300–301, 321, 333–334, 336, 341, 343, 345, 352–353, 360, 364, 366–367, 370, 375–376, 379–380, 382–383, 388, 390–391, 395–397, 400–401, 403, 410, 420–421, 438, 440, 484
Gastric ulcers, 129, 140, 164, 173, 186, 204, 289, 310, 425–429
Gastritis, 341
Gastrointestinal issues, 147, 151, 163, 183, 199, 201, 230, 237, 245, 257, 263, 282, 291, 344–345, 361, 374–376, 425, 455
Gelatin, 148, 403
Genital herpes or warts, 136, 150, 282, 329

Gentian violet, 345
Germanium, 170, 297, 379
Ginger, 139, 144, 162, 208, 275, 296–297, 352, 370, 374, 380, 434, 477
Ginkgo, 144–145, 288, 348, 433
Ginseng, 144–147, 149, 380, 394, 417
Glaucoma, 236, 240, 347, 376–378, 392, 487
Gluconate, 408, 421
Glucose, 102, 108, 130–131, 152, 162, 170, 183–185, 187, 189, 191–192, 237, 239, 264–266, 279–280, 288, 300, 309–310, 317–318, 357–358, 360–363, 393–395, 416, 478
Glucoside, 135, 153
Glutamate, 273, 300, 302, 307, 314, 388, 390, 433
Glutamine, 416
Glutathione, 282, 289, 346, 415
Gluten, 179, 284, 363, 474
Glycerol, 184, 207, 416
Glycine, 131, 346, 420
Glycogen, 102, 161, 184, 189, 239, 357, 478
Glycoside, 138, 140, 143, 238, 420
Goat's milk, 186, 192–193, 200, 217, 262, 298, 339, 360, 370, 399, 402, 404, 408, 428
Goiter, 147–148, 182, 230, 265, 322, 365, 443
Goldenseal, 144, 146, 280, 334–335, 353, 376–377, 380, 391, 396, 410, 420, 422–423, 425
Gonorrhea, 146, 160
Gotu kola, 147
Grains, 16, 36, 96, 115–117, 125, 130–131, 134, 160, 162, 174–175, 189, 198, 202–204, 213, 216–217, 220, 223, 231–233, 235, 237, 245–246, 258, 260, 265, 267, 270, 284, 289–290, 294, 313, 332, 334, 336, 339, 343, 346–347, 360–361, 366, 376, 379, 383, 391, 394, 402, 404, 412–413, 428, 436, 439, 480
Granola, 438
Grape juice, 150, 157, 160, 171–172, 215, 264, 335, 420
Grapefruit, 131–132, 172–173, 208, 228, 239, 263, 280, 296, 300, 333, 360, 370, 372, 377, 380

Halitosis, 48, 160; *see also Bad breath*
Hallucination, 233, 236, 291
Hanson's disease, 432
Hawthorn, 147, 366, 380, 383, 391
Headache, 14, 17, 48, 54, 56–57, 59–61, 83, 91–94, 98, 112–113, 122, 140, 144, 150, 153–154, 171, 183, 189, 191–192, 212, 233–234, 241, 267, 269, 272, 284, 309, 340, 348–350, 353, 364, 366, 368, 375, 387, 389, 391, 393, 405–406, 432–434, 436–438, 443–444, 449, 455, 463, 475, 478; see also Migraine
Heartburn, 183, 374, 376
Hemoglobin, 161, 184, 188, 229, 254, 265, 289, 335, 358, 396
Hemorrhage, 70, 139, 141, 151, 157, 184, 239, 245, 247, 250, 269, 274, 297, 343, 365, 367, 387, 389
Hemorrhoid, 143, 149, 161, 166, 175, 286, 294, 374, 376, 430, 480
Hepatitis, 142, 149, 236, 240, 275, 281–282, 372, 401–403
Herbicides, 54, 293
Hernia, 332
Heroin, 22

Herpes, 136, 150–151, 171, 227, 232, 282, 369
Herpes simplex, 136, 150, 171, 369
Hesperidin, 238
High blood pressure; *see Hypertension*
High blood sugar, 191, 300, 359, 393–394
Hippuric acid, 127, 131, 166, 213
Histamine, 150, 283, 286, 356, 428, 434
Hodgkins disease, 148, 269, 333
Homogenize, 116, 196, 200–201, 207, 225
Homosexuality, 127
Honeycomb, 2, 183
Hop tea, 155, 157
Horehound, 353, 370, 442
Hormones, 48, 68, 81, 92, 98, 102–105, 111, 127–128, 146–149, 152–153, 191, 194, 206, 214, 224, 230–231, 240, 243, 256, 260–261, 264, 279, 296, 299, 302, 313–314, 320, 322–324, 326, 330–333, 338, 340, 344, 354, 357, 359–360, 362, 364, 367, 369, 372, 390–391, 394, 400, 407, 415, 418–420, 423, 426, 434, 438, 441–443, 478
Horseradish, 275
Horsetail, 431
Hyaluronic acid, 143
Hydrocarbons, 91, 100, 309
Hydrochloric acid, 124, 199, 216, 233–234, 255, 257, 262–263, 266, 270, 272, 294, 307, 344, 374, 425, 480
Hydrocortisone, 296
Hydrogenated, 105, 209–211, 249, 279, 302, 313, 448
Hydrotherapy, 97, 396, 420, 441–442, 461
Hyperactive, 107, 231
Hypercalcemia, 103, 227, 243
Hyperinsulinism, 187, 403
Hyperplasia, 324
Hypertension, 128, 144, 175, 273–274, 386, 389–390, 409, 447, 455
Hyperthermia, 327
Hyperthyroidism, 275, 372
Hypertrophy, 149, 215, 419
Hypervitaminosis, 226, 228
Hypocalcemia, 474
Hypodermic, 64
Hypoglycemia, 149, 187, 191, 284, 355, 361, 383, 393–394, 425, 433, 447, 478, 483
Hypothalamus, 20, 369, 439
Hypothermia, 350
Hypothyroidism, 100, 344, 366
Hyssop, 136, 272, 442
Hysterectomy, 367

Ibuprofen, 291, 392
Ice water, 101, 122, 430
Immune system, 22, 47, 49–50, 57, 59, 63, 70, 82, 87, 89, 102–103, 105, 111, 116, 137, 140, 145–146, 154, 159–160, 170–171, 193, 199, 238, 255, 266, 269, 277–278, 281–283, 288–289, 292, 294, 296–297, 299, 304, 308–309, 320, 326, 331–332, 334, 338, 340, 344, 353, 383, 395, 414–417, 422, 438–439, 443–444, 446, 454, 469, 484
Immunize, 171, 186, 319, 331, 344, 356; *see also Vaccination*
Immunodeficiency, 281
Immunoglobulin, 292
Immunosuppressant, 309, 418
Impetigo, 103
Impotence, 94, 147, 152, 268, 314, 359, 392, 420–421
Incense, 33, 91, 135–136
Indigestion, 85, 123–124, 127, 132, 136, 144, 146, 150, 156, 176, 188, 198, 257, 289, 292, 349, 375–376, 387, 430, 433, 475
Infertile, 94, 119, 268, 342
Influenza, 49, 143, 170, 173, 199, 240, 350
Inoculation, 319, 329, 337Inositol, 164, 180, 215, 231, 236–237
Insecticide, 54, 71, 120, 160, 263, 303, 338, 403; *see also DDT*
Insomnia, 83, 129, 144, 147, 153, 160, 198, 233, 261, 273, 327, 375, 406–407, 411, 416, 429, 436
Insulin, 21, 75, 84, 129, 142, 145, 162, 168, 170, 174–175, 183, 187, 207, 216, 233, 252, 264, 266, 280, 295, 345, 357–363, 388, 393–394, 478
Intemperance, 15, 19, 28, 32, 34, 39, 42, 45, 62, 110, 113, 120, 124, 156, 433, 470, 472–475, 477, 482
Interferon, 102, 146, 149, 170, 200, 212, 237, 296, 299, 353–354, 369, 397, 415
Interleukin-1, 212
Intoxication, 118, 128, 161, 171, 190, 221, 258, 433, 477–479
Inulin, 360, 394
Iodine, 97, 147–148, 169, 184, 195, 254, 259, 262, 264–265, 275, 279, 311, 321–322, 363, 365, 431
Iodized, 148, 265, 275, 279, 342
Irradiation, 104, 193, 243
Islands of Langerhans, 187, 356, 393
Itching, 106, 140, 183, 283–284, 301, 346, 431

Jaundice, 112, 139, 142–143, 160, 228, 348, 403
Jefferson, Thomas, 88
Jewelweed, 423
Jojoba, 325
Juniper, 394, 420

Kale, 163, 180, 230, 263–264, 273, 290, 331
Kaopectate®, 160
Kefir, 131, 196, 198, 222, 339, 355, 360, 366, 375, 412, 418
Kelp, 93, 123, 131, 147–148, 198, 208, 235, 265–266, 268, 270, 274–275, 290, 297, 364, 367, 392, 406, 416, 420
Keratosis, 105
Kidney disease, 14, 16, 60, 175, 178, 185, 211–212, 214, 273, 287, 306, 332, 338, 357, 359, 398–400
Kidney stones, 96–97, 99, 149, 160, 166, 178, 180, 201, 234, 255, 259, 294, 362, 397–400, 409, 426
Kloss, Jethro, 115, 146, 150–151, 157, 335, 410, 485
Kneipp, Father, 95, 98, 152, 185, 428
Kohlrabi, 163, 331
Kumquat, 172
Kyolic®, 170, 280, 282, 301, 334, 383, 396

Lactaid®, 196
Lactase, 48, 123, 189, 195–196, 199, 284, 376, 482
Lactate, 92, 192, 202, 246, 255, 258, 355, 408
Lactic acid, 47–49, 83, 102, 125, 130–131, 164, 197–199, 226, 259, 309, 327, 339, 394, 404, 412, 418, 435

Lactobacillus, 197–199, 230, 277, 285, 345, 376
Lactose, 83, 189, 195–196, 198–200, 241, 284, 344, 376, 412, 482
Laetrile, 161, 174, 327–328, 342, 486
Lard, 194, 312
Lavender, 434, 441
Laxative, 68–69, 142, 144, 168, 172, 175, 180, 188, 235, 302, 307, 318, 348, 363, 375, 405, 439, 489
Learning disability, 231, 394
Lecithin, 75, 117, 140–141, 144, 179–180, 195, 207–211, 215–216, 222, 236–237, 239, 250, 264, 268, 287–288, 343, 346, 355, 371–373, 380–381, 386, 392–393, 395, 402, 406, 416–417, 423, 434
Leeks, 168, 480
Legume, 117, 162, 217, 221, 346, 361, 379, 392, 480
Lemons, 94, 101, 122, 129, 132, 153, 172–173, 178, 185, 221, 237, 260, 269, 271–272, 275, 283, 300, 333, 341, 352, 370, 372–373, 377, 380, 388, 401, 403, 415, 420, 423, 431, 441–442
Lentils, 130, 162, 219, 221, 231, 328, 360, 372, 421
Leprosy, 11, 50, 136, 147, 169, 247, 432, 443
Lettuce, 180, 187, 219, 238, 251, 262, 273
Leukemia, 91, 94, 99, 102, 143, 148, 165, 261, 269, 281–282, 289, 304, 310–311, 314, 321, 333, 340, 343, 397, 463
Leukocytosis, 96, 126
Leukoplakia, 229
Levulose, 183–184, 186, 226
Libido, 411, 420
Licorice, 139, 148–149, 301, 354–355, 376, 394, 410, 422, 427, 429, 442
Lightheadedness, 291
Lignin, 153, 323, 332
Lima beans, 130, 328, 372, 437
Limes, 97, 132, 172–173, 187–188, 225, 266, 275, 293, 300, 333, 397, 424
Linden leaves, 373, 441
Linoleic acid, 103, 166, 179, 211, 222, 295, 366, 392, 404, 419
Linolenic acid, 179, 192, 295, 366, 382, 403–404, 419
Linseed oil, 212, 295, 313, 419
Lipase, 133, 184, 195, 372, 441
Lipids, 93, 160, 246, 267
Lipoprotein, 162, 206, 363, 378, 382, 480
Liquor, 8, 36, 393, 405, 433, 470, 476–479
Lithium, 184
Loma Linda, 67, 77, 87, 170, 208, 321, 334, 383, 397, 429, 458, 460
Low blood sugar, 122, 191–192, 265, 272, 284, 300, 355, 360, 384, 393–394, 406, 447
Lumbago, 164, 177
Lung, 31, 54, 62, 81, 84–95, 98, 102, 106, 108, 112, 135, 141, 144, 149, 153, 157, 161, 163, 165, 168, 172, 180–181, 195, 206, 221, 230, 247, 251–252, 260, 263, 267, 288, 299–300, 303, 308, 318, 320, 323, 328, 333–334, 336, 340, 347–348, 350–351, 405, 409–411, 419, 424–425, 439, 444, 489
Lupus, 269
Lutein, 333
Lycopene, 333

Lymph, 143, 149, 152, 180, 191, 212, 277, 279, 281–282, 299, 313, 333, 388, 409, 415
Lymphocyte, 89, 102, 105, 140, 212, 233, 277–278, 282, 288, 299, 321, 334, 444, 469, 478
Lymphoma, 150
Lysine, 220, 358
Maalox®, 426
Mackerel, 211, 391
Macrobiotics, 414
Macronutrients, 255, 264
Macrophage, 140, 212, 229, 288, 299, 334, 369, 397
Macular degeneration, 145; see also Eyesight
Magnesium, 69, 96–97, 103, 140, 165–166, 172, 174, 181, 184, 221–222, 234, 243–244, 254–260, 262–263, 268, 273–275, 290, 311, 354–355, 364–366, 381–382, 384–386, 390, 392, 397–399, 404–408, 411, 426, 429, 437, 478
Malaria, 75, 129, 154, 273, 289, 327, 370
Malic acid, 50, 131, 160, 181, 373
Malondialdehyde, 305
Malt, 133
Maltase, 133, 189
Maltose, 133, 184, 189
Manganese, 125, 140, 170, 264, 266, 311, 362, 394
Mangoes, 386
Margarine, 103, 209–210, 216, 279
Marigold, 250, 431
Marjoram, 434, 442
Marriage, 171, 444, 449, 454, 479
Marrow, 2, 60, 231, 233, 235, 282, 288, 290, 415
Massage, 82–83, 137, 250, 405–406, 438, 440–442
Masticate, 121, 375
Mastitis, 194
Mayonnaise, 374
McCay, Dr. Clive, 117, 416
Measles, 142–143, 169, 173, 231
Medulla oblongata, 147
Melaleuca, 280
Melanin, 103, 256, 316
Melanoma, 141, 240, 308, 316, 334
Melatonin, 105
Melittin, 298, 436
Melons, 132, 168, 332, 360
Meningitis, 169–170
Menopause, 128, 147–148, 193, 256, 314, 324, 331, 340, 354–355, 365, 367, 406–408
Menorrhagia, 367
Menstrual, 48, 84, 140, 149–150, 192, 279, 289, 340, 354, 365–367, 433, 438
Premenstrual, 249, 364–367, 401
Menstruate, 55, 84, 112, 127, 129, 136, 252, 266, 289, 354–355, 365–367, 406, 489
Menthol, 150, 420
Mentholatum®, 150
Mercury, 75, 93, 99, 160, 178, 241, 268–269, 287, 294
Metabolic rate, 86, 265, 368

Metabolism, 12, 45, 54–55, 81–82, 84, 94, 96–97, 99–100, 102, 104, 109, 111, 122, 124, 141, 147, 150, 178, 188, 201, 206, 214, 221–223, 227, 229, 232–234, 236, 243, 256, 260, 264–266, 268, 272, 283, 291, 298, 307, 310–311, 325–328, 331, 337, 339, 341–342, 354, 356–358, 360–362, 365, 368, 377, 380, 382, 387, 401, 407, 411–412, 414, 440–442
Metastasize, 212, 323, 326, 335
Methacholine, 428
Methionine, 220, 358, 402, 427
Migraine, 48, 61, 98, 138–139, 145, 189, 204, 212, 234, 272, 284, 393, 406, 433–434, 438, 443–444; *see also Headache*
Milk, 16, 47–49, 58, 93, 96, 107, 116–117, 123, 125, 128, 130–131, 133, 135, 167, 178–179, 182–184, 188, 192–202, 206, 208–209, 211, 215, 217, 220, 222–223, 226, 228, 232–233, 235–237, 240–242, 244–245, 250, 256–259, 262, 265–268, 271–272, 274, 279, 282, 284, 289–292, 297–298, 300, 304, 306–307, 313, 321–322, 339, 341–345, 347, 352, 355–356, 360, 363–364, 366–367, 370–371, 374, 376, 379, 384, 387, 392, 396, 398–399, 402, 404, 407–408, 412–413, 418, 424, 426, 428, 437–440, 474, 482
Skim milk, 193, 198, 202, 208, 279, 289, 291, 313, 379, 437–438
Milkweed, 140, 250
Millet, 117, 130, 220, 258, 290, 322, 339, 355, 360, 366, 391
Mint, 48, 150, 355, 376, 391, 434
Miso, 179, 197, 235, 376
Mitochondria, 260, 316, 342
Molasses, 130, 184, 193, 234, 237, 257, 265–266, 279, 290, 360, 366, 375, 386, 392, 421–422
Moles, 105, 279–280
Mononeucleosis, 281
Monosaccharide, 133, 183–184, 189
Monosodium glutamate, 273, 300, 302, 307, 314, 388, 390, 433
Monounsaturated, 103, 176, 209, 211, 313, 382–383, 391
Morphine, 22, 437, 469
Mosquitoes, 48, 189, 327
Motherwort, 366
Mucilage, 144, 153, 285, 332, 480, 489
Mucin, 168, 428
Mucosa, 55, 285, 365, 428
Mucus, 54–56, 58, 70, 93–94, 111–112, 129–130, 144, 146, 168, 172, 193, 200–201, 229–230, 281, 283, 285, 299–300, 340, 343–344, 350–352, 363, 368, 375, 409, 424, 427–429, 463, 484, 489
Mullein, 285, 301, 396
Mumps, 142–143
Muriatic acid, 250
Muscular dystrophy, 99, 103, 240, 247, 250, 253
Mustard, 155, 157, 163, 168, 180, 230, 262, 275, 331, 348, 402, 435–436, 468, 477
Myasthenia, 236, 266, 274
Myelin, 236, 284, 403, 437, 439
Mylanta®, 426
Myocardial infarction, 379, 381, 385
Myopia, 230, 244, 347, 377, 464
Myrrh, 134–136, 288, 374, 423
Myrtle, 136

Narcotic, 257, 489
Naturopathy, 11–13, 48, 60, 75, 116, 149, 300, 305–306, 318, 325, 328, 343, 387, 390, 428, 465, 484
Nausea, 60, 66, 113, 122, 139, 141, 144, 150, 183, 226, 234, 340, 371, 398, 434
Nearsightedness, 230, 244, 264; *see also Eyesight*
Necrosis, 212
Nephritis, 195, 236, 306, 398, 406
Nephrons, 261, 416
Nettle, 149, 280, 373, 401, 423
Neuralgia, 154, 262, 297, 405, 425, 441
Neurasthenia, 16, 129, 233
Neuritis, 129, 160, 216, 262, 264, 340, 400
Neurosis, 191, 232, 394, 454
Neurotransmitter, 84, 107, 151, 273, 287, 415, 437–438
Neutrophils, 103, 288
Niacin, 90, 140, 163, 200, 207–208, 222, 225, 227, 231, 233–234, 257, 273, 291, 299, 326, 329, 358, 363, 385, 414, 417–418, 429, 433
Nicotine, 478
Nitrates, 99, 228, 230, 302, 315, 389
Nitric oxide, 93
Nitrite, 230, 239, 302, 315
Nitrogen, 47, 93, 203, 216, 252, 255, 263, 283–284, 318, 415, 489
Nitroglycerin, 383
Nitrosamine, 163, 172, 180, 199, 239, 248, 315, 331, 333–334
Norepinephrin, 81, 84
Nosebleed, 349, 352, 433
Noxzema®, 150
Nucleic acid, 235–236, 414, 418
Nutmeg, 336, 477
Nutrisweet®, 192
Nystatin, 345

Oat bran, 175, 208, 331, 373, 396, 480
Oatmeal, 153, 175, 202, 235, 246, 341, 360, 373, 481
Oats, 117, 174–175, 235, 257–258, 263, 279, 322, 332, 360, 366, 391, 404, 437
Obesity, 22, 97, 100, 104, 124, 128–129, 148, 160, 164, 166, 173, 192, 216, 237, 248, 273, 314–315, 332, 357–358, 371, 379–380, 384, 416, 474, 480–481
Okra, 262
Olive oil, 103, 156, 164, 175–177, 208–211, 278, 289, 334, 347, 363, 371–373, 375–376, 382–383, 391, 419, 425, 428, 430, 440–442
Omega-3, 179, 192, 194, 211–212, 295, 382, 391
Onion, 117, 145, 168, 170–171, 208, 264, 266–267, 271, 278, 283, 285, 289, 301, 308, 333–334, 336, 353, 360, 375, 379–380, 382, 390–391, 396, 430–431, 480
Opiate, 85, 479
Opium, 368, 478
Oral contraceptives, 106, 234, 266, 288, 305, 314, 324, 354, 371, 389, 392
Oregano, 288, 388
Osteoarthritis, 290–291, 299, 438–440
Osteomalacia, 243, 255, 257

Osteoporosis, 48, 84–85, 97, 222, 243–244, 255–256, 265, 298, 314, 365, 398–399, 407–409, 413, 416
Ovarian cancer, 304, 407
Overweight, 84, 119–121, 128, 148, 207, 217, 234, 291–292, 315–316, 358, 361, 371, 384, 387–389, 392, 416, 481
Ovulate, 129, 193
Oxalates, 188, 293, 397–400
Oxalic acid, 131, 180–182, 188, 256, 293–294, 397, 400
Oxidation, 90, 93, 95, 103, 105, 127, 130, 135, 154, 210, 212, 225, 228, 233, 240, 246–249, 251, 265–267, 269, 279, 283, 288, 295, 310, 316, 321, 329–330, 340, 342, 382, 394, 414–415, 428
Ozone, 91, 93, 165, 252, 282–283, 311, 342

PABA, 106, 229, 317
Palsy, 152, 443, 460
Pancreas, 84, 133, 137, 139, 142, 148–149, 161, 165, 170, 172, 187, 197, 214, 266, 308, 311, 328, 334, 342–344, 356–358, 360, 362, 393, 419, 426
Pantothenic acid, 94, 179, 222, 231, 234–236, 240, 270, 285, 291, 293, 299, 329, 418
Papain, 376, 441
Papaya, 124, 167, 198, 376, 386, 400, 416, 441
Papillomavirus, 329
Paprika, 151, 388
Papyrus ebers, 137
Paralyze, 14, 21, 59, 62, 68, 93, 112, 179, 221, 232, 250, 269, 291, 319, 358, 368, 386, 405, 422, 433, 467, 477
Parasites, 169, 292, 363
Parathyroid, 244–245, 256, 407
Parsley, 148–150, 230, 290, 355, 373, 380, 388, 392, 399–400, 403, 406, 416, 420
Parsnips, 131–132
Pasteurize, 48, 116, 127–128, 185, 193–196, 198–201, 225, 284, 313, 341, 370, 424, 440
Pau d'arco, 278, 282, 334–335, 345
Peanut, 117–118, 164, 174, 177, 179, 211, 220, 222–223, 234–235, 246, 284, 298, 339, 346, 375, 389, 391–392, 406, 438
Peanut oil, 174, 177, 391
Pears, 184, 372
Peas, 117–118, 132, 162–163, 191, 221, 231, 236, 238, 266, 284, 360, 372, 421
Pectin, 159–161, 168, 172–173, 175, 208, 332, 361, 364, 379, 480
Pellagra, 188, 225, 233, 328, 363
Penicillin, 49, 68–69, 72, 136, 168, 170, 185, 194, 199, 201, 225, 281, 284, 344, 363, 379, 395–397
Pennyroyal, 366, 376, 423
Peony, 297
Pepper, 151, 208, 238, 292, 296, 308, 348, 382, 388, 402, 435–436, 477
Peppermint, 150, 275, 297, 351, 353, 373–374, 376, 441
Pepsin, 54, 131–133, 141, 148, 374
Peptic ulcers, 128–129, 139, 148, 425–427, 446, 454
Periodontal disease, 189
Periosteum, 141
Peristalsis, 113, 128, 136, 144, 168, 184, 293, 374
Peroxide, 47, 92, 95, 106, 184–185, 201, 247, 249, 251–252, 305, 311–312, 345, 356, 415, 431

Perspiration, 70, 81–82, 95, 98–99, 101, 143, 156, 239, 261, 274–275, 349, 353, 421, 482, 489
Pertussis, 356
Pesticides, 99, 213, 219, 224, 293, 308, 326, 402, 415
Phagocytes, 238, 288, 299, 396
Phenol, 132, 171, 331, 353
Phenylacetic acid, 132
Phenylalanine, 192, 298, 438
Philodendrons, 92, 219
Phlebitis, 250, 380
Phlegm, 56, 172, 193
Phosphatase, 195, 225
Phosphate, 96, 257, 267, 286, 397, 400, 407, 409
Phospholipid, 141, 208, 373, 416
Phosphoric acid, 127, 131, 213, 407, 416
Phosphorus, 69, 96, 130, 148, 164, 166, 184, 189–190, 195, 200, 222, 233–234, 239, 242–245, 254–260, 290, 354, 398, 405, 407–408, 411, 427, 441
Photosensitivity, 106, 234
Photosynthesis, 92, 102
Pickles, 131–132, 197, 272, 307, 339, 348, 376, 404, 435, 477
Pimple, 54, 112, 137, 166, 198, 279–280, 348, 421
Pineapple, 124, 131–132, 167, 172, 265, 295–296, 298, 300, 360, 376, 380, 396
Pineapple juice, 295, 343, 400, 415
Pituitary gland, 20–22, 298, 367, 417, 436
Plantain, 161, 208, 366, 423, 428, 431
Plantar warts, 250
Pleurisy, 112, 172
Pneumonia, 47, 60, 71, 129, 173, 185, 199, 229, 240–241, 281, 301, 308, 352–353, 395, 409–410, 439
Polio, 49, 99, 159–160, 169, 171, 189, 191, 203, 240, 257, 259, 261, 327
Poliomyelitis, 169
Pollen, 94, 183, 185–186, 188, 235, 283, 285, 416, 420–421
Polyneuritis, 260, 405
Polysaccharides, 189
Polyunsaturated, 105–106, 127, 174, 176, 201, 208–212, 216, 246, 248–249, 279, 300, 305, 312–313, 322, 346, 356, 381–382, 403–404
Pork, 369, 432
Postum®, 313
Potash, 142, 258
Potatoes, 117, 119, 129, 131–132, 177–178, 219–220, 223, 262, 270, 284, 292, 295, 313, 317, 322, 331, 339, 341, 348, 364, 380, 388, 392, 422, 428
Poultice, 136, 139, 141–142, 144, 150–151, 153, 155–157, 162, 178, 278, 301, 364, 370, 374, 396, 423, 429–431, 437–438, 440, 489
Poultry, 212, 314, 324, 367
Pregnancy, 94, 227–228, 234, 243, 246, 258–259, 269, 273, 305, 314, 321, 324, 326, 329, 355, 365, 406
Preservative, 63, 120, 136, 197, 203, 219, 248, 288, 303, 309, 315, 326, 338, 360, 366, 389
Primrose, 365, 419
Probiotics, 199
Progesterone, 152–153, 340, 344, 400, 423

Prolactin, 128, 322
Propolis, 186, 423
Prostaglandin, 103, 154, 291, 295–296, 369, 391, 434–435, 439
Prostate, 143, 147–149, 154, 165, 181, 218, 266, 311–314, 328–329, 333, 335–336, 399, 419–421
Protease, 162, 174–175, 177, 179, 195, 331, 334
Prunes, 204, 262, 290, 355, 360, 363, 366, 375
Psoriasis, 54, 103–104, 112, 152, 175, 178, 212, 218, 231, 422–423, 430
Psyllium, 373
Ptyalin, 131–133, 189
Puberty, 84, 279, 307, 357
Pumpkin, 21, 220, 228, 420–421
Pumpkin seeds, 220, 299, 420–421
Purines, 221–222, 291
Putrefaction, 49, 81, 115, 120–121, 132, 168, 170, 196, 198–199, 221–223, 291, 308, 380, 412
Pyorrhea, 129, 160, 164, 222, 257, 341
Pyridoxine, 164, 231, 234, 299, 358, 418
Pyruvic acid, 394

Quinine, 75, 145

Rabies, 49, 143
Radiation, 60, 91, 103, 106, 139–140, 145–147, 163, 169, 171, 194, 248, 269–270, 288, 290, 303–304, 307, 321–322, 333, 342, 345, 396, 414–415, 430, 461, 464
Radish, 264, 273, 286, 300, 375
Radium, 303–304, 308, 321, 326
Raisins, 183, 290, 392, 436, 447
Rapeseed oil, 211–212, 391
Rash, 54, 106, 112, 151, 233, 280, 283, 340, 422–423
Raspberry, 290, 364, 370
Rauwolfia, 138
Raw food, 101, 109, 118–119, 121, 123, 126, 159, 197–198, 239, 280, 293, 295, 327, 331–332, 337, 342–343, 360, 404–405, 432, 485
Raw potato juice, 177, 295, 428
Rectum, 81, 163, 309, 373
Red blood cells, 60, 102, 206, 208, 234–235, 241, 246–248, 252, 254, 260, 266, 269, 289–290, 300, 310, 418, 444
Red clover, 75, 150, 155, 187, 280, 282, 335, 342, 348, 370, 391, 396, 421
Red pepper, 151–152, 208, 238, 388, 391, 428
Respiration, 70, 92, 98, 101, 250, 260, 305, 342, 368
Retin-A®, 106
Retinol, 224, 228, 279
Rheumatic fever, 168, 189, 191, 248, 370
Rheumatism, 14–15, 60, 97, 129, 135–136, 138, 141–143, 147, 149, 152, 154, 160, 164–166, 168, 171–172, 177, 186, 190, 262, 292–293, 297, 400, 405, 425, 429, 486
Rheumatoid arthritis, 70, 143, 167, 194, 212, 239, 290–292, 296–297, 299, 415, 438, 440
Rhinitis, 285, 353
Rhinovirus, 301
Rhubarb, 131, 180, 256, 293
Riboflavin, 163–164, 195, 227, 231–233, 257, 329, 346, 423

Rickets, 104, 111, 143, 149, 188, 195, 225–226, 243–244, 255, 257–258, 293
Ringworm, 135, 167, 431
Rolaids®, 426
Romaine lettuce, 262
Rosehips, 297, 353, 406, 409
Rosemary, 150, 152, 288
Roughage, 164, 166, 303, 341, 427, 481
Royal jelly, 186, 236, 296, 299
Rubella, 173
Runny nose, 351–352

Saccharin, 191–192, 285, 309
Safflower oil, 176, 179, 209, 211, 339, 386, 403–404
Saffron, 134, 275
Sage, 152, 288, 353, 370, 380, 391, 416
Salicin, 135, 154, 439
Salicylate, 70, 145, 440, 463
Salicylic acid, 68, 135, 154, 172, 439
Saliva, 101, 113, 121, 131–133, 135, 144, 151, 267, 273, 278, 375, 476
Salmonella, 146, 168, 185, 199
Sanitariums, 20, 62, 73, 76–77, 200, 278, 343, 347, 457–460, 462
Saponin, 139, 144, 297, 420
Sarcoma, 102, 281
Sardines, 403
Sarsaparilla, 149, 152–153, 348, 354, 400, 403, 423
Sassafras, 153, 348, 391, 423
Sauerkraut, 49, 131, 164, 197–198, 235, 289, 339, 376, 404, 413, 418
Sauna, 98–99, 298, 413
Saw palmetto, 396, 420
Schizophrenia, 113, 220–222, 233–234, 237, 242
Schlenz-bath, 99
Sciatica, 216, 232, 297, 440–441
Scrofula, 144, 149, 152, 432
Scurvy, 164, 173, 203, 225, 227–228, 237, 240, 305, 311, 328, 330, 343, 489
Seafood, 212, 346, 382
Seasickness, 144, 150
Seaweed, 147–148, 208, 235, 263, 265, 275, 297, 360, 362, 370, 388, 404, 410, 416
Sebaceous, 152, 231, 278–280
Seborrhea, 236
Sebum, 279
Sedative, 138, 140, 147, 150, 153, 257, 273, 383, 407, 489
Seizure, 136, 151, 153, 234
Selenium, 93, 103–104, 170, 229, 248, 264, 269, 288–289, 297, 322, 331, 334, 346, 355, 365, 379, 382–385, 402, 413, 415, 417, 422, 429
Selye, 87, 258, 320, 417
Senility, 145, 199, 229, 234, 258, 287, 345, 408, 413–414, 417–418
Sepsis, 168
Septic poisoning, 169
Serotonin, 84, 92, 107, 273, 391, 402, 438–439

Sesame, 117, 177, 209–210, 220, 257–258, 260, 279, 290, 312, 322, 355, 366, 386, 388, 402, 408, 420
Sex hormones, 105, 206, 246, 354, 365
Shavegrass, 431
Shelton, Dr. H. M., 306
Shigella, 146, 185
Shingles, 146, 151, 227, 232, 423, 430
SIDS, 201, 355–356; *see also Crib death*
Silica, 362
Silicon, 165
Sinus, 54, 112, 146, 150, 165, 168, 229, 240–241, 274, 343, 353, 397, 433
Sitz bath, 95, 401, 420
Skullcap, 301, 366, 374, 405
Slippery elm, 153, 370, 380, 406, 420, 423, 425, 431
Smallpox, 61, 143, 319
Smartweed, 353, 430, 437
Smog, 91, 93, 267, 301–302, 318, 352
Snakebite, 143, 431; *see also Venom*
Soda, 125, 191, 204, 232, 238, 262, 310, 358–359, 371, 435, 477
Sodium, 69–70, 97, 100, 129, 140, 142, 148–149, 161–162, 164, 166, 176, 181, 204, 219, 234, 240, 246, 254, 260–263, 268, 270–275, 286, 291, 294, 307–309, 311, 314–315, 318, 345, 358, 361, 384–386, 389–390, 392, 394, 406, 426, 478
Solanine, 292
Sorbitol, 163, 363
Sorrel, 180, 366
Soup, 22, 120, 178–179, 232, 238, 341, 364, 433
Sourdough, 125, 235
Sourgrass, 324
Soy, 132, 163, 179, 195, 200, 257, 279, 324, 339, 364, 372, 374, 392, 419, 474
Soy milk, 195, 200, 257, 364, 374
Soybean, 117, 119, 130, 163, 177, 179–180, 194, 208–209, 212, 216–217, 219–220, 222, 231, 234–236, 246, 257, 260, 264, 266, 287, 331, 333–334, 339–340, 360–361, 364, 370, 372–373, 382, 385, 391, 403, 406, 408, 420, 425, 439, 483
Soybean oil, 177, 194, 209, 222, 246, 382, 403
Soybean paste, 179
Spearmint, 150, 376
Sphincter, 374
Spikenard, 134, 136–137, 153, 423
Spinach, 125, 131, 142, 149, 163, 180, 187, 217, 228, 236, 256, 262, 265, 273, 280, 286, 290, 293–294, 380, 389–391, 423
Spine, 227, 329, 405, 440
Spleen, 142–144, 149, 152, 281, 360, 405, 415
Splenic leukemia, 165, 333
Sprains, 83, 177, 296, 431, 440
Sprue, 161, 200
Sputum, 409
St. John's Wort, 403
Staphylococcus, 49, 140, 143, 146, 170, 199
Stearic acid, 182, 358, 416
Sterility, 148, 195, 249, 251, 266, 314
Sterilization, 192, 194–196, 322, 431
Steroid, 70, 92, 103, 163, 206, 210, 230, 256, 280, 297, 307, 323, 331, 344–345, 418, 420, 422, 425

Sties, 423
Stillbirths, 249
Stimulant, 54, 102, 118, 143, 145, 147, 151, 161, 182–183, 186–187, 214, 272–273, 307, 376, 387, 416, 475–478
Stockpile, 322
Strawberry, 129, 131, 165, 180, 184, 238, 262, 273, 284–285, 290, 332, 368
Streptococcus, 143, 146, 168, 197, 199
Streptomycin, 185, 199
Strontium, 145, 148, 194, 294, 321
Strychnine, 156, 241
Sucrose, 183–184, 187, 189, 393
Suicide, 70, 369, 393
Sulfur, 59, 91, 95, 97, 130, 164, 167, 170, 181, 184, 186, 225, 241, 254, 260, 263–264, 283, 294, 310, 342, 346, 352, 379, 396, 420, 438
Sulfuric acid, 127, 130, 213, 260, 263
Sunbath, 102–103, 294, 325
Sunbathing, 102–104
Sunflower seeds, 183, 191, 220, 232, 235, 258, 260–261, 279, 290, 312, 365–366, 388, 392, 406, 408, 413, 421, 474
Sunlight, 12–13, 20, 31, 77, 79, 91–92, 101–106, 138, 156, 229, 234, 243–244, 248, 317, 345, 378, 404, 440, 459, 470, 482, 484
Sunscreen, 103, 106, 296–297
Sunshine, 13, 19–21, 30–31, 55, 74, 79, 89–90, 101–103, 105, 138, 242–245, 255–256, 316, 424, 440–441, 457–458, 469
Suntan, 105, 317
Superoxide dismutase, 282, 346, 415
Sweet potatoes, 21, 178, 228
Sweeteners, 163, 192, 302, 309, 361, 363, 402, 404
Swine, 33, 182, 432
Synovial fluid, 190, 290, 298
Syphilis, 49, 143, 146, 152, 289, 327
Systolic pressure, 171, 176, 387, 390–392

Tagamet®, 392, 427
Tahini, 257, 402
Tangerine, 132, 172
Tannic acid, 153
Tannins, 136, 147, 149, 152, 171, 266
Tapioca, 364
Tarragon, 275, 380
Tartaric acid, 131, 160, 373
Taurine, 386
Teeth, 100, 115, 143–144, 160, 162, 172, 174, 179–180, 182–183, 188–190, 193, 195, 198, 222, 231, 234, 237, 239, 244, 255, 257, 259, 269, 274, 305, 336, 341–342, 405, 409, 411
Temperance, 6, 28, 32, 34, 109–110, 459, 471–473, 475, 481, 487
Testes, 148
Testosterone, 105, 152–153, 279, 400, 423
Tetanus, 240, 242, 356
Tetracycline, 69, 106, 170, 260, 279
Thalamus, 435
The Pill, 68, 230, 234, 241, 272, 314, 324, 344, 367, 433, 444
Theobromine, 105, 182–183, 364, 374, 393
Theophylline, 105, 364, 374

Thiamin, 117, 168, 178, 200, 225, 227, 231–232, 234, 236, 250, 394, 423
Thistle, 36–37, 282, 335, 435
Throat, 136, 141, 144, 152–153, 160, 165, 167–168, 173, 182, 185–186, 283–284, 301, 343–344, 351–353, 368, 395–396, 409, 413
Thrombophlebitis, 314, 409
Thrombosis, 99, 145, 245, 380, 386, 480
Thyme, 352–353
Thymus, 21, 277, 281, 299, 388, 397, 409, 415
Thyroid, 21, 62, 102, 147–148, 150, 230, 235, 237, 253–254, 256, 265, 275, 289, 311, 321, 352, 359, 367
Thyroxin, 147, 265
Tilden, Dr. J. H., 53
Tincture, 136, 152, 366, 374, 423, 431, 439, 489
Tinnitis, 145
Tobacco, 8, 221, 225, 235, 283, 293, 302, 304, 309, 328, 343, 405, 415, 425, 433, 455, 472, 476–479
Tocopherol, 150, 224, 245, 250–251, 301
Tomato, 95, 131–132, 180–181, 187, 238, 263, 273, 284, 286, 289, 292, 332–333, 388, 396, 404
Tonsillitis, 112, 146, 152, 202, 395
Tonsils, 61, 152, 165, 188, 293, 342–343
Tooth, 97, 100, 142, 165, 173, 189, 234, 239, 257, 259, 274, 293, 409, 436
Toothache, 135, 167
Toxemia, 45, 129, 161, 164, 234, 273, 279, 283, 292, 294, 300, 326, 340, 348, 387, 422, 468
Trachoma, 186
Trall, Dr. R. T., 55, 270
Tranquilizers, 70, 75, 87, 91, 140, 144, 153, 174, 252, 260, 348, 355, 406, 428, 438, 447, 450
Tremors, 269, 406, 411
Trichloride, 203, 284
Trichomonas, 146
Trichosanthin, 282
Triglyceride, 83–84, 170, 193, 207, 211, 279, 315, 361, 363, 379, 382–385
Tryptophan, 100, 107, 140, 193, 220, 234, 273, 291, 306, 391, 402, 438–439
Tuberculosis, 45, 49, 89, 104, 112, 129, 141, 145, 150, 160–161, 164, 168–170, 187, 215, 226, 289, 306, 364, 422, 424–425
Tumors, 60, 100, 111, 116, 140–143, 150, 153, 163, 165, 170–173, 178, 189, 192, 195, 198, 200, 210, 212, 214–215, 229–230, 237, 240, 272, 280, 289, 303, 306–307, 310–312, 314–316, 318, 321, 323, 326, 329–331, 333–338, 340–343, 369, 373, 397, 424, 439
Tums®, 286, 426
Tungsten, 242
Turmeric, 296
Turnip, 180, 230, 264–265, 270, 273, 286, 346
Turpentine, 135, 431
Typhoid, 47, 50, 100, 157, 168–170, 185, 199, 201, 319, 327
Tyramine, 183

Ulcer, 59, 66, 71, 112, 128–129, 136, 139–142, 144, 148, 150–151, 153, 157, 161–164, 167–168, 173, 176, 179, 185–186, 191, 200, 218, 236–237, 247, 249–250, 262, 272, 277, 284, 289, 291, 307, 310, 342, 344, 359, 361, 376, 413, 422–423, 425–430, 432, 441, 443, 446, 449–450, 454, 477, 480
Ultraviolet light, 103, 165, 240, 243–245, 249, 288, 316–317, 330, 345, 414
Undigested, 124, 132, 162, 284, 376
Unfermented, 118, 171, 479
Unpasteurized, 196, 198, 200, 339, 363, 366, 424
Urea, 216, 221, 261, 397, 401
Urethra, 400, 419–420
Uric acid, 99, 111, 149–150, 152, 165–166, 172, 178, 181, 214–216, 221–222, 279, 291, 294–295, 384–385, 397, 399, 401
Urinary, 95, 139, 141, 149–150, 166, 180, 232, 259, 261, 263, 317, 349, 373, 398–401, 412, 419–420, 478
Urine, 69–70, 95, 99, 101, 103, 130–131, 141–142, 166, 178, 182, 187, 213, 221, 226, 232, 240, 242, 256, 260–261, 263, 266, 287, 296, 328, 357, 360, 362, 396–401, 419–420, 465, 489
Uterus, 112, 148, 309, 312, 314, 323–324, 331, 340, 365, 367, 373, 398, 407, 409

Vaccination, 47, 57, 60–61, 152, 171, 319, 321, 356, 467; *see also* Immunize
Vagina, 140–141, 199, 313–314, 329, 340, 344, 365, 367, 395
Vagus nerve, 299, 433
Valerian, 50, 136, 153, 374, 479
Valium®, 153
Vaporizer, 353
Varicose veins, 160, 171, 249, 252, 294
Vasoconstriction, 377, 454
Vasodilation, 233, 246, 489
Vegetarianism, 217, 270, 307
Veins, 82, 145, 160, 171, 179, 247, 249, 252, 294, 347–349, 379, 387, 433
Venom, 184, 241–242, 259, 431, 436; *see also* Snakebite
Vertigo, 144–145, 378
Vervain, 94, 353, 442
Vinegar, 30, 127–128, 132, 136, 197, 403, 409, 477
Viruses, 47–49, 57, 99, 102–103, 141, 160, 164, 168, 171, 175, 177, 215, 237, 241, 282, 292, 303, 306–307, 330, 335, 350–353, 368, 370, 396–397, 405, 409, 415, 423
Vitality, 14, 20, 40, 43, 56, 58–59, 68–69, 77, 82, 90, 111, 146–147, 167, 180, 182, 193, 229, 292, 326–327, 338, 367, 401, 410, 416–417, 424, 468, 478
Vitalized, 85, 89–90, 352
Vitamin A, 93, 103, 142, 149, 161, 164–165, 193, 196, 210, 224–231, 238, 243, 247, 267–268, 277, 279, 288, 311–313, 317, 328–329, 337, 342, 345, 353, 366, 380, 385, 397–399, 402, 409, 417–418, 420, 427, 431
Vitamin B_1, 168, 189–190, 203, 226–228, 231–232, 250, 394–395, 439, 474
Vitamin B_2, 195, 232, 314, 324, 346, 365
Vitamin B_3, 140, 207–208, 222, 233–234, 330, 429, 433
Vitamin B_6, 61, 107, 161, 222, 234, 260, 273, 293, 299, 354–355, 367, 370, 381, 385, 397–398, 400, 406, 419, 422, 433, 439, 484
Vitamin B_{12}, 127, 142, 179, 197, 231, 235, 265, 288, 290, 299, 328, 367, 439

Vitamin C, 75, 91, 93–94, 103, 105, 117, 125, 142, 147, 149, 159, 161, 163–164, 168–169, 172–173, 185, 191, 193, 195, 203, 206, 208, 215, 220, 225–228, 237–242, 250, 252, 265–266, 268–269, 275, 277, 281, 283, 285, 288, 292–293, 296, 299, 304–305, 308, 311, 315, 320, 322, 324, 326, 328, 330–331, 334, 336, 340, 342–343, 345–346, 350, 352–355, 358–359, 361, 366–367, 370, 372, 377–379, 382, 385, 392, 396–397, 400, 402, 406, 409, 411, 418, 420–421, 427, 439–440, 442, 483, 485

Vitamin D, 69, 93, 102–103, 105, 193–194, 206, 212, 224–227, 230, 242–245, 255–258, 262, 296, 317, 346, 355, 398, 404, 406–408, 411, 440–441

Vitamin E, 70, 90, 93, 96, 100, 103, 105–106, 117, 150, 153, 179, 190, 193, 201, 203, 208, 211, 216, 222, 224, 229, 232, 240, 245–253, 263, 266–267, 277, 280, 285, 289, 297, 299–301, 309, 311, 331, 346, 355–356, 359, 362, 365, 367, 371–372, 381–386, 392, 396, 399, 402–404, 406, 417–418, 427, 431, 439, 486

Walnut, 174, 192, 204, 212, 234, 258, 266, 339, 365, 382, 391, 438

Watercress, 230, 263, 265, 270, 285, 290, 295, 400

Watermelon, 152, 285, 333, 390–392, 400

Wheat, 36, 51, 117, 123, 125, 142, 161, 175, 178–179, 183, 187, 198, 202–204, 222, 231–233, 235–237, 245–246, 248, 250–251, 258, 260–261, 267–268, 278–279, 281, 283–284, 291, 299, 312, 314, 322, 324, 331, 336–337, 343, 346, 348, 358, 360–361, 364–365, 372–373, 379, 384–385, 391–392, 398–399, 404, 406, 421, 430, 432, 437–439, 474, 480–481

Wheat grass, 95–96

Wheatgerm, 246–247, 250

Wheezing, 301

Whey, 93–94, 198, 200, 262, 268, 404, 412

Whiplash, 438

White blood cells, 49, 60, 71, 84, 89, 103, 116, 140, 143, 146, 149, 159, 193, 238, 277, 281, 283, 285, 288, 310–311, 332, 343, 351, 353, 397, 405, 415, 439

White cedar, 173

White, Mrs. Ellen, 4, 9, 29, 41–44, 61, 65, 67, 73, 75–76, 98, 110, 122, 150, 155–157, 186, 194, 204, 211, 214–215, 264, 270, 307, 312, 319, 321, 335, 340, 350–351, 353, 358, 367–368, 370, 409–410, 416, 424, 437, 439, 450, 457–458, 460, 465, 469, 471, 476

Whooping cough, 58, 170, 301

Wigmore, Ann, 98, 343

Willow bark, 153–154, 439, 463

Wintergreen, 442

Witch hazel, 366

Wormwood, 366, 439

Wrinkles, 105–106, 230, 272, 348, 412, 416

Xanthine, 196

Yams, 117, 340, 428

Yarrow, 366–367, 380

Yeast, 94, 125, 140–141, 143, 146, 197, 199, 202, 222, 231–233, 235–236, 243, 260–261, 277–280, 297, 311, 324, 334, 336, 344–346, 355, 358, 360–361, 381, 395–397, 406, 418, 421, 423, 437, 439, 474, 484

Yogurt, 22, 47–49, 83, 93–94, 124, 128, 131, 164, 195–200, 208, 222, 230, 268, 278, 280, 285, 297, 323, 339, 342, 344–345, 355, 360, 363–364, 366, 369, 372, 375–376, 380, 395, 397, 407–408, 412–413, 418, 438–439

Yucca, 297

Zinc deficiency, 279, 419, 421

Zwieback, 202

We invite you to view the complete
selection of titles we publish at:
www.TEACHServices.com

We encourage you to write us
with your thoughts about this,
or any other book we publish at:
info@TEACHServices.com

TEACH Services' titles may be purchased in
bulk quantities for educational, fund-raising,
business, or promotional use.
bulksales@TEACHServices.com

Finally, if you are interested in seeing
your own book in print, please contact us at:
publishing@TEACHServices.com

We are happy to review your manuscript at no charge.

www.ingramcontent.com/pod-product-compliance
Lightning Source LLC
Chambersburg PA
CBHW081754300426
44116CB00014B/2112